AF677491

History of Nephrology 3

Reports from the Second Congress of the International Association for the History of Nephrology, Padova, Italy, October 4–7, 1998

Guest Editors
Garabed Eknoyan, Houston, Tex.
Augusto Antonello, Padova
Natale G. De Santo, Naples
Lorenzo Calò, Padova
Shaul G. Massry, Los Angeles, Calif.

163 figures, 16 in color and 27 tables, 1999

KARGER

Basel · Freiburg · Paris · London · New York · New Delhi · Bangkok · Singapore · Tokyo · Sydney

S. Karger
Medical and Scientific Publishers
Basel · Freiburg · Paris · London
New York · New Delhi · Bangkok
Singapore · Tokyo · Sydney

Drug Dosage
The authors and the publisher have exerted every effort to ensure that drug selection and dosage set forth in this text are in accord with current recommendations and practice at the time of publication. However, in view of ongoing research, changes in government regulations, and the constant flow of information relating to drug therapy and drug reactions, the reader is urged to check the package insert for each drug for any change in indications and dosage and for added warnings and precautions. This is particularly important when the recommended agent is a new and/or infrequently employed drug.

All rights reserved.
No part of this publication may be translated into other languages, reproduced or utilized in any form or by any means, electronic or mechanical, including photocopying, recording, microcopying, or by any information storage and retrieval system, without permission in writing from the publisher or, in the case of photocopying, direct payment of a specified fee to the Copyright Clearance Center (see 'General Information').

© Copyright 1999 by S. Karger AG,
P.O. Box, CH–4009 Basel (Switzerland)
Printed in Switzerland on acid-free paper by
Reinhardt Druck, Basel

KARGER

Fax+ 41 61 306 12 34
E-Mail karger@karger.ch
www.karger.com

Vol. 19, No. 2, 1999

American Journal of Nephrology

Contents

KARGER

Fax+41 61 306 12 34
E-Mail karger@karger.ch
www.karger.com

© 1999 S. Karger AG, Basel

Access to full text and tables of contents, including tentative ones for forthcoming issues:
www.karger.com/journals/ajn/ajn_bk.htm

Introduction

Am J Nephrol 1999;19:99–100

On Progress in the History of Nephrology

Garabed Eknoyan Augusto Antonello Natale G. De Santo Lorenzo Calò
Shaul G. Massry

The present volume represents the transactions of the Second Congress of the International Association for the History of Nephrology held in Padua, Italy, on October 4–7, 1998, under the auspices of the University of Padua Faculty of Medicine, the Italian Ministro dell'Università e della Ricerca Scientifica e Technologica, the City of Padua, the Province of Padua, and jointly sponsored by the Istituto Italiano per gli Studi Filosofici and the Arturo Borsatti Association for Nephrology.

The International Association for the History of Nephrology (IAHN) was founded in 1994 in response to expressed interest in continuing the tradition initiated at an International Congress on the History of Nephrology held in Naples, Italy, on October 28–30, 1993. The stated purpose of the IAHN is to foster, stimulate, encourage and promote investigation in the history of medicine as it pertains to all aspects related to the kidney and urinary tract. This is a more accurate statement of the objectives of the IAHN than its name implies, for nephrology was clearly foreign to the period of history encompassed in the publications of the IAHN under the title of History of Nephrology. Yet, by any other name, the conceptualization of the functions and diseases of the kidney had a past, developed over time, and continues to unfold as time goes by. After all, the kidney and urinary tract have served a vital function and their diseases have haunted mankind since its existence, while nephrology is but a toddler in the relatively brief history of compartmentalization of disciplines which have been constructed in medicine over the past two centuries. Now that nephrology is part of the accepted medical nomenclature, it does allow one to integrate the historiographic analysis of the conceptual evolution of our understanding of the function and diseases of the kidney and urinary tract.

Having said that, a question concerning the history of nephrology is surely, why do we need it at all? Why search the musty archives of medical history for references to the kidney and urinary tract? The answers are as simple or complicated as one wishes to make them. As individuals, literally everyone, sometime or another, and some more than others, wants to know how did 'it' all get started. As a discipline trained in the sciences, and therefore as seekers of truth, determining these origins is ingrained in the nature of every physician, and actively pursued by those amongst them who have a strong desire to extend intimacy with their discipline. As clinicians who have experienced the thrills of an accurate diagnosis within their practice, knowledge of the history of a disease allows for a strange but pleasing transposition of the other discoverer's world into one's own. As nephrologists operating in a technological age, using the last equipment we did not design, we need the intellectual escape into the humanities to explore by whom and why the equipment and our very discipline came into existence in the first place. It is to fulfil these, as well as a host of other reasons, that we need to know the history of nephrology. Unfortunately, there is an embarrassing disproportion between the meager reference to the kidney in available sources on the

KARGER
Fax + 41 61 306 12 34
E-Mail karger@karger.ch
www.karger.com

© 1999 S. Karger AG, Basel
0250–8095/99/0192–0099$17.50/0

Accessible online at:
http://BioMedNet.com/karger

history of medicine and the tremendous scientific achievements that have occurred in nephrology in the brief period of its existence as a discipline. That is why the search must continue to reconstruct our past. That is the purpose of the IAHN. *History of Nephrology 3* is another step in that direction.

The inaugural meeting of the IAHN was held on the Island of Kos, Greece, on October 14–16, 1996. In keeping with tradition, the site of the Second Congress was selected because of its historic importance as the home of the medical university which led the renaissance of medicine in the sixteenth century. The meeting would not have been possible without the efforts of the local Organizing Committee, consisting of A. Antonello, A. D'Angelo, S. Favaro, L. Calò, L. Bonfante, S. Cantaro, and the Department of Nephrology of the University of Padua. It was the relentless toil and boundless energy of Augusto Antonello and Lorenzo Calò in attending to every fine detail that ultimately determined the success of the meeting, and created the fond memories with which the congress participants departed. Obviously, individual memories are very personal experiences that even the best analytical psychologist may not be able to unravel. However, there were memorable events in which all participants shared. The first of these was the opening ceremony in the historic Aula Magna (Great Hall) of the University of Padua, lavishly decorated with the old coats of arms of its past illustrious alumni. Appropriately, it is in this august setting that an honorary membership in the IAHN was presented to Avvocato G. Marotta, President of the Istituto Italiano per gli Studi Filosofici, who has been a staunch supporter of the IAHN, beginning with his sponsorhip of the first International Congress on the History of Nephrology in Naples in 1993. Another memorable event that will be cherished by all was the visit to the Anatomy Theatre of Girolamo Fabrici d'Acquapendente (1594), an icon of renaissance medicine which decorates the cover of this volume. Equally memorable was the ambrosial gala dinner at the Ristorante Belle Parti, at which honorary memberships in the IAHN were presented to Professors George Schreiner and Klaus Hierholzer.

The layered depth to the understanding of the history of nephrology that has been generated by the meetings of the IAHN is evident from the contents of the present volume. The presentations made at the congress have been grouped topically for the edited volume. Two of these groupings were planned as special sessions for the meeting. The first is the section on the Contributions of Padua to Nephrology, dedicated to the memory of Professor Arturo Borsatti, Dean of the Medical School of the University of Padua. Professor Borsatti was instrumental in the inception of the IAHN and had issued the original invitation for its meeting in Padua. Unfortunately, he passed away in 1995, prior to the first meeting of the IAHN on Kos. His obituary appeared in *History of Nephrology 2*. The other section is the one on the Origins of Renal Physiology. The title and preliminary content of this session was conceived by Professor Carl Gottschalk, a founding Councillor of the IAHN. Unfortunately, Professor Gottschalk passed away unexpectedly two weeks after agreeing to organize the session on the History of Renal Physiology. Professor Klaus Hierholzer was kind enough to assume the responsibility of organizing the session, which is dedicated to the memory of Carl Gottschalk. The session was chaired jointly by its organizer, Klaus Hierholzer, and Professor Gottschalk's beloved wife, Susan Fellner. The list of participants in the session and its content speak for themselves. Professor Stewart Cameron gave the inaugural talk on 'Carl Gottschalk – Physiologist and Historian of Nephrology'. His presentation, eloquent as it was, is but a partial expression of the deep debt of gratitude that the IAHN owes Carl Gottschalk. He, before anyone else, had kindled everyone's interest in the history of nephrology and he, more than anyone else, nurtured its growth in his gentle but relentless support of the IAHN. His wise council on the Board will be missed, but remembered dearly.

At the closing business meeting of the Association, the Board of Directors announced that it had accepted the invitation of Shaul M. Shasha to host the next meeting of the IAHN in Jerusalem, Israel in October of 2000. Also at the business meeting, the following officers were elected to serve for 1998–2000: Shaul G. Massry, President; Spyros Marketos, Vice President; Garabed Eknoyan, Secretary-Treasurer and Luciana Angeletti, Marc E. De Broe, Athanasias Diamandapoulos, Charles George, Shaul M. Shasha, and Sandor Sonkodi as Councillors. In addition, Professor Natale G. De Santo, a founding officer of the IAHN, was elected an ex officio Councillor to serve on the Board of Directors.

In closing, acknowledgements are due to the following organizations, for their generous support of the Second Congress of the IAHN: Associazione Borsatti, Baxter Spa, CISA, Dompè Biotec, Gruppo Iniziative Culturali E Sociali Di Villafranca Padovana, Prodotti Hoechst, Istituto Gentili, Janssen-Cilag, Lofra Cucine, Merck Sharp & Dohme, Novartis Farma, Sangemini, and Sigma Tau.

American Journal of Nephrology

Am J Nephrol 1999;19:101–106

The Metaphorical and Mythical Use of the Kidney in Antiquity

Giovanni Maio

Institute for the History of Medicine and Science, University of Lübeck, Germany

Key Words
Kidney · Metaphor · Medical philosophy · Ancient history, medicine · Mythology · Bible

Abstract
While the Syrians and the Arabs viewed the liver as the center of life, the kidneys, in contrast, held a primary place of importance in Israel. In Hebrew tradition, they were considered to be the most important internal organs along with the heart. In the Old Testament most frequently the kidneys are associated with the most inner stirrings of emotional life. But they are also viewed as the seat of the secret thoughts of the human; they are used as an omen metaphor, as a metaphor for moral discernment, for reflection and inspiration. This field of tension in metaphoric usage is resolved under the conception of the kidneys as life center. In the Old Testament the kidneys thus are primarily used as metaphor for the core of the person, for the area of greatest vulnerability. For us today, this metaphorical use of the kidneys has lost its meaning. One reason for its disappearance is certainly the monopoly of causal-analytic rationality in science of today. The kidney has developed from myth to organ, and with this transition a variety of perspectives and ways of looking at knowledge inherent in imaginative thought have been lost. But the metaphor uncovers a deeper level of truth, it represents another form of reconstruction of reality which needs not necessarily be subordinate to the scientific rationality. Today as well, these imaginative ideas can provide an approach to an essential level of reality which may otherwise remain hidden.

Introduction

The mythical and metaphorical use of the kidney appears hardly to have been thought worthy of study up until now. There are entire libraries of works on the metaphoric and mythical use of the heart, but scarcely any discussion on the subject of the kidney as myth or metaphor. In offering a few thoughts on this subject, this fact alone unavoidably forces us to a more than fragmentary discussion of the topic. Our comments are based on the use of very heterogeneous material which can hardly be brought together in historical context, a disparate accumulation of material, that, beyond the mention of the object, kidney, has very little in common. Our approach to the mythical and metaphorical use of the kidney is thus of phenomenological-eclectic. Clearly, such a method of approach must be questioned. If we have nonetheless decided to take this path, it is mainly for the reason that this method seems to be most legitimate when general basis structures of anthropological conceptualizing are being sought, when a

KARGER
Fax + 41 61 306 12 34
E-Mail karger@karger.ch
www.karger.com

© 1999 S. Karger AG, Basel
0250–8095/99/0192–0101$17.50/0

Accessible online at:
http://BioMedNet.com/karger

Dr. Giovanni Maio
Institute for the History of Medicine and Science, University of Lübeck
Königstrasse 42
D–23552 Lübeck (Germany)
Tel. +49 451 70799814, Fax +49 451 74689, E-Mail maio@imwg.mu-luebeck.de

level of fundamental convictions and attitudes is being discussed which is less dependent upon historical change than some consciously formulated cultural characteristics [1]. Especially in the first section, in the discussion of the conceptualization of the kidney for primitive peoples, this deeper level appears to be given and in this we feel the legitimacy of the method to be confirmed.

The Kidney in Religious Cults of Antiquity

In his 'Elements of Folk Psychology' of 1920 the psychologist and philosopher Wilhelm Wundt [2] notes:

> 'The idea of the kidneys and their surrounding bed of fat as the bearer of life, of physical and spiritual power, seems to have been widely spread over the earth at an earlier time.'

Wundt explains this connection between the kidney and bearer of the soul with the central location of the organ, but in particular, with the fact that for many ancient primitive peoples – and not only for them – the kidney was brought into close association with the organs of reproduction. Rituals and cultic practices of the so-called ancient primitive people offer numerous clues that the kidney was viewed as a bearer of the spirit and lender of power. For example, it has been reported that aborigines of Australia wore a piece of kidney as an amulet around the neck. They attributed to it a spiritual power capable of working at a distance, able to protect them from harmful magic.

It is primarily in the sacrificial cults of the primitive peoples that the kidney plays an important role as bearer of the soul. Thus, in the ancient Indian rites of cremation, the kidney of the sacrificial animal is placed in the hands of the deceased, in order to – as interpreted by well known anthropologists – protect the soul of the dead on its way into the hereafter through the spiritual power residing in the kidney [3]. Frazer [4] reports that amongst the tribes of Southeast Australia the belief was universal that diseases were caused by medicine men of hostile tribes who abstract the kidney (and kidney fat) magically from living people and then stuff a handful of grass into the wound.

There are numerous sacrificial rituals in which the kidneys in particular are sacrified – so to speak as the best portion, as the soul of the sacrificial animal. These rituals are also repeatedly mentioned in the Old Testament, although here no underlying animism may be expected, but rather for which numerous other interpretations are under discussion. Wilhelm Wundt [5] even saw the origin of cannibalism in the interconnection between kidney and soul, in his postulation that the anthropophages were led by the idea that they, through ingestion of the kidneys, could acquire ownership of the soul of the victim. It may be that these last thoughts are disputed today [6], but, in any case, these – although very disparate observations – make it clear that for some ancient primitive peoples a special importance was attached to the kidney.

This reverence for the kidney is not limited to primitive peoples. In ancient Egypt as well, there are indications of the special position of the kidney. Thus, at the beginning of this century, the archeologist Elliot Smith [7] discovered that it was especially the heart and the kidneys which were left in the body in embalming of the mummies. Following Smith, it was the intention of the embalmers to leave the kidneys, like the heart, in position of the body, because some special significance was attached to these two organs which made it undesirable that they should be removed from the body along with the other viscera.

Not only the kidney itself, but also the surrounding fat, was thought to possess the characteristics of a carrier of power and spirit. Thus it was the custom in various archaic cultures, as part of the sacrificial rites, to rub the sacrificial altar and the body of those participating in the sacrifice with kidney fat to protect these from magic or in order to sanctify it. For some primitive peoples, anointing with kidney fat was a ceremony of initiation at the entrance to manhood [8]. Referring to Australian tribes, the anthropologist Howitt [9] states:

> 'The fat is greatly prized, and is divided among the adults, who anoint their bodies with it and carry some of it about, as they believe the prowess and virtues of the victim will pass to those who use the fat.'

Again, this idea is not limited to primitive peoples. Even in Homer – who never mentions the kidney itself – we find indications of the particular importance of kidney fat in culling the favor of the Gods. The following passage can be found in the Iliad [10]:

> 'With this he (Achilles) drew his bronze spear out of the bank, and now that he had killed Asteropaeus, he let him lie where he was on the sand, with the dark water flowing over him and the eels and fishes busy nibbling and gnawing the fat that was about his kidneys. Then he went in chase of the Paeonians, who were flying along the bank of the river in panic when they saw their leader slain by the hands of the son of Peleus. Therein he slew Thersilochus, Mydon, Astypylus, Mnesus, Thrasius, Oeneus, and Ophelestes, and he would have slain yet others, had not the river in anger taken human form [...]'.

The idea of the kidney as bearer of spirit and power was very early superseded by other motives, although in part it has survived in popular belief for centuries. Here, one only needs mention the widespread use of the kidney as aphrodisiac even in modern times, by, for example, the old Prussians [11].

The View of the Kidney in the Semitic Tradition

As an introduction, we would like to make a few etymological remarks on the Hebrew word for kidney. There is much evidence in favor of the idea that the word 'kidney' can be viewed as a borrowing from the Semitic language family. Therefore, there is a remarkable resemblance between the Hebrew 'kelayot', the Assyrian 'kalitu', and the Arabic 'kulyat'. Concentrating on the Hebrew word 'kelayot' (singular: kiliah), the question of its derivation is particularly informative. Although this is still a subject of scientific discussion, some thoughts can nonetheless be considered here. The Old Testament expert Kellermann [12] offers three models of explanation for its origin. One possible root could be the Hebrew 'kl' or the indogermanic 'kel', both of which mean approximately 'capsuled, enclosed, embedded'. Another possible origin could be the root 'klj' or 'kll', which means approximately 'something round' or 'sound of rolling'. Others [13], on the other hand, connect the Semitic word with the verb 'kalah', to confine, obviously referring to the capsule and fat. Thus, it can be emphasized that it was primarily the shape and position of the kidney which played the most important role in its naming in Hebrew. Its use as a metaphor plays no decisive role here. Interestingly, however, as Kottek [14] has pointed out, a further possible Hebrew meaning for kidney could be the word 'tuchoth', a word which means approximately 'to be hidden'. But opinions are divided as to whether this term really refers to the kidneys at all.

While the Syrians and the Arabs viewed the liver as the center of life, the kidneys, in contrast, held a primary place of importance in Israel. Next to the heart, they were considered to be the most important internal organ. It is the expression of this idea which becomes particularly clear in the Old Testament which we would like to discuss in somewhat more detail. The kidneys are mentioned 31 times altogether in the Old Testament, in every instance appearing in the plural, even when the context is referring to the singular. Of the 31 biblical references in the Old Testament, 16 deal with the parts of sacrificial animals to be burned in offerings at the Temple. Of these references, 2 can be found in Exodus (Ex 29, 13.22) and 14 in Leviticus (Lev 3, 4.10.15; 4, 9; 7,4; 8, 16.25; 9, 10.19). Kidney fat is also mentioned twice (Deut 32, 14 and Isa 34, 6), where it, interestingly, is used in a metaphorical sense in both instances. Thus, in Deuteronomy 32 'with the fat of the kidney of wheat' which is to be understood as a reference to the future world in which the grains of wheat shall be as large as the kidney of an ox. In Isaiah, the knife of the sacrificial offering, called the sword of Yahweh, is full of the blood and fat of the sacrificial animals, particularly the fat of the kidney of the ram [15].

With the exception of the lobes of the liver, which, according to recent studies, only later came to be viewed as parts worthy of sacrifice, one may state that the sacrifices which were originally burned on the altar as the Lord's portion consisted only of the two kidneys, the kidney fat and the net. This manifests as well the particular importance of the kidneys in the Old Testament. Explanatory models for this fact are diverse and remain the subject of controversial discussion. While some view this special position as being due to 'their color and density', regarding them in a particular sense as the seat of life, others refer to the fact that the kidneys were viewed as reproductive organs which one did not want to disturb [16]. However, it is undoubtable that the most frequent references to kidneys in the Old Testament pertain to the physical organs of sacrificial beasts. At this juncture, it is remarked that kidney fat gained independent status as an offering material at a very early stage. In the course of history, blood and fat came to represent the epitome of an offering. While the fat of the kidney was a delicacy among primitive peoples, it was tabooed in Israel where it was reserved as a meal only for Yahweh. As for the the kidneys, they were still counted within traditional sacrificial material, but this custom soon lost its special meaning [17].

The Metaphorical Use of Kidney in the Old Testament

At a first glance, the kidney is mentioned nine times in all in direct connection with the heart in the ancient Hebrew writings. No other combination of internal bodily organs appears with similar frequency in the Old Testament as that of kidneys and heart. In three passages, the expression 'reins and heart' occurs (Jer 11, 20; Jer 20, 12; Ps 26, 215), while the combination but once appears in the inverted order of 'hearts and reins' (Ps 7, 10) [18]. Finally, in five passages, the two organs are mentioned in a parallel pattern in consecutive clauses; in four instances, the heart is mentioned first (Ps 73, 21; 1 Mac 2, 24; Prov 23, 15.16; Jer 17, 10), and in one instance the kidney appears before the heart (Wisd 1, 6).

The expression 'heart and kidneys' may be interpreted as a reference to 'the whole personality'. This wholeness carries a double meaning. It signifies wholeness with respect to the two cavities of the body: the heart as representative of the upper, the kidneys as representative of the lower body cavity. It also refers to wholeness in the metaphorical sense as well: wholeness as the connection between the intellectual and emotional sides. While in the Old Testament, as for the ancient Egyptians, the heart is regarded as the seat of reason, of thought and deliberation, the kidney is associated with the most inner stirrings of the emotional life. The range of emotional metaphors occurring in conjunction with the kidney in the Old Testament is truly very broad: the kidney as the seat of joy (Prov 23, 15.16) [19], as the seat of rage (1 Mac 2, 24) [20], as the seat of desire (Job 19, 27) [21], as the seat of sorrow and discontent (Ps 73, 21) [22], and as the seat of deepest spiritual need and suffering (Job 16, 13; Lam 3, 13; Prov 7, 23).

This is the most frequently occurring metaphorical use of the kidney in the Old Testament. It is clearly regarded as the seat of human emotion. It would be too limited, however, to view these metaphorical uses as being in reference only to the emotions. Much more, the kidneys were regarded as the global seat of the most secret and inner portions of the human soul. In the old Christian tradition, it was viewed as the seat of the most secret thoughts of the human, the stirrings which are today attributed to the conscience.

There are also numerous indications of this view in the Old Testament and in the Talmud. In this sense, returning to observation of the use of the combination of heart and kidney, a precise analysis makes clear that the sequence of the wording is not without importance. While the symbolization of the emotional is only found in the passages in which the heart is mentioned prior to the kidney, the Bible verses in which the kidney is named first, with but two exceptions, makes its association to reflection and to conscience clear: thus, in Jeremias 20, 12 ('But, O Lord of hosts, that triest the righteous, and seest the reins and the heart') and similarly in Psalm 26, 2 ('Examine me, O Lord, and prove me; try my reins and my heart'). Here the kidney functions as the seat of 'discernment', as an object of testing, as an omen metaphor [23]. This function of discernment between good and evil and of impulse to right action becomes even more apparent in Psalm 16, 7 ('My reins also instruct me in the night seasons'), and similarly in Prov 23, 16 ('And my kidneys exult when thy lips speak right things'). The kidneys are not only the seat of the emotion, but, as it were, a metaphor for moral discernment, of reflection, understanding, and inspiration.

Of course there are parallels in use of the heart as metaphor in most ancient traditions [24]. The heart is viewed as the organ of intellect, of feeling, and of understanding. Research on the metaphoric use of the kidney is relatively new, although one thing can be said at least for the Semitic tradition. More than the heart, in the Bible as well as in the Talmud, the kidney appears as symbol for that which is secret, that which is hidden in the most inner part of the body. The metaphors of the kidney pick up those innermost sources of thought and desire which are barely available to humans, but can be judged by God.

This may be one of the possible reasons for the combination of heart and kidneys. The kidneys may have been associated with the heart (as the metaphor for conscience) because they were regarded as the seat of feelings which instructed the conscience [25]. It is this association which has also been articulated by the Syrian Father Ephraem (306–378) who explains: 'In the kidneys are seated reasoning, and there dwells in them the faculty of discernment; they distinguish truth from falsehood, and judge what is base and what is noble' [26].

In the Talmud as well the relationship of the kidney to reflection is particularly clearly emphasized. At numerous places the kidneys appear in the Talmudic metaphoric physiology as counselors of the heart, as has been convincingly discussed by the Israeli medical historian Samuel S. Kottek [27]. Characteristic for this connotation is the verse from Berakhot 61a in which the process of human speech is described in the following manner: 'The kidneys give advice (kelayot yo'azot), the heart comprehends, the tongue articulates, the mouth concludes.' It is characteristic here that the kidneys are mentioned first and also that the next reference to the kidney appears on the same page of the Talmud. Here it is said: 'There are in man two kidneys, one gives good advice, the other one provides bad counsel. It seems logical to conclude that the right side is good whereas the left side is bad' [28]. In the Talmud, we can conclude, the kidneys are associated with the good and evil impulses in man.

The kidney as the seat of emotion – the kidney as the seat of reason, this field of tension in metaphoric usage leads us to the final metaphor which is at the same time the most central and which again leads us back to the beginning of our thoughts. Then, it is the metaphor of the kidney as 'lifecenter' under which this field of tension is resolved. Three verses (all of them are the 13th) can be found in the Old Testament which are rooted in such ideas (Job 16, 13; Ps 139, 13; Lam 3, 13) [29].

The kidneys thus are used here as metaphors of the core of the person, the implication being that this core is understood to consist of not only the emotional area, but also the area of reason, the location of the most inner stirrings and of greatest vulnerability.

In conclusion, just a few basic reflections on the concept of the organ and the metaphoric use of the kidney which suggest a carefully differentiated handling of the results up to now. The question arises as to whether in the references, in which the kidney is mentioned, truly pertain to the organ itself. As our modern concept of the organ is rooted in an anatomical-physiological perspective, this concept cannot be transferred to the ancient traditions. Philosophers of the body speak, in referring to antiquity of 'Leibesinseln' (islands of the body) [30], just as the German language differentiates between the 'Leib' (living body) and the 'Körper' (thing body). The word organ as used today refers to the body as object while ancient use refers to the concept of 'Leib' or living body including the soul. Thus, all references to the kidney cannot be understood in the anatomical- physiological sense which is usual today.

A further restriction to what has been stated must be mentioned. From a philological perspective, we cannot with certainty state that at an earlier stage in the history of the word kelayot, it had a wider and more general meaning than that mentioned above. Based on the fact that the kidney is often used as a metaphor in the Old Testament, the question must be posed as to whether the anatomical concept was first and later extended by the metaphorical or whether the metaphor may also be a parallel survival of a vaguer, more general, earlier meaning. At least there are some indications that this may be so [31]. Independent of whether the anatomical term came first and then was secondarily used a metaphor or whether the metaphor appeared first and was later brought into relationship with the physical organ, we can say nothing about the consciousness of the physical basis of the metaphor.

Concluding Remarks or: What Does All This Tell Us Today?

The fate of the metaphorical use of the kidney in the Middle Ages and Modernity would be worth a study of its own and cannot be presented here. One thing appears to be certain, however. For us today, the connections between kidney and center of the soul, between kidney and innermost feelings, and between kidney and discernment have lost their meaning. This becomes clear, for example, in the modern translations of the Bible in which the original word 'kidney' is replaced by 'secret thoughts', 'soul', 'innermost', or even 'heart'. Of the original connection between heart and kidney as a metaphorical phrase, only the heart has retained its metaphorical meaning, while the kidney has disappeared from these phrases. This makes it appear to be even more important for the application of historical research to uncover the reasons for the appearance of the metaphorical use of the kidney as well as the reasons for its gradual loss. One reason for its disappearance is certainly the monopoly of causal-analytic rationality in science of today. The kidney has developed from myth to organ and with this transition a variety of perspectives and ways of looking at knowledge inherent in imaginative thought have been lost. In recent philosophy and theology the metaphor has been 'valued as a peculiarity of human speech which uncovers in a pictorial manner a deeper level of truth, which can only be spoken of in metaphorical rather than discursive, conceptual diction' [32]. It is thus a level of reality which may be beyond the consciousness, but the metaphor represents another form of reconstruction of reality which needs not necessarily be subordinate to the scientific causal-analytic rationality. From this perspective, it seemed to us essential to remember us of the high position of importance that the metaphor of the kidney had in the ancient cultures. Today as well, these imaginative ideas can provide an approach to an essential level of reality which may otherwise remain hidden.

References

1 Assmann J: Zur Geschichte des Herzens im Alten Ägypten; in Berkemer G, Rappe G (eds): Das Herz im Kulturvergleich. Berlin, Akademie-Verlag, 1996, pp 143–172.
2 Wundt W: Völkerpsychologie. Eine Untersuchung der Entwicklungsgesetze von Sprache, Mythus und Sitte, ed. 3. Leipzig, 1920, vol 4, p 88.
3 Oldenberg H: Religion des Veda, ed 2. Stuttgart, Cotta, 1917, p 577.
4 Frazer JG: 'Heart and Reins' and ideas of uncultured races. J Manchester Egyptian Oriental Soc 1911;1:107–108.
5 Wundt, p 242.
6 Arens W: The Man-Eating myth. Oxford, Oxford University Press, 1979.
7 Smith GE: 'Heart and reins' in mummification. J Manchester Egyptian Oriental Soc 1911; 1:41–44.
8 Wundt, p 89.
9 Howitt AW: The native tribes of Southeast Australia. Facsim. ed. Canberra, Aboriginal Studies Press for the Australian Institute of Aboriginal and Torres Strait Islander Studies, 1996, p 367.
10 Homerus: Iliad. Rendered into English prose by Samuel Butler. London, Cape, 1925, p 204.
11 Galling K: Die Religion in Geschichte und Gegenwart. Handwörterbuch für Theologie und Religionswissenschaft, ed 3. Tübingen, Mohr, 1960, p 1474.
12 Kellermann D: Kelayot; in Botterweck GJ, Ringgren H, Fabry HJ (eds): Theologisches Wörterbuch zum Alten Testament. Stuttgart, Kohlhammer, 1973, vol. 4, pp 185–192.
13 Hogg HW: 'Heart and Reins' in the Ancient Literatures of the nearer East. J Manchester Egyptian Oriental Soc 1911;1:49–91.
14 Kottek SS: 'The kidneys give advice'. Some thoughts on nephrology in the Talmud and Midrash. Koroth 1993–1994;10:44–53.
15 All citations of the Old Testament are from: The Holy Bible containing the Old and New Testaments (King James version). New York, American Bible Society, 1963.
16 Kellermann.
17 Münderlein G: Holoeb; in Botterweck JG, Ringgren H (eds): Theologisches Wörterbuch zum Alten Testament, vol 2. Stuttgart, Kohlhammer, 1977, p 956.
18 This expression of 'hearts and reins' is the only one passage with the word kidney which appears in the New Testament (Rev 2, 23).
19 'My son, if thy hear is wise, my heart shall rejoice, even mine. Yea, my reins shall refoice, when thy lips speak right things.'
20 'He became filled with zeal, and his reins trembled.'
21 'Whom I shall see for myself, and mine eyes shall behold, and not another; though my reins be consumed within me.' Another translation is:
22 'Thus my heart was grieved, and I was pricked in my reins.'
23 Durant T: The 'Kidneys', organs of discernement. Eternity 1971;Jan:17–18.
24 Dhorme P: L'emploi métaphorique des noms de parties du corps en Hébreu et en Akkadien. Rev Bibli 1922;31:489–517.
25 Canney MA: 'Heart and Reins'. Further notes on Hebrew idioms. J Manchester Egyptian Oriental Soc 1911;1:93–94.
26 Cited in Hogg, p 63.
27 Kottek SS: The kidneys give advice. Some thoughts on nephrology in the Talmud and Midrash. Koroth 1993–1994;10:44–53.
28 The association of left and bad is a topographic topos which was widely accepted in Antiquity and which has even survived in English language which uses the word 'sinister' to describe (evil) badness.
29 Job 16, 13: 'His archers compass me round about, he cleaveth my reins asunder, and doth not spare'. Ps 139, 13: 'For thou hast possessed my reins: thou hast covered me in my mother's womb.' Lam 3, 13: 'He hath caused the arrows of his quiver to enter into my reins.'
30 Rappe G: Archaische Leiberfahrung. Der Leib in der frühgriechischen Philosophie und in aussereuropäischen Kulturen. Berlin, Akademie-Verlag, 1995, p 20.
31 Hogg, p 54.
32 Kartelege K (ed): Metaphorik und Mythos im neuen Testament. Freiburg, Herder, 1990, p 86.

Origins of Nephrology – Magic, Myth and Science

American Journal of Nephrology

Am J Nephrol 1999;19:107–110

Saint Marina: The Protectress of Nephrology

A.C. Eftychiadis S.G. Marketos

Department of History of Medicine, Athens University Medical School, Athens, and the International Hippocratic Foundation of Kos, Greece

Key Words
Saint Marina · Patron Saint · Miracle · Cure · Relic

Abstract
Saint virgin and martyr Marina (Margarita) of Antioch in Pisidia (255–270) is recognized as the patron saint of kidney sufferers and the protectress of nephrology. Beginning in the 13th century she heals in particular patients suffering from nephropathies, pregnant women having a difficult childbirth, barren women and sickly children. She protects the patients from every side effect and complication. Saint Marina is represented in hagiography as a victor, defeating the dragon satan, holding a hammer or a cross and wearing a belt around her back in the area of kidneys. According to writers, artists and sculptors the belt is the perceivable means of Saint Marina for the miraculous recovery from and healing of kidney diseases. Therefore, kidney sufferers and pregnant women put belts upon her relics for blessing and then wore them. From the Middle Ages and Renaissance and up to the contemporary period Saint Marina (Margarita) was considered the patron saint of kidney sufferers. Justifiably she is recognized by the modern medical world as the protectress of nephrology.

Medical science, in general, and every speciality, in particular, have protectors and patron saints of the patients. In the former category are the Evangelist Luke, Cosmas and Damian, Panteleimon, the women physicians Zenais and Philonilla, and Hermione as protectors of medicine. In the latter category are Saint Physician and Bishop Blasius protector of laryngology and throat diseases, and Saint Bishop Erasmus patron of gastroenterology. Saint virgin and martyr Marina (Margarita) of Antioch in Pisidia (255–270) is recognized as the patron saint of kidney sufferers and the protectress of nephrology (fig. 1).

The 'saint child Marina' [1] is represented in hagiography as a victor, encroaching upon the dragon satan, holding a hammer or a cross and wearing a belt around her back in the area of the kidneys (fig. 2).

According to *Acta Sanctorum, Martyrologium Romanum, Menologium* [2] and *Synaxarium* [1] Marina and Margarita are the same person: 'Marina virgo martyr Antiochena, Aedesii filia sub Olybrio praeside passa, quae nescio quo metamorphosi in Margarita a Latinis transformata' (the virgin martyr Marina of Antioch, daughter of Aedesius, who suffered martyrdom during the domination of Olybrius, I know not by which way the Latins altered her name to Margarita). 'Graeci quippe eam memorant die XVII Julii sub nomine Marinae; Latini vero di

KARGER

Fax +41 61 306 12 34
E-Mail karger@karger.ch
www.karger.com

© 1999 S. Karger AG, Basel
0250–8095/99/0192–0107$17.50/0

Accessible online at:
http://BioMedNet.com/karger

Dr. Aristotelis C. Eftychiadis
15 Georgaki Olympiou Str., Koukaki
GR–11741 Athens (Greece)
Tel./Fax + 30 1 9230136

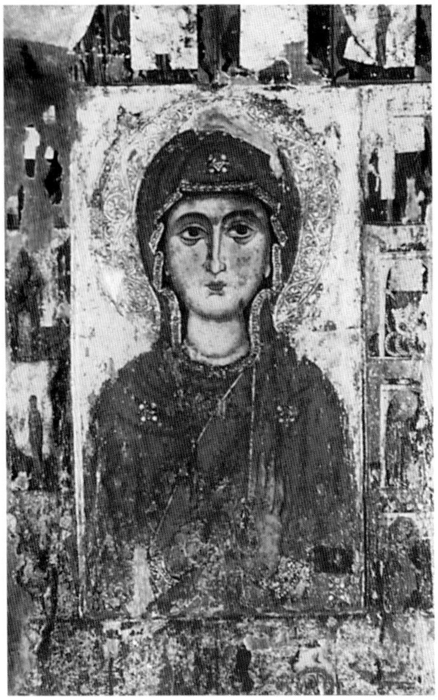

Fig. 1. Saint Marina, Church of Holy Cross in Pedoula, Cyprus (13th century).

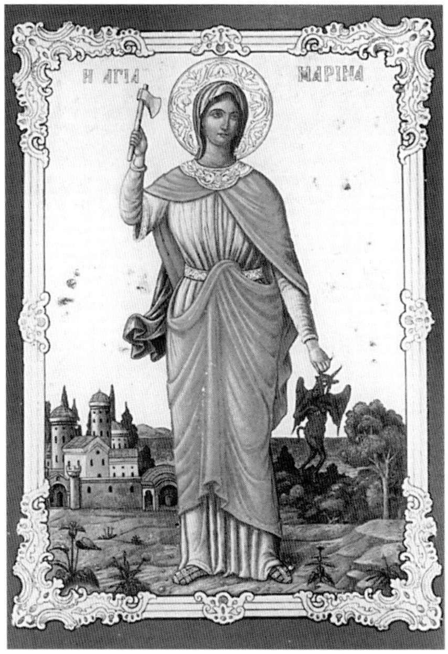

Fig. 2. Saint Marina, Church in Theseion, Athens.

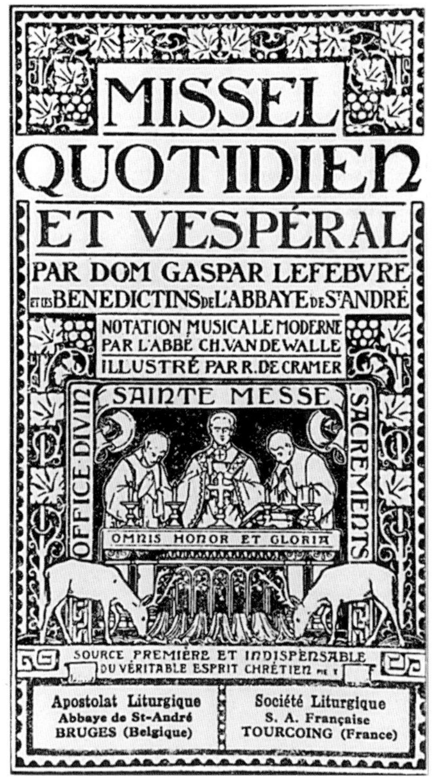

Fig. 3. Title page of *Missel quotidien et vespéral* by G. Lefebvre [8].

XVII et XX sub nomine Margaritae vel Margaretae' (Greeks commemorate her on the 17th of July under the name Marina; while the Latins on the 17th and 20th of July under the name Margarita or Margareta). Moreover the Russian Orthodox Calendar uses on '17 Juillet' the names 'Marina (Margarita)' [3].

The etymology of the name has various versions: according to *Acta Sanctorum* Marina originates probably from a transformation of Maria. 'Margarita origine vox Graeca ... deducitur a margaritis' [2] (Margarita comes from the Greek word Pearl); in Latin Marina means marine, of the sea, and Margarita the pearl. Therefore Marina Margarita signifies a pearl of the sea; it is possible that Marina also derives from Marianna, who is another saint with appellation of Marina or Marianna [4].

Saint Marina was born in Antioch, a small village in Pisidia [1, 2, 5] of Asia Minor during the 3rd century (255). Her father Aedesius was a pagan priest. Her mother died, when she was twelve. For her upbringing Aedesius found a nurse, who was Christian and taught Marina the true faith. After that the father disinherited her. When Marina, the little shepherdess was fifteen, the pagan prince Olybrius saw her, asked her to refuse Christ and to marry him. But she refused the offer and invoked the name of Jesus Christ. For this reason Marina suffered many torments with admirable endurance. While she was in prison an earthquake occurred and Satan, as an enormous dragon vomiting fire and whizzing frightfully, appeared and menaced to swallow her. At this terrible moment she made the sign of the Cross, which killed the wild beast dragon.

According to the *Synaxarium Ecclesiae Constantinopolitanae* [5] 'in prison she tore praying the attacker dragon'. After which the Devil converted to a furious black dog, but Marina beat it with a hammer [6, 7]. Satan for a third time was transformed to a prodigious black man. Saint Marina grabbed him by the hair, struck down and killed him [7]. Immediately the prison was engulfed by a luminous Cross and a white pigeon congratulated her on the victory, crowned her with an indestructible garland and announced the end of her torments. Repulsed, Olybrius ordered her decapitation [4].

Saint Marina is said to have worked many miracles and cures for the patients who invoked her faithfully. In

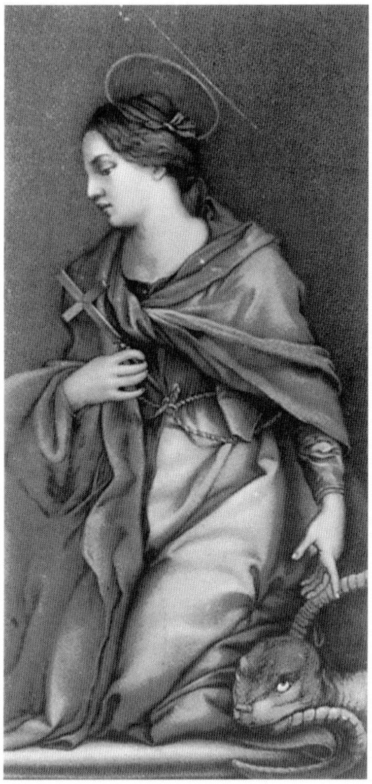

Fig. 4. Saint Marina, Andrea del Sarto (Vannucchi), Pisa (16th century).

particular, she heales the kidney sufferers, pregnant women having a difficult childbirth, barren women, and sickly children. She is honoured as a healer 'glorious because of most mights', 'shining from miracles of cures', and 'taking grace to expel every disease' [7]. The *Bibliotheca Hagiographica Graeca* notes miracles, 'which she every day performs and benefits us' [1]. A special preventive ability by Saint Marina is mentioned in *Acta Sanctorum* concerning the avoidance of congenital diseases: 'in domo illis non nascatur infans claudus aut caecus vel mutus' (in the house of faithful parents not one infant is born neither lame nor blind nor dumb) [2].

Saint Marina (Margarita) was considered as the patron saint of patients suffering from nephropathies, beginning in the 13th century [8] (fig. 3). First Jacobus de Voragine in 1298 in Genova described the golden and sacred legends, according to which saint Marina (Margarita) cures the kidney sufferers [4, 9]. He also mentioned the belt and the robe of the saint and mainly the use of belts by nephritic patients as a sign of miraculous healing [4, 9]. Moreover the orthodox faith and the Catholic tradition accept this characteristic: 'they represented her holding a belt because they considered her as protectress of pregnant women having difficult childbirth and of kidney sufferers ... the nephritic patients and pregnant women in order to avoid any complication wore belts' [4]. 'Sainte Marguerite 20 Juillet au dragon qu'elle tient enchaînnée. Invoquée contre les maux de reins et par les femmes qui doivent être mères' (Saint Margarita 20 July with the dragon, which she holds in chains. She is invoked against diseases of the kidneys and by women who are going to become mothers) [8].

Saint Marina's mass notes that 'drops of her blood wove a valuable greatcoat and robe', 'she dressed up a robe of virginity and eternity' [7]. According to the writers, artists and sculptors the belt is the perceivable means for healing kidney disease by saint Marina-Margarita, as she is represented wearing a robe and a belt around her back in the area of the kidneys, or holding a belt: 'The kidney sufferers and the pregnant women put belts upon her relics for blessing and then took and wore them' [4]. The belt as the intellectual evidence of miraculous treatment and a symbol of therapy is also offered to women by Physician Saints Zenais and Philonilla for blessing of women suffering from menorrhagia. The Saint Belt (Aghia Zone) of Theotocos (Mother of God) constitutes according to Byzantine faith a spring of healing and teems with cures, particularly against pestilence. In accordance with the Orthodox and Catholic Church the relics of the saints send forth spiritual divine grace and the bones become a spring of miraculous treatment. The patients confess that they 'embrace the case of Marina's relics and take the grace of healing' [7]. Therefore a crowd of people and especially kidney sufferers respect and honour the relics and adore saint Marina-Margarita every time and particularly on the day of her memory, to obtain a recovery from their disease. Saint Marina-Margarita heals the renal diseases 'raining always upon faithful divine waters of healing'. She practices preventive medicine 'preserving us unhurt from diseases' and 'granting health of body and soul continually'. Moreover she protects the patients from various complications: 'keep us from illnesses and arduous symptoms, curing horrid weaknesses and sicknesses, preserving us safe always from every side effect and complication' [7].

During the centuries, the events of saint Marina's life were represented in hagiography by different painters, artists and also by sculptors. Some of the most important are: Andrea del Sarto (Vannucchi; 1486–1531), Pisa (fig. 4); Francesco Guercino (1591–1660), Basilica San Pietro in Vincoli, Roma; Francisco Zurbarán (1598–1664), London, National Art Gallery and Sevilla Museum of Arts; Tiziano Vecelli (1488–1576), Prado Museum, Madrid.

Jeanne d'Arc invoked the force of Saint Margarita for her achievement.

Saint Marina's relics are found in several countries, both in the East and then in the West after the crusades (13th century), such as France, Italy, Germany, England and Belgium. Her head is kept in the Cathedral of Montefalcione near Napoli and a part in the Collège d'Andrelec in Bruxelles. The lower jaw bone with one of her belts are preserved in Paris Saint-Germain-des-Prés. In Greece her right hand is preserved in the Monastery Xenophon of Saint Mountain, a leg in the Monastery of Saint Stephanus in Meteor, other relics lie in Saint Marina's churches, such as in Theseion of Athens. The Church of Saint Marina in Theseion, the oldest in Greece, was built originally into a cave in the hill opposite the Acropolis [4]. In this location there were ancient temples of Diana and Zeus.

Conclusion

From the Middle Ages and Renaissance and up to the contemporary period, Saint Marina (Margarita) was considered as the patron saint of kidney sufferers. She heals diseases of the kidneys, provides preventive medicine and preserves the patients from complications and side effects of pregnancy. Justifiably, she is recognized by the modern medical world as the protectress of nephrology.

References

1 Halkin F: Bibliotheca Hagiographica Graeca. Subsidia Hagiographica 8a, Bruxelles, 1957, vol 1–3, vol 1, pp 80, 83, 86.
2 Acta Sanctorum Julii, Venetiis, 1748, in J. Baptistam Albrizzi, vol 4, pp 278, 279, 280, 297, vol 5, pp 24, 25, 31.
3 Russian Orthodox Calendar, Patriarcat de Moscou, Paris, 1997.
4 Tassoula M: Aghia Marina. Athens, 1994, pp 20, 22, 76.
5 Delehaye H: Synaxarium Ecclesiae Constantinopolitanae. Acta Sanctorum, Paris, 1902, p 825.
6 Nicodemou Aghioreitou: Synaxarion dodeca menon eniautou. Athens, Spanou, 1868, vol 2, pp 265–266.
7 Gerasimou monachou Micraghiannanitou: Bios cai acolouthia aghias endoxou Megalomartyros Marinas. Athens, Aghias Marinas Theseiou, 1992, pp 25–78.
8 Lefebvre G: Missel quotidien et vespéral. Abbaye de S. André, Bruges, 1947, pp 1882, 1899, 1901.
9 Jacobus de Voragine: Legenda sacra vel legenda aurea. Genova, 1298.

Origins of Nephrology – Magic, Myth and Science

American Journal of Nephrology

Am J Nephrol 1999;19:111–113

The Medicinal Use of Urine

Walter H. Hörl

Division of Nephrology, Department of Medicine, University of Vienna, Austria

Key Words
Urine · Urea · Uric acid · Autotherapy · Urine therapy

Abstract
Oral intake of freshly voided morning urine has been recommended for many diseases such as viral or bacterial infections. Symptoms reported during the first days of oral intake of urine include nausea, vomiting, headache, palpitations, diarrhea or fever. Several substances in the urine are believed to be important for oral intake such as urea, uric acid, cytokines, hormones or urokinase. Local urine therapies include embrocations, compresses for local tumors, whole body bath or foot bath in the urine, use of urine as eye drops, ear drops or nose drops and the use of urine for wound cleaning.

Many diseases have been treated by the oral intake of one's own urine. Urine has also been used for local therapies [1, 2]. These possible therapies are summarized in table 1.

During the past, oral intake of urine has been recomended for many diseases. For oral therapy, only freshly voided morning urine should be taken whereas 3- to 4-day (in extreme cases 10- to 12-day)-old urine can be used for local therapies. Cooking inactivates the urine for both local and oral treatment. In order to get used to the bitter taste of urine, the following prescription has been suggested: 1–5 drops of fresh morning urine on day 1, then 5–10 drops on day 2 followed by 5–10 drops twice daily. From day 4 a daily increase of the oral intake of urine is recommended until an improvement of the symptoms occurs.

Advantages of the oral intake of one's own freshly voided urine include experience over many centuries and the fact that this kind of therapy is free of major side effects and completely inexpensive. Symptoms reported during the first 2–3 days of the oral intake of urine include nausea, vomiting, headache, palpitations, diarrhea or fever. It has been argued that a high amount of urea may cause gastric ulcers. Indeed, some patients may develop gastrointestinal symptoms for months during and after the intake of urine.

The kind of urine used for specific symptoms or diseases for external or internal treatment depends on localization of symptoms or diseases within the body. It has

Table 1. Local urine therapies

Embrocations
Compresses for local tumors
Whole body bath or foot bath in the urine
Use of urine as eye drops, ear drops or nose drops
Use of urea crystals for wound cleaning

KARGER
Fax + 41 61 306 12 34
E-Mail karger@karger.ch
www.karger.com

© 1999 S. Karger AG, Basel
0250–8095/99/0192–0111$17.50/0

Accessible online at:
http://BioMedNet.com/karger

Prof. Walter H. Hörl, MD, PhD, FRCP
Med. Univ.-Klinik III
Währinger Gürtel 18–20
A–1090 Wien (Austria)
Tel. +43 1 40400/4390, Fax +43 1 40400/4392

Table 2. Reasons for oral intake of one's own urine

Interindividual differences in composition of urine
Urine of every subject is unique
Every subject's own urine contains elements important to solve individual health problems
Substances such as antibodies, hormones and/or enzymes involved in protection against diseases and regulation of host defense

Table 3. Potential effects of urea

Nitrogen donor
Support of protein synthesis
Excellent effectivity against bacterial and viral pathogens
Best natural diuretic substance

Table 4. Medical products obtained from urine and urea

Medical products obtained
Diuretic substances derived from urea
Fertility drugs obtained from urine
Ointment containing urea for local therapy
Estrogens obtained from urine
Ointments containing urea and papain for burn injures and wound infections
Further pharmacological benefits suggested from oral intake of urine due to presence of
Insulin or insulin-like activity
Growth hormones
Urokinase
Ovulation-inducing hormone(s)
Urea

been believed that there is a relationship between four body regions and the four urinary slices of the flasks used for the collection of the urine: the upper slice for symptoms and diseases of the head, the next two slices for thoracical and abdominal symptoms and diseases, and the lower one for diseases of the lower part of the body.

In the absence of any symptoms and diseases, the daily oral intake of one's freshly voided urine should prevent several diseases such as certain viral infections. The theory behind this therapeutic concept is that shortly after an unrecognized infection during the incubation period undetermined but specific defending substances may be produced and would – at least in part – be excreted via the urine. Milder courses of the disease can be expected according to this theory due to reingestion of defending substances present in the urine. Reasons for oral intake of one's own urine are summarized in table 2.

There are speculations that millions of people worldwide are regularly using their urine either for local therapy or oral intake. One of those was the earlier Indian prime minister Desai who throughout his life daily drank a glass of his morning urine even in his old age of more than 90 years.

Urine as an autotherapeutic remedy was recommended for patients with cystitis and prostatitis by Ch.H. Duncan in 1918. He gave his patients their own morning urine half an hour before breakfast. He noticed that this therapy might result in rapid recovery from symptoms, mostly within 48 h and he reported on relapses in cases where this autotherapeutic remedy was stopped too early.

Urine autotherapy was recommended since more than 1,000 different substances present in the urine were identified (at least in part) and/or suggested. Furthermore, inhibition of the growth of different microorganisms responsible for tuberculosis, rabies or poliomyelitis has been observed in vitro. Some people with daily oral intake of urine also believe that urine contains natural antibodies/inhibitors against HIV in AIDS patients.

A bacteriostatic activity of urine has been observed according to the inhibition of growth of gonococci by urea. It has been calculated that approximately 100 mg urea/ml are necessary to inhibit this growth in vitro. Oral intake of urine enhances urea concentration and acidifies the urine. Both maneuvers may be able to reduce microorganisms. Potential effects of urea discussed for autotherapeutic remedy are summarized in table 3.

Another substance in the urine which is believed to be important for oral intake of urine is uric acid. It is suggested that uric acid protects against malignancies and ageing. This substance is also thought to have beneficial effects by destroying free radicals.

Some drops of their freshly voided urine are believed to be of benefit for sick children. Frequent small doses (1–10 drops) per day have been recommended, particularly in children with influenza, respiratory tract infection, and viral infections such as measles, mumps or small pox. Urine therapy has been used in children and adults with pharyngeal and pulmonary diseases. Gargling with urine has been recommended for patients with pertussis, pharyngitis and/or angina tonsillaris. Oral intake of urine was believed to be effective during epidemic diphtheria among students during 1931/1932 and among soldiers during the Second World War. In patients with bronchial infections the thorax was rubbed with urine.

Interleukin-1 (IL-1) and IL-1 inhibitors are found in the urine of healthy subjects. People who advocate the oral intake of urine argue that this kind of therapy may reduce fever during infection, since IL-1 inhibitors increase in the urine during infection and/or inflammation. However, nobody has shown that oral therapy with IL-1 inhibitors is effective.

Medical products obtained from the urine and urea are summarized in table 4.

A clear-cut conclusion for the oral intake of urine comes from the fact that every fetus drinks urine in the amniotic fluid during pregnancy. Therefore, it cannot do any harm.

References

1 Thomas C: Ein ganz besonderer Saft – Urin, ed 37. Köln, Verlagsgesellschaft, 1997.
2 Christy MM: Selbstheilung mit Urin. Unsere eigene perfekte Medizin. Steyr, Ennsthaler Verlag, 1997.

Origins of Nephrology – Magic, Myth and Science

American Journal of Nephrology

Am J Nephrol 1999;19:114–124

Exorcisms Used for Treatment of Urinary Tract Diseases in Greece during the Middle Ages and Renaissance

Athanasios Diamandopoulos

Renal Unit, St. Andrew's Regional Hospital, Patras, Greece

Key Words

Icon · Demon · Acedia · Magic · Christianity

Abstract

Using an unpublished 16th century manuscript as a pilot case, we examined the role of the formal Christian rituals and of hybrid semi-Christian semi-pagan exorcistic writings in curing renal ailments. It was found that in spite of the changing religious and cultural orthodoxy in the lands around the Eastern Mediterranean Basin, people did adhere to their belief in divine intervention when they were suffering from renal and/or other afflictions. We traced the origin of these beliefs at least to the pre-classical period, and its continuation well beyond the Renaissance. The same practice applied both to nephrological diseases of humans (clergy and laymen alike) and of animals. We also present several interesting works of art from the palaeo-Christian to the post-Byzantine era supporting our theses.

The aim of this paper is to present some evidence on the use of blessings and exorcisms in patients with renal problems during the early post-Byzantine era (15th to 17th century AD) in Greece. Incantations, prayers, and wishes, either purely religious or in a framework of magic and demonology, had been in use for many diseases since at least the Babylonian and the Egyptian era. Hence, the presentation of yet another manuscript containing similar examples would not suffice for an article on the history of nephrology. Our extended aim is to use our evidence as a basis for a discussion on the cultural background for such treatments. Our material consists of two manuscripts, one from the 16th and the other from the 17th century, found in the Library of the Holy Transfiguration Monastery near Naupactos in southwestern Greece. Both were brought to my attention by Father Ereneous of the same Brotherhood, whom I cordially thank. Both are similar in context and have remained unpublished and forgotten for centuries. In this article, I will proceed to a more detailed description of the 16th century one and will discuss the latter in a future publication.

This manuscript is written on thick cream-colored paper with three whitish vertical lines as laid marks, probably made in Germany. Its dimensions are 14 cm long by 10 cm wide, and it has 148 written original pages, 6 unwritten pages, while 8 blue pages were added to it some time before it was leather bound. It is written in Greek minuscules, black ink is used throughout except for a few simple ornaments and some capital letters for which red ink was used. On the second page (fig. 1), we can see the most ornate part, i.e., the title page. On the top, below a simple floral ornament, we read the year '1204 of Our Lord', the supposed date of its creation. However, due to

KARGER

Fax + 41 61 306 12 34
E-Mail karger@karger.ch
www.karger.com

© 1999 S. Karger AG, Basel

0250–8095/99/0192–0114$17.50/0

Accessible online at:
http://BioMedNet.com/karger

Prof. A. Diamandopoulos
Renal Unit
St. Andrew's Regional Hospital
GR–26001 Patras (Greece)
Tel. +30 61 641 364, Fax +30 61 622 227

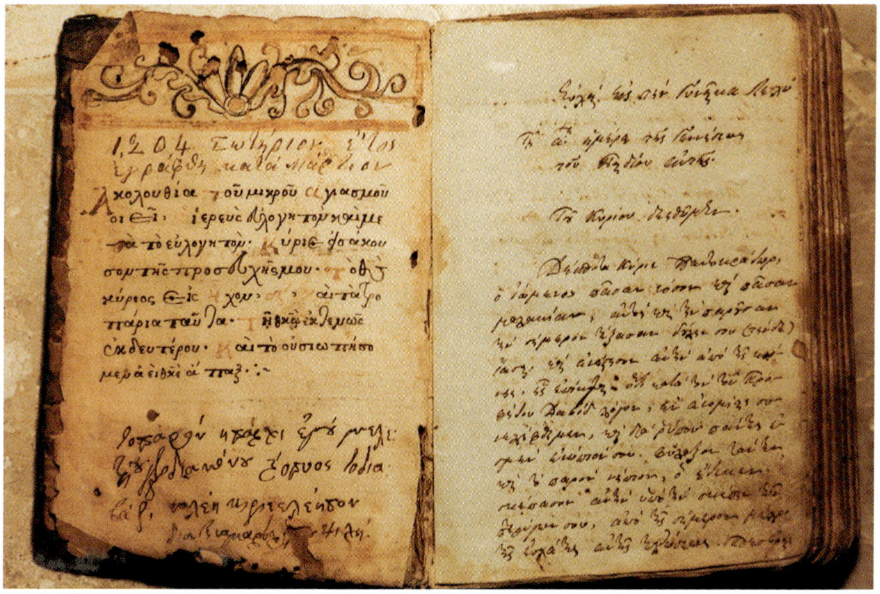

Fig. 1. Title page of the manuscript (fol. 1[v]).

internal palaeographic evidence, i.e., language, style of the script, paper used, etc., we dated it to the beginning of the 16th century. Obviously the date in the inscription is a false one. Before we dismiss it as yet another postmedieval fraud by monks, I find it relevant to my subject to extend the discussion of what was false and what was authentic in Byzantium. Many writings were falsified intentionally for an illegal act to be accomplished, e.g., acquiring the land of another person. However, many manuscripts, although false according to modern legal terminology, were not the result of deceit. Rather, they were compiled with a genuine respect towards antiquity in Byzantine society. The late empire had ceased long ago to be the super Roman power of the past; however, its people chose to ignore it and to continue to consider it as the only *real* empire and its head the only *real* emperor. Even the political descendants of the Byzantine Empire, e.g., the Russian Monarchy and the Romanian feudal aristocracy claimed – falsely but seriously – their ancestry from the Imperial Byzantine Houses. Holy monasteries which did not *happen* to have genuine saints' relics or miraculous icons or ancient books like their more lucky neighbors were *furnished* with them by pious men who considered it only an act of justice to rectify what an unjust luck had deprived them of. Even closer to our subject, many medical writings claimed to be the works of Hippocrates, Galen, or other famous writers, but at best contained only fractions of their works. During the following period, i.e., the first two or three centuries that Greece was under Ottoman conquest, several books on remedies were circulating. They were intended to be used by wandering quasi-doctors or the wise men of the village. All of them boast an ancient and illustrious lineage. Still, it was not considered wrong to claim a false authorship. It was a tribute to the glory of antiquity. Even if these were not genuine, they were definitely useful. And this is what counts [1]. In contrast to the modern hysteria of how recent any discovery in the pharmaceutical industry is, in Byzantium the older was the better. Hence, our manuscript claiming a longer life, did not do anything more than *prove* that it was as serious as its copyist intended it to be. Anyway, it was declared by Gregorius Akindynus in the 14th century, that

> 'There is only one body of the Church, made from everything, as the [works] of everyone are considered the property of everyone else because of the Holy Ghost which is acting in everyone and in everything ... and according to the God-loving opinion [we] should appropriate to ourselves everything good' [2].

Hence, plagiarism had a theoretical and moral basis.

Below the date, there is the title of the book, which in an English translation reads: *The Service of the Short Sanctification*. Hence, it looks that in belongs to the category of 'prayers book' (Euchologion, in Greek: Ευχολόγιον). Three such books exist in the Christian service: one for priests, one for bishops, and a short book – the Sanctification (Missale, Pontificare, and Rituale in the Latin Church). Our manuscript reminds us of the last kind. The oldest existing manuscript of an Euchologion is the Sera-

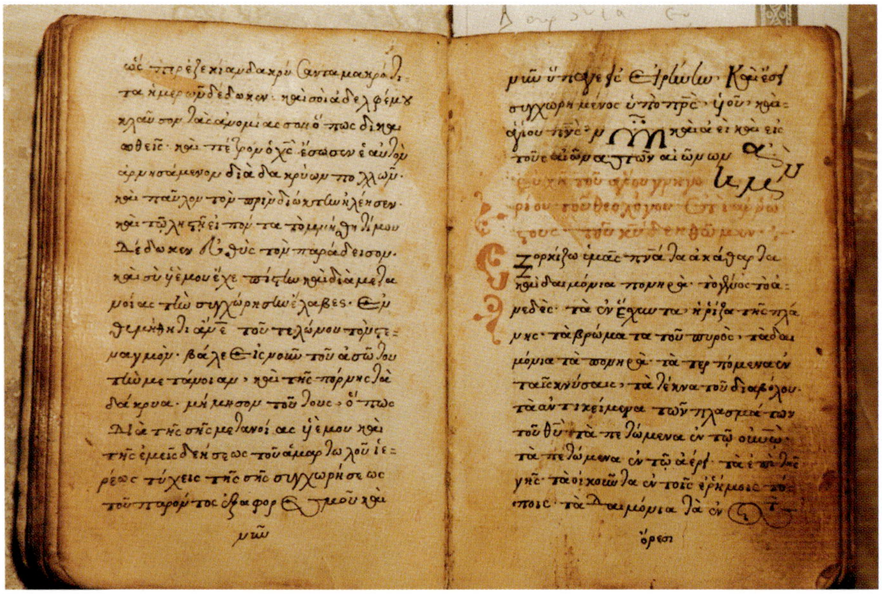

Fig. 2. On the verso, a prayer by St. Gregory Theologus, written for sick people: 'I exorcise you dirty and cunning demons, having the root of the fallacy ... children of the devil ... living in houses, flying in the air, residing over the mountains ...'

pion manuscript (4th century AD, Egypt). The principal edition of these books was the Goar Edition (Paris 1687). After the title follows the beginning of the service. At the bottom, there is the provenance inscription. The owner had once been the deacon Meletios, who – in typical medieval humility – asks future readers to pray for the salvation of his sinful soul. The prayer is addressed to the Almighty God who is expected to cure the patient by just touching him with his hand. This is a very ancient therapeutical gesture, and till modern times patients in Great Britain were cured by the Royal Touch. The invocation of God is further justified because he is *the doctor of our souls and of our bodies.* In all religions God was the all-curing power. Christianity in particular was aptly named the religion of miracles. And henceforth, the manuscript continues by exorcising the dirty demons to leave the body of the patient (fig. 2). By naming them, the priest or the sorcerer acquires a power over them. The naming of the demons recalls all the names used for them in ancient pagan cults. It has to be stressed that pagan and Christian worship and attitudes toward the appearances of angelic and demonic supernatural beings coexisted for at least 6 centuries in Greek lands during Late Antiquity [3], mutually influencing one another. People were carrying their *spiritual luggage* [4] and did not abandon it at the next station when they were turned to Christianity. Conversely, practicing Christians influenced via their piety and forms of rituals some pagan groups in their society [5]. Hence, when we notice similarities between pagan and Christian worship, we cannot automatically conclude that it was always the former that influenced the latter. The most obvious aspect in which Greco-Roman pagan culture influenced the originally abstract Jewish-Cristian art is the visual methods of representing divinity in an anthropomorphic form. This eventually led in the 7th century to the conflict between the iconodules and the iconomachs. Conventionally, the former were superstitious lower fanatical classes, while the latter were the enlightened progressive forces of the Empire. In reality, in spite of the many decrees of the iconomach emperors that economically helped the impoverished people and also in spite of the progress made then in science and technology, in reality the conflict was between the Eastern tendency towards abstract forms of worship and the Hellenistic love for the human person and form. We are justified to draw a parallel with the conflict between Protestants and Catholics during the Reformation. It is characteristic that the Protestant writer Reginald Scot (1584) attacks the Catholic tradition (that had eventually incorporated a great part of the pagan lore), using the same arguments that St. Augustine, a notable anti-Hellenist, had used against the pagans. Scot went even further in explaining that basically idolatrous practices were made possible 'with certain charms and popish praiers' [6]. It is well known which impact the Protestantism versus Catholicism conflict had on the way of thinking of medical writers after the Renaissance. My suggestion then, that even the study of the History of Nephrology is an attempt to bridge the apparent gap between pure science and admiration of personalities and beauty, may not be an arbitrary one.

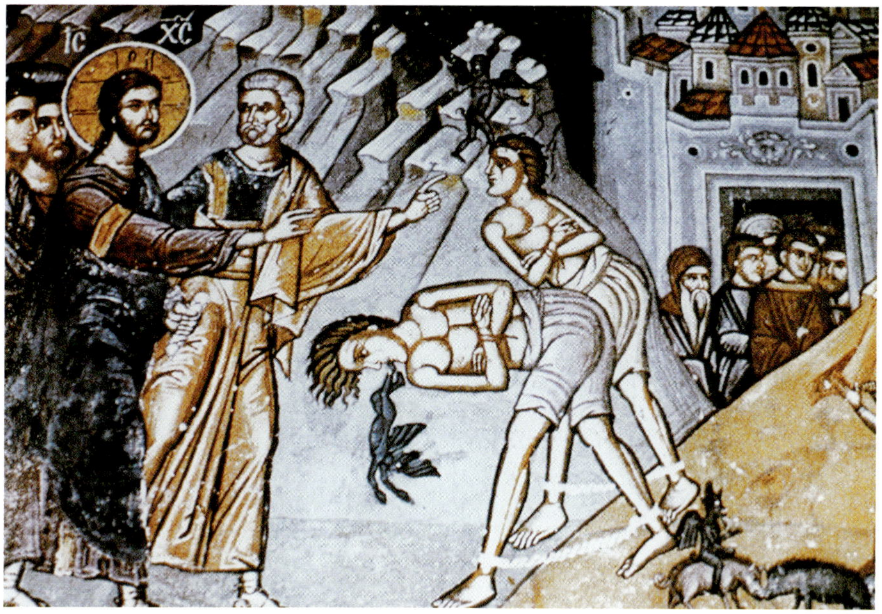

Fig. 3. A 16th-century icon from the Dionysios Monastery in Mount Athos. Christ curing the possessed Gadarene by exorcising the demons (black little creatures) to leave his body. The departing demons are entering the bodies of some wild pigs depicted at the lower right-hand corner of the icon.

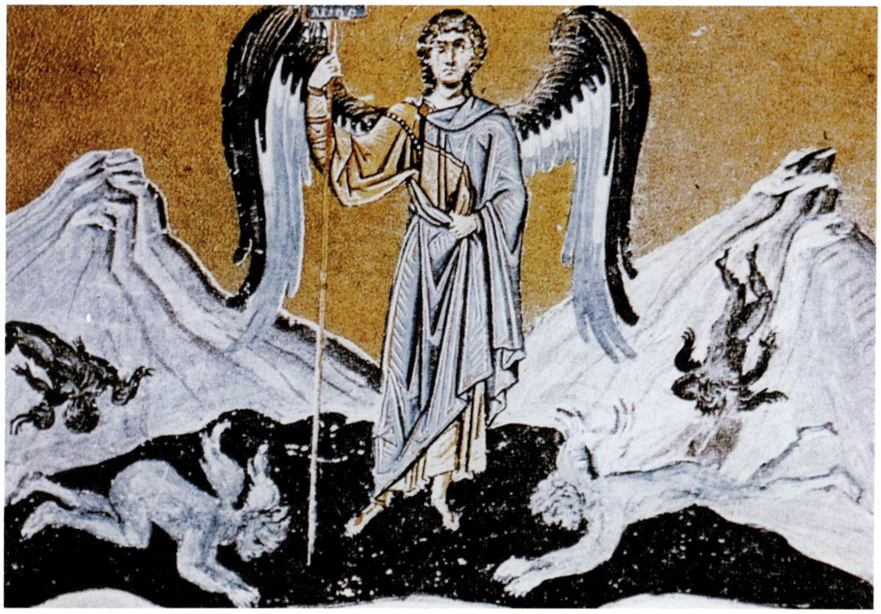

Fig. 4. Archangel Michael defeats the demons. Manuscript illumination ca. 1000 AD (Vat. gr. 1613, f. 168).

Interfering in the clash between iconoduls and iconomachs in a conciliatory way, St. John Damascene declared in the 7th century that 'The icon is the theology of the illiterate'. Consequently, there are many icons that express artistically what our manuscript does with the written word (fig. 3). After the defeat of the demons, the angelic good will reign supreme (fig. 4).

An interesting question is whether this kind of beliefs belongs to the formal Christian rite or to the realm of sorcerers and magicians. The answer is a difficult one. Demons were present in Babylonian and Egyptian religions, and they were responsible for causing many disasters including diseases. Greeks – who coined the name demon – also believed in them. However, they did not think of them as ever ugly and evil creatures. They thought of them as the escorts of each person who might be benign or malicious. Hebrews believed in demons, and there are several references about them in the Old Testament. Seventy-five references to demons are included in the New Testament (e.g., Matt. 8:31, Mark 5:12, Apoca-

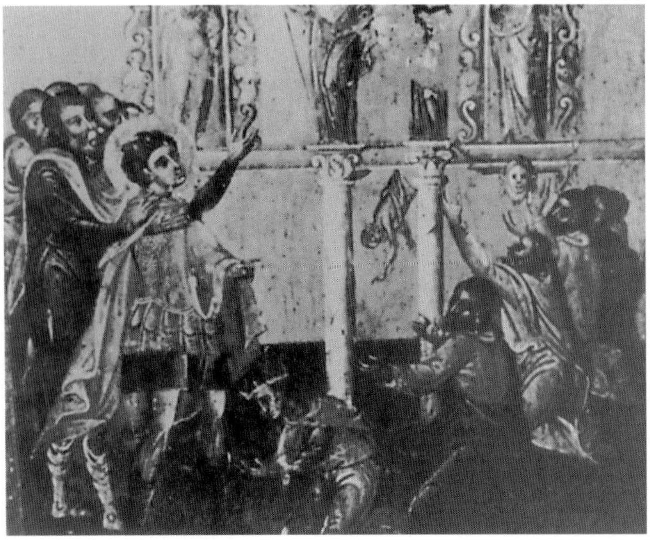

Fig. 5. St. George crushes down the idols of the pagan gods. The devils inside them are flying away in terror. Detail of an 18th-century portable icon. Pinacotheque of the Leucada Island, West Greece.

lypse 16:14 and 18:2, John 6:70). In spite of this abundance of demonic references, the early Christian Fathers were influenced towards accepting the existence of these spirits, and mainly their form and mode of action, through the writings of pagan philosophers of the Neoplatonic movement. It was in this era that stories about demons, chthonic rituals, and offerings to the souls of the dead were very popular. Even the most logical down-to-earth medical doctor, Hippocrates, who fought hard against superstition, was given a protagonistic role in these notions. Lucianus (Philòpseudes: 21), relates that

> '... Hippocrates the doctor demands sacrificies to be made in his honour, and he is vexed if he is not regularly fed by the sacred and perfect offerings ...'

It was mainly in North Africa that this amalgamation of Hellenistic, Neoplatonic, Jewish, and Christian notions of demons took place. Its product is the appearance of demons as we came to know them. St. Augustine, referred to earlier in this article, elaborated on Psalm 96, which said '... for all the gods are idols dumb, which blinded nations' fear ...', by introducing the notion that the gods of the nations were diabolic [7]. A further step was then taken by the apologetic and apocryphal philosophers and thus the declaration that demons were inhabiting the inside of every pagan statue and altar [8, 9] (fig. 5), thus enhancing the acceptance of demons by the Christian dogma. Moreover Christians in that era were attacked from all sides and frequently tortured and executed. It was only natural for them to believe that all their misfortunes were the works of demons [10]. In parallel, Origen, Tertillianus, and Hermas wrote on the actions of demons in detail. Hermas, known mainly via his book 'The Shepherd', was the founder of a long-lived school of monastic philosophers, the hermetics. I will expand on them later. The formal Church doctrine only assigned to demons the power that God gave them in order to test the faithful's power to resist temptation. Exorcism was successful and acceptable only in the name of Christ. One of the weapons of demons was to cause disease. On the other hand, sorcerers believed that Satan had a power in his own right, and the sorcerers exorcised him with his own power. However, the distinction was a very thin one. Laymen did not hesitate to visit consecutively a sorcerer and a clergyman, shopping around for the best cure. The Church strongly condemned the practice, but it did not succeed in destroying it. It was a kind of vicious circle. The more pagans were turned to Christianity, frequently illiterate and somehow pushed by the Byzantine state authorities, the more pagan beliefs of demons were incorporated into the Christian flock. On the other hand, the educated aristocracy never resigned absolutely from its elitistic hellenophilia that incorporated demonic beliefs. On top of all that, the Fathers of the Church taught feverishly against demons and the ways to exorcise them, thus accepting their existence [11]. In late Byzantium, that is after the 11th century, prominent members of the educated classes, even Emperors themselves, held a rather tolerant stance towards magicians and even trusted them. An example is Michael Psellus, the famous politician, poet, philosopher, and medical doctor of the 12th century, who wrote a treatise on kidney diseases and uroscopy [12] which has been translated in English with commentaries [13]. He also believed in demonic powers and wrote a treatise on them [14]. However, when challenged, he took all his talent as a successful courtier to theoretically balance his knowledge of Greek science and his interest in magic, with his orthodox Christian faith [15, 16].

In the manuscript we are presenting, there are exorcisms against various demons causing altogether 72 different diseases and ailments. In the next picture we see what is for us the most interesting part of the manuscript. Here, the devils are asked *to leave* the kidneys of ill persons (fig. 6). But how could devils cause a renal symptom? Usually it happened by the patient's own fault. We read for example in the writings of the 6th century hermetic philosophers (the cultural descendants of Hermas) that when a monk is reluctant to perform his duties in the ser-

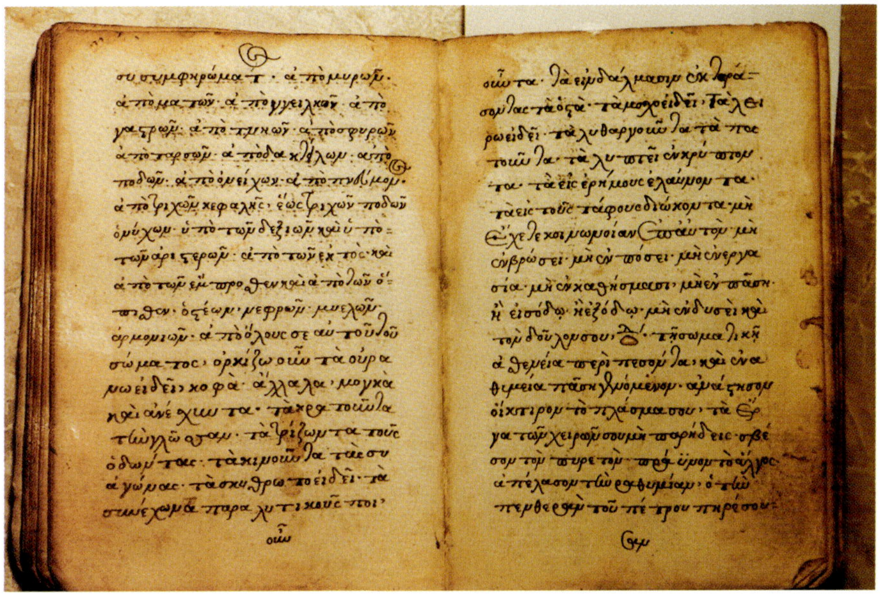

Fig. 6. On the verso: '(sent away the demons) from the stomach, the ankles, the feet, ... the kidneys, and exorcise you pseudo-celestial, deaf, dumb ... creatures ... who grind your teeth ...'

vice, he will be attacked by the demon of reluctance, of heaviness, called Acedia in Greek (Ακηδεία). This demon causes many bodily symptoms, one of them being a colic (of any organ) (fig. 7). The first to mention such a spirit of heaviness (Ακηδεία in the Greek translation) is Prophet Isaiah: '... to give unto them ..., the garment of praise for the spirit of heaviness' (61:3). And from the Greek sources, we meet the same in the writings of the prosocratic philosopher Empedocles in the 6th century AD. But it was through the hermetic monk writers that the idea expanded. From the hermetics John of the Climax (of the Ladder), a monk in the Monastery of St. Catherine in Sinai, wrote an extensive treatise on the several stages of a monk's strife in perfecting himself. He likened a monk's spiritual evolution to a ladder (climax). Each step brings the monk closer to God. Unfortunately, in each step there are waiting for him particular demons causing all kinds of hardship, with the goal to overturn him from his spiritual ascent and to prevent him from reaching paradise (fig. 8). The monastery stands in the Arabian peninsula, surrounded from the early years of its foundation (6th century) by Islamic populations. Islam inherited the Greek/Jewish/Christian tradition of demons, and the Koran has many references to them [17]. Hence, it was only natural in this cultural *milieu* for the native Arab-Christians to accept John of Climax' ideas about demons (fig. 9). John names one of these demons as the demon of acedia, the 'all embracing death for monks who is causing colics' [18]. The same idea is promoted by the 6th-century hermetic philosopher Meletios Homologetes:

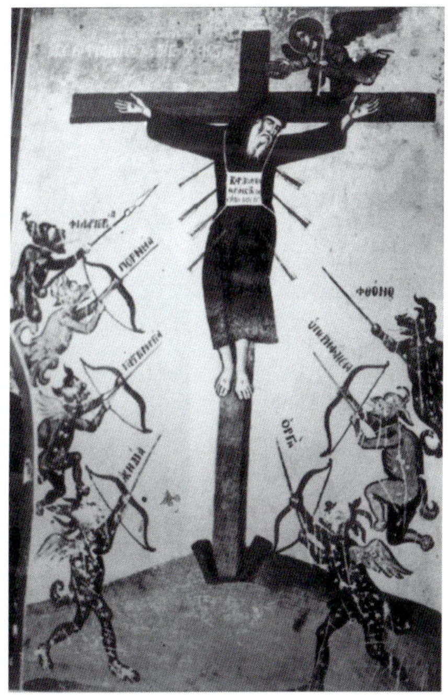

Fig. 7. A 16th-century mural from the outer narthex of the Philotheos Monastery in Mount Athos. It depicts the difficulties facing the life of a 'true monk'. He is crucified, and several demons are shooting their arrows at him. The one at the left-hand lower corner is the demon of acedia, the one causing colics.

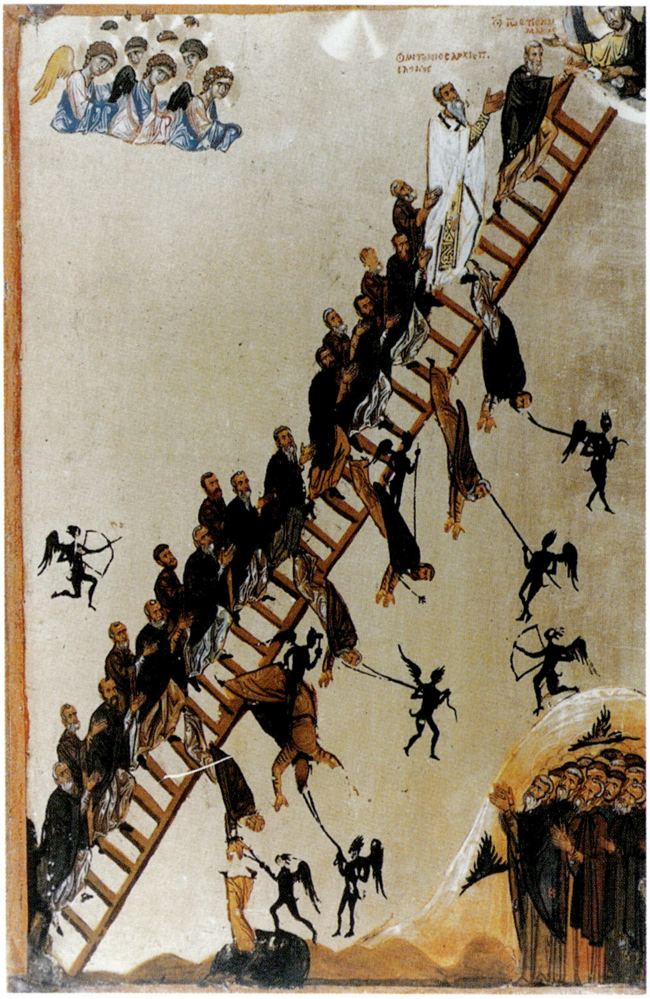

Fig. 8. A 12th-century icon (tempera on wood) in St. Catherine's museum, Mount Sinai, depicting the struggle of monks towards reaching Christ. Demons are overturning them.

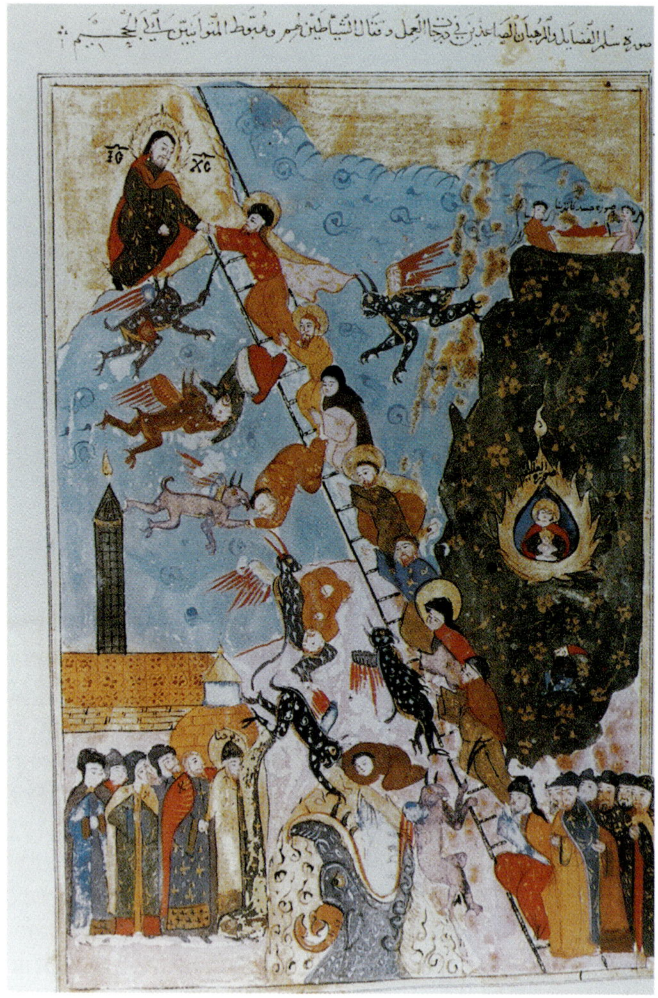

Fig. 9. An Arabic paper codex in St. Catherine's library, Mount Sinai. Old collection No 343, fol. 13^{v}. It depicts the same subject as shown in figure 7, but in an Arabic artistic manner. It was made probably between the 9th and 12th centuries and was meant for use by the Arabic-speaking Christians of the Middle East.

'Terrible meanness of spirit, the father of the dreadful third-hour fever, of headache and of *colic* in monks, the demon of acedia attacks ascetics at midday and moves those whose souls are small to go away despairing ...' [19].

We can compare this demon of acedia which attacks at midday, with the 'daemonium meridianum' in Greek and Latin patristic literature. The idea was repeated again by another famous hermetic, Maximos Homologetes [20]. Greenfield [21] cites an extended list of writers on the demon of acedia. The notion continued in later ages (fig. 10). Many theories have been put forward to explain the proliferation of demonic literature and befliefs in the hermetic circles, initially in Egypt and from it to the great monastic centers of the Middle East and Asia Minor. One of them is that the extreme climatic conditions in the Sahara were favorable for the appearance of imaginative scenes, especially before the rich cultural background of demonic Egyptian traditions. Another one is that the early Christian anchorite monks, reared in the socioreligious culture of their pagan society, who now felt isolated and had a guilt for betraying the faith of their ancestors, imagined the spirits of the pagan gods as devils who now attacked them bodily, for revenge [22]. It is interesting though to note that during the same period that the Greek hermetic writers were describing the demon of colic, at the other end of Europe, in Ireland, Saint Fiacre

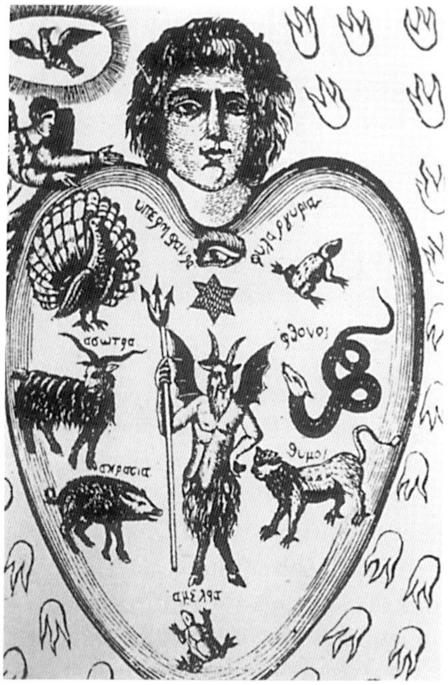

Fig. 10. A 19th-century etching depicts the seven deadly sins personified as animals. The culprit of colic, the demon of acedia, amelia ('αμέλεια' in its modern Greek name), is depicted in the middle of the lower zone.

was born in the 7th century. He sailed to France, became abbot of Breuil, and was acclaimed as the saint to be invoked against colic. Independent of their source, demons having arrived stayed for good in the Christian world.

In the Late Byzantine Empire, when Psellus wrote his treatises and John Actuarius, another believer in demons, his famous books on uroscopy, the ancient story of the Testament of Solomon was very popular. According to it, King Solomon the Wise left a kind of spiritual will in which he named several hundreds or even thousands of demons responsible for many diseases. The eponymous demons Kourtael, Rex Audemoeth, and Rex Anoster, were blamed for symptoms of the urinary tract. A special amulet was used against all three. Even the high clergy were not immune to such practices. Nicephoros Gregoras (14th century) maintained that the patriarch John Kalekas promised eternal rewards to anyone who should destroy Emperor John the 6th Kantakouzenos by poisonous medicines or deceitful exorcisms [23]. The Empire was then in decline, and, as was usual in times of crisis, the general feeling was to ask for supernatural assistance, hence magic and magicians were called for. Magicians, however, had not entirely disappeared before that period, nor have they stopped to exist in our times. We know of their existence since the Turanian people (5000 BC) inhabited the lands that later became the home of the Babylonians and Assyrians. We read their exorcisms against diseases in the Turanian language, inscribed on the Assurbanipal stone tablets. They continued to exist in the Persian Empire where medicine was not very much in use [24]. They were flourishing in Ancient Egypt, and we know from the Iliad that bleeding from one of Ulysses' wounds was stopped when the sons of Autolycus performed a special exorcism for it [25]. Classic Greek and especially Roman societies were infested by magicians of all sorts. Christianity did not succeed in extinguishing them, although during the Middle Ages in the Latin West the Catholic Church attempted magicide on a huge scale. Nowadays public performances of magic rituals do not exist, at least in Western societies. However, the less popular public magic becomes, the more widespread the private practice of magic is. Europe and the USA witness a revival of apocryphal magic societies. As a result, the formal Christian Church continues its rhetoric against them. It is characteristic that at the same time that our second Congress on the History of Nephrology took place in Padua, an article contrasting private magic practises was published in Greece, in the most prestigious of the Church's magazines [26]. It contained, amongst its many arguments, the old story of St. Cyprian, the ex-magician (fig. 11). It was the magicians' luck since their early appearance in history to be trusted, revered, looked at with awe, and prosecuted, according to the prevailing cultural climate [27]. They tried to understand the laws of nature and the irregularities of the living human body and tried to influence them towards their goals. Hence, they were the spiritual ancestors of priests, alchemists, medical doctors, and the modern breed of alternative therapists. Their reputation fluctuated inversely to that of the scientists and of formal priesthood. Yet in several cases the same person was using both scientific and magical methods. A well-known example is the medical writer Alexander of Trailles (6th century AD) who was the most eminent doctor of the early Byzantine period. He still believed in amulets and exorcisms [28]. While these events were taking place in the Orthodox East, in the Latin West the frenzy for magic and the pogrom against magicians had declined. Early Rennaissance was appearing and with it the love for the ancient logic, science, and art. However, it also brought the love for Neoplatonic and Neopythagorean ideas. Consequently, magic that was thrown out of the

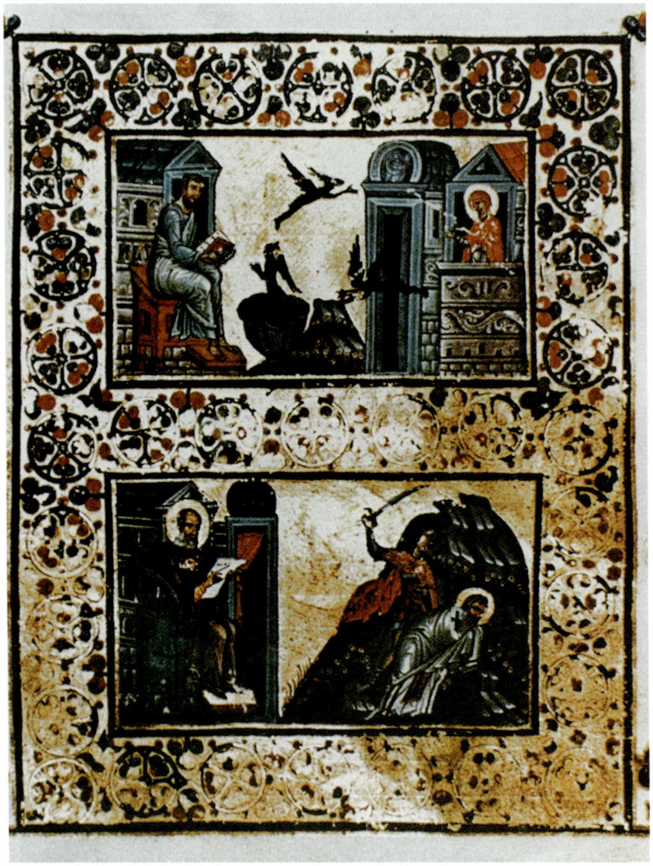

Fig. 11. At the upper zone St. Cyprian is depicted as a pagan magician sending demons against St. Justin. In the lower zone he is depicted as a Saint martyr, ready to be beheaded, after his conversion to Christianity. Manuscript illumination, ca. 12th century (Par. gr. 543, f. 87).

door returned back via the window. The ideas of Paracelsus, Campanella and Cornelius Agrippa testify to this mixture of progressive science and deeply rooted magic in the West. As already mentioned in the Byzantine East, there was no distinct separation between scientific thought and belief in demons.

Also, no tight separation existed between humans and animals. The latter, if unblessed by God, could also be affected by renal problems. Hence, a prayer for the health of the flock was a suitable chapter in our manuscript (fig. 12). The Almighty is asked to bless the flock, as the God of the Old Testament had already done for the sheep of Patriarch Jacob, in a basically agricultural society. The early Christian Fathers of the Church, and paleochristian art emphasized the role of Christ as the Good Shepherd (fig. 13). Up to this point the manuscript we present is identical with the formal Book of Prayers still in use in the Greek Orthodox Church [29]. The passages that follow are very interesting, but not included in the authorized version of the Book of Prayers. Apparently, they are false additions in the form of magical exorcisms and ancient pagan rituals that found their was into a deacon's Book of Prayers. So we read in the manuscript that:

> The sheep were brought inside the church, they stood in front of the altar, were sprinkled with holy water, and then the priest was asking the Lord to purify the sheep – (among other symptoms) – from dysuria and trisuria (frequency).

The zoological ailments just referred to were serious problems for the sheep – and the flock owners –, and any prayer against them was useful, if not genuinely religious and dogmatically Christian. We return back to the discussion at the beginning of this article, about what was false and what was authentic in Byzantium and the post-Byzantine era. It looks that our manuscript represents a hybrid book – semireligious semisorcery –, aiming at a hybrid society that was semidevotedly Christian with some bucolic-paganistic memories.

The last question that arises is why God, in His benign and all-loving nature, should wait for mankind, or even animals, to suffer for long from any diseases – renal problems, dysuria, trisuria, cystitis, in our case – before he interferes to cure them. Joseph Bryennios (15th century) provides an interesting explanation: God had never forgotten man in his tribulation, but, in a medically correct way, waited for this moment, because

> 'Just as a good doctor does not put the poultice on when the pain is increasing but when all the pus has burst forth, so also he who is long suffering by nature, withdrawing, waiting for every evil to come complete and, like a boil, to have come to a head and swelled up, and (only) then brought healing' [30].

In conclusion, I hope that sufficient evidence has been presented that renal diseases were faced in a familiar setting. Ancient and reverent traditions, from a pagan and/or Christian background, going as far back as the prophets of the Old Testament, the Hellenistic mystic deity of Hermes Trismegistus, the 4th century AD 'Books of Prayers' (Ευχολόγια), and the post medieval exorcistic remedies were amalgamated in an attempt to cure the patient. In this kind of cultural time capsule, renal – and other – diseases were looked on as a fact of life, and as a temporary hardship, before serenity and eternal life were won. Even urinary tract symptoms from the zoological realm had a parallel treatment, in a very modern, ecologically correct, I dare say, perspective. As I have emphasized in a previous paper on the history of natural mem-

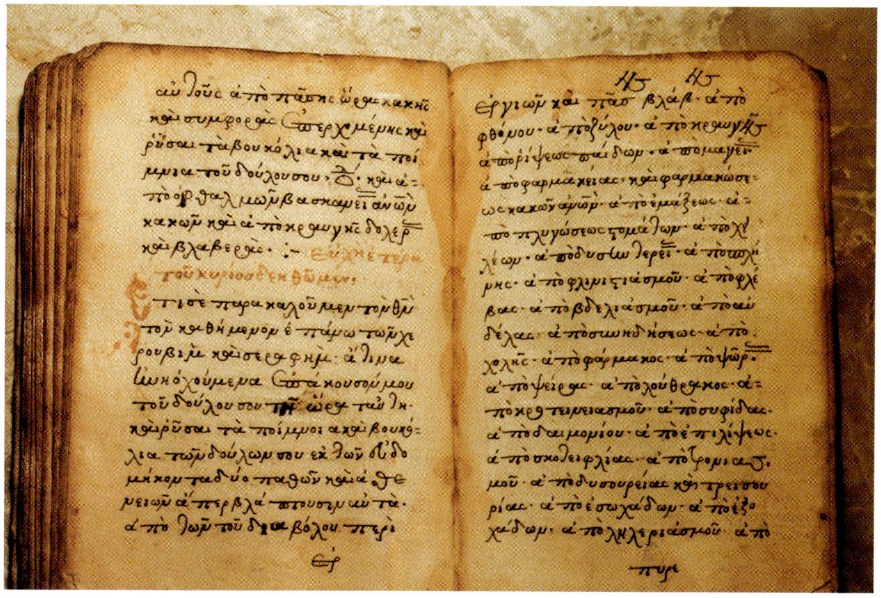

Fig. 12. On the recto: 'We pray to You Lord, the one sitting above the Cherubim and Seraphim ... and listen now to your servant and purify his flock ...' On the verso: 'from ... dysuria, trisuria'.

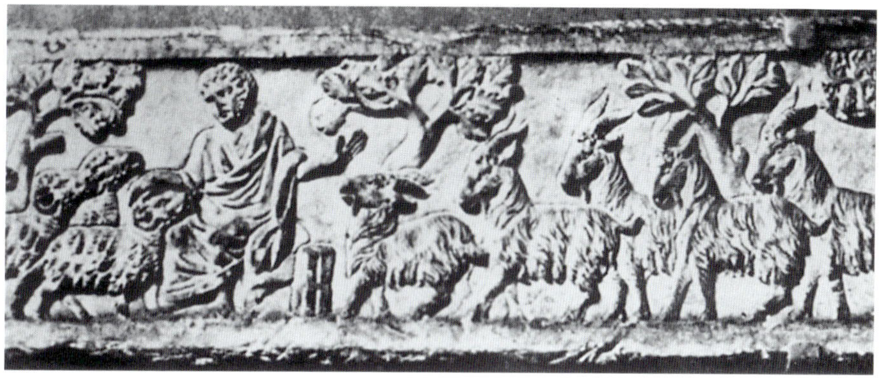

Fig. 13. A marble relief from a Paleochristian sarcophagus in the Metropolitan Museum of New York. Christ is blessing the sheep. The scene is a symbolic representation of the Last Judgement.

branes in dialysis [31], people in the medieval period did not separate themselves from the cosmos, the polis, the psyche. It is fit to add now a similar explanation for the action of prayers and exorcisms against the demons of renal diseases. It was written by the aforementioned Nicephoros Gregoras [32] in the 14th century, in his commentary on *de Insomniis*:

'The parts of the cosmos must be linked and have a share in each other just as in the case with the limbs of an animal, and (they must) have a sympathy with each other and some sort of symbiosis, as it were. Having said these things, (Synesios), as though taking himself up, raises a question and asks himself 'Perhaps the spells of magicians are like this?' For the wise man, who knows the relationship of things to each other, seeing that some things are charmed by others, attracts one thing by another. Thus, just as iron is (attracted) by a magnet, so also this or that is (attracted) by this or that material, this or that design, or this or that speech ... Not only are trees charmed by tress ... plants by plants, and animals by animals, but even the terrible fish (is charmed) by garlic and other things by other things; (finally), what is even more amazing is that demons from the air and from the land are charmed by certain stones, certain plants, certain speech, or certain designs which are called characters and which, I think, were first discovered by the Chaldeans and Egyptians, each capable of making each demon known' [32].

It looks then from the pages of our manuscript that, in patients' and healers' minds alike, the same holistic approach existed towards the cosmos, the polis, the psyche, and their effect on diseases. That is the acceptance of an unseverable link between the macrocosm and the microcosm. Thus, patients felt more comfortable with their renal problems in a cultural environment they could understand and accept.

References

1 Pitsakis KG: Crime without punishment; in Troianos S (ed): Crime and Punishment in Byzantium. Athens, Goulandri-Horn, 1997, p 337.
2 Pitsakis KG: Gregorious' Akindynus: An unpublished essay about (Constantine?) Armenopoulos. Ann Res Centre Acad Athens Hist Greek Law 1972;19:111–216.
3 Lane-Fox R: Pagans and Christians. Suffolk, Viking, 1986.
4 Perdrizet P: Feuilles de l'Université Foud à Hermoupolis Ouest, 1994, p 97.
5 Bowersock G: Hellenism in Late Antiquity. Ann Arbor, University of Michigan Press, 1990, p 35.
6 Scot R: The Discoveries of Witchcraft. London, 1930, p 178.
7 Augustine St: City of God, 8:24, 9:23, and 19:23.
8 Thomas' Acts; in James R (ed): Apocrypha Anekdota. Cambridge, 1987, vol 2, chap XXIII, p 33.
9 Athenagoras: Delegation about Christians; in Migne JP (ed): Patrologia cursus completus, series graeca. Paris 1844–1890, vol 6, p 949.
10 Eusebius: History of the church; in Migne JP (ed): Patrologia cursus completus, series graeca. Paris 1844–1890, vol 31, p 316.
11 Provataki Th: The Devil in the Byzantine Art. Salonika, Rekos, 1980, p 35.
12 Ψελλού του σοφωτάτου καί υπερτίμου, πόνημα ιατρικόν άριστον δι' ιάμβων; in Ideler IL (ed): Physici et medici Graeci minores. Berolini, 1841, vol 1, p 202.
13 Diamandopoulos A: Musical Uroscopy, on Urines: By the Wisest Vlemydes. An Excellent Medical Work in the Iambic Manner: by the Wisest Pseullus. Athens, Achaikes Ekdoseis, 1996, p 14.
14 Psellus M: Τίνα Περί δαιμόνων δοξάζουσιν Ελληνες; in Migne JP (ed): Patrologia cursus completus, series graeca. Paris 1844–1890, vol 122, pp 876–882.
15 Grisuolo U: Michele Psello, epistola a Giovanni Xiphilino. Testo critico, introduzione, traduzione e commentario. Naples, 1973.
16 Garzya A (ed): On Michael Psellus's Admission of Faith. EEBS 1966/67;35:45.
17 Arberry A (translator): The Koran Interpreted Oxford, Oxford University Press, 1982. The Cow, sections 30 and 95.
18 Clim J: The ladder of our Father John, who is amongst the Saints; in Migne JP (ed): Patrologia cursus completus, series graeca. Paris 1844–1890, vol 13, pp 857–861.
19 Homologetes M: Alphabetalphabetos (in Greek). Athos, Lavriotes, 1928, vols 8, 9.
20 Ceresa-Gastaldo A (ed): Rome, Massimo Confessore Capitoli sulla Carita, 1963, Keph. 1.49, p 66.
21 Greenfield R: Traditions of beliefs in Late Byzantine Demonology. Amsterdam, Hakkert, 1988, p 104.
22 MacDermot V: The Cult of the Seer in the Ancient Middle East: A Contribution to Current Research on Hallucinations Drawn from Coptic and Other Texts. London 1971.
23 Schopeni L, Bekker et al: Gregoras Nikephoros: Ρωμαική ιστορία. Bonn, CSHB, 1829–1855.
24 Hude C (ed): Herodoti Historiae. Oxford Classical Texts. Oxonii 1970, vol I, p 197.
25 Homer: Iliad, pp 457–458.
26 Panouses E (monk): You can defeat magic! (In Greek.) Church Piraeus, October 1998, p 24.
27 Hude C (ed): Herodoti Historiae. Oxford Classical Texts. Oxonii 1970, vol III, pp 77–79.
28 Hunger H: Die hochsprachliche profane Literatur der Byzantiner. Athens, Educational Foundation of the National Bank of Greece, 1994, p 122.
29 Zervos S (monk): The Great Book of Prayers, ed 3; based on the 1862 Venice edition (in Greek). Astir Publishing, 1986, p 503.
30 Voulgaris and Mandrakases, 1768–1794, Bryenniou logoi (in Greek). Leipzig, vol 2, p 10.
31 Diamandopoulos A: A history of natural membranes in dialysis. Am J Nephrol 1997;17:304.
32 Gregoras N: De insomniis: Ερμηνεία ειζ τον Συνέσιον Περί ενυπνίου λόγον; in Migne JP (ed): Patrologia cursus completus, series graeca. Paris 1844–1890, vol 149, pp 521–642.

Origins of Nephrology – Magic, Myth and Science

American Journal of Nephrology

Am J Nephrol 1999;19:125–132

The Contribution of Nephrology to the Development of Current Concepts of Disease

C.R.P. George

Department of Medicine and Unit for the History and Philosophy of Science, University of Sydney, Australia

Key Words

Renal disease, history · Causation · Pathogenesis · Symptoms

Abstract

Historians and philosophers of science rarely comment upon nephrological contributions to the development of general concepts of disease. In the present study, I examine this topic by starting from the premises that an idea of disease pervades most human societies, that received explanations of disease vary between people, societies and eras, and that an understanding of renal disease has often reflected general explanatory trends. Traditionally, most students of disease have belonged to one of four schools: descriptive, causal, mechanistic, or statistical. Descriptivists have tended to focus on manifestations, be these of a symptomatic, a structural, or a functional type. Causationists have focussed upon identification of the origins of diseases. Mechanists have emphasised pathogenetic processes. Statisticians have calculated mathematical differences of parameters from the mean ('the normal'), without explaining the reasons for these. Mechanists currently appear to hold the ascendancy in nephrology through their focus upon the links that connect causes with manifestations. As, however, all schools of thought have historically waxed and waned, I question the wisdom of granting any of them hegemony. Rather, I promote an event idea of disease that encompasses the causal, mechanistic and descriptive schools. Such considerations should assist nephrologists both to treat disease and to identify those of their predecessors who most advanced knowledge.

Introduction

A belief in the existence of disease is an article of faith in the religion of medicine. Without disease, our faith lacks foundation. Yet how do we know that there is disease? What do we mean when we speak of disease? Do we all mean the same thing by this word? Do *diseases* differ from *disease*? Have nephrologists contributed to the general idea of disease and, if so, which of them made the great contributions? If we truly wish to understand our patients' afflictions, then we must answer these questions.

To many doctors, schooled in the hard science of medicine and over-whelmed by the fulminating problems of the sick, such philosophical discussion must seem irrelevant. I note, however, that hardly any two people give the same definition of disease, and I suggest that if people are unclear about what they mean by something, then they are unlikely to control it. So, in order to improve our abili-

KARGER

Fax + 41 61 306 12 34
E-Mail karger@karger.ch
www.karger.com

© 1999 S. Karger AG, Basel
0250–8095/99/0192–0125$17.50/0

Accessible online at:
http://BioMedNet.com/karger

C.R.P. George, MD
Renal Unit, Concord Hospital
Sydney, NSW 2139 (Australia)
Tel. +61 2 9767 5000, Fax +61 2 9449 3212
E-Mail georgec@crgmail.crg.cs.nsw.gov.au

ty to solve ourpatients' problems, I propose to examine the ideas of disease in general and renal disease in particular.

The focus of this article is on the history of nephrology. I have set myself the task of examining the development of ideas about renal disease and their contribution to the development of universal ideas. I believe that one can best understand ideas about any subject if one understands their historical development. Hence I shall examine in turn the universality of the idea of disease, some possible explanations for this, the development of ideas about renal disease, and the place within them of much contemporary nephrological research. On the basis of this, I shall hazard a comprehensive account of the idea of disease.

The Universality of the Idea of Disease

People often speak of *disease* and *diseases* with an implication that these phenomena exist and that we do not need to justify that implication. In the present study, I too shall start from this premise and justify my action on the grounds that the literature in the fields of linguistics, anthropology, sociology, philosophy, medicine, biography and fiction contains a wealth of supportive data. Lest anyone questions this, and in deference to the venue of this meeting, I shall merely quote three literary references from works written or set near Padua two of which specifically refer to renal disease.

Dante spent much of his exile in this locality. In Canto Thirty of *The Divine Comedy*, during the journey through Hell, he wrote about an unfortunate man [1]:

> And when the furious pair had gone away
> At whom I had been gazing so intent,
> I turned towards the other luckless souls
> And saw one who was fashioned like a lute,
> If at the groins his legs had been cut off.
> The heavy dropsy, which so swells the limbs
> With ill-digested humours, that the face
> No longer fits the belly, made him hold
> His lips apart, as hectic fever makes
> A man curl one lip up, the other down.
> 'You who are free from punishment', he said,
> 'And in this dismal grim world I know not why,
> Consider Master Adam's misery.
> While living I had all that I could wish.
> And now alas I crave a drop to drink.
> The rivulets, that from the grassy hills
> Of Casentino into Arno flow,
> Making their little channels cool and moist,
> Stand ever in my sight, and not in vain –
> The image of them parches me far more
> Than this disease that robs my face of flesh'.

Shakespeare, in *The Two Gentlemen of Verona* (Act II, Scene 1), had the clownish servant, Speed, explain to Valentine, why he knew that Valentine was in love [2]:

> ... these follies are within you, and shine through you like the water in an urinal, that not an eye that sees you, but is a physician to comment on your malady.

Elsewhere Shakespeare described the universality of disease. Shylock, the Jewish hero of *The Merchant of Venice* exclaimed to a Christian acquaintance (Act II, Scene 1):

> He hath disgraced me, and hindered me half a million, laughed at my losses, mocked at my gains, scorned my nation, thwarted my bargains, cooled my friends, heated mine enemies; and what is his reason? I am a Jew. Hath not a Jew eyes? hath not a Jew hands, organs, dimensions, senses, affections, passions? Fed with the same food, hurt with the same weapons, subject to the same diseases, healed by the same means, warmed and cooled by the same winter and summer, as a Christian is? If you prick us do we not bleed? If you tickle us do we not laugh? If you poison us, do we not die? And if you wrong us shall we not revenge? If we are like you in the rest, we will resemble you in that.

These, and many similar passages, persuade me that disease both exists and is universally recognised as doing so.

Possible Explanations for Disease

People writing about disease have, at various times, advanced diverse theories to account for its nature. Examples of the many definitions that have appeared for this word include:

> Morbid condition of body, plant, or some part of them, illness, sickness; any particular kind of this with special symptoms and name; deranged or depraved state of mind or morals [3]
>
> Illness, disorder of health [4]
>
> A specific state of malfunctioning of a plant or animal body [5]
>
> An interruption, cessation, or disorder of bodily functions, systems, or organs. A morbid entity characterized usually by at least two of these criteria: recognized etiologic agent(s), identifiable group of signs and symptoms, or consistent anatomical alterations [6]
>
> Literally, the lack of ease; a pathological condition of the body that presents a group of clinical signs and symptoms and laboratory findings peculiar to it and that sets the condition apart as an abnormal entity differing from other normal or pathological body states [7]
>
> In general, a departure from the normal state of health. More specifically, a disease is the sum total of the reactions, physical and mental, made by a person to a noxious agent entering his body from without or arising within [8]

Alteration of the state of health; perturbation of the normal functions of one or more organs, of which the causes are in general known and which express themselves by some signs and symptoms [translated from 9]

These definitions have huge differences. They range from emphasis on morbidity to malfunction, from structural abnormality to definitive cause, from manifestations to statistical variation, from a single phenomenon to a multiplicity of phenomena, and from one diagnostic criterion to a combination of criteria. Different people obviously mean different things by the word *disease*. Elsewhere I have attempted a classification of the principal theories under the major headings of manifestation theories, internal imbalance (pathogenetic mechanism) theories, external causal theories and an event theory [10].

It is also obvious that various explanations have gained favour at various times. Acceptance has varied from society to society and from era to era. Many of them, interestingly, correlate with beliefs espoused by the competing medical schools ('sects') of classical Greece and Rome [11]: the Hippocratic physicians who followed the practices of the Asclepiads (they observed the patient and his symptoms carefully, reflected soberly upon these, adhered to the accumulated corpus of medical wisdom about classes of disease, and placed the patient's best interests ahead of all other considerations); the empiricists, who only accepted evidence that they could elicit by careful history taking and physical examination of the individual patient, and who denied an ability to generalise about classes of disease; the dogmatists, who emphasised imbalance of various postulated internal 'humours' as the mechanism of disease; the methodists, who believed that imbalance of fluids traversing microscopic pores in tissues caused disease; the pneumatists, who emphasised physical mechanisms, especially of 'vital air', in the mediation of disease; the sceptics, who, whilst accepting the eventual possibility of knowing something about the nature of disease, considered this impossible at that time, and the eclectics, who saw some merit in the claims of each of the other sects, but stood aloof from all of them.

An outstanding feature of these classical schools was that they reflected into medicine general philosophical ideas that circulated in the contemporary world. Indeed, one can speculate as to what had the greater influence – attempts to explain disease upon general Graeco-Roman philosophy, or general philosophy upon medical ideas. Regardless of which pertained, close interaction has persisted ever since.

Later, during the Renaissance, the revival of anatomical dissection extended the field of vision of physicians to structural abnormalities of internal organs. These emphasised a manifestation-type understanding of disease. Soon afterwards, the development of Newtonian physics, followed by a clearer understanding of chemistry encouraged further manifestation thinking by emphasising the idea of internal malfunction associated with disease.

Superimposed upon each of these manifestation ideas, however, was the idea of causation. From the earliest times, people had thought about causes. The ancient Egyptians (to whom gastrointestinal parasites loomed large) emphasised them, as did members of the Cnidian school in classical Greece. Factors such as air, water and climate received special aetiological emphasis. With the invention in the late 18th century of new intellectual and physical tools of investigation, discussion again flourished. David Hume's innovative analysis of causation coincided with the application of new physical, chemical and microscopical techniques. Means then existed by which to associate causes with observed manifestations. Searching for deterministic pathways became an important exercise in medicine, and rose to new heights of influence with the discovery of pathogenic micro-organisms during the late 19th century. Well into the 20th century, the prospect of causal explanation continued to drive research powerfully by its implication that, once the cause of a disease was known, nothing further remained for investigators to discover. Thus the great medical historian and philosopher, Lester S. King [12], claimed in 1965 that: 'Twentieth century medicine revolves around the notion of cause'. Along similar lines, the authors of many current textbooks seek to classify most diseases into causally based categories [13, 14].

Nevertheless, however clearly the causes and the manifestations were delineated, their mere enunciation failed to explain how one transformed into the other. Each, in its own right, was an important component of the total disease process, but neither alone nor together explained the link between them. In some way, the instigating cause (what Aristotle would have called *the efficient cause*) acted on the patient (whose presence was also causally necessary) to induce some change within the patient. The fact that interaction had occurred then became apparent as manifestations. In this schema of disease, not only were the causes and the manifestations important, but also the interaction that linked them together – its physical position within the body, its timing, and the details of its mechanism.

One might develop a new idea of a disease by invoking a combination of all of these factors – the causes, the interaction and the manifestations – as a composite description of the total event. In contemporary medicine, such possibilities particularly appeal to researchers who focus upon the mechanisms that link causes with manifestations. On this analysis, each event is a unique disease and there are as many diseases as there are events. However, many such disease descriptions then resemble other disease descriptions, such that when a similar cause acts upon a similar individual then a similar event probably occurs conforming to a typical disease pattern. Expressed otherwise, whenever a cause of type X acts on an individual of type Y, then an X-Y event occurs and produces an example of X-Y disease. This encompasses the ideas of the causal, the mechanistic and the descriptive schools of thought. The statistical school emphasises recognition of the difference of X-Y disease from normal, but does not explain the origin of that difference from normal.

The Development of Ideas about Renal Disease

Symptomatic Description

Much understanding of renal disease followed the development of knowledge about renal anatomy and physiology. Without the latter, most ideation equated to symptomatic explanation and avoided speculation. Thus the Bible, the Hippocratic corpus, Arabic and medieval writings contained many references to the urine and the kidneys that emphasised urinary symptoms. These included the passage of stones or blood, changes in the appearance of the urine ('uroscopy'), and symptomatic associations of purported prognostic significance [15–18]. Such descriptions of kidney disease correlated closely with descriptions of diseases of other organ systems of the body.

Lesion Theories

By the late 16th century, however, the occasional performance of autopsies transformed manifestation perceptions from a symptomatically based to a lesion-based level. An early example of this occurred in the studies of Francisco Diaz, a Spanish physician who in 1588 published reports of patients with urinary symptoms [19].

A few other writers before the early 19th century described patients with grossly damaged kidneys. William Charles Wells [20] in 1812 was one of the more important of these because of his integration of observations of clinical and anatomical abnormalities with causal considerations and speculation about the mechanisms that linked the various aspects. Fifteen years later, Richard Bright [21], in his beautifully illustrated *Reports of Medical Cases Selected with a View of Illustrating the Symptoms and Cure of Diseases by a Reference to Morbid Anatomy*, enhanced the intellectual link between symptomatic manifestation and anatomical abnormality. He distinguished between yellow, mottled 'degenerate' kidneys, kidneys with a granulated white deposit, and hard contracted kidneys. He also sought correlations between the anatomical abnormalities and the clinical manifestations from which the patients had suffered before death.

Bright's work stimulated many others to investigate the structural abnormalities present in renal disease. An outstanding early investigator was the Frenchman, Pierre Rayer [22], who published his comprehensive *Traité des maladies des reins* in 1839. The classification of renal disease that he proposed provides considerable insight into contemporary ideation. He suggested two major categories, with further subdivisions: diseases of the kidneys and special alterations of urinary secretion. He then subdivided diseases of the kidneys into eleven groups with further subdivisions of those:

A Diseases of the kidneys
1 Wounds, contusions or tears
2 Inflammations attacking the substance of the kidneys: nephritis (simple, gouty, rheumatic, from purulent resorption, or albuminous), pyelitis (simple, mucous, calculous, or haemorrhagic), pyelonephritis, idiopathic perinephritis (idiopathic, or symptomatic), and renal fistulae (to the loins, duodenum, colon, peritoneum, or lungs)
3 Haemorrhages: idiopathic, symptomatic (of wounds, pelvic calculi, cancer, or purpura), or endemic
4 Hyperaemia, or anaemia
5 Hypertrophy, or atrophy (congenital, or accidental)
6 Hydronephrosis, or cysts
7 The elementary renal tissues: of veins, arteries, lymphatics, or nerves
8 Tissues and dead materials: homologous (fibrous, cartilaginous, bony, erectile, or fat), or heterologous (tubercles, cancer, yellow material, or melanosis)
9 Foreign bodies: animate (Strongylus, or spiral organisms), or inanimate (pseudohelminths, or balls)
10 Gangrene
11 Anomalies: of number (supernumerary kidneys, absence of one or two kidneys), of situation (in the pelvis, or fusion), or configuration (congenital, or accidental).

B Special alterations of urinary secretion
1 Abnormalities of quantity: anuria, dysuria (by which he meant diminution of the secretion of urine), or polyuria
2 Abnormalities of composition: by reduction of one or more natural substances, by increase of some natural substances (of water, urea, acid, or phosphate), by the presence of abnormal substances (gravel or stones due to carbonate of chalk, oxalate, silica, cystic oxide, xanthic acid, or hair, phosphorus, chyle, sugar, blue material, or black material)
3 Abnormalities of the method of excretion.

Rayer based his extensive classification on symptomatic and anatomical manifestations. His rare forays beyond those bounds, included some cases of nephritis that he associated with such infections as scarlet fever and typhoid fever. In these, he introduced the idea of causality.

Similar ideas prevailed throughout the 19th century. Thus, Henry Morris [23], in his *Surgical Diseases of the Kidney* in 1885 gave a classification that closely resembled that of Rayer. Regarding Bright's disease, Carl Wedl [24] in his *Rudiments of Pathological Histology* of 1855 attributed that condition predominantly to exudation into the renal tubules, although he did mention that in some cases a fibrinous exudate also occurred on the surfaces of the glomerular capillary tufts. A new era of anatomical precision dawned in 1870, however, when Edwin Klebs [25] coined the term *glomerulonephritis* to emphasise glomerular involvement by targeting the glomerular inflammation that he observed to occur in postscarlatinal nephritis. Others were slow to accept his ideas, with the result that for most of the next decade authors such as Loomis [26] continued to emphasise the tubules as the principal site of damage in 'nephritis'. Nevertheless, in amyloid disease, they did accept that the glomeruli suffered severe damage. Most discussion throughout the 19th and early 20th centuries remained about symptomatic and lesion-based manifestations with some speculation about aetiology, especially previous streptococcal infection [27].

Progressively during the 20th century – and especially with the increasing use of percutaneous renal biopsy after 1951 [28] – nephrologists adopted histological classifications to allocate patients to a range of disease categories based primarily upon light microscopical observations [29–32]. The introduction of electron microscopy later enhanced their ability to categorise these on histological grounds [33]. The consequence was development of a hierarchy of glomerular diseases classified on histological grounds, including such entities as lipoid nephrosis (later known as minimal lesion nephrotic syndrome) [34, 35], focal sclerosing glomerulonephritis (focal segmental glomerulosclerosis) [36, 37], membranous glomerulonephritis (membranous nephropathy) [38], mesangiocapillary glomerulonephritis (lobular glomerulonephritis, membranoproliferative glomerulonephritis) [39], focal proliferative glomerulonephritis [40], diffuse proliferative and exudative glomerulonephritis, and crescentic glomerulonephritis [40]. Almost every year, investigators have added additional entities to this burgeoning manifestation-based list, with the result that clinicians have found themselves working with a primarily histological classification of glomerular diseases. This has inevitably served to perpetuate a lesion-based idea of the nature of disease in the minds of many nephrologists, although concomitant developments have tended to challenge this.

Theories of Disordered Function

William Charles Wells, to whose observations on clinical and anatomical abnormalities of the kidneys I have already alluded, drew attention in his 1812 papers to the associated functional abnormality of excessive excretion of protein. Richard Bright [21] and John Bostock developed this theme further, with the latter describing a reduction of urinary excretion of urea in some cases. Shortly afterwards, Robert Christison [41] in Edinburgh demonstrated the accumulation of urea in the blood of such patients and attributed these changes to failure of excretion of urea that, he postulated, was formed elsewhere in the body than the kidneys. In this he confirmed in humans observations that Prevost and Dumas had made a short time previously in France in animals subjected to bilateral nephrectomy. Many more years passed before nephrologists gained further insights into the functional abnormalities associated with renal diseases. In the first two decades of the 20th century, however, with the improvement of micro-analytical techniques in chemistry, observers noted that substances such as creatinine, hydrogen ions, potassium, phosphate, and urate accumulated in renal failure. Then – in the mid-20th century following upon the identification of various hormones secreted by the endocrine glands – perturbed endocrine function associated with uraemia also claimed attention.

Patients suffering from chronic glomerular diseases formed the majority of those upon whom nephrologists had made these observations. Despite an earlier awareness that renal function could deteriorate rapidly in many victims of glomerulonephritis, the clear recognition of acute renal failure as a syndrome most commonly associated with damage to the renal tubules did not develop until the observations made by Bywaters [42] and others on previously healthy people who suffered from crush injuries in the air raids of World War II.

Awareness of the existence of other functional defects of the kidneys – especially the renal tubules – gradually accumulated, especially in the mid-20th century [43]. Most often this arose through intensive testing with newly developed biochemical methods of occasional patients who presented with bizarre clinical features. Urinary stone formers comprised another large group whom investigators subjected to intensive biochemical analysis at about the same time in attempts to identify the functional abnormalities associated with their disease.

The reality that much of the everyday work of renal medicine involves the supervision of dialysis and transplant treatment for acute and chronic renal failure emphasises the practical implications of functional deficit as the crucial manifestation of disease. Just as the current system of histological classification magnifies the importance of a lesion-based manifestation theory of disease, so the therapeutic imperatives of renal failure emphasise the idea of a functionally based theory.

Causal Theories

In nephrology, one of the earliest positive identifications of a causal condition for kidney disease is found in William Charles Wells's 1812 paper [44], in which he associated scarlet fever with proteinuria and underlying renal disease. With the identification, towards the end of the 19th century, of streptococcal infection as the cause of scarlet fever, many people gained the impression that most or all cases of glomerulonephritis resulted from previous streptococcal infection. Subsequently, however, the development of serological markers (by which previous exposure to streptococcal infection became provable) destroyed that hypothesis. Many investigators searched intensely for other causes, usually unsuccessfully. Thus, although renal involvement secondary to a range of other febrile illnesses and bacterial infections had received attention during the 19th century – triggered especially by the microbiological revolution that occurred between 1880 and 1900 – for most renal conditions ultimate causation remained, and still remains, unclear.

Although this situation applies to glomerulonephritis and many other renal diseases, some obvious exceptions include analgesic nephropathy, heavy metal poisoning, drug-induced renal diseases, urinary tract tuberculosis, schistosomiasis and other parasitic diseases, Hantavirus, many cases of acute renal failure, and some cases of stone disease. In other situations – such as diabetic nephropathy and atherosclerotic renal and renovascular disease – the manifestations in the urinary tract are merely part of a broader clinical picture in which the ultimate causal details remain obscure. In some other cases, the renal disease is inherited but the cause of the original genetic mutation remains unclear. In still others, the urinary tract disease is associated with infection to which anatomical abnormalities that themselves have an unclear cause have predisposed.

In summary, therefore, all cases of renal disease are assumed to have causes, however most of these causes remain partially or completely unidentifiable. Nephrology does not, in this regard, differ greatly from many other medical disciplines. Causation seems in practice to fail as a useful paradigm for disease when causes are so difficult to identify.

Mechanistic Theories

One of the distinguishing characteristics of twentieth century nephrology has been the burgeoning of mechanistic investigations into the processes involved in the development of disease. The creation of animal models of human diseases and the development of progressively improving techniques for animal experimentation have stimulated these events. Their development has occurred in close conjunction with the evolution of the fields of immunology and molecular biology.

The discovery of the phenomenon now known as serum sickness was of outstanding significance to these developments [45]. The observations of Claude Bernard (1869), Lindemann (who first induced nephrotoxic nephritis in 1900), Pearce (1903), von Pirquet (who postulated the possibility of circulating immune complexes in 1911), Longcope (who studied the renal pathology in detail in 1913), Masugi (in 1931–1932), Pressman (who employed radiolabelled antibodies in 1949) all culminated in the proposal by Germuth in 1953 that acute serum sickness is an immune-complex-mediated disease. Other animal models followed rapidly. Heymann (1959) and Steblay (1962) developed important examples, soon followed by many others.

Another major advance occurred in 1914 when Gunn [46] observed that the serum level of haemolytic complement fell markedly in acute post-streptococcal glomerulonephritis. This information in turn led to many subsequent investigations into the role that the complement system plays in the mediation of glomerular injury. More recently, many additional mediators have attracted attention. They include leucocytes, monocytes, macrophages, platelets, fibrinogen, cytokines and adhesion molecules. The families of the latter two of these in particular have grown rapidly over the past decade as investigators have identified new substances and examined their roles in the mediation of disease, especially of the glomeruli [47].

In other types of renal disease apart from glomerulonephritis, corresponding advances have occurred in recent years in the identification of mechanisms of injury. Examples of these include polycystic kidney disease, for which the genetic basis of the condition has now been identified (although the original cause of the damaged gene remains unknown) and Alport's syndrome, where researchers have not only identified the genetic abnormalities, but also derived information about the biochemical processes with which these interfere [48].

The mechanisms and mediators mentioned above form only a few of the many that have attracted attention and investigation over recent decades. Each of these mediators of injury serves to link the cause of a disease with its manifestations. The roles of such mediators extend to many diseases beyond those of interest to the nephrologist. Clearly any idea of disease as a whole cannot rely solely upon them since they neither arise spontaneously nor perform their actions entirely without manifestations. Since, however, they do command considerable attention in current assessments of individually diseased animals and patients, they are fundamental to any contemporary ideation about the nature of disease.

An Event Concept of Disease

The evidence presented above suggests that ideas about disease change from era to era. Similar evidence suggests that they change also from society to society. Running through many of the ideas, however, and waxing and waning with time, are the three major themes – of causes, of mechanisms, and of manifestations. All of them recur in any consideration of any individual disease, and of disease as a generic whole. Presumably, then, if one wishes to capture the essence of the idea of disease one should attempt to capture elements of each of these themes.

One might manage to achieve that goal by postulating that (at least at the present time) people understand by disease something that attacks the body from outside (hence the attacker and the body are both necessary causes) leading to an internal event (the pathogenetic mechanism of the disease) that often is manifested by observable stigmata. In that the latter differ from normal, they accord with statistical views of disease. In this theory, all three elements are necessary for the occurrence of disease. A key element, however, that distinguishes this case of disease from that similar case is that the mechanistic event at the centre of the link between cause and manifestation is unique to the individual in which it occurs. As such, it differs from the external element of the causal component (which may be identical between many individuals), but not from the manifestations, which are also unique to this individual. Thus the interaction of the external cause and the individual occurs in a unique person at a unique time and so distinguishes each case from the next.

In the above analysis, developments in nephrology have contributed significantly to the current understanding of disease, although they have often moved closely in parallel with developments in other organ systems. These developments have not occurred spontaneously, but rather have arisen out of insights expounded by particular research workers. Their identification should, then, enable historians to identify those researchers who contributed most to the development of the field.

References

1 Dante Alighieri: The Divine Comedy. Translated by Kenneth Mackenzie. London, Folio Society, 1979.
2 Shakespeare W: The Illustrated Stratford Shakespeare. London, Chancellor Press, 1985.
3 Fowler HW, Fowler FG: The Concise Oxford Dictionary of Current English. Oxford, Clarendon Press, 1954.
4 Makins M (ed): Collins Concise Dictionary and Thesaurus. Glasgow, Harper Collins, 1991.
5 Husted J: Dorland's Pocket Medical Dictionary, ed 20. Philadelphia, Saunders, 1959.
6 Spraycar M (ed): Stedman's Medical Dictionary, ed 26. Baltimore, Williams & Wilkins, 1995.
7 Thomas CL (ed): Taber's Cyclopedic Medical Dictionary, ed 17. Philadelphia, Davis, 1993.
8 Critchley M (ed): Butterworths Medical Dictionary, ed 2. London, Butterworths, 1984.
9 Grünfeld J-P (ed): Dictionnaire de Médecine Flammarion, ed 5. Paris, Flammarion, 1994.
10 George CRP: The philosophy of disease. Bull Postgrad Comm Med Univ Sydney 1988;44: 83–93.
11 Sarton G: Galen of Pergamon. Lawrence, University of Kansas Press, 1954.
12 King LS: Some problems of causality in eighteenth century medicine. Bull Hist Med 1963; 37:15–24.
13 Weatherall DJ, Ledingham JGG, Warrell DA (eds): Oxford Textbook of Medicine, ed 3. Oxford, Oxford University Press, 1996.
14 Wilson JD, Braunwald E, Isselbacher KJ, Petersdorf RG, Martin JB, Fauci AS, Root RK (eds): Harrison's Principles of Internal Medicine, ed 12. New York, McGraw-Hill, 1991.
15 Kopple JD: The Biblical View of the Kidney. Am J Nephrol 1994;14:279–281.
16 Eknoyan G: Origins of nephrology: Hippocrates, the father of clinical nephrology. Am J Nephrol 1988;8:498–507.
17 Eknoyan G: Arabic medicine and nephrology. Am J Nephrol 1994;14:270–278.
18 Angeletti LR, Caavarra B: Critical and historical approach to Theophilus' *De Urinis*. Urine as blood's percolation made by the kidney and uroscopy in the Middle Ages. Am J Nephrol 1994;14:282–289.
19 Palmero JR: Nephrology from the Middle Ages to humanism: The Italian influence in Spain (12th–16th centuries). Am J Nephrol 1994;14: 282–289.
20 Wells WC: On the presence of the red matter and serum of blood in the urine of dropsy, which has not originated from scarlet fever. Trans Improvement Med Chir Knowledge 1812;3:194–240.

21 Bright R: Reports of Medical Cases, Selected with a View of Illustrating the Symptoms and Cure of Diseases by a Reference to Morbid Anatomy. London, Longman, Rees, Orme, Brown & Green, 1827.
22 Rayer P: Traité des maladies des reins, et des altérations de la sécrétion urinaire étudiés en elles-mêmes et dans leurs rapports avec les maladies des uretère, de la vessie, de la prostate, de l'urètre, etc. Paris, Baillière, 1839.
23 Morris H: Surgical Diseases of the Kidney. London, Cassell, 1885.
24 Wedl C: Rudiments of Pathological Histology. London, Sydenham Society, 1855, pp 257–268.
25 Klebs TAE: Handbuch der pathologischen Anatomie. 1. Abt. Berlin, Hirschwald, 1870, pp 644–648.
26 Loomis AL: Lectures on Diseases of the Respiratory Organs, Heart and Kidneys. New York, William Wood, 1878, pp 452–475.
27 Heptinstall RH: Pathology of the Kidney. Boston, Little, Brown, 1966.
28 Kark RM: Renal biopsy and the modern era; in Cameron JS, Glassock RJ (eds): The Nephrotic Syndrome. New York, Dekker, 1988, pp 57–86.
29 Russell DS: A Classification of Bright's Disease. London, His Majesty's Stationary Office, 1929.
30 Brewer DB: Renal Biopsy. London, Arnold, 1964.
31 Kincaid-Smith P, Mathew TH, Becker EL: Glomerulonephritis: Morphology, Natural History and Treatment (2 vols). New York, Wiley, 1973.
32 Striker LJ, Olson JL, Striker GE: The Renal Biopsy, ed 2. Philadelphia, Saunders, 1990.
33 Farquhar MG, Vernier RL, Good RA: An electron microscope study of the glomerulus in nephrosis, glomerulonephritis and lupus erythematosus. J Exp Med 1957;106:640–660.
34 Müller F: Morbus Brighti. Verh Dtsch Pathol Ges 1905;9:64–99.
35 Kark RM, Pirani CL, Pollak VE, Muehrcke RC, Blainey JD: The nephrotic syndrome in adults: A common disorder with many causes. Ann Intern Med 1958;49:751–774.
36 Rich AR: A hitherto undescribed vulnerability of the juxta-medullary glomeruli in lipoid nephrosis. Bull Johns Hopkins Hosp 1957;100: 173–186.
37 McGovern VJ: Focal sclerosing glomerulonephritis. Bull Postgraduate Comm Med Univ Sydney 1964;20:116–120.
38 Bell ET: Clinical and pathological study of subacute and chronic glomerulonephritis, including lipoid nephrosis. Am J Pathol 1938;14: 691–736.
39 West CD, McAdams AJ, McConville JM, Davis NC, Holland NH: Hypocomplementemic and normocomplementemic persistent (chronic) glomerulonephritis, clinical and pathological characteristics. J Pediatrics 1965; 67:1089–1112.
40 Volhard F, Fahr TH: Die Bright'sche Nierenkrankheit. Berlin, Springer, 1914.
41 Christison R: Observations on the variety of dropsy which depends on diseased kidney. Edinburgh Med Surg J 1829;32:262–291.
42 Bywaters EGL: Crush injuries with impairment of renal function. Br Med J 1941;1:427–432.
43 Woolf LI: Renal Tubular Dysfunction. Springfield, Thomas, 1966, pp 71–74.
44 Wells WC: Observations on the dropsy, which succeeds scarlet fever. Trans Soc Improvement Med Chir Knowledge 1812;3:167–186.
45 Albini B, Brentjens JR, Andres GA: The Immunopathology of the Kidney. London, Arnold, 1979.
46 Gunn WC: Variation in amount of complement in blood in some infectious diseases and its relation to clinical features. J Pathol Bacteriol 1914;19:155.
47 Savill J, Rees AJ: Mechanisms of glomerular injury; in Davison AM, Cameron JS, Grünfeld J-P, Kerr DNS, Ritz E, Winnearls CG (eds): Oxford Textbook of Clinical Nephrology, ed 2. Oxford, Oxford University Press, 1998, vol 1, pp 403–439.
48 Tryggvason K: Molecular Pathology and Genetics of Alport Syndrome. Basel, Karger, 1996.

American Journal of Nephrology

Am J Nephrol 1999;19:133–139

The Future of the Realm: Medicine and Divination in Ancient Syro-Mesopotamia

Salim Mujais

Renal Division, Baxter Healthcare Corp., Deerfield, Ill., USA

Key Words
Legislation · Divination · Omen · Extispicy

Abstract
The contributions of Syro-Mesopotamian cultures to the understanding of illnesses and organ functions have been sought in examination of medical and therapeutic texts. These provide a wealth of knowledge on prevalent diseases and nascent empirical therapeutics. There are, however, other sources of information relevant to this topic that have not been as thoroughly explored. Examination of representative arts, for example, provides documentations of the breadth of anatomical knowledge in these cultures. Study of the omen literature is useful in illustrating beliefs in disease etiology as well as documentation of prevalent diseases and observations on anatomical variations. In the present article we explore the various sources for information relevant to the kidney and related diseases.

Introduction

The contributions of the cultures of Syro-Mesopotamia to the medical field have remained largely unrecognized [1]. This can be ascribed to multilayered difficulties emanating from several sources. Primary among the latter is the ubiquitous presence of what the Palestinian scholar Edward Said has termed 'Orientalism' which is the tendency of Western authors to view the Near East (ancient and modern) through the prismal distortions of preconceived ideas and notions. In the case of ancient Syro-Mesopotamia, the major distorting prism is the Old Testament that created the impression of militarism and pagan depravity of these cultures. Additional difficulties arise from the dispersion of primary sources of information and the difficulties inherent in the understanding of ancient languages. The literary and intellectual heritage of Syro-Mesopotamia is not as readily available for examination as that of Ancient Egypt for its material evidence was preserved on clay tablets that required for their preservation firing which is energy demanding. Further, clay tablets are easier to disperse and loose, and those relating to medical issues are not as likely to elicit the enthusiasm of Assyriologists as would historical or mythical narratives.

In the early 1920s, Campbell Thompson published 660 medical tablets from the library of Asshurbanipal. More recently, Franz Kocher has published a series of volumes called 'Die Babylonisch-Assyrische Medizin'. The first four of these contain 420 tablets found from sites other than Assurbanipal's library, including the library of a medical practitioner from Neo-Assyrian Assur, as well as Middle Assyrian and Middle Babylonian texts. The remaining two volumes of Kocher's work augment Camp-

KARGER
Fax + 41 61 306 12 34
E-Mail karger@karger.ch
www.karger.com

© 1999 S. Karger AG, Basel
0250–8095/99/0192–0133$17.50/0

Accessible online at:
http://BioMedNet.com/karger

Salim Mujais, MD
Renal Division, Baxter Healthcare Corp.
1 Baxter Parkway
Deerfield, IL 60015 (USA)
Tel. +1 847 948 3610, Fax +1 847 948 3694, E-Mail mujaiss@baxter.com

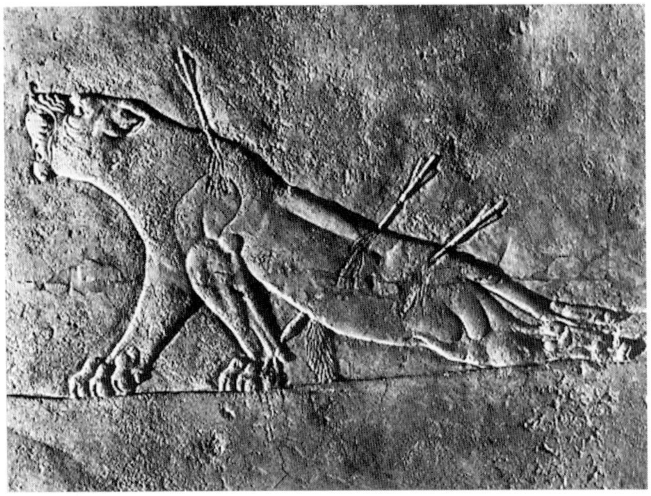

Fig. 1. Representation from a lion hunt, illustrating paraplegia of the lower extremities from arrow injury to the spinal cord. The accurate depiction of surface anatomy for which Assyrian artists are famed for is coupled with correct observation of the effects of injuries.

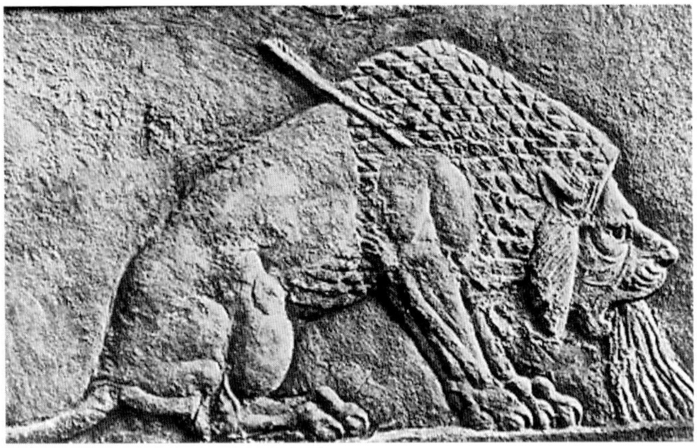

Fig. 2. Another representation from a lion hunt, depicting hemoptysis from a perforating chest injury.

bell Thompson, providing new joints of broken fragments and much material uncovered in the British Museum. The vast majority of these tablets are prescriptions, but there are a few series of tablets that contain entries that were directly related to each other and have been labeled 'treatises'. The largest surviving such medical treatise from ancient Mesopotamia is known as 'Treatise of Medical Diagnosis and Prognoses'. The text of this treatise consists of 40 tablets collected and studied by the French scholar R. Labat. Although the oldest surviving copy of this treatise dates to around 1600 BCE, the information contained in the text is an amalgamation of several centuries of Mesopotamian medical knowledge. The diagnostic treatise is organized anatomically from head to toe, with separate subsections covering convulsive disorders, gynecology, and pediatrics.

It is unfortunate that the antiquated translations available at present to the non specialist make ancient Mesopotamian medical texts sound like excerpts from a sorcerer's handbook. In fact, as recent research is showing, the descriptions of diseases contained in the diagnostic treatise demonstrate a keen ability to observe and are usually quite astute [1–6]. Virtually all expected diseases can be found described in parts of the diagnostic treatise, when those parts are fully restored, as they are for neurology, fevers, worms and flukes, sexually transmitted diseases, and skin lesions. The medical texts are, moreover, essentially rational, and some of the treatments may be shown to have an empiric basis.

To restrict the examination of medical knowledge to 'medical' texts, however, is to underestimate the achievements of these ancient cultures in the areas of anatomic observations and disease manifestation (fig. 1, 2). The sources of this knowledge may lie in 'nonmedical' texts such as omen and divination texts. Further, the concepts of disease etiologies may be better appreciated against the background of religious thought, particularly when no mundane event could explain the pathology for ancient observers. In the present article we will attempt to shed light on the various sources of medical-anatomical-pathologic observations, focusing whenever possible on conditions affecting the urogenital system.

Medical Practitioners

Two categories of Syro-Mesopotamian medical practice may be identified: The first can be labeled 'therapeutic medicine' and was practiced by the *Asu*. It was focused on surgery and the use of either simple herbal or complex herbal therapies, administered orally, rectally, percutaneously, or by instillation into the bladder. Many of the plants incorporated into the *Asu* medicinal repertoire had antibiotic properties, while several resins and many spices have some antiseptic value and would mask the smell of a malodorous wound. The second category can be labeled 'divinatory medicine' and was practiced by the *Asipu*. It was focused on incantations, amulets, and prognostication. Several gods were associated with the work of both types of physicians: (1) *Ninib* (*Enlil*'s son) and his consort *Gula*, the great female physician who resuscitated the dead by touching them with her pure hands. The temples of Gula have been identified as healing spaces to which the sick were brought. (2) *Ninazu* (Lord of Physicians) and his son *Ningishzida* whose emblem was a double-headed snake and may be the original source of the modern emblem of the medical sciences. (3) *Ea* (Lord of Water) worshiped as ancestor of physicians.

Legislation for Therapeutic Medicine

As indicated in the Introduction, the assessment of Syro-Mesopotamian medical achievements can be expanded by examination of 'nonmedical' texts. Legal texts from the rule of Ur-Namu (3rd millennium BCE) establish monetary penalties for bodily injuries (whether resulting from medical practice or not), a practice that continues in many current penal codes [7].

A more elaborate handling of the legal aspects of medical practice is found in the laws of Hammurabi promulgated in the early part of the 2nd millennium BCE. Two examples will suffice:

(1) If a physician operates on a man for a severe wound with a bronze lancet and saves the man's life; or if he opens an abscess of a man with a bronze lancet and saves that man's eye, he shall receive ten shekels of silver.

(2) If a physician operates on a man for a severe wound with a bronze lancet and causes the man's death; or if he opens an abscess of a man with a bronze lancet and destroys the man's eye, they shall cut off his fingers.

It can be argued from these and similar texts that these laws already established the concept of managed care for the practice of medicine [8]. Codex Hammurabi described a sliding fee schedule for services, promoted outcome measurements, which if not met resulted in harsh penalties, required medical records to document diseases and therapies, included prescription benefits, fully explained patient's rights, and marketing and advertising publicized in the edicts of the King. The laws were inscribed on large pillars and erected in most cities under this ruler's hegemony. Even though the managed care was authoritarian, there were legal actions to insure justice and equity particular to each social class in the kingdom. Spiegel and Springer [8] have argued that, tempered by time, the managed care mandates of Codex Hammurabi can still be considered the genesis of the current concepts of managed care.

Divine Causes of Illness

Illnesses for which no obvious event or directly observed causation could be identified were ascribed to divine causes. Spirits (gods, ghosts, demons etc.) were held responsible in an anatomically specific scheme, i.e., each spirit was responsible for disease in a well-defined body part as illustrated by the following incantation (fig. 3, 4):

'*Ashakku* has approached the head of the man
Namtar has approached the throat of the man
The evil *Utukku* has approached his neck
The evil *Alu* has approached his breast
The evil *Etimmu* has approached his stomach
The evil *Gallu* has approached his hand
The evil god has approached his foot.
The seven together have seized him:
They have burned his body like a glowing-fire.'

Presumably specific offerings were made to a particular god or ghost when it was considered to be a causative factor, but these offerings are not indicated in the medical texts and must have been found in other texts. The plants used in treatment were generally used to treat the symptoms of the disease and were not the sorts of things generally given for magical purposes to such a spirit. This would imply that while divine causes were thought to be operative, empiric solutions were devised. It also suggests that they may have had an understanding that various organs could simply malfunction, causing illness.

Diseases of the Urogenital System

Diseases of bladder and urethra were well known and can easily be related to modern-language renditions of similar conditions: *Aban mustinni*: bladder stone (compare with *mathanna* – bladder – in Arabic); *Musu*: bladder schistosomiasis with hematuria, calculi, and painful micturition, and *Hiniqtu*: urethral stricture (compare with *khiniqtu* in Arabic). Geller and Cohen [1] have described similar aspects. It is more relevant at this point to revisit the prognostic texts mentioned above and examine the manifestations of renal diseases in them in the light of novel interpretations of certain words. In particular, modern Assyriologists have indicated that Labat [9] overutilized the term 'inflammation' in segments of the text where a more accurate rendition would have been swelling.

The following segment from the 12th tablet is immediately evident to nephrologists [9]:

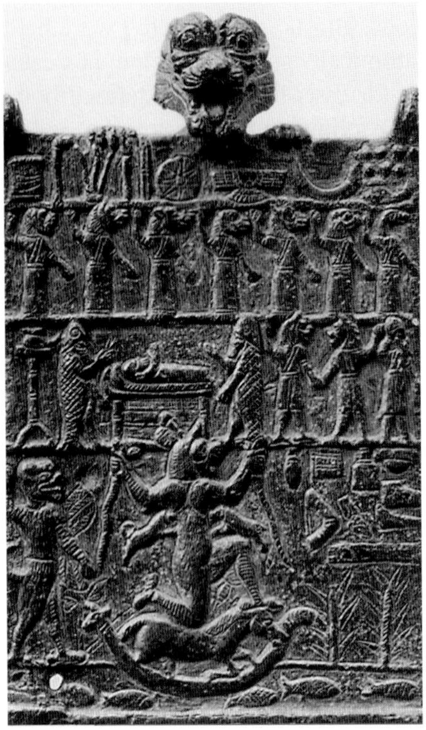

Fig. 3. A metal amulet depicting in the upper panel the Seven Gods related to illnesses that are mentioned in the incantation (see text). The middle panel shows the sick on a bed flanked by two priests in fish garb.

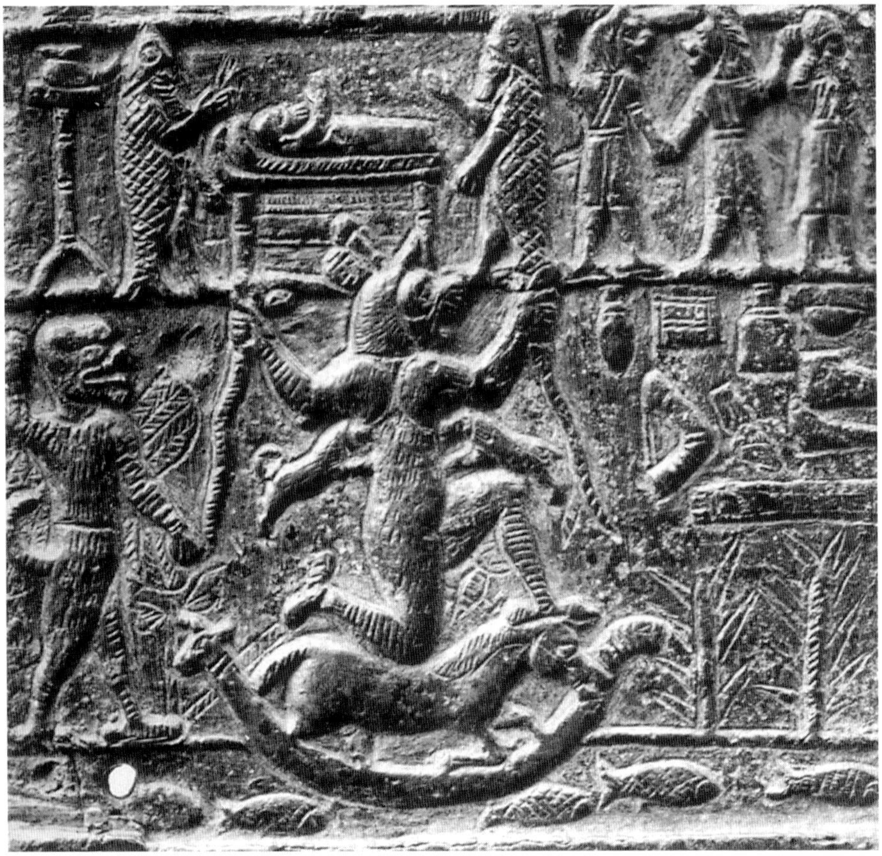

Fig. 4. Detail of the amulet presented in figure 3 showing the sick person flanked by the two priests and below the demon on a barge crossing the river leading to the underworld (symbolized by the fish below the boat).

'If his right kidney hurts, yet he is able to lie on his rightside, he will be cured.

If his left kidney hurts, yet he is able to lie on his left side, he will be cured.

If both his kidneys hurt, and if he is unable to lie on either side, he will die.

If he is 'seized' in the right kidney and he becomes confused, he will die.

If he is 'seized' in the left kidney and urinates blood, he will die.'

Several possible diseases can be suggested to explain the syndromes described that fit the suggested prognosis. Unilateral pain may represent nephrolithiasis. Bilateral pain may represent bilateral pyelonephritis with or without papillary necrosis. Confusion in the context of unilateral renal pain may be indicative of uremia secondary to obstruction of a solitary functioning kidney. The associated prognosis indicated in the tablets parallels the gravity of the conditions if left untreated. Diagnostic possibilities are also clear from descriptions of the urine [9]:

'If his urine is constantly retained, he will die.

If his urine is like water, his illness shall be long, but he will survive.

If his urine is like wine, his illness shall be painful, but he will survive.

If his urine is like milk, he will survive.

If his urine is normal, even if the illness is long, he will survive.'

Clearly, anuria is seen as prelude to certain death. Watery urine may be referring to dilute polyuria from either diabetes or vasopressin deficiency/resistance. Wine-colored urine may represent acute post-infectious glomerulonephritis, and 'milky' urine may be a manifestation of severe nephrosis. The following from tablet 14 may be a description of the manifestations of advanced anasarca [9]:

'If his legs are swollen and cold, his eyelids swollen, his penis swollen, and his umbilicus protruding: 'hand of mamit', his illness will drag then he will die.'

The following two prognostications may be describing the cardiac manifestations of fluid overload, and preeclampsia/toxemia [9]:

'If the skin of his feet is 'elevated', his head affected, and his heart 'trembles' vigorously, he will die.'

'If the pregnant woman's face becomes 'deformed' (swells), because of her pregnancy, she will die.'

Conteneau [10] has quoted a series of prescriptions on urogenital diseases, previously translated by Campbell Thompson, which reflect a keen sense of observation and deductive reasoning. The following examples are illustrative:

'If a man's urine is white ... and blood comes after he has finished urination, through a bronze tube introduced in his penis pour a mixture of ...' (terminal hematuria treated by intrabladder instillation of therapeutic mixture).

'If a man looses his urine drop by drop without being able to hold it, examine him with the finger ... he suffers from urinary retention' (dribbling and urinary retention of prostatic hypertrophy diagnosed by rectal examination).

'If a man suffers from his kidneys, if he is weak, confused, has painful dreams ... if his heart beats fast with no reason, if he can not rest night or day, he suffers from urinary retention. To cure him ...' (symptoms of uremia from urinary obstruction).

'If a man is unable to urinate ... crush some myrrh, mix with oil and blow it in his urethra with a bronze tube ... Boil in oil the resin of galbanum, filter it, and blow it in his urethra with a bronze tube' (intraurethral instillation of mixture by bronze tubes for urethral obstruction).

Divination

Divination, while very ancient, has nevertheless never been abandoned. Official divination was practiced in Rome well into the Christianized Byzantine Empire and in one way or another continues until our time. Several types of divination have been described including oil omens, incense omens, birth omens, dreams, speech omens, physiognomic omens, extispicy, necromancy, celestial omens, and the river ordeal. Of these, only birth omens and extispicy are relevant to our topic. The only relevance of celestial omens is to indicate that the zodiac sign Capricorn was associated with the urogenital system [11].

Rationale for Divination

Organs were believed to be the seats of specific psychic functions. The heart was the site of intellect, the liver, affectivity, the stomach, cunning, the kidneys, vigor, the uterus, compassion, the eyes and ears, attention. The liver, the largest and bloodiest organ, was also the seat of the soul. As the soul left the body at the time of sacrifice, it mirrored the disposition of the deity. By careful inspection of variations in form, the priests could read the intentions of the god to whom the sacrifice was made. Cicero in his *De divinatione* gives this interpretation of the reason divination works:

'In every field of inquiry great length of time is employed in continued observation begets extraordinary fund of knowledge, which may be acquired even without the intervention or inspiration of the gods, since repeated observation makes it clear what effect follows any given cause, and what sign precedes any given event.'

Statistical Validation of Omens

With repeated observations, specific procedural refinements were possible. Primary among them was insuring proper interpretation. In the case of extispicy, as many organs were examined during a sacrifice, and differing indications may be read in the various organs, a method of synthesis of the rite was necessary. The training text explains [12]:

'If the good signs are many and the bad few, that omen is favorable

If bad signs are many and the good few, that omen is unfavorable

If your first inspection is confused and does not agree with its countercheck, you do it a third time and if that is good you make a statement; if your countercheck is confused and does not agree with your first inspection, you do not make a statement.'

Linguistic Rationale for Omens

The implications of the omens need not always have derived from repetitive observations. A more mundane origin is sometimes identified, such as the occurrence of homonyms [12]:

'If the gallbladder is enclosed *(kussat)* in fat, there will be cold weather *(kussu)*.

If the diaphragm clings *(emid)*, there will be divine support *(imid ili)*. If there are two fingers on the liver, there will be rival pretenders to the throne. If the lung is red, there will be conflagration.'

Birth Omens

These allow for the identification of some congenital abnormalities. Siamese twins of various types, hermaphroditism, cleft lip/cleft palate with possible hydrocephalus can all be identified in the following [13]:

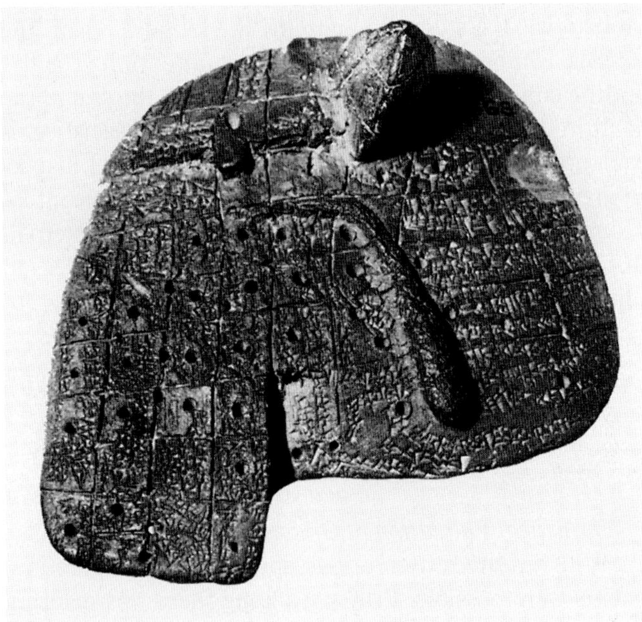

Fig. 5. A clay model of a liver with annotations in cuneiform script relating abnormalities in different segment to their relevance. This is a representational guide to interpretation. It should be noted that these were models of animal livers.

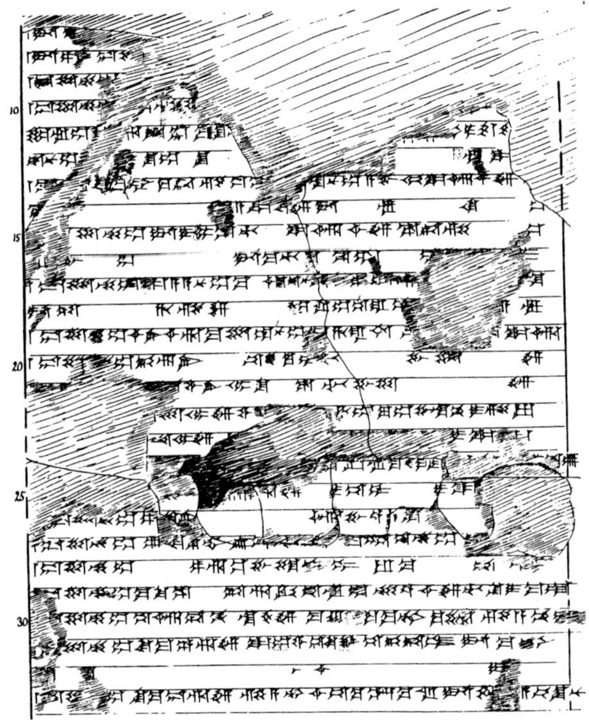

Fig. 6. An omen text related to the appearance of the kidneys and the significance of abnormalities observed. Note the lacunae in the text, one of the difficulties inherent in reconstruction of such writings.

'If a woman gives birth to twin male children and their *libbu (heart)* is common to both ...

If a woman gives birth to twin male children and they are joined at their backbone ...

If a woman gives birth to twins and they are attached at the ribs ...

If a fetus is male and female, without testicles, a son in the palace will rule the land or will assert himself against the king;

If a woman gives birth to a lion, that city will be taken, the king will be captured.'

Extispicy

This was an elaborate procedure that has more complexity than the simple aspect of hepatoscopy. The survival of many liver models in clay (fig. 5) has given for a while the impression that the liver was the only major organ examined. Discovery of omen texts (fig. 6) has significantly altered this picture. The animal (usually a lamb) was sacrificed and then the skin was cut along the midventral line. The ribs were separated from the sternum by cutting the cartilage and folded back so that all the internal viscera could be seen. The organs were examined in situ sequentially and observations made. They were subjected to a second detailed examination after removal. The initial overall 'topographic' examination has given us the representations of the face of the monster Humbaba as seen in the convolutions of the small intestines [14]. While significant anatomic detail can be derived from the texts written as 'procedure guides', it should be remembered that the anatomy in question is not human. This may explain some of the difficulties in textual interpretation faced by early researchers. Nevertheless, these texts have value as identifying an awareness of anatomico-pathologic alteration in organ structure and topography or position that may have been linked to the idea of disease. Goetze [15] has published a series of omen texts from the early part of the second millennium BCE that offer descriptions of multiple organs allowing detection of which organ anomalies had been observed. Duplication of the collecting system, unilateral dysgenesis with contralateral hypertrophy, cystic disease, and horseshoe kidneys are likely identifications in the text related to the kidneys.

References

1 Geller MJ, Cohen SL: Kidney and urinary tract disease in ancient Babylonia, with translations of the cuneiform sources. Kidney Int 1995;47: 1811–1815.

2 Parmeggiani A: Surgical pathophysiology and disease management during the centuries. J Invest Surg 1998;11:159–162.

3 Coleman M, Scurlock J: Viral haemorrhagic fevers in ancient Mesopotamia. Trop Med Int Health 1997;2:603–606.

4 Rose FC: The history of migraine from Mesopotamian to medieval times. Cephalalgia 1995; 15 (suppl 15): 1–3.

5 Adamson PB: Surgery in ancient Mesopotamia. Med Hist 1991;35:428–435.

6 Eadie MJ: The understanding of epilepsy across three millennia. Clin Exp Neurol 1994; 31:1–12.

7 Feenstra O, Roll P, Seybold I: The Austrian penal code and the Codex Ur-nammu: A comparison from the forensic medicine viewpoint. Beitr Gerichtl Med 1991;49:289–295.

8 Spiegel AD, Springer CR: Babylonian medicine, managed care and Codex Hammurabi, circa 1700 B.C. J Community Health 1997;22: 69–89.

9 Labat R: Traité Akkadien de diagnostics et prognostics médicaux. Leiden, Bill, 1951.

10 Contenau G: La médecine en Assyrie et en Babylonie. Paris, Maloine, 1938.

11 Thorwald J: Science and Secrets of Early Medicine. London, Thames & Hudson, 1962.

12 Gurney OR: The Babylonians and Hittites; in Loewe M, Blacker C (eds): Divination and Oracles. London, Allen & Unwin, 1981.

13 Boyd E: Origins of the Study of Human Growth. Eugene, University of Oregon Press, 1980.

14 Cryer F: Divination in Ancient Israel and Its Near Eastern Environment. Sheffield, Sheffield Academic Press, 1994.

15 Goetze A: Old Babylonian Omen Texts. New Haven, Yale University Press, 1947.

American Journal of Nephrology

Am J Nephrol 1999;19:140–147

The Kidney in Ancient Egyptian Medicine: Where Does It Stand?

Mohamed E. Salem[a] Garabed Eknoyan[b]

[a]Cairo University Pediatric Hospital, Cairo University, School of Medicine, Cairo, Egypt;
[b]Department of Medicine, Baylor College of Medicine, Houston, Tex., USA

Key Words

Mummy · Medical papyri · Sounou · Symptomatology

Abstract

Driven by their deep-seated desire for eternal life in a healthy body, ancient Egyptians were one of the first civilizations to begin collecting and recording medical lore and medicinals that were effective for a healthy body. With its religious origins, medical care was initially provided by priests, but evolved over time into an independent discipline practiced by the swnw (sounou) or physician. What has been preserved of their knowledge in extant medical papyri reflects the great capacity of Egyptians for practical achievement in treating symptoms, but lacks the abstract thought that was to come with the advent of the more rational Greek medicine. The number of prescriptions and incantations for the management of urinary disorders (hematuria, retention, frequency, infection) and dropsy that are mentioned in extant medical papyri likely reflect the frequency with which these problems were encountered. Urine was thought to be formed in the region of the bladder, by a process considered akin to purification. Available studies on preserved mummies indicate that kidney disease was not uncommon. Whether a functional role of the kidney was appreciated at all is highly doubtful. On the other hand, the available evidence suggests an awareness of the kidney (ggt) to which was ascribed a mythological role that may well account for why the kidneys and the heart were the only organs not removed during the process of mummification.

According to Aristotle: 'The Ignorant ... affirms; the Scientist ... doubts; the Sapient ... reflects.' He was certainly right about our topic, for who, that we know of, has the knowledge to vouch for what the ancients thought? And, if it is an offense to the learned mind to listen to pedants foretelling the origins of medical knowledge with any degree of confidence, it is a consolation to observe the wise reflect on the past, with prudence. On the other hand, what we now consider a subspeciality (nephrology) may well be considered exceptionable, since ailments of the kidney did occur in ancient times and seem to have changed little over time. Hence the need to reflect on the past, with prudence.

KARGER

Fax + 41 61 306 12 34
E-Mail karger@karger.ch
www.karger.com

© 1999 S. Karger AG, Basel
0250–8095/99/0192–0140$17.50/0

Accessible online at:
http://BioMedNet.com/karger

Mohamed E. Salem, MD
Cairo Medical Tower (808)
55 Abdel Moneim Riad St.
Agouza 12311 Cairo (Egypt)
Tel. +20 2 303 0535, Fax +20 2 302 6020, E-Mail medsalem@intouch.com.eg

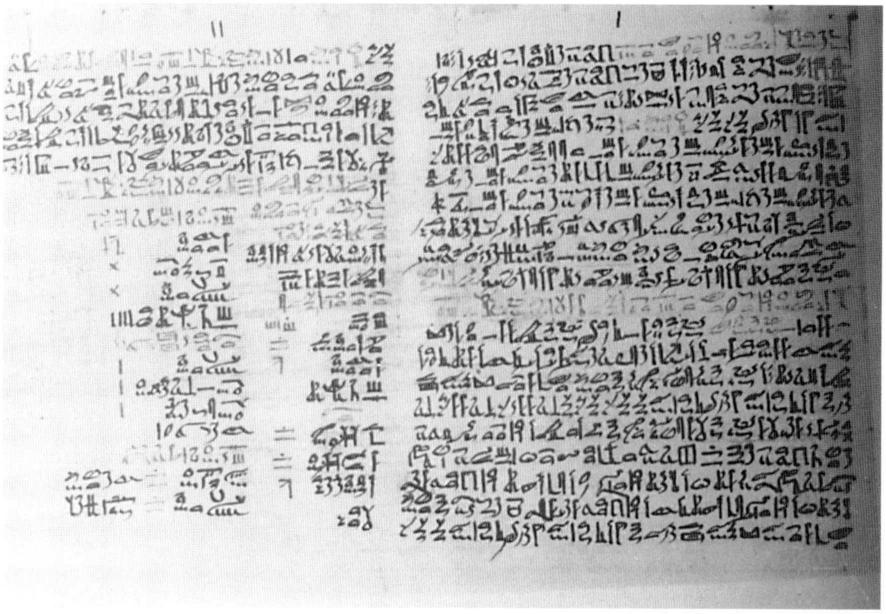

Fig. 1. Medical hieroglyphs from the *Ebers Papyrus.*

From the earliest beginnings of recorded history, the body of knowledge and practice we now term medicine has been a center of human concerns. For it is the basic human desire to be alive and well, coupled with our eternal subconscious wish for immortality that led to the emergence of medicine as the route to achieve them. The ancient Egyptians were no exception. They seem to have cherished life to such a degree that living forever became an obsession and then a religion. It was only natural then that in early Egypt it was the priests who were the initial providers of health care. It is only in later dynasties, when sufficient medical lore had accrued, that medical practioners dissociated themselves from priests, although the discipline retained its religious roots and remained shrouded in magic and myths. Much of their medical knowledge was forged on how to live happily, healthily and eventually to cure rapidly should ailment prevail.

Ultimately, the ancient Egyptians may have achieved some semblance of the eternity they so avidly sought, for their silent tombs utter the messages which they dug in for us to dig out and interpret. As we read their inscriptions they live again. Other civilizations which attempted to achieve the same may have been successful for a brief span in history, but only the ancient Egyptians have been able to accomplish it at least for the past 40 centuries. Chapter 31 of the *Book of the Dead* sums it up quite well: 'He shall come forth by day. He shall rise up to walk upon the earth among the living and he shall never fail or come to an end, never, never, never ...' [1].

Traces and Indices

Academically, the understanding of ancient Egyptian medicine in general, and the kidney in particular is complicated by several factors: (1) the diversity and variety of sources; (2) the accuracy and attribution of those sources; (3) the long span of 40 centuries over which those sources have been collected and transmitted; (4) the convoluted transcription modes, i.e. the hieroglyphs with their inherent difficulty of interpretation (fig. 1), and (5) the destructive hands of man through time: the erasers, plunderers, thieves, pretentious antique dealers, and sometimes even pharmacists of the recent past who used the mummies to treat disease. Still, considerable medical information can be gleaned from preserved mummies and extant papyri.

Mummies

Although mummies have been a principal source of medical information on ancient Egypt, that certainly was not their original purpose. It was religion, magic, and only a form of protomedicine that were components of mummification. The name derives from the arabic word 'mummia', i.e. a waxy dried reddish material [2]. As centuries folded, mummification evolved from that of a magical fancy to that of a mandatory necessity, since destruction of the body was thought to result in its soul erring and decaying in turn. Mummification appears to have served three main purposes: purification, immortalization and preservation of supremacy. The technique of mummifica-

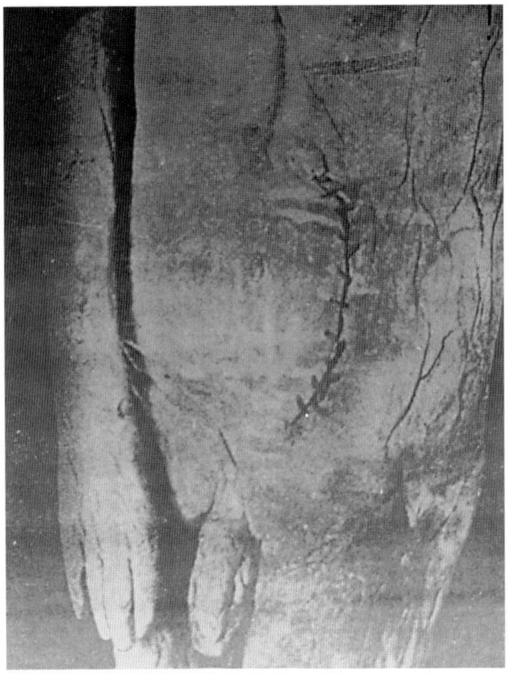

Fig. 2. Site and size of incision from which the floating viscera were removed during mummification.

tion, first practiced in the Old Kingdom, developed steadily during subsequent dynasties until it attained its highest degree, just before the Ptolemaic period. Following the spread of Christianity, it endured for a few centuries but gradually vanished, [3–6].

Shortly after death, the body was brought to the 'Per Nefer', the Beautiful House, to be cleansed from its impurities [7]. In brief, the mummification process may be summarized as follows: wash – dehydrate – sterilize – perfume – seal – tag and stock. All done ceremoniously and with due respect to the dead body. The viscera were extracted through an incision about 10 inches long, usually made in the left side of the abdomen, (fig. 2). Through this incision, all the 'floating' contents of the abdominal cavity, namely, the stomach, the liver, the spleen, and the intestines, were removed but the kidneys were left in place. The diaphragm was then cut and the thoracic contents removed through the abdominal incision. The heart, which was considered the center of emotions and the seat of conscience, was left in place. They seem to have attached no importance to the brain, which was removed through the ethmoid bone. Following this begun the slow process of sterilization and dehydration of the body, accomplished by osmosis with dry natron. Resterilization of the cavities, perfuming, closing the incision (fig. 2), and wrapping the body with linen and with beeswax completed the process. Molten resin was used to seal the body and its wrappings, providing a barrier against insects and anaerobes.

Although the removed organs were potentially available for study, they do not seem to have been accessible to practitioners of medicine who were a totally separate discipline (swnw) from that of the official embalmers (wt).

Medical Papyri

Another source of knowledge of Egyptian medicine derives from their medical papyri (fig. 1). Unfortunately, many medical papyri are lost or else not yet found. Written over a period of 800 years, extant manuscripts add up to a little less than 200 translated and printed pages [3–15].

The texts consist mainly of short paragraphs – about 1,200 in all – which are either prescriptions and incantations for specific symptoms, descriptions of diagnostic criteria of assumed diseases, or technical information on a substantial number of surgical procedures. They provide very little or no data on prognosis as indicated in the following example: 'If a newborn baby cries "ny" he will live, if "ba" he will die' [9, 10]. Their anatomic and physiologic subject matter is limited and has been summed in some 10 pages on the subject by Grapow et al. [9] who describes 200 anatomical terms, and in the 72 pages devoted to human parts by Lefebvre [8].

Invaluable as they are in understanding ancient Egyptian medicine, medical papyri are frustratingly incomplete and many of their technical terms, symptoms and drugs await definite interpretation and translation. The *Kahun Papyrus* is the first known medical text and appears to have been written during the Middle Kingdom (1900 BC). Better known are the *Ebers* and *Smith Papyri.*

Ebers Papyrus (Medical). Translated and classified in 1937 Ebbell, the only medical doctor among egyptologists, the *Ebers Papyrus* dates to 1550 BC. It is the first known medical papyrus and the longest, being over 20 m in length. Several blank spaces have been left in the extant text – why is not known. Its interpretation is subject to considerable divergence of opinion, to say the least. It contains extracts on anatomy, physiology, a section on the heart and vessels, and several medicinal prescriptions. It can be considered a sort of primary medical protoencyclopedia, though by no means complete or fully clear [4, 5, 9, 13–16].

Smith Papyrus (Surgical). In its outstanding Breasted edition of 1930, detailed yet simple and lucid, the *Smith*

Papyrus is quite engaging to read and provides a wealth of information. It is often referred to as the 'surgical papyrus' because of the number of pedagogic surgical treatises it contains quasi no magical spells [5, 9, 14].

The available medical texts suggest specialization. Indeed, Herodotus, in his *History*, describes the Egyptians as being the most religious of men and reports a novelty, subspecialty: 'In Egypt, every physician treats one and only one disease ... this is why the country is full of medical specialists of the eye, the head, the teeth, the belly and also for unsettled (indefinite) diseases' [Her. II. 84]. It is buried in the latter that the kidney and its diseases fall.

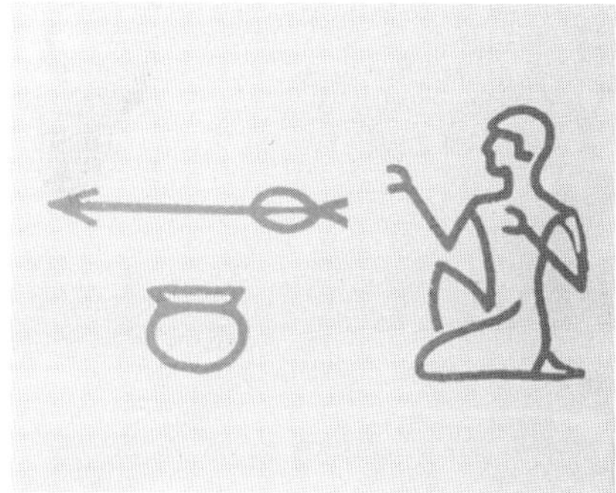

Fig. 3. Pictogram of the (SwnW) or physician.

Caregivers, Physicians and the Sounou (SwnW)

Hieroglyphic representation of the physician or the sounou is shown in figure 3. Healing was traditionally intertwined with myths and rooted in religion. Disease was not considered inevitable, but felt to be imposed on humans by a hostile force. The role of the sounou was to eject the intruders with incantations, spells and drugs. He was expected to provide protection from the evil external forces that caused disease, as well as control over the natural internal ones [3–13]. Health was considered the balance between equal forces: Good and Evil, Gods and Demons, Life and Death. The all-in-one physician, magician, priest, and apothecary was expected through his skills, potions, and spells, to tip the balance in favor of the Good, the Gods, and Life. Accordingly, a prospective caregiver was obliged to bear an amazing bouquet of knowledge that consisted of a mixture of priesthood, craftsmanship, magical expertise and philosophical wisdom. In other words a man for all seasons, who had to impress but not transgress. A rather difficult situation since there is mention of the 'good sounou' to be rewarded and the 'bad sounou' to be rebuked. Malpractice seems to have its roots as well.

'Per Ankh', the House of Life, was the place where medical aphorisms and remedies accrued over the years were preserved as part of medical culture [5, 7]. They were meant as rules, directives and instructions for the practice of medicine. Physicians went there to study and copy the medical wisdom and potions of their predecessors. Some extant examples of these aphorisms are: 'Malady takes place when the heart (IB) silences (when you can't feel the pulse)', and 'When blood inundates the lungs, the (IB) vessels become filled with blood' [EB 855 V], which probably corresponds to the 'plethora' of Greek medicine. Clinical diagnosis entailed history taking and a systematic examination, which included general and special examinations. Distinction between various modes of management was quite clear. The sounou was trained to recognize: 'An ailment which I will treat; an ailment with which I will contend; an ailment not to be treated' [5, 9]. Diagnosis of a given disease does not seem to have always been established in the course of a single encounter. In such cases, empirical management was often initiated and, as the text implies, the patient was left 'moored to his moors' awaiting further reassessment. In retrospect this is no different than that of the current 'conservative treatment' of an experienced physician who is quite aware of the resources and limitations of medical science.

Practically speaking, the main role of the sounou was to rid the body from noxious materials and influences, the major representative of which was the 'whdw' (ukhedu) or morbus peccans (morbid matter) [3–14]. Extrusion of the evil ukhedu would expectedly be through the all too natural exit route: the anus (phwyt), which acquired a significant standing in matters of health and purging became a principal component of therapy. The ukhedu, which may be related to fecal matter, is referred to sometimes as disease, sometimes as evil matter, and sometimes as a vehicle of good riddance. The circulation of ukhedu from its entry into the body to its exit was considered to take place in the 'Mtw' (metou) [3, 5, 9, 13].

The 'metou', a generic term for vessel, encompassed the vasculature, lymphatics, tendons, muscle, nerves and the excretory canals. Being a conduit system, the metou was an omnivehicle for lymph, bile, stool, urine, mucus, phlegm, vomitus, milk, semen and air; all circulating across the body under control of the heart (IB). 'Regarding man, there are 22 vessels in him belonging to his heart. It is them that deliver to all his members' [EB 656J a]. The

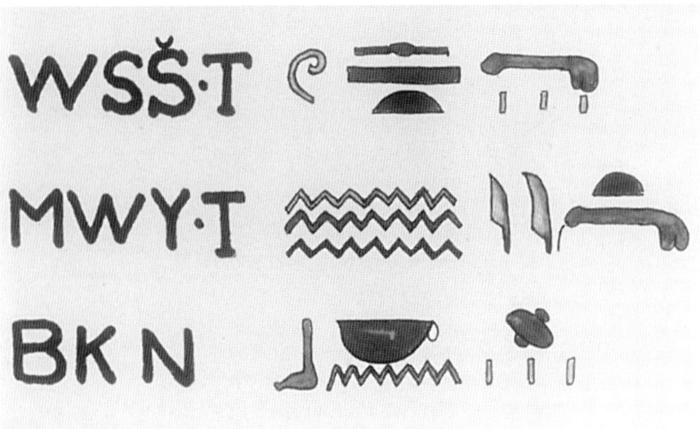

Fig. 4. Hieroglyphic inscriptions representing the various Egyptian terms for urine.

importance of the metou can be gleaned from one of the incantations for the dead: 'May his metou flourish. May his metou be sound. May his metou be excellent. May his metou be comfortable' [3].

Being a totipotent attribute, the 'metou-ib complex' was, in a pathologic context, considered to contribute to the production of disease by transporting the ukhedu to the sites where it localized and produced the ailment. Damage or injury was considered an inundation by ukhedu and other noxious materials of desiccation which extracted the elements of viability. It has been suggested that the ancient Egyptians drew such concepts from the river Nile which was not always beneficent and 'refused to return those who embraced it' (i.e. drowned), and how both inundation and draught ruined agriculture. Such plurality of views complicates interpretation even further rendering any accurate translation tenuous [12].

The Kidney: Where Does It Stand?

The metou included the ureters which in occasional scripts are named 'MT' (mat) = flute or hollow tube. According to the *Ebers Papyrus*, two metous go to the bladder [4, 13, 15]. The *Berlin Medical Papyrus* provides further insight on the subjects: 'There are two metous (vessels) to the bladder, it is they which give the urine' [14]. While this may well be reference to the ureters, it is equally applicable to the iliac arteries or other metous in the region [14]. The formation of urine was considered to be through 'the power that is inherent in the parts about the region of the bladder' and a result of putrefaction: 'when it goes into the bladder, it changes for the worse' [*Papyrus Londinesis* 29, 49; 30, 15]. Commonly referred to as 'mwyt' urine was also dubbed 'wsst' or 'bkn', the hieroglyphic renderings of which use an undulating line for water and a phallus for its source (fig. 4).

Concerning the kidney, why is it out of focus in Egyptian medicine and, if not, where does it stand? Description of organs, symptoms, signs, diseases, syndromes, prognostics, and prescribed medicinals of ancient Egypt have reached us only in fragmentary fashion. To sort out what would now be considered nephrology without attributing presumed thoughts to ancient Egyptians is rather difficult, but possible. A review of some of their nomenclatures would be helpful in assessing where the kidney stands [3–16]:

Shepetyet	Urinary bladder
Mwyt	Urine
Mat	Ureter
Hennen	Phallus as an anatomical sign
Met	Phallus as phonetic sign
Bah	Phallus as functioning organ emitting urine or semen
Depet	Loin, lumbar
Ourmyt	Seems to indicate calculi
Geget	Is the name hesitantly suggested by Egyptologists to designate the kidney

The 'geget' – or if one is so inclined the kidney – does not seem to have been adequately recognized or described. An overshadowed organ, residing in the back, it was not removed during the process of mummification. Its retroperitoneal position surrounded by perinephric fat and fascia is considered the reason, since only the 'floating organs' were removed (liver, spleen, bladder, pancreas, intestines, stomach and lungs). To accept this rather simple explanation underestimates the skill of the embalmers, who so assiduously removed the brain. The fact that the heart and kidneys were left in place may have been intentional. This was clearly the case for the heart. That there might be some significance to leaving the kidneys in place might be gleaned from the article by Maio in this issue and from several incantations in the *Book of the Dead* such as: 'May naught be against me in the presence of the great god, the lord Amentet. Homage to thee, O my heart. Homage to thee, O my kidneys' [chap. 30], and another, 'Art thou a servant?, come out in vomit. Art thou a noble?, come out in his urine'. Thus, the kidney was recognized, but the word geget (ggt) does not appear in extant medical papyri [13].

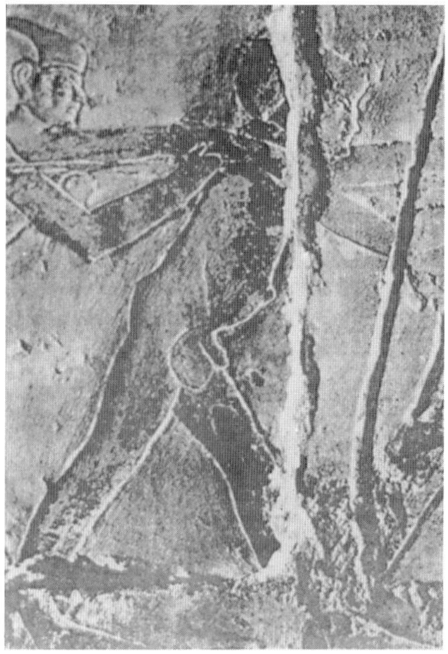

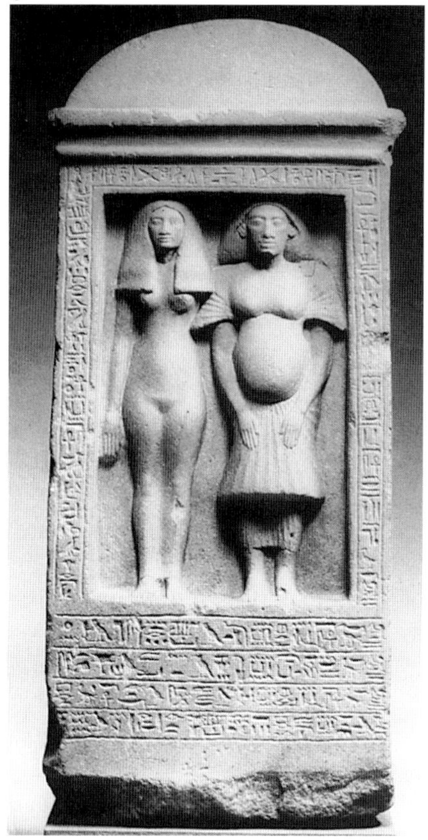

Fig. 5. Engraving depicting edema of the abdominal wall, scrotum and legs.
Fig. 6. 18th dynasty stele (14th century BC). Egyptian Museum, Berlin. While the man represented in the figure may be considered plain obese, closer scrutiny reveals what may well be ascites, gynecomastia and relatively more clearly but not upper extremity edema.

Pathophysiological Profiles and Symptomatologies

Uroscopy and coproscopy seem to have been used in the everyday practice of medicine [4–15]. The *Ebers Papyrus* contains recipes for the treatment of different micturition disorders, grouped in some 24 paragraphs under the heading of: 'Starting Remedies to Make Disappear the Retention of Urine when the Lower Hypogastrium Is Full' [EB 261]. It lists several treatments such as: 'Another remedy to make disappear a burning pain in the bladder, in the same time when (the patient) suffers while urinating' [EB 278], which could be considered a reference to cystoureteritis, and 'Another remedy when to make disappear a violent pain during micturition', which could well be a reference to ureteritis or prostatitis [EB 43]. Paragraphs 69 and 70 of the *Hearst Papyrus* recommend a 'burning hat(?) at the bladder'. The *Ebers Papyrus* reports on a patient who suffered 'henaou (?) in his urine' [EB 267]. What disease 'henaou' implies is not known, though it is mentioned in conjunction with a treatment for apparent symptoms of cystitis.

Urinary retention was termed urine accumulation due to failure to 'expel all of the urine which is in the intestine' [EB 24], for which is prescribed, 'Another (remedy) to regularize urine when the lower hypogastrium is painful. This potion will be prepared in the morning before the coming time of breakfast, then it is to be drunk in such a way that he (the patient) will be immediately cured.'

The *Ebers Papyrus* also prescribes 'Another remedy to stop escape of urine when it is too frequent' [EB 274] and to 'Regularize urine when it is no more regular'[EB 266]. Whether these refer to polyuria or frequency cannot be ascertained. Enuresis and incontinence did not have a particular nomenclature, but there are designed 'remedies to stop the escape of urine' [EB 276] and 'to hold urine' [EB 264]. Cases of enuresis related to sacrovertebral trauma are described [4, 5].

Essentially, retention of urine and what we may consider enuresis or cystitis seem to have been recognized. Management was aimed mainly at relieving the symptoms and consisted of decongestion and disinfection [3–7, 13–19]. Some remedies were given orally or rectally with the apparent goal of decongestion. Other remedies still were applied directly on the penis with the apparent goal of disinfection. As a rule, these were compounds of oily nature.

Hematuria, mentioned 50 times, is likely related to schistosoma, whose eggs have been discovered in mummies [11]. Hematuria was said to be painful in some instances and painless in others. It is also reported in association with stones [EB 20]. The expulsion of calculi (ourmyt) is said to be associated with dysuria and hematuria or (âaâ) [4, 5]. Actually, (âaâ) is a mysterious entity which, according to Jonckheere [11] is characterized by abdominal distension, pain, escape, of the heart or palpitations, and blood-stained evacuations (urine and/or stools). Its exact nature is debatable. It has been linked to worms, or 'hrrt', engaged in a constant 'battle' each trying to 'kill' the other. The term worms is also used in connection with hematuria and might be ascribed to the vermiform clots of blood that form in standing urine, which the text likens to 'worms formed inside the fractured nose' [p. 12].

Edema of the scrotum and penis (fig. 5), and of the legs in conjunction with abdominal distension (fig. 6) has been pictographed and linked to hematuria (âaâ). Whether some of these were cases of kidney disease requires a giant leap of imagination. Of course, the relation between edema and a 'renal' etiology was not and could not have been considered. That edema was a common problem can be gleaned from the *Hearst Medical Papyrus* which gives one prescription for hematuria, eleven for urinary disorders, and nine for dropsy or fluid accumulation [14]. One remedy prescribed for the accumulation of urine in the body is: 'An old book cooked in oil. Smear on his body' [15]. The diuretic properties of papyrus cooked in oil remain to be tested.

Pathologic examination of 28th dynasty mummies reveal pyonephrosis and multiple abscesses in both kidneys, which have been shown to be due to gram-negative coccobacilli [13–19]. Kidney stones have also been identified. Three calculi, weighing 3, 12, and 24 g, and containing leukocytes, epithelial cells and a nonidentifiable central inorganic substance, as well as a mixture of pus and uric acid have been identified by Ruffer [20].

The frequency of nephrolithiasis is not known. Dawson and others [4, 21, 22], who examined numerous mummies, could identify only 3 cases of calculi.

Ruffer [20] discovered the ova of bilharzia in two mummies, Jonckheere, Ebbel and others have associated bilharziasis with the (âaâ). Histological examination of several mumifieds kidneys reveal little parenchymal distortion and a single case of congenital renal atrophy [15–20]. A case of apparent nephrosclerosis has been described in a mummy with atherosclerosis [23].

Conclusion

Symptomatology is, and has always been, the core of the matter. Ancient Egyptians described and, to a certain extent, managed those frank urinary symptoms.

It took 17 centuries until Marcello Malpighi discovered the famous corpuscle, and even 2 further centuries until Claude Bernard recognized the importance of the 'Milieu Intérieur', seven thousand years in all since the dawn of known history, and uncounted millennia since Creation. This controlling-monitoring interrelationship escaped primordial medical understanding. Indeed, it has continued in this way for only a few decades.

Disturbance of the 'homeostasis' is a faithful index of the kidney's state of function. The discrete manifestations of such renal dysfunction including electrolyte imbalance, acid-base disturbance, mineral alterations, azotemia, hypertension, anemia and maybe failure to thrive are all well disguised by the cloaks of other disorders or symptoms. The kidney, too, has its own hieroglyphs, being a pluripotent, sophisticated organ belonging more to the understanding and facilities of modern times.

Acknowledgments

The authors are grateful to the staff of the Cairo Museum, especially that of its library, and to the Supreme Council of Antiquities in the Egyptian Ministry of Culture for their support of the research for this report.

References

1 Mummification Museum, Royal Mummies Egyptian Museum, Luxor 77, Supreme Council of Antiquities, Ministry of Culture, Egypt, 1997.

2 Webster's Third New International Dictionary (English Language). (Merriam-Webster). London, Encyclopaedia Britannica, 1981.

3 Majno G: The Healing Hand Man and Wound in the Ancient World. Cambridge, Harvard University Press, 1975.

4 Leca AP: La Médecine Egyptienne. Paris, Editions Roger Dacosta, 1983.

5 Ghalioungi P: La médecine des pharaons. Les énigmes de l'univers. Paris, Laffont, 1983.

6 Ghalioungi P: The Spiral Course of Medical Thinking. J Egypt Public Health Assoc 1966; 41:127–131.

7 Ghalioungi P: The House of Life: Per Ankh. Magic and Medical Science in Ancient Egypt. Amsterdam, Israel, Boekhandel en Antiquariaat NV, 1974.

8 Lefebvre G: Tableau des parties du corps humain mentionnées par les égyptiens. Supplément aux ASAE, Le Caire, 1950.

9 Grapow H, Von Deines H, Westendorf W: Grundriss der Medizin der alten Ägypter. Berlin, Akademie-Verlag, 1954–1962, vol 1–8.

10 Withington ET: Medical History from the Earliest Times. A Popular History of the Healing Art. London, Holland Press, 1964.

11 Jonckheere F: Les médecins de l'Egypte pharaonique. Bruxelles, Fondation Egypt Reine Elisabeth, 1958.

12 Gardiner A: Egyptian Grammar. London, Oxford University Press, 1973.

13 Nunn JF: Ancient Egyptian Medicine. Norman, University of Oklahoma Press, 1996.

14 Dawson WR: The Egyptian Medical Papyri in Diseases in Antiquity. Springfield, Thomas, 1952, pp 98–111.

15 Rawling JP: Urology in Egypt in Diseases in Antiquity. Springfield, Thomas, 1952, pp 532–537.

16 Bryan CP: The Papyrus Ebers New York, Appleton, 1931.

17 Ghalioungi P: Some body swellings in two tombs of the Ancient Empire and their possible relation to *aaa*. ZAS 1962;87:108–114.

18 Jonckheere F: Pathologie pharaonique et diagnostic 'ex arte'. Hist Méd 1952;11:3–7.

19 Jonckheere F: 'Le préparateur de remèdes' dans l'organisation de la pharmacie égyptienne. Ägypt St. 149161, 1955.

20 Ruffer MA: Studies in the Paleontology of Egypt. Chicago, University of Chicago Press, 1921.

21 Dawson WR, Gray PR: Catalogue of Egyptian Antiquities. British Museum, London, 1988.

22 Gray PHK: Radiological aspects of the mummies of ancient Egyptians in the Rijksmuseum van Oudheden, Leuden. Oudheidkidge Meded 1966;97:1–29.

23 Long AR: Cardiovascular renal disease: Report of a case of 3000 years ago. Arch Pathol 1931; 12:92–94.

Origins of Nephrology – Antiquity

American Journal of Nephrology

Am J Nephrol 1999;19:148–154

Pre-Columbian Medicine and the Kidney

José Carlos Peña

Hospital Mocel y Hospital Angeles del Pedregal, México D.F., México

Key Words
Olmecs · Aztecs · Religion · Kidney disease · Bone disease

Abstract
Medicine in Mesoamerican cultures began in the year 1500 BC and ended with the conquest and destruction of Mexico-Tenochtitlan in 1521 by Spain. Mesoamerica started with the Olmec civilization followed by the Teoitihuacanes, Toltecs, and Mayas and perished with the Nahoa Empire. The medicine used by the Aztecs *(ticiotl)* is undoubtedly the sum of all Mesoamerican medicine. The medical history of the ticiotl was recovered in the years that followed the conquest from the works of Bernardino de Sahagún and Francisco Hernández and the Cruz-Badiano codex. All these works describe the use of plants and herbs in the treatment of diseases, including, edema, urinary retention, kidney stones, and podagra. The Aztec doctors (titicih) were also well acquainted with innumerable diseases and were excellent healers of wounds and fractures. The works of modern historians confirm the theory of the *ticiotl* medicine and its application by the titicih and define the differences between the hippocratic-galenic medicine and the ticiotl medicine. The latter used a complex and philosophically elaborated medical theory based on the polarity cold/warm, different from the four-humor theory. They demonstrate that every culture is capable to understand and 'invent' the meaning of disease and its cure, even when it is different from our modern medical views.

Introduction

The medical history of Mesoamerica constitutes one more chapter of the universal medical history. Pre-Columbian medicine in Mexico is richer in working materials than in other territories conquered by the Spaniards in the 16th century, including Peru.

In that century, the fusion of European and Indian medical roots occurred, and some form of medical syncretism was born. Hospitals and medical schools were established, and a new medical conscience developed in the New World.

Medicine was practiced in most ancient cultures of Mexico [1]. Although the chronology of the original cultures in Mexico is not well established, the first human emigration to the Anahuac or Valle de México (Mexican Valley), seems to have occurred some 12,000–15,000 years ago. The medicine used by these groups was prehistoric and no doubt very primitive, but there is no reliable information in this regard.

A more formal art to cure appeared during the Olmec culture, some 1,500–600 years BC [2]. The Olmecs occu-

KARGER

Fax + 41 61 306 12 34
E-Mail karger@karger.ch
www.karger.com

© 1999 S. Karger AG, Basel
0250–8095/99/0192–0148$17.50/0

Accessible online at:
http://BioMedNet.com/karger

Dr. José Carlos Peña
Monte Pichincha 29
Lomas de Chapultepec
11020 México DF (México)
Tel. +52 525 596 0279, Fax +52 525 251 2996

pied the rivers in the states of Veracruz, Tabasco, Campeche, Chiapas, and the Mexican Valley; the giant heads of La Venta are some of the remains of this great civilization. The Olmecs and after them the Theotihuacans, Toltecs, Mayas and Mexicas gave form to the Mesoamerican culture that lasted 3,000 years, until the arrival of the Spanish conquistadores in 1519 [1, 2].

The Ticiotl or Aztec Medicine

Information on the medicine used by the Aztecs or Mexicas *(Ticiotl)* at the time of the conquest 1519–1521 and long before that was obtained during the following 40–50 years by the priests, Aztec doctors *(ticitl)*, and the protomedical of Philip II of Spain, Francisco Hernández, in his monumental work *Natural History of New Spain* [3]. Other sources came from the works of Brother Bernardino de Sahagún [4] and Brother Alonso de Molina. de Sahagún produced a collection of rich texts between 1529 and 1590 related not only to the anatomy of the body parts, but also to different diseases of the human body and their treatments. His works were published in two important codices, the *Florentine* [5] and the *Matritense* [6], and in the *General History of the Things of the New Spain* [4]. The complete version is the one included in the *Florentine* codex [5]. This information derives from the second version of the *Matritense* codex [6], with the following running title: 'From the intestines and all that is inside man, of everything that is on the surface and the joints and of what belongs to males and of what belongs to females'. The subtitles of all the different paragraphs are written in *Náhuatl language*, in Bernardino de Sahagún handwriting. The Sahagún texts [4] directly involved in medicine were divided in three parts: one dedicated to diseases, the second to treatment, and the third to the anatomy of the different parts of the human body.

Another important document is the Cruz-Badiano codex [7], which was written in Náhuatl by Martín de la Cruz, an Aztec doctor (*ticitl*), in the early part of the 16th century and translated into Latin by Juan Badiano, better known by its Latin name: 'Libellus de medicinalibus indorum herbis' [7]. In this fascinating work the botanic and medical knowledge was mixed with religious and magic believes, coupled to treatment with plants and herbs of the Mexicas. Both authors belonged to the School of Santa Cruz de Tlatelolco. Originally, the manuscript was dedicated to Francisco de Mendoza, the son of the first Viceroy of New Spain, Antonio de Mendoza. For this reason no copy was left behind in Mexico, and the manuscript, taken to Spain between 1626 and 1628 was acquired by Cardinal Francisco Barberini, nephew of Pope Urbano VIII; Barberini also recovered innumerable works, among them, part of the writings of Francisco Hernández [3]. This last monumental work, severely damaged and reduced, was in part recovered, out of five copies left behind in the Imperial College of Madrid, by the same Hernández before his death. The Cruz Badiano codex was lost in the Vatican Library for almost 400 years, until 1929, when it was rediscovered by Charles Upson Clark [cited in ref. 7].

The magnificent work of these three codices plus the work of Francisco Hernández [4–6], all with elegant iconography, summarize the use of the local plants in Mexico-Tenochtitlán and probably in all the Aztec domains. The Aztec emperors maintained botanical gardens for plants collected throughout the empire. One of the purposes of these gardens was to provide doctors with new plants to use in the cure of diseases [4]. The codex and writings contained the medicine, surgery, and anatomy used by the Mexicas and are the result of knowledge accumulated from all Mesoamerican medical cultures.

Even when a great number of the Indian codex, hieroglyphics, and writings of the Mexica empire and remains of other Mesoamerican cultures were destroyed, works by priests, historians, anthropologists, and medical doctors [2–7], in the past 500 years, have provided new meaning and form to the medical practice and philosophy of the *ticiotl*, Aztec medicine, and its application by the *ticitl*, the Aztec doctor.

The Florentine and Matritense codices [5, 6], compiled by Brother Benardino de Sahagún, include the history and costumes and social, political, and philosophical organization of the Aztecs obtained from the Indian codex and the oral tradition kept alive in the communal schools of Mexico-Tenochtitlán: the *Calmécacl* (the school of the *pipiltin*, the Mexican nobility of Mexico-Tenochtitlán) and the *Telpuchcalli* (education centers for the *macehualtin*, common people). This oral tradition added to the study of the written codices, on *amate* paper (obtained from the crust of the tree known as the amate) or on deer skin, ceramic figures, and hieroglyphics, was fundamental in the education of students in the Aztec schools. Education was the charge of old wise men called *tlamatini* who maintained the traditions and the history of the Mexicas.

The difference among the *ticiotl* (Aztec medicine) and the hippocratic-galenic medicine brought by the Spaniards is fundamental to understand pre-Columbian medicine. There is no doubt that the *ticiotl* identified and cured many diseases quite beyond their empirical accomplishments recognized by men such as Bernardino de

Sahagún and the protomedical Francisco Hernández [3]. The questions addressed were: Was it really possible to pretend the existence of a náhuatl medical theory? And in this case: How it was conceptually structured? What interrelationship it may have with the world vision and the social and cultural spectra of the nahuas?

Even the conquistadores, including Hernan Cortés [8], soldiers, captains, priests and doctors, recognized that the *ticiotl* possessed a wide knowledge of herbs and plants, treatment of fractures and wounds, and identification of innumerable diseases and that they had a great ability in general to heal and cure wounded and sick patients.

Accordingly, with the analysis and findings of the Spanish doctors that came to New Spain, including Francisco Hernández [3], they were convinced that the *titcih (plural of ticitl)* ignored completely the nature and the etiology of diseases – simply because they were not acquainted with the hippocratic-galenic concepts of medicine. They thought that the *ticiotl* was only the consequence of empirical practice with repetitive applications of certain remedies for certain diseases. However, recent analyses and findings of López-Austin [9], Ortiz de Montellano [cited in refs. 9 and 10], and Viesca [10] provided evidence that practice and medical conceptions of the *titicih* were infinitely more complex and philosophically more elaborated than originally conceived. They, the *titicih*, possessed a medical theory as vulnerable ad efficacious as the hippocratic-galenic theory brought to Mexico-Tenochtitlán by the Spaniards. It was considered 'scientific' and separate from the religious beliefs, even when it was based on aphoristic conceptions like the theory of the four humors.

The *ticiotl* recognized the polarity of cold/warm considered as a concept of the pre-Hispanic Mesoamerican culture, as has been clearly analyzed by the Mexican investigators such as López-Austin [9, 11], Ortiz de Montellano [cited in ref. 10], and Viesca [10]. The objections of Foster [12], in this matter, trying to relate this conception of warm/cold to the hippocratic-galenic theory of the humors, have been clearly analyzed and discarded by López-Austin [9, 11] in a long and well-documented argumentation. Presently, it is well established that in Aztec medicine exist two elements and not four. It is important to appreciate that the concepts of warm and cold are not humors or physical elements. López-Austin [9], based on his investigations, identified these concepts in the following manner: Everything that was masculine, celestial, or came from above was considered warm; on the contrary all that was feminine came from below, and the infraworld was considered cold.

In the celestial cosmos of the Aztecs, the horizontal plane of the surface of the earth, the warm will be oriented southeast and cold northwest. With this division we can build a universe in which we could locate warmer and colder parts. Also we can find colder and warmer bodies by their essence, like the heart and the sun. Sometimes the coldness or warmness might depend on the relative position they maintain inside the cosmos. The stars are colder than the sun, for example. In the same way, the human body replicates the universe: the tip of the head is hotter than the feet that belong to the infraworld. The heart, the body's sun, participates in the celestial heat and is warmer than the liver. It is important to emphasize that human beings are equilibrated and keep a relation with heaven and infraworld. Their influence is reproduced or duplicated in their own body, and warm and cold are maintained graduated in the interior of the organism. As we can see, this concept is a characteristic of the *ticiotl* and is different from the four-humor theory of hippocratic-galenic medicine.

Cosmic and Religious Views of the Aztecs and Their Relation to Medicine

The *ticiotl* took into account a great number of external influences according to circumstantial and temporal variations. These influences were attributed to deities and creatures and the goddesses of medicine: *Tlazeoteotl* and *Tzapotlatenan*. It is in this very wide context that the *ticiotl* conceived diseases *(cocoliztli)* and their treatments (medicines and other remedies, *pahtli*).

In summary, *ticiotl* was much more than just empirical knowledge [10]. Behind it, a whole 'theory' existed, conformed by structured information and an integrated vision of the world including the cultural and social behavior of the *Aztec* people. What Viesca [10] and Lopez-Austin [9, 11] propose is that every culture understands and 'invents' the meaning of disease and its cure.

The vision of the Aztec and the Mesoamerican world was an anthropocentric one. It projects everyday experience to the distant spheres of all that is reachable. Men depart the natural representations of their natural and social realities, to divide, animate, structure, and regulate the cosmos.

It is also important to analyze the triple division of the cosmos: a superior heaven, a inferior heaven, and the infraworld. This division belongs to the integration of the nuclear family, above the Great Telluric Mother is the Great Celestial Father and between them their children.

These beliefs have survived until our times in *nahuas* of the northern Sierra of Puebla. The Aztec priests, as well as the *ticitl*, recognized three spiritual entities: The *tonalli* corresponds to 'the star' and the air, the *teyolia* to the central world or Talocan and the water, and the *ihíyotl* to the infraworld and the land.

The *tonalli* was located inside the head, in the brain on the 'tip of the head'. The *tonalli* came from outside, it descended from heaven like jade, like a precious feather in the moment of conception. It came from the highest of heaven, the Omeyocan.

> 'There, where men were created, from there, comes our *tonalli*. Falls like a drop into the baby, inside the woman's womb. From there comes our *tonalli*, penetrates his or her interior and is sent by Ometecuhtl.'

The *teyolía*, a second entity, was located in the heart *(toyollo)*. It came from the center, not from the superior heavens. – The Aztecs conceived the universe as a vertical axis that led to the highest heaven (the *Ometéotl*), consisting of 22 floors located in different heights. That vertical axis was cut by a horizontal plane, the surface of the earth, where the humans live. Below they counted 9 floors and above 13 (the 13 heavens). The main characteristic of this entity is the vitality, expressed in the constant movement transmitted by the blood *(iztil)*, a substance intimately related with the *teyolía*. Accordingly life could not exist in its absence.

That was the reason that heart and blood were considered the nourishment of the solar gods of the fifth sun. – The Aztecs had no knowledge of the circulation of the blood. In the *teyolía* resided the organized and rational thinking, the capacity to interpret nature, and to structure the data for divination and those products of the imagination. In funerals, the heart was represented by a precious stone [9–11, 13].

Finally, the last of the entities is the *ihíyotl*, an emanation from the inside of the earth and localized in the liver. It is the spiritual entity that corresponds to the lower part of the body and was the symbol of the infraworld. The meaning of this word is 'breath' originated in the inferior regions. It was considered as luminous air constantly fed by the inhaled air and through the energy provided by food, transformed in the liver. The term was related to the emotional life firmly linked to the liver. A strong liver with a well-integrated *ihíyotl* was considered sane, equilibrated, the source of joy and pleasure, as well as a defense against witchcraft and maleficent influences.

Kidney and Urinary Tract Diseases

Something striking in the texts of de Sahagún [4–6] is the lack of a description of the testicles, its place is occupied by the kidneys (*ceyotl* or *cuitlapanaatetl*, testicles from the posterior part of the body; *cuitlapantheutli*, testicles of the back; *pactli*, the gay ones, the joyful; *yoyomoctli*, the itchy, the voluptuous). The kidneys were considered sexual organs similar to the testicles, but located in the inside.

The name of the different diseases involving the urinary system and the cure for them are depicted in different codices and texts [3–7, 14, 15]. They had a name for nephritic colic, bladder pain or discomfort, hematuria, pyuria, and urinary retention. Urinary and biliary stones were not very common in Mesoamerica, even though they had medicines (herbs) for its cure.

Edematous afflictions were probably frequent judging from the great number of representations of dropsy in pre-Columbian art. Peruvian Incas used a very descriptive expression for this syndrome: 'the current of the source is exhausted'. This revealed an interesting explanation for the pathogenesis of the swelling. The Aztecs put patients with dropsy under the protection of *Tlaloc*, the god of rain; those who succumbed went to the *Tlalocan* heaven. The tears of children and the presence of patients with dropsy in the festivities dedicated to *Tlaloc* determined abundance or lack of rain. When the swelled skin became red and infected, they proceeded to make incisions to alleviate the pain and drain the water retained.

One of the most impressive pieces that I have found [16] is one discovered in Nayarit on the west coast of Mexico in 'mine shaft like tombs' and belongs to the classical period (4th century BC to 7th century AD). It is a grotesque figure of a man deformed by the presence of disseminated gummas, severe dropsy, ascites, swelling of the genitalia, and impressive edema of the face mainly around the eyes and cheeks. Since the first time I saw this piece, my impression was: secondary syphilis with nephrotic syndrome. This ceramic man was profusely decorated with arm bracelets, big gold earrings, and painted body typical of the figures discovered in this region and from this period. Syphilis was a common disease in Mesoamerica (fig. 1).

As already mentioned, there are other figures with dropsy, found in different parts of the Mesoamerican world, in all probability this was a common manifestation of disease among these peoples and secondary to different medical conditions: cardiac failure, cirrhosis with ascites (a Jaina figure from the Mayan early postclassical culture,

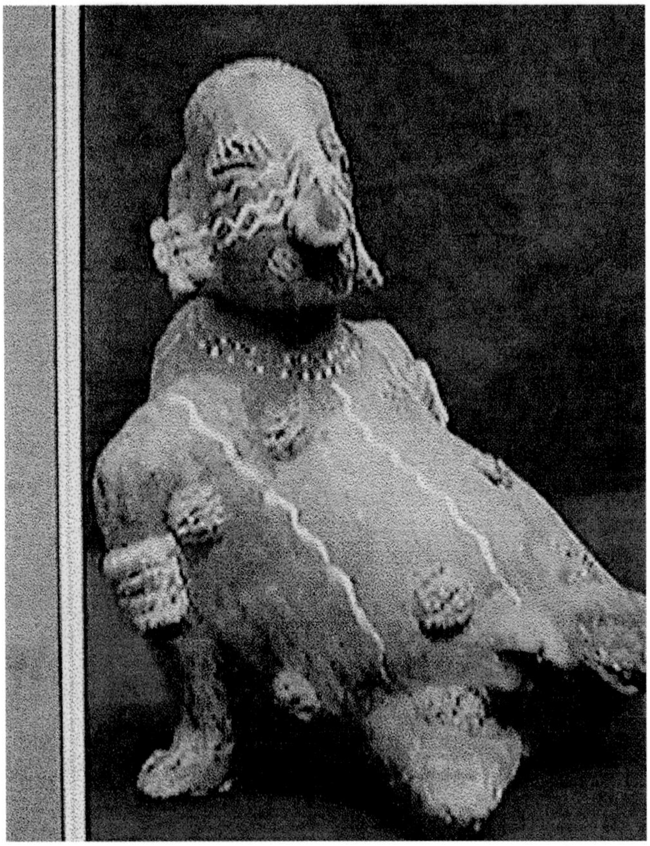

1

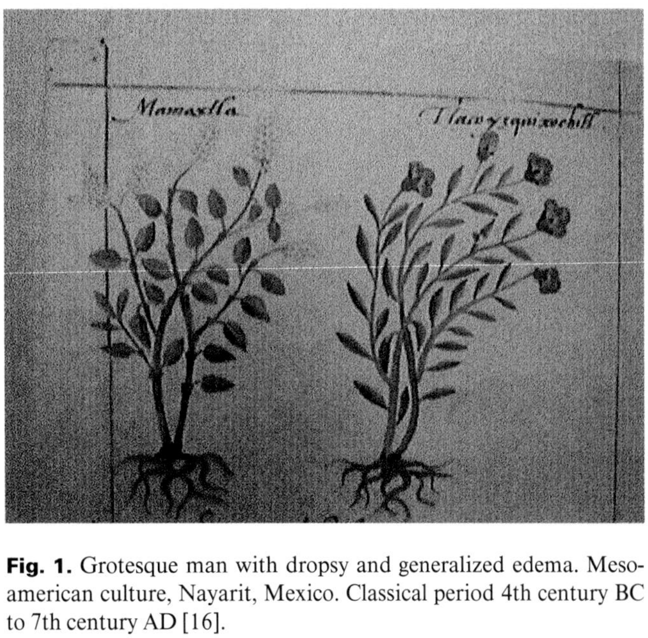

2

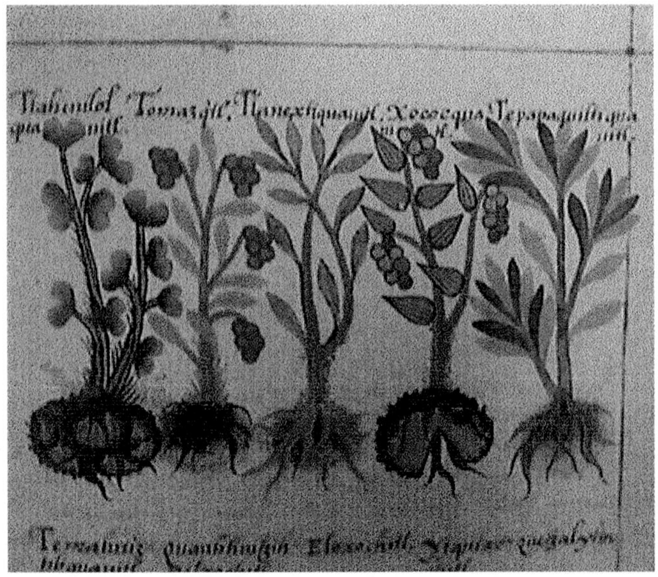

3

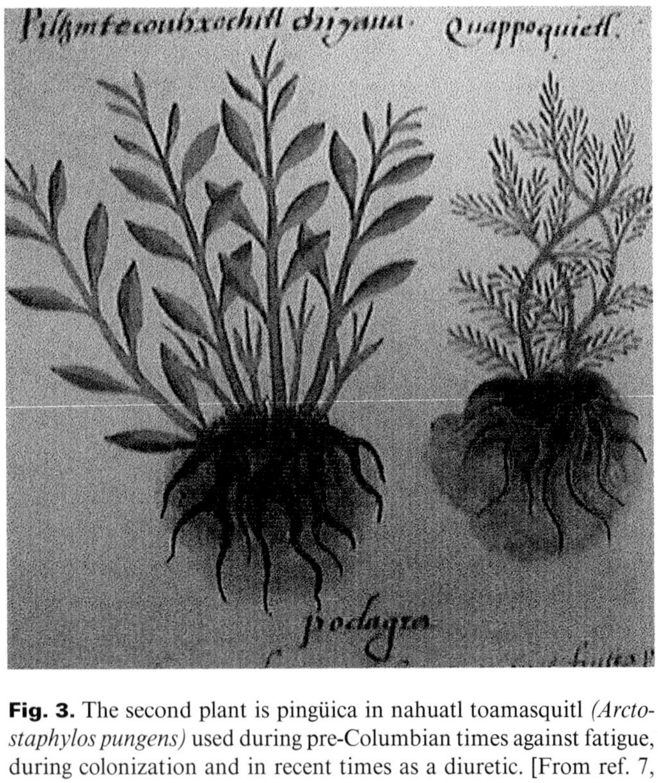

4

Fig. 1. Grotesque man with dropsy and generalized edema. Mesoamerican culture, Nayarit, Mexico. Classical period 4th century BC to 7th century AD [16].

Fig. 2. Root of mamaxtla *(Rumex mexicanus)* on the left and the flower tlacoizquixochitl *(Cordia alba)* on the right. [From ref. 7, p 34 v.]

Fig. 3. The second plant is pingüica in nahuatl toamasquitl *(Arctostaphylos pungens)* used during pre-Columbian times against fatigue, during colonization and in recent times as a diuretic. [From ref. 7, p. 39.]

Fig. 4. For the treatment of podagra (gout) the shrub on the left side is pitzintecouhxochitl chiyaua *(Zinnia pauciflora)* and on the left the plant cuappoquietl (has not been identified clearly by Emmart; Reko believes is some kind of Schkuhria). [From ref. 7, p. 35 v.]

900– to 1200 AD, is suggestive of this disease), nephrotic syndrome, and probably eclampsia.

Diuretic plants were well known and amply used by the Mexicas. We will mention them in the following paragraphs.

The pale urine as is mentioned in the Cruz-Badiano codex [7] in a febrile patient is a sign of renal insufficiency. (Quod si urina albicat, ni statim periculo obuietur, sero medicina parabitur.) So they accepted that the urine came from the kidneys, and this relationship was clearly analyzed in the codex.

Bladder obstruction and stenosis of the urethra were treated [7, fig. 34] with dilatation to improve the urine flow, with the use of a very thin and delicate leave of a palm tree, covered with cotton, coated with honey and the ground root of the herb *huihuitzmallotic*. This stick was introduced with great care in the urethra until the obstruction is relieved.

The root of the *mamaxtla (Rumex mexicanus)* and the flower *tlacoizquixochitl (Cordia alba)* are mentioned for diuresis (fig. 2). The patient drank with water a mixture of flowers, mamaxtla root, red earth, *eztetl* (blood flower), and white earth. With this mixture diuresis was reestablished. Other plants and remedies utilized as diuretics were: (1) *eloquiltic* [4, book XI, No. 79], the leaves of this plant ground and drank produced urine; (2) *iztaquíltic* is a bush, the branches of which were used to improve the flow of urine [6, book XI, No. 108]; (3) *xalatómatl*, the root of this herb purifies and clears the urine [4, book XI, No. 125]; (4) *aitztoli*, this green hard leave produces a heavy gravy considered excellent for those who could not urinate, and when drank before breakfast increased the urine flow and eliminated sandy urine and small stones [4, book XI, No. 139]; (5) leaves of the *ahuéhuetl (Cupressus moctezumae);* (6) bulbs of *zozoyátiv (Veratrum albae);* (7) *cihuapatli (Monatonoa hemionitica);* (8) the crust of *ulquáhuitl (Castilloa elastica);* (9) *tianquizppetla (Illecebrum achyrantha);* (10) *xocoxochitl (Myrtus pimenta);* (11) root of *tepetómatl (Archostaphylos tomentosa);* (12) *cempoaxochitl (Tagetes erecta);* (13) the fruits of *tlilxochitl (Epidendrum vanilla);* (14) *tlalquequétzal (Adiantum trapecifirme);* (15) *jaltómatl (Saracha jaltomata);* (16) *yoloxóchitl (Magnolia glauca)*, and (17) *phehuame* (*Aristolichia* sp?). The plants 5–16 all were utilized as diuretics and are described by Ocaranza [14]. Another interesting plant is *pingüica*, nahuátl name *tomasquitl (Arctostaphylos pungens)* which is depicted in the Cruz-Badiano codex [7] (fig. 3) and was used during pre-Columbian times against fatigue and during colonization and in recent times as a diuretic [17]. Another plant used as a diuretic and aphrodisiac was *tlaolli (Zea mays L.)*, common name corn silk [17].

For the treatment of podagra, the shrubs called *piltzintecouhxochitl chiyaua* and *cuappoquietl* were used [7, p. F35 v.] (fig. 4). The leaves of the first shrub mixed with cypress and laurel branches were located outside an ant hole, and the patiently waited for the ants' dejections. Then everything was mixed with other leaves and added to blood of different animals (rabbit, hare, fox, snake, and others). If the foot hurt because the mixture was very hot, they soaked the soft plaster with cold fluids until it reached a tolerable temperature.

Bone Diseases

The osteopathology in ancient Mexico has been widely studied in bones obtained from the mixteco Zapoteco in Oaxaca and the Valley of Mexico [18]. A typical case of osteitis fibrosa cystica, suggesting the existence of primary or secondary (renal osteodystrophy) hyperparathyroidism, has been reported. These bones came from the classical period and were described in bones excavated in Oaxaca. Osteoporosis was also described in innumerable bones of different parts of Mesoamerica [19]. This entire subject could be the purpose of another communication.

Acknowledgments

Thanks go to my wife, Adela Benitez-Brito, for her suggestions and patiently reviewing the manuscript, and to Dr. Carlos Viesca, Head Departamento de Historia de la Medicina UNAM, and Prof. Enrique Serrano, Director of Physical Anthropology, Museo Nacional de Antropología, Mexico City, for use of the facilities offered to the author.

References

1 D'Ardois S: La medicina en las culturas Mesoamericanas anteriores a la conquista. Edición de la Sociedad Mexicana de Historia y Filosofía de la Medicina, México D.F. 1978.
2 Bernal I: El mundo Olmeca, ed 2. México D.F., Porrúa, 1991.
3 Hernández F: Historia natural de la Nueva España. México D.F., y UNAM, 1959–1960, vol II–III.
4 de Sahagún, B: Historia general de la Nueva España. México D.F., Porrúa, 1991.
5 Florentine Codex: Book X, chap xxvii and xxviii; book XI, chap vii, paragraph 5. Consulted in the Library of the Anthropological Museum, México D.F.
6 Matritense Codex: Book X, chap xxvii, pp 146r–148r; pp 148r–162v divided in 14 paragraphs in Spanish by Brother Bernardino de Sahagún. Consulted in the Library of the Anthropological Museum, México D.F.
7 de la Cruz M: Libellus de medicinalibus indorum herbis. Also known as the Cruz-Badiano Codex. Manuscrito Azteca de 1552. Traducción latina de Juan Badiano, traducción al Español por Angel Ma Garibay K. Fondo de Cultura Económica, Instituto Mexicano del Seguro Social, México D.F., 1991.
8 Cortés H: Cartas de relación. México D.F. Porrúa, 1978.
9 López-Austin A: Cuerpo humano e ideología. Las concepciones de los antiguos nahoas. México D.F., UNAM, 1980.
10 Viesca C: Ticiotl: Conceptos médicos de los antiguos mexicanos. México D.F., Facultad de Medicina de México UNAM, 1997.
11 López-Austin A: Textos de medicina Náhuatl, ed 3. México D.F., UNAM, 1996.
12 Foster G: On the origin of humoral medicine in Latin America. Med Anthropol Q 1987;1:355–392.
13 Lopez-Austin A, López-Luján L: El pasado indigena. México D.F., Fondo de Cultura Económico, 1996.
14 Ocaranza F: Historia de la medicina en México. México D.F., Direccion General de Publicaciones del Consejo Nacional para la Cultura y las Artes, 1995.
15 Trabulse E: Historia de las ciencias en México, ed 1. México D.F., Conacyt y Fondo de Cultura Económica, 1983, pp 291–316.
16 Velut D: Pre-Columbian Dermatology and Cosmetology in Mexico. New York, Chanticleer Press, 1973.
17 Plantas medicinales de México: Usos y remedios tradicionales. Medicinal plants of Mexico. Traditional uses and remedies. Xochimilco, Centro de Tecnología Electronica e Informática, 1995.
18 Jaén Esquivel MT, Bautista J, Hernández PO: Evidencias patológicas en restos óseos antiguos de México. Rev Méx Antropol 1991;36:171–195.
19 Jaén Esquivel MT: Osteoporosis en cráneos de las cuevas de las momias. Bol Inst Nac Antropol Hist 1970;41:5–7.

Origins of Nephrology – Antiquity

American Journal of Nephrology

Am J Nephrol 1999;19:155–158

Edema in the *Corpus Hippocraticum*

Alain Touwaide[a] Natale Gaspare De Santo[b]

[a]Consejo Superior de Investigaciones Científicas, Instituto de Filología, Madrid, Spain;
[b]Servizio di Nefrologia, Seconda Università di Napoli, Policlinico, Napoli, Italy

Key Words
Hippocrates · Dropsy · Edema · Four humours

Abstract
In this paper, we analyze the collection of ancient Greek treatises ascribed to Hippocrates (460; between 371 and 350 BC), in order to determine whether or not edema can be traced. As a result of reading these works on the Greek text, we recognize some symptoms of edema in those called *oidêma* (swelling) and *udrôps* (dropsy) in the oldest treatises of the *Corpus*; in some cases, it seems also possible to recognize its description as the uremic coma. The dysfunction of edema had not been identified as such, however, even though the phenomena associated with the above symptoms received a specific explanation, which was fully hypothetical. This theoretical explanation also justifies the therapies prescribed for the treatment of the phenomena among which edema appears. Significantly enough, the treatment changed during a period which corresponds to that of Hippocrates' life: it changes from the four-quality system to that one of the four humors, but not necessarily under the infuence of Hippocrates himself.

Introduction

In this paper we trace the edema in the 60 treatises which are attributed to Hippocrates (460; between 371 and 350 BC), but constitute, in reality, the so-called *Hippocratic Corpus*, i.e. a collection of works of different authors and epochs, falsely presented as written by the Father of Medicine. We will try to reconstruct, if possible, the medical thinking at the time and examine therapies prescribed.

Sources and Method

In the *Corpus Hippocraticum*, edema may be identified, as we shall see, in the following treatises, listed here according to their possible chronological sequence (in parentheses we note their possible origin, if any)[1]:

[1] Bibliographical Remarks: Edition of Hippocrates' text: Hippocrates. Edited and translated (in English), 8 vol. (*Loeb Classical Library*, No. 147–150, 472, 473, 477, 482), London and Cambridge (Mass.), 1923–1995 (edition by W.H.S. Jones [designated J in our text], E.T. Withington [=W] and P. Potter [=P]). For the treatises *Nature of Woman, Prenotions of Cos* and *Prorrhetic II*, see: E. Littré, *Œuvres complètes d'Hippocrate*, 10 vol., Paris, 1839–1861 (L in our text). General study on Hippocrates and the *Corpus Hippocraticum*: J. Jouanna, *Hippocrate*, Paris, 1992. On the edema: G. Eknoyan, A history of edema and its management, *Kidney Int* 1997;51(suppl 59):118–126.

KARGER

Fax +41 61 306 12 34
E-Mail karger@karger.ch
www.karger.com

© 1999 S. Karger AG, Basel

0250–8095/99/0192–0155$17.50/0

Accessible online at:
http://BioMedNet.com/karger

Natale G. De Santo, MD
Servizio di Nefrologia, Università di Napoli
Policlinico, Padiglione 17, Via Pansini, 5
I-80131 Napoli (Italy)
Tel. +39 81 566 6650, Fax +39 81 566 6655

Diseases II: ancient data (5th century BC, 2nd half), further reelaborated (school of Cnidus [?])

Prognostic and Prorrhetic II: 2nd half of 5th century BC (Hippocrates or a member of his school)

Epidemics III: end 5th century BC (Hippocrates or a member of his school)

Regimen in Acute Diseases (Appendix): end 5th century BC (?) (school of Cos [?])

Regimen: end 5th/1st half 4th century BC (independent author, unknown)

Internal Affections: 400–390 BC approximately (school of Cnidus)

Affections: approximately 380 (origin unknown)

Prenotions of Cos: 4th century BC approximately (summary of Prognostic)

We also quote the following Hippocratic treatises:

Nature of Woman: ancient data (mid 5th century BC [?]), recently reelaborated (school of Cnidus)

Diseases III: ancient data (5th century BC, 2nd half), further reelaborated (school of Cnidus [?])

Airs, Waters, Places: 2nd half of 5th century BC (school of Cos)

Epidemics II and *VI:* end 5th/beginning 4th century BC (unknown author)

On Wounds in the Head: end 5th/beginning 4th century BC (school of Cos)

Aphorisms: 4th century BC approximately (reelaboration of Hippocratic material)

Epidemics V and *VII:* approximately 358–348 BC (Hippocrates' school, after his death)

The method used is the so-called *retrospective diagnosis.* Albeit highly productive, it is extremely difficult, because signs considered to be characteristic by ancient physicians turned out not to be so and, instead, our characteristic signs were not noted or not observed by the doctors of Antiquity. Moreover, diseases were confused in certain cases, due to the possible external identity of some signs, as it is the case, for example, in *Int. Aff.* 40 (6.202–205P): the authors describe a tertian fever, which could correspond to malaria because of the swelling of the spleen, but this symptom gave rise to the association of the pathology with another phenomenon of swelling, which could be an edema; there is thus a superimposition of two pathologies due to a common symptom.

Possible Descriptions of Edema

The Greek word οἴδημα *(oidêma)* seems to be studied in the first instance because it means the *swelling,* which could correspond to what contemporary medicine calls edema. Analysis of the text reveals, however, the fragility of this hypothesis, as οἴδημα *(oidêma)* manifestly corresponds to several types of swelling, including gout, malaria and edema: undetermined swelling, for example in the heart (e.g. *Ep. II* 2.5 = 7.32–33P; *Pren.* 159 = 5.618.9–11L), internal swelling, not precisely identified (e.g. *Ep. II* 3.4 = 7.52–53P; *Pren.* 274 = 5.644.1–10L), swelling of the chest (e.g. *Dis. II* 26 = 5.238–239P.; ibid. 27 = 5.240–241P), internal swelling due to pus (e.g. *Dis. III* 47 = 5.274–275P), swelling of wounds (e.g. *Ep. II* 3.17 and 18 = 7.64–65P; *Wounds* 13 = 3.28–33W; *Aph.* 5.66 = 4.178–178J), or, for example, gynecological swellings (e.g. *Ep. V* 11 = 7.162–163P; *Ep. VI* 1.1 = 7.218–219P; *Pren.* 522 = 5.704.13L) and even swelling of the eyes (e.g. *Ep. VI* 8.18 = 7.284–285P; *Prorr. II* 18 = 9.44.4, 6, 10 and 21L) or of the joints (*Ep. VII* 47 = 7.352–353P).

All these types of swelling are attributed to several hypothetic causes: phlegm in the head (e.g. *Dis. III* 1 = 6.6–7P), pus (e.g. *Dis. III* 47 = 5.274–275P) or internal affection of the female reproductive organs (e.g. *Nat. Wom. II* 174bis = 8.354–357L).

Though polysemous, the meaning of the word may be structured as follows (fig. 1):

In some passages, swelling is linked with dropsy (ὕδρωψ/*udrôps*), so that we may include this term in our search for edema, all the more because the clinical portrait given in one passage seems to correspond quite well to our edema (*Int. Aff.* 24 = 6.152–153P): '... dropsy arises from the liver ... and gives rise to tympanites, and then, after a time, it fills up with fluid. After that, gnawing pains attack the body, and swelling occupies the legs below the knees, and the feet; the liver is hard and swollen, and the collarbones become lean'. Polysemous as *oidêma,* the term *udrôps* has, however, a more unitary meaning than this: dropsy is said to be provoked by the liver, the spleen, white phlegm, dysentery or lientery, as well as by a lack of katharsis (e.g. *Aff.* 22 = 5.38–41P), but it could also arise in the lung (e.g. *Dis. II* 61 = 5.306–307P; *Int. Aff.* 23 = 6.146–149P), from the phlegm (e.g. *Int. Aff.* 22 and 24 = 6.144–145 and 152–153P) or from climaticogeographical causes (e.g. *Int. Aff.* 23 and 26 = 6.146–149 and 158–159P; *Airs* 7 = 1.84–85J). But, in all the cases, its symptoms are of the following type: '... the belly is filled with water, the feet and the legs below the knees swell up ...' (*Aff.* 22 = 5.38–41P); '... the patient respires rapidly, his feet swell ...' (*Dis. II* 61 = 5.306–307P); '... he becomes very lean ... in most cases swelling occupies his whole body; the emaciated patient's skin becomes livid, his belly large, and he has a violent thirst ...' (*Int. Aff.* 26 = 6.158–161P).

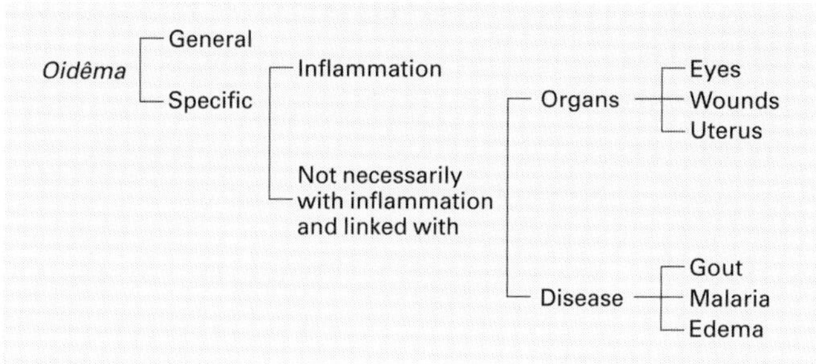

Fig. 1. The meaning of the word 'edema'.

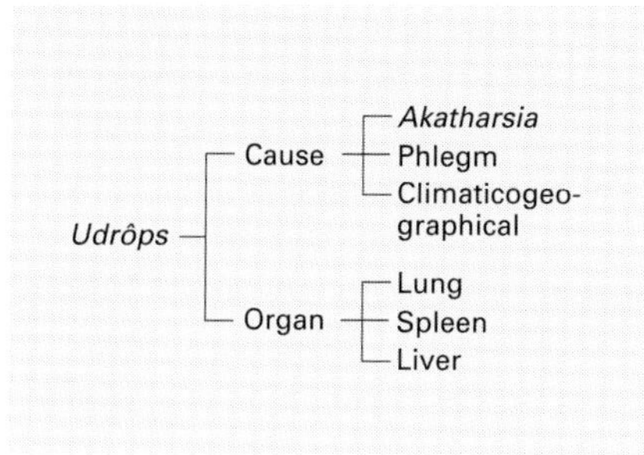

Fig. 2. The meaning of the word 'dropsy'.

As for *oidêma,* we can structure the different meanings according to the following tree (fig. 2):

If we link this tree with the previous one, they appear to be partially superimposable, at least for the following semantic areas: *oidêma*/specific/not necessarily with inflammation/linked with a disease/edema, on the one hand, and, on the other, *udrôps*/cause/*akatharsia.* This correspondence is extremely interesting because it makes apparent the etiology attributed to the phenomenon of edema: a lack of *katharsis,* i.e. a lack of elimination of one of the 4 humors which constitute the components of the body. Precisely, the presence of phlegm as the neighbor of akatharsia in the semantic tree of udrôps, as well as that of malaria in the one of oidêma indicates that phlegm and spleen (characterized by its swelling in case of malaria) are considered to be if not the direct causes of the phenomenon of *oidêma/udrôps,* at least factors linked with it. In this way, we identify an etiological mechanism which is typical in the *Hippocratic Corpus*, as the pathologies of the urinary tract (which includes liver, spleen, kidneys and the bladder) are frequently attributed to the action of phlegm (see e.g.: *Int. Aff.* 14 = 6.118–119P).

This link with the urinary system helps us to discover another possible description of edema, with the uremic coma: what is considered to be numbness of the head (νάρκη/*narkê*) linked with strangury in one case (*Dis. II* 12 = 5.206–207P; see also *Pren.* 60 = 5.596–598L; *Prorr. II* 40 = 9.68.19–70.9L). The presence of both *oidêma* and *udrôps* in clinical portraits (e.g. *Ep. III* 12 = 1.252–253J; *Pron.* 8 = 2.18–21J), also with weight of the body, *kôma* and burning, could probably be considered as edema, although it is identified as anorexia in the Hippocratic treatise (*Ep. III* 13 = 1.254–255J). This may be the best description of edema in the *Corpus.*

Through the words *oidêma, udrôps* and *narkê,* we reach a series of symptoms which seem to include our edema (see also *Pren.* 443 and 471 = 5.584.1–9 and 688.23–690–6L), even though they are polysemous and also encompass pathologies with externally similar signs such as gout (e.g. *Pron.* 17 and 18 = 1.34–35 and 38–39J; *Aph.* 5.25 = 4.164–165J) and malaria (e.g. *Prorr. II* 37 = 9.68.3–6L).

Etiological Mechanism of the Pathology

As for the pathogenesis, it is attributed to the phlegm, as we learn in *Dis. II* 71 = 5.324–325P: '... the whole body swells up with a white swelling, the belly feels stout to the touch, and the feet and thighs swell, the legs below the knees, and the scrotum. The patient breathes rapidly, his face becomes flushed, and his mouth is dry ...'. This is a highly hypothetical explanation of the phenomenon, according to the physics of solids: within the body conceived as a closed circuit, swelling results from an overflow of matter, which comes from the head, going down through the whole body; hence the swelling of the excretory organs and, further, of the lower parts of the body, due to the principle of heaviness which regulates movement downwards.

Therapy of Dropsy/Edema

On the question of the treatment of dropsy, the significant passages appear in 3 treatises: *Reg. II, Aff.* and in the *Reg. Ac. (App.)*, in each of which the theoretical principles underlying the recipes are specific. We examine them according to their possible chronological order.

In *Reg. Ac. (App.)* (52 = 56.312–313P), the drugs prescribed have to be dry and sharp, so as to be extremely diuretic. Although the fact is not explicit, this double action aims at absorbing an excess of moisture on one hand (this is the role of dryness) and, on the other, at opening the structure of matter in order to facilitate the elimination of moisture (this is the one of sharpness).

In *Reg. II,* we have three main types of action, which appear in the following order: animal's flesh is believed to moisten and to provoke diuresis for this reason (46 = 2.318–319J), while, in the same chapter, the flesh of other animals is considered to be dry, probably according to the mechanism that we met above. A little further, leek, garlic and wild vegetables (54 = 4.328–331J) are presented as diuretics because they are warm and sharp and have a pleasant smell, according to a logic not uncommon in the Ancient World which links flavor and warmth, while sharpness procures an opening of matter, as we saw.

In *Aff.* there are also three types of action, which are the following, according to their order of appearance: sharpness of onions (54 = 5.82–83P) and saltiness of some foods (55 = ibid.), sweetness of wines especially if they are dry and, among the dry ones, above all the thin, old and white ones (55 = ibid.), and *katharsis* and thinning provoked by honey (58 = 5.84–87P).

We have thus a progressive evolution in the four main steps, with, in the first one, warmth linked with pleasant flavor and sweetness; on the other hand, dryness and sharpness in the second, with the variant of saltiness, in order to eliminate moisture in both these two mechanisms; in the third, the mechanism is no longer the same: moisture to wash the organism, and, in the fourth, it is a new one: *katharsis,* which presents some similarity with the previous one.

These therapeutic agents and principles give rise to the following considerations: first, they confirm the etiology we saw for the dropsy/edema, i.e. the lacking of physiology due to phlegm; second, they appear only in the oldest treatises of the *Corpus Hippocraticum*, in a way which is probably significant of a possible evolution of the conception of dropsy/edema; third, they result in metaphoric thinking which expresses the action of therapeutics by means of images, transformed further by theoretical justification; fourth and finally, the concepts are associated with subjective values of a cultural nature as is the case with wine: the most active is not only the dry one (which eliminates moisture), but the old, thin and white one, with a series of relations between these qualities: it is thin because it is old (in elderly the moisture of the body has been eliminated) and it is white because, as old and thin, it has positive connotations; consequently, it transmits its qualities to the body into which it is administered.

Conclusions

Some of the symptoms of dropsy/edema seem to have been perceived correctly, including its presence in the uremic coma. The specificity of the disease, however, does not appear to have been clearly identified; instead, it was confused with other pathologies presenting similar external signs. Chronologically, the first elements of description appear in the earliest pathological treatises of the *Hippocratic Corpus*, i.e. from the 2nd half of the 5th century BC, and probably before Hippocrates himself, in the so-called Cnidian School. Further, the disease seems to have been well known if not by Hippocrates himself, at least in his milieu.

As for therapy, the specific one seems to be a little more recent than the clinical portrait of the disease, as it does not appear before the end of the 5th century BC. Significantly enough, its principles correspond to the one attributed to the pathology, which is highly speculative. Therapy changed, however, during the period at the end of the 5th century BC and 380 approximately, i.e. during Hippocrates' own life, and passed from the four-quality system (warmth and dryness, here) to the humoral one (the *katharsis* in our case). We cannot conclude that this modification was initiated by the Father of Medicine, as the chronology might suggest, because the treatises in which this change occurs are of unknown origin and do not seem to be strictly from the School of Cos.

Origins of Nephrology – Antiquity

American Journal of Nephrology

Am J Nephrol 1999;19:159–162

Uroporphyria: Some Notes on Its Ancient Historical Background

Valentina Gazzaniga

Section of History of Medicine, Department of Experimental Medicine and Pathology, University of Rome 'La Sapienza', Rome, Italy

Key Words
Black urine · Acute intermittent porphyria · Inherited porphyria · Acute hepatic porphyria

Abstract
Black urine is recorded in all ancient urology as a negative prognostic sign, often linked with the presence of blood; its presence can also be considered as a sign of massive hemolytic crisis, especially if associated with specific nosological patterns. The Hippocratic case of Epidemics III, 11 has recently been diagnosed as an intermittent acute porphyria. Despite the difficult 'retrospective' diagnosis of an ancient case, it seems likely that the Hippocratic physicians empirically knew clinical associations of symptoms that modern medicine could consider as the first descriptions of porphyria.

Black Urine in Medical History

In the sign-based medicine, which has been the medicine before the revolution of experimental medicine, diseases were recognized according to certain findings, such as the urine. Characterization of black urine as a negative, almost always lethal, prognostic sign is constantly recorded in ancient urology. Celsus, repeating a Hippocratic idea, in the second book, sixth issue of *De medicina* states: 'pessima tamen est, praecipuaque mortifera, nigra, crassa, mali odoris. Atque in viris quidem et mulieribus talis deterrima est' (II. 6.11), that is 'the worst and especially lethal urine ... is that which is black, thick, malodorous ...'. Galen adds: 'In the presence of cloudy appearance *(nephelos)* or particles in suspension *(enaiorema)* or black sediment *(ypostasis),* or in the case urine is uniformly dark, all these features are lethal' [1].

As for the color of urine, Hippocrates and Galen, although not attaining the chromatic wealth of Byzantine texts (Theophilus), suggest various gradations, ranging from dark *(zophodes)* to livid *(pelion),* ashy *(kolodeon)* and black *(melan).* The voiding of dark or black urine is reported in ancient medicine as an important component of many clinical patterns. Sometimes, in acceptable contexts, this observation should be interpreted as a mere indication of the presence of variable amounts of blood. Although bloody urines are clearly described in the *Hippocratic Corpus*, in many instances the adjective *melan* may similarly indicate the presence of blood in urine: this is likely the case of almost all black or dark urines reported in gynecological treatises as postpartum complications. On the other hand, black or dark urine may be considered as a sign of a massive hemolytic crisis, associated with nosological patterns such as those described in Epidemics I and III, mainly referring to hemoglobinuria, myoglobinuria or Falciparum-induced hemolytic crisis. The ancient

KARGER

Fax + 41 61 306 12 34
E-Mail karger@karger.ch
www.karger.com

© 1999 S. Karger AG, Basel
0250–8095/99/0192–0159$17.50/0

Accessible online at:
http://BioMedNet.com/karger

Valentina Gazzaniga
Viale dell' Università 34/A
I-00185 Rome (Italy)
Tel. +39 06 354 960 39, Fax +39 06 499 708 56

authors (see for instance the pseudogalenic lore on urines) generally explain both the dark color and the unfavorable prognosis on the basis of the presence of black bile or very cooked blood, in a theory destined to be maintained almost unchanged up to Theophilus and later authors [2, 3].

However, the dual etiology is clearly discriminated, as the presence of blood is generally considered as an indication of local pathology [4]; moreover, the *melan oura* (*melan* is translated as 'black' by 'traditional' authors such as Daremberg, Littré or Jones) may comprise a wide range of shades, according to the translations of Diller or Martiny, with which Grmek [5, pp 504–508] agrees on some passages. Therefore, the differentiating criterion should probably be represented by the gravity of the prognosis.

Acute Intermittent Porphyria in Antiquity: A Hypotesis

Rimington [6], in 1993, in a paper published in the *International Journal of Biochemistry*, stressed an interpretation given by Voswinckle [7] of a passage of the Hippocratic Epidemic III. The reported case, treated according to the clinical and semiological scheme typical of the ancient core of Epidemics, deals with a Thásos woman who, during 3 days preceding the onset of menstruation, showed severe neurological and psychiatric symptoms, such as convulsive attacks, fits of terror, lipothymia, progressive loss of consciousness up to a semicomatose state, accompanied by increasing fever – a slight increase in temperature on the first day, a little higher on the second, very high fever during the third night – and finally voiding of black urine, at once followed by a complete resolution.

The Hippocratic author stresses that the usual temperament of this woman was *dusanios,* which Galen, in his commentary on the third book of Epidemics, specifies as a *semeion* of particular interest, also in the light of the rarity with which this word is used in the *Corpus* [8]. *Dusanios* is therefore, according to Cryzia as reported by Galen, the temperament of subjects distressed by insignificant episodes and severely depressed, more and longer than others, by more serious circumstances. The Galenic passage ascribes the Thásos case to the accumulation of black bile due to scarce or lacking menstruation.

Rimington [6] classifies the case as an episode of intermittent acute porphyria – a disease sometimes named Swedish porphyria, the 'variegate' variant of which was extensively analyzed by Waldenstrom [9]. This is one of the most common syndromes characterized by an inborn error of heme synthesis, i.e. the so-called porphyrias. They are classified as hepatic or hematopoietic, according to clinical data and to the main site of expression of the specific enzymatic defect, involving in the case of intermittent acute porphyria (IAP) the porphobilinogen deaminase enzyme. IAP is characterized by the urinary excretion of a large amount of porphobilinogen and usually its immediate precursors δ-aminolevulinic acid without a significant overproduction of porphyrins of any type. This syndrome is a typical case of autosomal dominant inheritance and can be present in a latent form for an indefinite length of time, the main clinical features being characterized by global or focal central nervous system involvement, accompanied by motor polyneuropathy and dysautonomic symptomatology. The initial and most prominent symptom of the crisis is a diffuse or localized abdominal pain, usually colicky and associated with vomiting and diarrhea or constipation. Neurological manifestations are largely variable, involving peripheral nerves, the autonomic nervous system as well as cranial nerves or cerebral functions; about one third of the patients with IAP show significant signs of mental disturbances during the crisis; psychiatric manifestations may vary from mild (e.g. irritability, anxiety, confusion, restlessness) to severe (e.g. delirium, hallucinations, psychoses). Sometimes convulsive seizures occur followed by alterations in consciousness [10–13].

Pathological Reality or 'Modern' Lecture of Ancient Medical Thought?

As regards Rimington's idea that the Hippocratic patient was a case of IAP, some observations should be considered. Undoubtedly, the clinical history of the Thásos woman begins with important mental disturbances accompanied by acute and vaguely localized pains. It is noteworthy that the psychiatric syndrome of the Thásos patient is not attributed to a confusional state such as that characterizing toxic infectious states, since the fever was low on the first and second day (pyreton lepton-pyreton oxuteros) and only during the third day did it reach a really high level. This seems in disagreement with Grmek's idea that the psychotic changes so often cited in Epidemics I and III are always linked only to malarial attacks, typhoid fever or shigellosis [5, pp 488–489]. Another point that supports a possible diagnosis of IAP is the apparent complete resolution of the clinical symptomatology after the beginning of the menstrual bleeding, which is not the case in infectious diseases. Rimington [6] stresses the importance of menstruation, because IAP often occurs in females, in whom – as the crises are often activated by exogenous and/or endogenous factors, such as diet or drugs – the hormonal cycle plays a fundamental role.

However, what Joly [14] writes about the objectivity of ancient physicians in recording symptoms of the clinical cases reported in Epidemics I and III provides a tool for critical evaluation of Rimington's [6] 'modern' retrospective analysis. In fact, it is noteworthy that the Hippocratic physician records and emphasizes only what he knows and can justify on theoretical grounds. Therefore, the female poisoned by the well-known accumulation of corrupted humors, retained because of the intrinsic coldness of the female body, eliminates them by means of the menstruation as well as of postdelivery purification [15]. By examinating the subsequent case of the clinical list of Epidemics III, there is another example of a pathology of females relieved by the onset of the menstrual flux [16]. This point is stressed by Galen himself, in the above cited commentary on the Epidemics, when he is astonished by the fact that no irregular or lacking menstrual cycle is reported as a cause of the accumulation of black bile, which could explain the manic and depressive temperament, the voiding of dark urine and the appearance of menstruation concomitantly with the crisis. In other words, the voiding of black urine, which is generally a sign of fatal disease according to Erasistratus, should be of favorable significance only in the case of feverish female patients, as this phenomenon might replace the menstrual flux, which is generally suppressed in the presence of significant fever [17].

Another point that deserves discussion is the black color of the urine on the third day. We have already seen that the term *melan oura* could sometimes be translated only as dark, especially when linked to nonfatal illnesses. Porphobilinogen and δ-aminolevulinic acid, quantitatively excreted with the urine during an IAP crisis, are colorless compounds, which can be partially converted to red-color porphyrins after exposure to air, or to porphobilin, a brown oxidation product of BPG. It is noteworthy that the Hippocratic physicians examined urines left for some time in the *matula* (a glass vase to contain urine) and not immediately after voiding.

On the other hand, Gunther [18] decribes the color of IAP urine as 'red wine, port, malaga, magenta, cherries and occasionally almost black'.

Nevertheless, three features of the Thásos case are in disagreement with the hypothesis of IAP. The first one is that only in some patients acute episodes are associated with low fever, in contrast with the high fever of the Thásos woman on the third day, followed by a complete resolution. A second point is that acute episodes of IAP generally last from several days to several months; from this perspective, a 3-day crisis seems to be quite short. Third, and most importantly, it is always dangerous to look for a rare medical explanation of a clinical symptomatology – especially in a tentative reinterpretation of an ancient medical text [19] – when the context suggests other, more likely diseases characterized by high prevalence; this is similar to a recent attempt to diagnose Vincent van Gogh's illness, suggested by Loftus and Arnold [20] to be a case of IAP triggered by absynthism, when, according to Jamison and Wyatt [21], his mental disturbance could easily have been diagnosed as a manic-depressive disorder, especially on account of the absence of colored urine [22].

Conclusions

What Rimington [6] does not write is that at least two other passages of the *Hippocratic Corpus* are likely descriptions of porphyrias: *Prorrheticum* refers to reddish feces, similar in their color to fire, which are a clear prognostic sign of manic delirium and paralysis, and red feces are sometimes linked to phrenitis, abdominal pains, stomach ache and mania, but, in particular, *Coacae Praenotiones 2*, XXIV: 'Dysenteric feces, *uperutra* (reddish) ... which, when dispersed, get kindled, intensely red colours *(epi flogodesin exeputroisi chromasi luomena)* then mania may occur' [23].

The correlation between clearly red feces and mania (in this case, semantically, manic disorder, independent of a febrile context, as widely testified by the ancient medical literature that distinguishes mania from phrenitis; see Celsus Aurelianus) may refer to another form of porphyria, the inherited coproporphyria [24–28], an acute hepatic porphyria with autosomal dominant inheritance, due to the deficient activity of the coproporphyrinogen III oxidase enzyme, and therefore by the excretion of large amounts of red-colored coproporphyrin III in the feces and also in the urine. This syndrome, as IAP, involves acute attacks of neurological and psychiatric disorders, indistinguishable from the clinical manifestation of IAP. In conclusion, apart from the case of the Thásos woman which could or could not be an IAP, it seems likely that Hippocratic physicians empirically knew other clinical associations of symptoms that modern medicine considers as different forms of porphyrias.

References

1 Celsus: *De medicina* II, 6.11; Galen: *De cris.* I, XII.
2 Angeletti LR, Cavarra B: Critical and historical approach to Theophilus' *De urinis*. Am J Nephrol 1994;14:282–289.
3 Gazzaniga V, De Angelis E: L'oncologia ginecologica dai papiri egiziani ai testi ippocratici. Med Secoli 1994;6:117–138.
4 Celsus: De medicina II, 7: 'at si sanguis aut pus in urina est, vel vesica vel renes exulcerati sunt'.
5 Grmek MD: Le malattie all'alba della civiltà occidentale. Bologna, Il Mulino, 1985, pp 488–489, 504–508.
6 Rimington C: Was Hippocrates the first to describe a case of acute porphyria? Int J Biochem 1993;10:1351–1352.
7 Voswinckel P: A constant source of surprises: Acute porphyria. Two cases reported by Hippocrates and Sigmund Freud. Hist Psychiatry 1990;1:159–168.
8 Galen: *Comm. in Hipp. Epid.* III, III,LXXXII.
9 Waldenstrom J: Studien über Porphyrie. Acta Med Scand 1937(suppl 82).
10 With TK: Thirty years with biochemistry and clinic of porphyrias in man and animals. Int J Biochem 1980;12:985–988.
11 Ratnaike S, Blake D: The diagnosis and follow-up of porphyria. Pathology 1995;27:142–153.
12 Wetterberg L, et al: Estrogen treatment caused acute attacks of porphyria. Lakartidningen 1995;92:2197–2198.
13 Goldberg A: The porphyrias. Historical perspective. Clin Dermatol 1998;16:189–193.
14 Joly R: Le niveau de la science hippocratique. Paris, Les Belles Lettres, 1966, p 220.
15 Gazzaniga V: Phlegm and pregnancy in ancient Greek medicine. Increased erythrocyte sedimentation rate as a marker of impurity of pregnant women in Ancient Greece? Forum 1998; 8:188–193.
16 Corpus Hippocraticum, *Epid.* III, 12.
17 Galen: *De atra bile* 8.
18 Gunther H. Die Haematoporphyrie. Dtsch Arch Klin Med 1911;105:89–146.
19 Grmek MD: Le diagnostic rétrospectif des cas décrits dans le livre V des épidémies hippocratiques. Actas VII Colloque Intern Hipp. Universitad Nacional de Educación a distancia, Madrid, 1990, pp 187–200.
20 Loftus LS, Arnold WN: Vincent van Gogh's illness: Acute intermittent porphyria? BMJ 1991; 303:1589–1591.
21 Jamison KR, Wyatt RJ: Vincent van Gogh's illness. BMJ 1992;304:577.
22 Strik WK: The psychiatric illness of Vincent van Gogh. Nervenarzt 1997;68:401–409.
23 Corpus Hippocraticum, *Coa. Prae.* 2, XXIV; *Prorr.* 1, 85; *Coa. Prae.* 175, 476.
24 Kiso S, et al: Hereditary coproporphyria. Nippon Rinsho 1995;53:1433–1437.
25 Schoenfeld N, et al: Relation between uroporphyrin excretion, acute attacks of hereditary coproporphyria and successful treatment with haem arginate. Clin Sci 1995;88:365–369.
26 Bont A, Steck AJ, Meyer UA: Acute hepatic porphyria and its neurological syndrome. Schweiz Med Wochenschr 1996;126:6–14.
27 Schreiben WE, et al: Hereditary coproporphyria. Hum Mutat 1997;10:196–200.
28 Martasek P: Hereditary coproporphyria. Semin Liver Dis 1998;18:25–32.

American Journal of Nephrology

Am J Nephrol 1999;19:163–164

Treatment of Renal Stones in Bulgaria in Ancient Times ('Hissarya' Baths)

D. Nenov[a] V. Nenov[a] G. Lazarov[b] A. Tchepilev[b]

[a]Medical University, Varna and [b]Ministry of Health, Sofia, Bulgaria

Key Words
Hissarya baths · Renal stones · Mineral water

Abstract
Well-known mineral baths in Bulgaria, 'Hissarya', are described. Their existence dates back more than 25 centuries. 'Hissarya' is an Arabic word meaning 'siege of a castle'. Remains of castle walls are the symbol of 'Hissarya' today. Every year more than 100,000 patients from Bulgaria and other countries visit 'Hissarya'. From the time of the Thracians and the Roman Empire until now renal stones have been successfully treated by drinking the mineral water and by taking baths. The Roman Emperor Septimius Severus (193–211) visited 'Hissarya' every spring to treat his renal disease.

'Hissarya' baths, where urolithiasis therapy has been popular since ancient times, are among the oldest resorts in the world. Their existence dates back to more than 25 centuries. Discovered remains of a village date back to the New Stone Age, 3,000–4,000 years BC [1]. 'Hissar' is an Arabic word meaning 'siege of a castle'. Remains of the wall of the fortress are the symbol of Hissarya today. The resort is of national importance in Bulgaria, with more than 100,000 patients visiting it yearly. Beside renal diseases, mostly urolithiasis, other diseases such as gastrointestinal disorders are also treated. Geographically Hissarya is located at 58° east and 42° 30′ north, in the middle of Bulgaria, on the southern slopes of the Sredna Gora mountain, facing the wide Thracian valley. Its altitude is 365 m above sea level and the mean atmospheric pressure is 734 mm Hg.

In ancient times the vicinity of Hissarya was controlled by the Thracians. These inhabitants from the tribe 'Bessy' used to express their thankfulness for the healing mineral springs by making dedications to Heros, Aesculapius, Hygia, Telesfora and other gods, and by building the so-called nymfecia – sanctuaries for the water nymphs around the mineral springs. Votive tablets are still discovered nowadays during archaeological works in those areas. Coins and a bronze head of Nike from Roman times have also been discovered.

In the 1st century AD Thrace was a Roman province and Hissarya being a famous resort frequented by emperors was named 'Augusta'. Members of imperial dynasties and patients from the Balkan peninsula and from the islands of the Aegean sea, from Lesser Asia and Egypt vis-

KARGER

Fax + 41 61 306 12 34
E-Mail karger@karger.ch
www.karger.com

© 1999 S. Karger AG, Basel
0250–8095/99/0192–0163$17.50/0

Accessible online at:
http://BioMedNet.com/karger

Dimitre Nenov
Bld. Osmi Primorski Polk 137B
Varna 9010 (Bulgaria)
Tel./Fax +359 52 30 28 84

ited the resort. The Romans took special care as regards the growth of the resort, among them especially Severus [2]. According to some historical sources emperor Septimius Severus (193–211) came to Hissarya every spring to treat his renal disease and to enjoy the song of the Hissaryan nightingales. This is the origin of his nickname 'friend of the nightingales' [3].

One of the baths, 'Momina Banya', was built in 306 AD in the epoch of tetrarchs and under the rule of the emperors Maximilian Herkul (293–311) and Licinius (308–324). It had a large size and a complex structure, with a high internal wall, 4 m high and 16 m long with a stone script on it. The bath was equipped with a tepidarium (room with moderately warm air), caldarium (room for hot bath), frigidarium (room for cold bath) and hippocaust (heating installation under the floor of the bath, where hot water was running).

In addition to the exquisite marble baths there were a large number of public and private buildings, and paved streets with drains. A silver-plated surgical instrument has been discovered during archaeological work. 5 necropoles (Roman cemeteries) were discovered outside the walls of the town. The Romans used 7 out of 22 springs in Hissarya. The resort continued to be wealthy later during the Byzantine epoch. The village was then (3rd to 7th century) named 'Sevastopolis', 'Dioclecianos' and 'Alektopolis'. In medieval times under Bulgarian rule the resort was called 'Toplitza' [3].

Nowadays the total amount of water of all springs is 4,000 liters/min. The water has a low mineral content (≈230 mg/l) with the temperature ranging between 37 and 51 °C, radioactivity 10–165 emans and a pH of 8.13-9.12. It contains hydrocarbons, fluorides and radon [4]. About 5,000 patients with renal diseases are treated yearly in Hissarya. It is indicated in patients with uric acid and oxalate stones, but contraindicated for those with phosphate stones. Drinking mineral water helps eliminate urate and oxalate stones and bacteria, and the urine pH rises. 8% of patients excrete stones during the therapy. 83% have a subjective and 70% an objective improvement. The texture of the skin improves when bathing in mineral water, with the perspiration increasing, i.e. the excretory function of the skin is enforced. Bathing is done at 37–39 °C for 7–15 min 2–3 times with 1 day of rest. One course of therapy includes 15–20 baths. Water is drunk 3–4 times daily, 30 min to 1 h before meals, 300–500 ml of water at a time, a maximum in the morning and a minimum in the evening [4].

Hissarya water was blessed by a modern Bulgarian woman with extrasensory perception called Vanga. It is widely distributed on the Bulgarian market as bottled oligomineral drinking water with perfect organoleptic properties.

References

1 Malinov T, Madjarov K: Hissar. Sofia, Medicina I fizkultura, 1974, pp 1–80.
2 Najdenov G: Balneotherapy in Hissarya. Sofia, Medicina I fizkultura, 1959, pp 1–62.
3 Kostadinov D, Karakolev D: Major Balneological Resorts. Sofia, Medicina I fizkultura, 1983, pp 1–218.
4 Shterev K: Mineral Waters in Bulgaria. Sofia, Nauka I Izkustwo, 1964, pp 1–172.

Origins of Nephrology – Middle Ages, Renaissance

American Journal of Nephrology

Am J Nephrol 1999;19:165–171

Theophilus' *Auctoritas:* The Role of *De urinis* in the Medical Curriculum of the 12th–13th Centuries

Luciana Rita Angeletti Valentina Gazzaniga

Section of History of Medicine, Department of Experimental Medicine, University of Rome 'La Sapienza', Rome, Italy

Key Words
Theophilus · *Articella* · Blood-urine relationship · Salerno medical school

Abstract
The three principles *to know, to know how* and *to know how to be* are already condensed in the works of Theophilos (7th–9th centuries). Theophilus' *De urinis* was included in Latin translation in the *Articella*, probably because of its intermediate position between the texts of high doctrinal value by Hippocrates and Galen (lacking, however, a unifying 'theory of urine') and the *epitomes*, short manuals without any theoretical background. It thus forms an excellent synthesis of a cultural approach reconciling *iatrosophia* and *techne* and offers to the reader a text reconciling the theory and the practice, useful to health workers in hospitals, novice beginners and medical scholars. Thanks to his strong attention to the correlation between symptoms and pathology and to his search for assessment scales, Theophilus became the author on whom the birth of medical medieval studies was founded.

Introduction

According to current medical pedagogy the three objectives which the student must aim for by means of a carefully planned and specifically prepared didactic activity are: *to know, to know how* and *to know how to be.* These three principles are found already condensed in the works of Theophilus, a Byzantine doctor and writer who lived some time between the 7th and 9th centuries AD and who was an important figure in Greek medicine, particularly concerning uroscopy. He treats topics which are based on objective evidence (urine, pulse, etc.) and provides a doctrinal outline, in a constant effort to pick out the characteristics *(semeia)* which allow the observer to move from theory (how urine is formed) to its clinical application (to detect the type of illness according to the color of the urine).

To Theophilus is attributed a treatise called *Perì ouron* [1] which thanks to these features enjoyed great fame during the Middle Ages and was included in Latin translation in the medical canon called in the Renaissance *Articella* or 'little art'. This *corpus,* published in the 15th to the 16th centuries, was developed gradually in the medical school at Salerno from the 12th century onward and was used by the School as a textbook at the end of the 12th century and during the 13th century. The original *corpus* usually contained five texts, in the following order: *Isagoge* by Johan-

KARGER
Fax + 41 61 306 12 34
E-Mail karger@karger.ch
www.karger.com

© 1999 S. Karger AG, Basel
0250–8095/99/0192–0165$17.50/0

Accessible online at:
http://BioMedNet.com/karger

Prof. Luciana Rita Angeletti
Section of History of Medicine
Department of Experimental Medicine and Pathology
University of Rome 'La Sapienza', Viale dell'Università 34A
I–00185 Rome (Italy), Tel./Fax +39 06 4451721

nitius (an Arab-Jewish author of the 9th century); Hippocrates' *Aphorisms* and *Prognostics; De urinis* by Theophilus and *De pulsibus* by Philaretus; the sixth document, Galen's *Ars parva* or *Tegni*, does not appear in the ancient manuscripts and commentaries of the *Articella* until after the middle of the 12th century, usually at the end of the collection.

The *corpus* originates from the translation of medical works done by Constantine the African (1015–1087). He was a prominent figure who arrived in Salerno in 1077 and then went to live at the Monastery of Montecassino, where he carried on an intense activity, translating texts from Arabic into Latin, spreading both Greek and Arab medicine widely in the West, especially at the school of Salerno, and favoring a closer link between medicine and natural philosophy, which the Arabs were particularly dedicated to, with the development of both clinical medicine and mathematics, astronomy, alchemy. The use of the term *physicus* for *medicus* at the school of Salerno indicates that doctors were expected to have a theoretical preparation in the natural sciences as well as practical training. In fact, among classical authors a knowledge of Aristotle's naturalistic works becomes fundamental. Constantine almost certainly translated *Isagoge,* the *Aphorisms* and the *Prognosticon*, while *De urinis* and *De pulsibus* were presumably translated directly from Greek into Latin after 1100 [2]. Galen's *Ars parva* was also translated directly from Greek. This is not the place to go into the difficult and complex problems concerning the sources used for the translation of these texts: many of these problems have still not been solved, partly because they are related to another issue: that of the transmission of these texts along the double route of Greek to Latin on the one hand and Greek-Arabian-Latin on the other [3]. This topic would require a more ample and detailed treatment than is possible in this paper.

Theophilus, the Teaching of Urology and the *Articella*

Regarding the inclusion of Theophilus' text in the key textbook of the Salernitan medical school (the *Articella*), it must be remembered that the late Byzantine literature, following a model of citing 'ancient' authors partly owing to prevalent tastes in scholarly writing and partly to a principle of ritual respect for a culture which is above all a fruit of tradition, considers Oribase, Aetius, Nicolaus Mirepsus, Psichrestus and Theophilus himself among those who might be compared with Hippocrates and Galen [3]. Especially Theophilus' works, as well as those of Magnus and Stephen of Athens – interrelated, whatever the relationship might be between Magnus and Stephen, whether intellectual or didactic [5] – represent textual models for the ancient world which consolidates and integrates a tradition which classical medicine in many ways had left incomplete.

In fact, as we will see later, the *Corpus Hippocraticum* does not set the study of urine in a complex, orderly system, but looks upon it only as one of the many signs at the disposal of the physician for the formulation of an exact prognosis. On the other hand, the tracts on urine transmitted under the name of Galen, as transmitted by Kühn [6], are definitely spurious. Classical antiquity from the great master of Kos to his most famous commentator does not elaborate texts which are able to provide a unitarian theory on urine similar to that proposed by Galen, e.g., on the examination of the pulse.

It is worth noting that only with Stephen, Magnus and Theophilus [7] the classical humoral theory is used as a substrate for the examination of the physiologic and pathologic emission of urine in a theoretical context underlying the notion of humoral *cotion*, for example. Thus the works of these authors are collocated automatically in an intermediate position between the texts of high doctrinal value produced by Hippocrates and Galen – which, however, lack a unifying and systematic treatment of urine – and those of *epitomes*, the short manuals in which there is little space for any theoretical background, but which in simple language provide the practicing physician with the constant correlation obtained between the state of urine and pathology according to a cause-effect relationship.

These *epitomes* on urine soon find their selected audience in Western Europe, where they are translated into vulgar Latin from the 6th to the 7th century on and integrated with parts taken from a urological practice which is probably less sophisticated than that prevalent in Byzantium and spread among physicians who are in need of texts which can be consulted easily and quickly, just to formulate a diagnosis [8]. These doctors did not need the theoretical integration offered by the Byzantine *compendia*, at the disposal of those who wished to complete this practical approach with the justifications furnished by the *logos* [9]; at the most, this medical audience required manuals with low theory content, like the texts modelled, especially in Northern Italy between the 8th and 15th centuries, on the pseudo-Galenic treatises on urine or the ones by a certain Alexander, based on Galenic texts, among which *Ad Glauconem de methodo medendi*, from which the author takes the passages on semeiology (while cutting out their accompanying theoretical sections), a text which was translated into vulgar Latin as early as the Middle Ages.

Theophilus' text was to have a different destiny: neither scientific treatise nor simple epitome, it lacks any complex pathophysiological theory, but is also free of the epitomes' naive attempts to provide each visible appearance of urine with a corresponding pathologic reference. It thus forms an excellent synthesis of a cultural approach – which is typical of Byzantine society and its scientific mentality – in a constant effort to reconcile *iatrosophia* and *techne* or theoretical knowledge inherited from the Alexandrian world and everyday medical practice [10].

The oscillation of the Byzantine world between *logos* and *praxis* is, in fact, already evident during the early phases of elaboration of its medical thought: on the one hand, the Galenic *corpus* provides, with the Aristotelian finalism of its *De usu partium*, a model which is absolutely permeable to Christian teleogy, on the other hand, a more empiric form of knowledge begins to come to the fore which is strongly conditioned by anatomical traditions inherited from Alexandria and well expressed in hospital practice [11]. While the study of the human body is abandoned entirely in the West, at least until the experiments reproposed by Mondino de' Liuzzi, there is evidence in the Christian East of a survival of anatomical practice as early as the 4th century with St. Eustazio, in the 8th with Theophanus who records the practice of vivisection and in the 11th century with St. Simeon, the New Theologist [12].

The Byzantine tendency to choose pharmacological texts is another sign of this oscillation between professional training destined for practice in imperial hospitals or at the patient's bedside and the establishment of a concept of medicine which goes beyond its status as *techne* to claim a wider statute and a role defined by the cultural formation of those who dedicate themselves to it. Dioscorides' textual tradition is emblematic in this sense, because it is structured in texts which are not illustrated but with a firm theoretical underpinning (*Paris gr* 2179; *Marc gr* 273; *Laur* 74.17), and it also gives rise to alphabetical and illustrated publications, inspired perhaps by manuals such as Crateuas (1st century BC) and well represented by Dioscorides of Vienna and Naples (*Vindob med gr* 1; *Neapol gr* 1) [13].

Oribasius himself, although structurally anchored to the galenic approach, brings it up-to-date and integrates it in line with other authors in an attempt to render credible and useful a vast theoretic 'congerie' which was methodologically disordered and to coordinate it so as to extract a text, such as the *Synopsis* for Eustace, for practical purposes. Also Alexander of Tralles presents himself as a practitioner who integrates the theoretic aspects of classical tradition with his own experience, preferring to present truth rather than bowing obsequiously to the ancients [14, 15].

Similarly, Theophilus thus intended to write a treatise which would fill the gap left by Hippocrates and Galen on the topic of urology and would be rich in semeiotic detail bringing it close to minor medical texts (but the description of the color, consistency and suspensions of urine is much richer than anything found in the *epitomes*), while at the same time supported by a precise theory – that of urine as *'colamentum sanguinis'* which makes it distinctive and characteristic [7].

The Byzantine texts on urology thus follow two routes in the West: the vulgar Latin of Northern Italy, unsuitable for the translation of technical concepts, chooses simple texts also in the field of urology, whereas Salerno, after Alfano's translation of Nemesius' works [16], created a technical and scholarly language which was able to express the complicated system of galenic physiology in accordance with a teleology of Byzantine, and more marginally Christian, stamp [17].

In this context and thanks to this new linguistic resource, Theophilus' work is included among the works of the *Articella* [18] as the only document translated from Greek apart from the treatise on the pulse by Philaretes. This group of writings is meant to be used for practical and didactic purposes, but in a medical context which is far broader than in the North and for which the scarce epitomes with their oversimplifications would never have been adequate, on the other hand there were no works by the classical masters of antiquity containing a complete theory on urine [19].

Theophilus as *Auctoritas* in Medieval Teaching

The medical school of Salerno, already famous in the 10th century because of the competence of its physicians, constituted the important premise for the introduction of the study of medicine at the Universities of Montpellier, Paris and Bologna, which, organized generally round the *studium juris*, in the 13th century are found to have regular and organized medical courses, attested by the statutes and early official documents listing the texts on which the courses were based. These were listed not only with their table of contents but also with the texts of Greek and

Arabic origin which the student was expected to have heard read and commented on by his masters. These texts were submitted to two different reading methods:

'ordinary' and 'cursive' (ordinary-cursory).

The former was performed only by the teachers, with a general comment to solve any questions arising during the reading, the latter was performed by the student and accompanied by a detailed, literal explanation. Once the literal reading was completed, the *lectio* appealed to the *questio* to solve semantic difficulties and compare the author's opinion with that of similar works by other masters. Independently of the *lectio*, university instruction made use of the *disputatio* [20], an exercise in which various participants, masters or students, presented contradictory arguments on a set problem.

Moreover, the number of readings of the texts was established. For instance, we know from the list of texts of the medical diploma syllabus at Paris in the years 1270–1274, designated by the general term *ars medicine* [21], that Theophilus' *De urinis* was given a cursive reading, while it was also the object of both an ordinary and a cursive reading according to the Neapolitan statutes of 1278.

From 11th- and 12th-century Salerno, therefore, works with widely different aims have been handed down to us: besides brief anatomical tracts based on the dissection of animals, antidotaries and collections of prescriptions, *Regimi* and *Practiche* describing different illnesses and illustrating their treatment, we have a series of comments dating from the second half of the 11th century. At that time, in fact, the Salernitan School underwent an important transformation in which it lost its character as an eminently practical medical center and began to become more and more a center for the elaboration of theory.

The teaching methods based on the reading and comment of authoritative texts were confirmed and became characteristic in subsequent centuries in all universities. The appearance of the form of commentary marks the final switch from practical to theoretical teaching, and the most significant moment was when theoretical instruction started to be based not on the first products of Salernitan medical literature, but on classical works of Greek and Arabic medicine translated by Constantine the African. The first examples of Salernitan commentaries on classical medical texts are those by Maestro Bartolomeo and Maestro Mauro, one of the most important medical writers of Salerno who died in 1214 [22]. Maestro Mauro also wrote a commentary on Theophilus' *De urinis* which is found in a Parisian manuscript of the 13th century together with commentaries on the other texts of the *Articella*. It is important to note that the final version of the medical curriculum which is subsequently transferred from Salerno to Paris is attributed to him. The influence of Salerno on Paris is clearly apparent in the figure of Egidius of Corbeil who studied at Salerno and became the first medical teacher in Paris at the end of the 12th century.

The comments probably reflect the lessons held by the *magistri salernitani* and are based on a series of texts – a kind of medical *canon* – which they built up bit-by-bit and which became a real didactic program and curriculum also in other universities. Montpellier, Paris and Bologna had only to continue the exegesis of the Salernitan masters (at least during the 13th century) whose works they knew and who had proposed teaching methods which were precursors of university scholarship.

As mentioned above, it must be remembered that the core of the *Articella* is composed of translations done in the 9th century, from Greek or Arabic: *Ysagoge* by Joannizius, Hippocrates' *Aphorisms, Prognosticum, On the regimen of acute diseases* (added, as mentioned above, during the 13th century in the translation from Arabic by Gherardo da Cremona), Galen's *On the art of medicine,* a treatise *On the pulse* which under the name of a certain Filarete is derived mainly from a pseudo-Galenic leaflet, and lastly the treatise *On urine* by Theophilus Protospatarius which we will concentrate on here to show its *auctoritas.* We know about the wide-ranging importance of Theophilus from the Parisian statute of 1270–1274: as demonstrated by the Neapolitan statutes of 1278, students had to give *De urinis* a cursive reading for the medical diploma. Theophilus is, therefore, an authority, one of those figures whom the physician cannot ignore, on a par with Hippocrates and Galen. Moreover, whereas the *Corpus Hippocraticum* is a collated collection of the Alexandrian period, of the school rather than of the author, and the works of Galen were largely developed also as *commentaria* on the Hippocratic works, this is not the case regarding Theophilus; it seems to be the work of a single author written for a specific purpose. With Theophilus, in fact, uroscopy takes on a preeminent role in Byzantine medicine which through an intensified medical practice assigned a central role to *semeiotica.* As already noted, attention is focused on objective clinical findings which constitute a reliable guide for diagnosis and subsequent clinical treatment. In this sense, Theophilus is a real master whose *auctoritas* is equal to that of Hippocrates and Galen, especially if we consider that the work attributed to Filarete is a pseudo-Galenic text.

Uroscopy from the Hippocratic Medicine to the *Auctoritas* of Theophilus

Hippocratic medicine had assigned great importance to the search for signs and prognostic evaluation which serve to establish the rationality of medicine in general and of each disease in particular, including the so-called sacred disease which in no way differs from the others – as stressed at the beginning of *De morbo sacro* [23]. On the other hand, Hippocratic medicine had not attributed semeiologic value to urine, nor had it correlated the features of urine with any precise illness, except in the obvious case of urinary infections. It served rather to help determine the prognosis in terms of duration and outcome, like other physical signs of excretory products such as feces, vomit or sweat or pathognomonic signs such as facies, breathing, etc.

It is only with Byzantine medicine that texts are devoted to the detailed study of signs and in particular of pulse and urine. These texts – treatises, textbooks or epitomes according to the use to be made of them – also became part of Arab medicine and the medieval school of Salerno which in turn produced numerous works on these subjects. And obviously every important author is anxious to show his medical culture by addressing these topics: thus urology and uroscopy become a privileged sector of study which from Theophilus on is imitated starting from Salerno and then in Chartres, Montpellier, Paris and everywhere, in Bartolomeus, Maurus, Petrus Ispanus, Egidius of Corbeil and so on in any work aspiring to play an important role in Western medicine. It was as if, to become a professor, it was necessary to produce a commentary on Theophilus and possibly even one's own modest treatise on uroscopy. This is what happened with Magister Maurus *(Regulae urinarum)*, Magister Ursus *(Compendium de urinis)* and Egidius of Corbeil who wrote the *Carmina de urinarum judiciis* [24]. Thus, in Theophilus we find an *auctoritas maxima.*

The historical identity of Theophilus is uncertain. It is almost impossible to trace a biography on the basis of the historical sources, and it is also difficult to place him in a well-defined chronological period [25]. Theophilus has been conventionally placed in the 7th century AD, but he may have lived in the 9th and perhaps even in the 10th century. He is recorded in manuscript traditions as a *prothospa thàrios* or imperial official and also with the titles of *archiatròs, monachòs* and *philosophòs.* His historical identity can be defined with certainty only when the chronological collocation has been better established, in relation to some indications which we are currently working on. Was he an imperial official of the 9th century who retired at some point of his career to a monastery *(monachòs)* to meditate on divine mysteries and also on medicine? Or was he a learned scholar of medical science and as such holding an important position at the Byzantine court?

Theophilus was certainly Christian, as emerges clearly from his *De humani corporis fabrica libri V*; the introduction, with its passage from the Book of *Genesis* (2, 6–7), according to which man was created by God out of clay, definitely marks the boundary between the author and his galenic doctrinal source which, although rich in scientific arguments, did not offer the incomparable truth of the Christian faith. Man, as described by Theophilus, is made up of matter, but is the fruit of a divine miracle which reflects the four universal elements in the four humors. It is a concept which fits well in the traditions of Byzantine Christian anthropology, represented by Nemesius of Emesa (4th century AD) and Meletius the Monk (9th century AD) [26]. Theophilus links this tradition still further with that of Aristotle and Galen, as shown by the fact that he does not respect the exposition of the parts of the body *a capite ad calcem,* but stresses the role of the extremities which distinguish man as a rational, superior animal.

Theophilus presents himself as the paradigmatic representative of Byzantine medicine. He is capable of reconciling the gifts of theorist and scientist loyal to tradition, iatrosophist and learned commentator with those of practical physician, writer of handbooks and textbooks, the former written for health workers in Byzantine hospitals, the latter for novice beginners in the field. In this light, we ought to read and interpret on the one hand the *Scholia* on Hippocrates' aphorisms and the *De humani corporis fabrica* which stem from the attempt to theorize and re-elaborate the sources and on the other hand *De urinis, De excrementis, De pulsibus* and finally the *Apotherapeutikà*, a manual on therapeutic procedures compiled following Greek and Byzantine sources (Galen, Aetius of Amida, Paul of Egina). This text is found in only one codex of the 14th century kept in the Biblioteca Laurenziana in Florence: the *ms plut* 75, 19 which is followed immediately after by Theophilus' *De urinis. De urinis, De excrementis* and *De pulsibus* show similar features. In style and structure they seem destined for a student readership, anyway for beginners or doctors for whom a clear, brief consultation manual might offer the basic essentials of the discipline. The first two in particular seem complementary and follow the same rules of style and composition. Their syntax is straightforward, and the technical terminology is repetitive, elements which reveal their didactic function.

It is interesting to note that the expository technique in many paragraphs of the treatise is that of the *Erotapokriseis*, treatises consisting of question-answer dialogues used for scientific writing. This literary dialectic style was used for beginners, whether aspiring philosophers, rhetors or doctors, in antiquity and late antiquity. Thus, the use of nouns and adjectives in Theophilus is never casual, but each term has its own rigorous meaning which the author adheres to constantly, especially as regards technical terms. What is given priority is the detection of a paradigmatic doctrine of signs and the treatment of subjects with immediate practical implications. No wonder Theophilus criticizes one of his principal sources, the same Magnus iatrosophist who is cited together with the ancient masters Hippocrates and Galen. The latter and also Magnus, says Theophilus, had not treated the subject of urology thoroughly enough. *De urinis*, therefore, represents an attempt, as noted by Theophilus in the introduction, to offer a coherent interpretation of the significance of different types of urine and of the role of uroscopy. In this, he was fully aware that he was introducing a doctrinal innovation and teaching all those who wanted to learn the discipline of urology which was essential, because urine is a basic sign of health or illness of hidden parts of the body and helps to understand how blood is formed:

'Such is urine ... Urine is blood percolation' [27].

Urine is considered, in fact, the secretion of blood, because the perfect formation of blood by hemopoiesis also determines that of urine. If this does not occur, the urine will have the same characteristics as blood.

Particular attention is devoted to the different colors of urine, distinguished according to a conventional chromatic scale which is stressed also by the masters of Salerno. Theophilus dedicates an ample and detailed treatise to these practical color scale systems at various points in the text, in an attempt to assess the different evaluations so as to make a comparison between past experience and each new clinical case and to compare the assessments of different doctors. This is not yet the quantitative measurement of biomedical phenomena, but it is at least an attempt to render their evaluation more objective.

The Theophilus' Recognized *Auctoritas*, from 'Relationship' to Blood-Urine 'Derivation'

The author reflects on the fact that the long journey of medical science toward objectivity was limited for centuries by the fundamental absence of the 'quantitative' dimension. Since ancient times people have measured fields and buildings, weighed foodstuffs and used measuring containers for oil and wine. But the human organism was looked upon as a collection of humors and qualities, and hot and cold are two qualities, not the measure of the same physical phenomenon. Only in the 16th and 17th centuries will scholars acquire the concept of measure applied to the human body. Thus Harvey discovered the nature of the cardiac function in the circulation of the blood, because the blood which enters the heart is equal in quantity to that which goes out. It is not until the 19th century, in particular with Claude Bernard, that medicine passes from experience to experiment [28].

He claims that experience is the fruit of knowledge acquired through the observation of phenomena, while experiment is testing by means of data and reasoning of the facts which the experimenter compares, investigates and rationalizes. In a philosophical sense, we might say that observation reveals and experiment instructs. The true scientist goes through a series of stages: (1) he ascertains a fact; (2) on the basis of this fact he formulates a hypothesis; (3) to test this hypothesis he applies logical reasoning, then devises an experiment and invents the conditions to carry it out, and (4) from the experiment there arise new problems which he observes, and so on.

First there is observation, and here the milestone is set by whoever attributes to the observation the value of a correlation with a clinical symptom, a pathology or the development of a clinical manifestation. In this, Theophilos, with his *De urinis*, in which he searches for assessment scales, is truly an indisputable *maestro di auctoritas.* For this reason and not by chance Theophilos became, together with Hippocrates and Galen and the Arab-Jewish Joannitio, the author on whom the birth of medical studies in the medieval universities was founded.

References

1 Ideler IL (ed): Theophili *De urinis*; in: Physici et medici graeci minores. Amsterdam, Hakkert, 1963, p 261.
2 Kristeller PO: Studi sulla scuola medica Salernitana. Napoli, Istituto per gli Studi Filosofici, 1986, p 112. Jacquard D: Principales étapes dans la transmission des textes de médecine (XIe–XIVe siècle); in Hamesse J, Fattori M (eds): Rencontres de cultures dans la philosophie médiévale. Traductions et traducteurs de l'antiquité tardive au XIVe siècle. Louvain-la-Neuve-Cassino, Publications de l'Institut d'Etudes Médiévales, 1990, pp 251–271.
3 Angeletti LR: Transmission of classical medical texts through languages of Middle East. Med Sècoli 1990;2:293–329.
4 Nutton V: Aspects of Byzantine materia medica. Dumbarton Oaks Pap 1984;38:205–213. See, in particular, p 205.
5 Angeletti LR, Cavarra B: The *Peri ouron* treatise of Stephanus of Athens: Byzantine uroscopy of the 6th–7th centuries AD. Am J Nephrol 1997;17:228–232.
6 *De urinis liber, De urinis compendium, De urinis ex Hippocrate, Galeno et aliis quibusdam*; in Kühn KG (ed): Medicorum Graecorum Opera quae extant. Hildesheim, Olms, 1965, vol XIX, pp 574–628.
7 Angeletti LR, Cavarra B: Critical and historical approach to Theophilus' *De urinis*. Am J Nephrol 1994;14:282–289.
8 Baader G: Early medieval Latin adaptations of Byzantine medicine; in Scarborough J (ed): Symposium on Byzantine Medicine. Dumbarton Oaks Pap 1984;38:251–259. See p 253.
9 Strohmaier G: La ricezione e la tradizione: La medicina nel mondo bizantino e àrabo; in Grmek MD (ed): Storia del pensiero medico occidentale. 1. Antichità e medioèvo. Roma-Bari, Laterza, 1993, pp 167–215.
10 Baader G: Early medieval Latin adaptations of Byzantine medicine; in Scarborough J (ed): Symposium on Byzantine Medicine. Dumbarton Oaks Pap 1984;38:251–259.
11 Temkin O: Hippocrates in a World of Pagans and Christians. Baltimore, Johns Hopkins University Press, 1991.
12 Bliquez LJ: Two lists of Greek surgical instruments and the state of surgery in Byzantine times; in Scarborough J (ed): Symposium on Byzantine Medicine. Dumbarton Oaks Pap 1984;38:187–194.
13 Cavallo G: I libri di medicina, gli usi di un sapere; in Patlagéan E (ed): Maladie et société à Byzance. Spoleto, Centro Italiano di Studi sull'Alto Medioèvo, 1993, pp 45–46.
14 Nutton V: From Galen to Alexander: Aspects of medicine and medical practice in late antiquity; in Scarborough J (ed): Symposium on Byzantine Medicine. Dumbarton Oaks Pap 1984;38:1–14.
15 Temkin O: Hippocrates in a World of Pagans and Christians. Baltimore, Johns Hopkins University Press, 1991, p 232.
16 Montenero Cartelle E: Encuentro de culturas en Salerno. Costantino el Africano, traductor; in Hamesse J, Fattori M (eds): Rencontres de cultures dans la philosophie médiévale. Traductions et traducteurs de l'Antiquité tardive au XIVe siècle. Louvain-la-Neuve-Cassino, Publications de l'Institut d'Etudes Médiévales, 1990, pp 65–89. See p 84.
17 Baader G: Early medieval Latin adaptations of Byzantine medicine; in Scarborough J (ed): Symposium on Byzantine Medicine. Dumbarton Oaks Pap 1984;38:259. Jacquard D: Principales étapes dans la transmission des textes de médecine (XIe–XIVe siècle); in Hamesse J, Fattori M (eds): Rencontres de cultures dans la philosophie médiévale. Traductions et traducteurs de l'Antiquité tardive au XIVe siècle. Louvain-la-Neuve-Cassino, Publications de l'Institut d'Etudes Médiévales, 1990, pp 251–271.
18 Kristeller PO: Studi sulla scuola medica Salernitana. Napoli, Istituto Italiano per gli Studi Filosofici, 1986, pp 97–119.
19 Baader G: Die Schule von Salerno. Medizinhist J 1978;13:124–145. See p 130.
20 Agrimi J, Crisciani C: Edocere medicos. Medicina scolastica nei secoli XIII–XV. Napoli, Guerini e Associati-Istituto Italiano per gli Study Filosofici, 1988, pp 11–20. Agrimi J, Crisciani C: Malato, medico e medicina nel medioèvo. Torino, Loescher, 1980, pp 142–143.
21 Jacquard D: Principales étapes dans la transmission des textes de médecine (XIe–XIVe siècle); in Hamesse J, Fattori M (eds): Rencontres de cultures dans la philosophie médiévale. Traductions et traducteurs de l'Antiquité tardive au XIVe siècle. Louvain-la-Neuve-Cassino, Publications de l'Institut d'Etudes Médiévales, 1990, p 263.
22 Kristeller O: Studi sulla scuola medica Salernitana. Napoli, Istituto Italiano per gli Studi Filosofici, 1986, pp 97–121.
23 De morbo sacro; in Littré E (ed): Œuvres complètes d'Hippocrate. Paris, Baillière 6, pp 350–397.
24 De Renzi S: Collectio Salernitana, Napoli, Tipografia del Filiatre-Sebezio 1852–1859.
25 Angeletti LR, Cavarra B: Critical and historical approach to Theophilus' *De urinis*. Am J Nephrol 1994;14:282–289.
26 Cramer JA: Meletius the Monk on the Constitution of Man. Anedocta Graeca e Codicibus manuscriptis bibliothecarum Oxoniensium. Oxford, Clarendon Press, 1836. Reproduction: Amsterdam, Rodopi, 1963.
27 Ideler IL (ed): *Theophili De urinis*; in: Physici et medici graeci minores. Amsterdam, Hakkert, 1963.
28 Bernard C: Introduction à l'étude de la médecine expérimentale. Paris, Baillière, 1865.

American Journal of Nephrology

Am J Nephrol 1999;19:172–176

Kidney Disease in Byzantine Medical Texts

Effie Poulakou-Rebelakou Spyros G. Marketos

Department of History of Medicine, Athens University Medical School, Athens, and the International Hippocratic Foundation of Kos, Greece

Key Words

Early Byzantine medicine · History of nephrology · Medical encyclopedists

Abstract

The most significant contribution of the great Byzantine physicians to the evolution of medicine is their effort to summarize all the medical knowledge of the Greco-Roman world, which included earlier sources in antiquity, lost forever in our days. The transition from ancient to medieval medicine included the adoption of Christian spiritual values, which took place in the early Byzantine period (4th to 7th century). In the field of nephrology, under the influence of Hippocratic and Galenic doctrines, the most prominent medical personalities, Oribasius of Pergamum, Aetius of Amida, Alexander of Tralles and Paul of Aegina, performed the role of the researcher and healer, as well as that of the encyclopedist. Their works on kidney disease are presented in this paper.

The history of Byzantine medicine is usually divided into three periods, early, middle and late, generally corresponding to the historical division of the empire's millennium. Early Byzantine medicine (4th to 7th century) is considered to be a continuation of the Greco-Roman medical tradition and Alexandria still remained synonymous with its doctors and research and played a dominant cultural role until the Arab conquest [1]. It is not a coincidence that the four great medical personalities of this period studied in Alexandria as did the majority of students from all corners of the east and west [2]. Another common element is their origin from Asia Minor (table 1).

Oribasius, court physician of the Emperor Julian (4th century), honored with the title of Quaestor, was born in Pergamum, also the birthplace of Galen, and had been a student of the famous iatrosophist Zeno of Cyprus [3]. At Julian's request he prepared a synopsis of Galen's works and a second, more extended text summarizing other medical authorities, altogether totalling 70 books with the title *Medical Collection*, half of which is lost today. His other writings are: *Synopsis for Eustathius* (his son, also a physician) and *Book for Eunapius*, both translated into Latin. His whole work proves that he had read and assimilated many medical authors of the past but much personal experience is also included.

Aetius, court physician of the Emperor Justinian I (6th century) was born in the eastern region of Asia Minor, near the river Tigris, in the city of Amida, today Dijarbekir. He lived and practiced his profession in Constantinople, having the official title of 'comes obsequii'. His works named *Tetrabiblon* (fig. 1) are based on different ancient sources, mainly Rufus of Ephesus and his compiler Philagrius.

KARGER

Fax + 41 61 306 12 34
E-Mail karger@karger.ch
www.karger.com

© 1999 S. Karger AG, Basel

0250–8095/99/0192–0172$17.50/0

Accessible online at:
http://BioMedNet.com/karger

Effie Poulakou-Rebelakou, MD
51, Themidos Street
GR–15124 Athens (Greece)
Tel./Fax +30 1 8025547

1

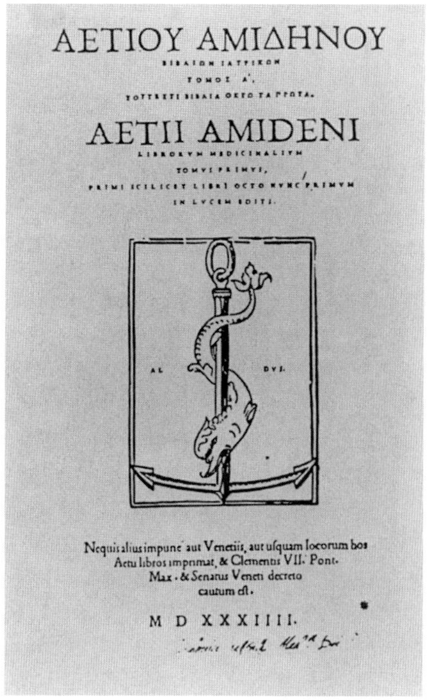

2

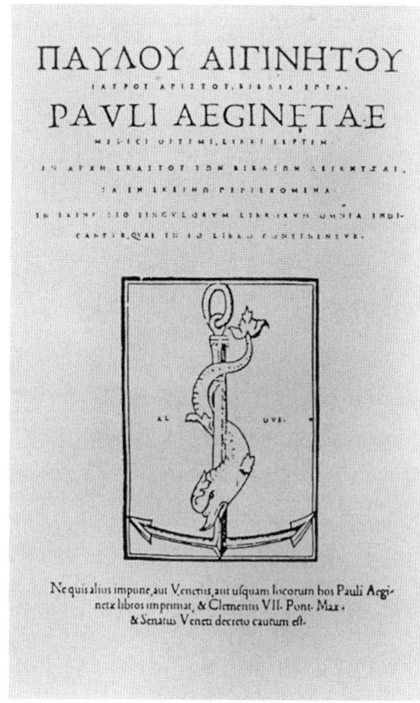

Fig. 1. Title page of the first edition of Aetius' *Tetrabiblos* published in Venice in 1534.
Fig. 2. Title page of the first edition of Paul of Aegina's *Seven Books* published in Venice in 1528.

Table 1. The four great medical encyclopedists of early Byzantium

Century	Name	Birthplace	Place of studies	Place of practice
4th	Oribasius	Pergamum	Alexandria	Constantinople
6th	Aetius	Amida	Alexandria	Constantinople
6th	Alexander	Tralles	Alexandria	Rome
7th	Paul	Aegina	Alexandria	Alexandria

Alexander of Tralles, today Aidin, was born 30 years after Aetius and was the son of the physician Stephen. His brother Dioscurus was also a physician, another brother, Olympius, was a famous lawyer, a third, Metrodorus, was a great mathematician, and the most eminent son of this significant family was Anthemius, the architect-engineer of the Saint Sophia Church in Constantinople. Alexander's best friend was the son of the great navigator Cosmas Indicopleustis. They traveled together in Galatia, Spain and Africa [4]. He practiced his profession in Rome until his death at the age of 80. Towards the end of his life he wrote a therapeutic handbook for doctors, telling us that, unable to practice anymore, he was writing down the cures and the treatments which he had found to be most effective. This work, entitled *Therapeutica*, was highly valued throughout the following centuries.

The last of the four encyclopedists was Paul of Aegina, who not only studied in Alexandria but also practiced there, even after the Arab conquest of the city, and was known by the Arabs as Al Qawabilly (= the Gynecologist). Translated 200 years later by Hunain Ibn Ishaq into Arab and in 800 AD into Latin, his *Seven Books* combined ancient traditional knowledge with direct clinical experience (fig. 2).

Nephrology in the Work of the Encyclopedists

The period of the great encyclopedists starts with the founding of Constantinople by the Emperor Constantine the Great (330 AD) and practically ends with the conquest of Alexandria by the Arabs (641 AD). Their most significant contributions to nephrology were: Oribasius was the first to use the term 'ureter', he treated dysuria and recommended lithotriptic substances; Aetius and Alexander promoted the differential diagnosis of bowel and

3

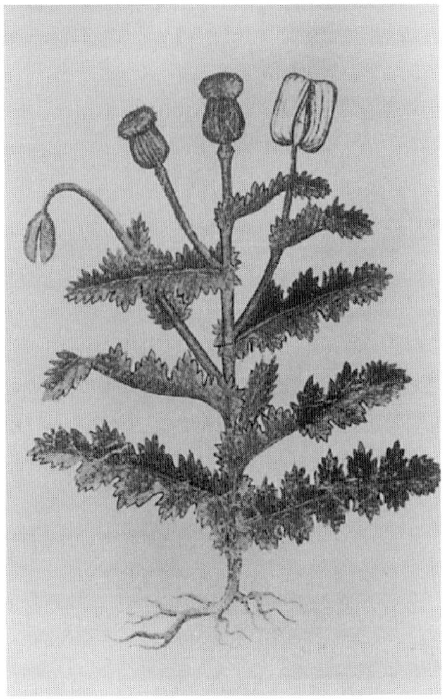

4

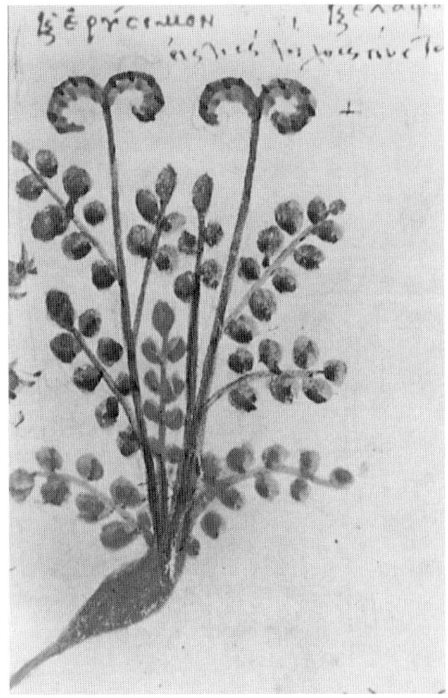

Fig. 3. The medicinal plant *Papaver somniferum* (mecon hypnophoros) poppy according to a Dioscorides codex is recommended for relief of renal pain.
Fig. 4. The plant *Sisymbrium polyceratum* (eryssimon), commonly London rocket, is believed to have lithotriptic and analgetic action. From a 12th century codex of Saint Lavra's Monastery, Holy Mountain (Athos).

renal colic; Aetius first introduced a new classification of renal stones according to their color, and supported the surgical drainage of renal abscesses; both Paul and Alexander worked on lithiasis and the latter theorized that stone formation was due to thick humors accumulating in the kidneys [5]. Several renal diseases are mentioned by the Byzantine compilers of the early period.

Acute Renal Nephritis – Pyelonephritis

Aetius and Oribasius used the term 'nephritis' [6] and 'nephritic' patient [7]. The symptoms as well as the treatment were described by Paul [8]:

> 'If there is an inflammation of the kidneys it is to be recognized by the heat in the place, attended with heaviness and pain, fever, delirium, vomiting of pure bile and inability to make water. Wherefore we must have recourse immediately to venesection, and use soothing fomentations and cataplasms from rue, dill, fenugreek and root of marshmallow, also emolient clysters and injections consisting of poppies ... They must abstain from the strong diuretics and much drink ... they must abstain from very cold applications, for thereby the kidney will become scirrhous.'

Aetius prescribed the seed of the aromatic plant crocodilian for oral intake, because of its warm, dissolving and drying force [9]. Also a decoction of cinnamon orally and the coating of the renal area with valerian and camomile were recommended. Oribasius [10] added some more decoctions for acute nephritis: high mallow, sagebrush, Cretan spikenard, sweet flag and baldmoney. Finally he suggested a mixture of several herbs he called 'nephritic', containing common dill, wild celery, parsley, black and white pepper, cinnamon, poppy (fig. 3), fennel flower, Alexanders, white henbane, all diluted in honey from Attica. Alexander noticed that pus was ejected by the kidneys or ureters [11].

Necrotic Renal Diseases – Crush Syndrome
Aetius attributed the reasons for the kidney's destruction to the toxic influence of remedies and poisons, and external pressure [6]. He suggested drugs to relieve the pain: a concoction of poppy and a poultice of turpentine and flour.

Acute Renal Failure
A general instruction was to forbid the use of diuretics during the acute period. Aetius recommended clysters with mallow, peeled barley, linseed oil, dill, camomile and reed. At the next polyuric phase diuretics were recommended: parsley, cinnamon, amaranth and a diet of bread, birds, sea urchins, egg, vegetables, fennel, celery and carrots [12].

Ulcer of the Kidney

The term 'ulcer' includes various nephropathies such as tuberculosis, tumors, chronic nephritis, 'weakness' of the kidney and sclerosis. Oribasius described the sclerosis as 'painless oliguria' and the 'weakness' as incontinence [13]. Aetius described the symptoms of the ulcer: pyuria, hematuria, strong smell, and recommended an antidote called Andromachus, a formula consisting of thirty-two ingredients such as costus, licorice, iris, rose, cinnamon, and bluestem. Dioscorides had been one of the first Greco-Roman physicians to recognize the usefulness of the traditional Egyptian multiingredient incense recipes, which soon occupied an important place in Byzantine pharmacology [14] and assumed a knowledge of numerous medicinal plants and minerals.

Diabetes

It is believed that Aretaeus is the creator of the term 'diabetes', signifying a syphon [15]. It is classified among the renal diseases by all the Byzantine encyclopedists [16]. There is no evidence of a distinction between diabetes mellitus and diabetes insipidus. For the common symptoms of the disease, Alexander recommended overfeeding if the patient lost weight and Oribasius, Aetius and Paul recommended hydration [17].

Lithiasis

The four great medical authors agreed on the calculus formation theory. They supported the hypothesis that the coexistence of two factors is necessary for the manifestation of the symptoms: (1) thick material passing through the kidneys and (2) increased temperature. Furthermore, Aetius compared this process with the porous stone formation in the copper tubes and boilers of a bathroom and Alexander with ceramic construction [16]. Both suggested methods of differential diagnosis between bowel and renal colic, including always a urine examination.

The therapeutic methods aimed at pain relief, the expulsion of the stone and the avoidance of new stone formation.

Oribasius described some mixtures of soothing plants such as dropwort, myrrh tree, London rocket (fig. 4), cardamon, saffron crocus, nut grass, iris, aloe, valerian, cassia in rose and fragrant wine for the relief of pain. Another mixture included wormwood, pennyroyal, white pepper, fennel flower and laurel. For lithotriptic action the four writers suggested althea, chick pea, black pepper, baldmoney and cinnamon. Alexander treated the colic and the stone's movement with male goat's blood, Paul with asparagus [18]. Aetius attempted to perform a pharmaceutical lithotripsy with a Persian poultice consisting of thirty-one ingredients [19]. On the other hand, the patients had to follow a diet to prevent new stone formation and avoid spices, alcohol, milk and milk products. They also had to use diuretics like absinthium and the calculus-preventive plant, paeonia.

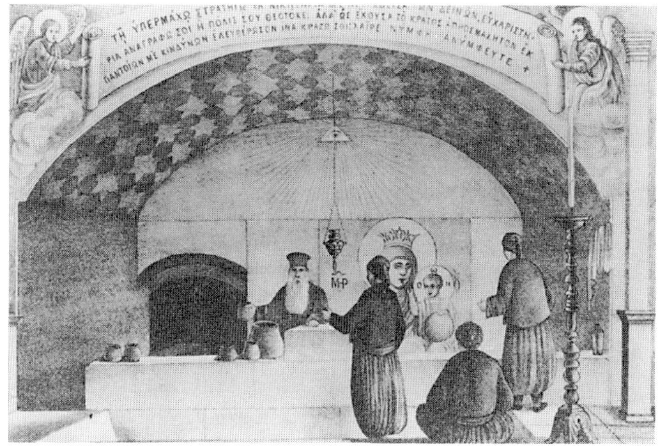

Fig. 5. A general view of the Fountain of the Holy Water (Agiasma) of Life-Giving Spring in Vlaherna, Constantinople, near the Imperial Palace.

In parallel with rational medicine, belief in miraculous healings also figured in Byzantine society. Nephrological diseases were generally considered as difficult to cure, so that supernatural intervention was often the only hope. Especially the Agiasma (= Fountain of Holy Water) was a place of miracles [20]. Two of them became famous in Constantinople: (1) the Fountain of Holy Water of Life-Giving Spring close to the Imperial Palace of Vlaherna (fig. 5) and (2) the Fountain of Holy Water of Life-Giving Spring at the village of Baloukli. One of the famous patients who was miraculously cured from a renal stone associated with infection was the Emperor Justinian I [21, 22]. Suffering from severe dysuria which the doctors failed to cure, he was cured simply by drinking the Holy Water in Vlaherna and since then the location became famous [23] for the treatment of dysuria and lithiasis.

Conclusion

Oribasius, Aetius, Alexander and Paul, the four great medical encyclopedists of the early Byzantine period, also preserved the knowledge and tradition of antiquity in the field of nephrology. Their writings are not a simple repetition of Hippocratic and Galenic doctrines, but also a successful attempt to incorporate their personal experience.

References

1 Duffy J: Byzantine medicine in the Sixth and Seventh centuries: Aspects of teaching and practice. Dumbarton Oaks Papers 1984;38:21–27.
2 Hunger H: Die hochsprachliche profane Literatur der Byzantiner. München, Beck'sche Verlagsbuchhandlung, 1978 (Greek translation ed MIET, Athens, 1994, vol 3, pp 107–153).
3 Baldwin B: Beyond the house call: Doctors in early Byzantine History and Politics. Dumbarton Oaks Papers 1984;38:15–19.
4 Bitschai J, Brodny L: A History of Urology in Egypt. Chicago, Riverside Press, 1956.
5 Marketos SG, Diamandopoulos AA, Poulakou-Rebelakou E, Dimopoulos C: Highlights from the history of Greek urology. De Historia Urologiae Europaeae 1996;3:35–64.
6 Froben I: Aetius Amidenus Libri XIV, Sermo undecimus, Basiliae, 1535, pp 268–269.
7 Bussemaker C, Daremberg C: Œuvres d'Oribase, Paris, 1851–1862, vol 4, p 571.
8 Adams F for the Sydenham Society: Paul of Aegina: The Seven Books. London, 1844, vol 1, pp 543–544.
9 Olivieri A: Aetius Amidenus Libri Medicinales, Lipsiae, 1935, vol 1, p 97, vol 3, p 278.
10 Raeder I: Oribasii Collectionum Medicarum Reliquiae, Lipsiae, 1933, vol 4, p 225.
11 Alexandrus Trallianus Therapeutica, Basiliae, 1556, p 269.
12 Eftychiades AC: Diseases in the Byzantine world with special emphasis on the nephropathies. Am J Nephrol 1997;17:217–221.
13 Raeder I: Oribasii Synopsis ad Eustathium. Libri ad Eunapium, Lipsiae, 1926, p 295.
14 Scarborough J: Early Byzantine Pharmacology. Dumbarton Oaks Papers 1984;38:213–232.
15 Poulakou-Rebelakou E: Aretaeus on the kidney and urinary tract diseases. Am J Nephrol 1997; 17:209–213.
16 Malakates S: Urology during the Byzantine Era (in Greek); doctoral thesis Athens University, 1993, pp 51–52.
17 See Ref. No. 11, p 496.
18 See Ref. No. 8, p 541.
19 See Ref. No. 6, pp 254–258.
20 Atzemoglou N: Fountains of Holy Water in Constantinople (in Greek). Athens, Ressos, 1990.
21 Lascaratos J, Poulakou-Rebelakou E, Rebelakos A: Urolithiasis in non-medical Byzantine texts. De Historia Urologiae Europaeae 1998; 4:155–162.
22 Lascaratos J: Diseases of the Byzantine Emperors; PhD thesis Ionian University, 1995, pp 92–95.
23 See Ref. No. 5, pp 50–51.

Origins of Nephrology – Middle Ages, Renaissance

American Journal of Nephrology

Am J Nephrol 1999;19:177–181

The Academy of Science of Bologna and the Kidney

V. Bonomini[a] C. Campieri[a] M. Zuccoli[b]

[a]Department of Nephrology, St. Orsola University Hospital, Bologna, and
[b]Department of Astronomy, University of Bologna, Italy

Key Words
Bologna Academy of Science · *Commentarii* · 18th century medicine

Abstract
The Academy of Science of Bologna, founded in 1711, played an important role in the development of medicine. Receiving the heritage of Malpighi's and Morgagni's researches, the academy encouraged nephrological studies, which produced articles published in its journal, the *Commentarii*. Since the *Commentarii* were widely distributed all over Europe, the nephrological research practiced in Bologna reached all the main academies of science, in a fruitful circulation of knowledge. The paper presents the nephrological contributions to the *Commentarii* in the 18th century, thus introducing physicians, like Domenico Galeazzi and Luigi Galvani, who were both professors at the University of Bologna and at the Academy of Science. In their work three main topics can be identified: uroscopy, anatomy of the kidney and renal pathologies.

Introduction

During the 17th century, Bologna was a medium-sized town, under the Pope's rule. Its economy was based mainly upon two activities: trade (especially the silk trade) and the university. The latter, attracting several thousand students and promoting the activity of about 13 printers, made Bologna a center of paramount importance for the spread of culture in Italy and all over Europe.

A typical phenomenon, which arose at the end of the 17th and continued during the 18th century, was the flourishing of several private academies which gathered the most brilliant minds of the time. Among them, the Accademia degli Inquieti was particularly devoted to the development of science. In 1711 it was to become the original nucleus of the Institute of Science, when the Bolognese nobleman Luigi Ferdinando Marsili (1958–1739) promoted it, against the decay of the university in the scientific field. The teaching method, consisting of lectures and strictly following the Aristotelian and Thomistic tradition, did not involve research which was practiced at the scientists' private homes.

At the end of the 17th century, this proved to be rather unsatisfactory, although the activity of scientists, such as Marcello Malpighi and Giovanni Battista Morgagni, still gave lustre to the university. Malpighi and Morgagni laid the foundations of the medical research practices in Bo-

KARGER
Fax + 41 61 306 12 34
E-Mail karger@karger.ch
www.karger.com

© 1999 S. Karger AG, Basel
0250–8095/99/0192–0177$17.50/0

Accessible online at:
http://BioMedNet.com/karger

Prof. Vittorio Bonomini
Institute of Nephrology and Dialysis, St. Orsola University Hospital
Via Massarenti, 9
I-40138 Bologna (Italy)
Tel./Fax +39 051 391 336

logna during the 18th century which culminated in the outstanding personality of Luigi Galvani.

Malpighi, who may be considered the father of microscopy, discovered the structure of the lungs as air cells surrounded by blood vessels. He also applied his method to the study of the kidney, trying to explain secretion in mechanical terms. Malphighi discovered the tufts of vessels attached to the branches of the interlobular arteries and showed the renal tubules. He located the filtering unit of the kidney in the ampullar extremities of the tubules (the Malpighi corpuscles). In 1669 Malpighi was the first Italian to become a member of the Royal Society of London.

Morgagni followed Malpighi's idea of rational medicine and became a great anatomist, although he made a lesser use of the microscope. In his *De sedibus et causis morborum per anatomen indagati* (1761), Morgagni used the reports of 640 autopsies in order to investigate the causes of breakdowns in the human organism. Here, Morgagni, who considered the kidneys as glands that secreted the urine, exposed the renal pathologies: he presented cases of tumors, pyonephrosis and uropyonephrosis, abscesses, wounds, hypoplasty, hydronephrosis and nephrolithiasis. In 1704 Morgagni became persident of the Accademia degli Inquieti and reformed it according to the Paris Académie Royale des Sciences, thus giving his imprint to the following Institute of Science of Bologna.

As an alternative to the university method, a new approach in teaching had been experimented at the Jesuit schools, while research found its renovation at the Institute of Science. It was divided into two branches, the Academy of Science and the Accademia Clementina (named after Pope Clemens XII), dedicated to painting.

The same scientists were usually professors at the university and researchers at the Academy laboratories, called *camere* (rooms). Marsili had planned a laboratory for each discipline, wanting the Academy to be a place 'made more for eyes than for ears'. The method practiced at the Institute coupled theory and experience, deriving theoretical explanation of phenomena from observations and experiments. The importance of such an approach to medical studies can be easily argued, although the 'medicine room' was not among the first to be established. In any case, the famous anatomist Domenico Galeazzi was invited by Marsili to the reunions in the physics room starting from 1714.

Medicine was introduced to the Academy by Pope Benedict XIV in 1747, with his Motu proprio, opening an anatomical room and a collection of wax models.

The Pope, born in Bologna as Prospero Lambertini (1675–1758), was particularly generous towards the Institute of Science which he supplied with an impressive library (now called the Biblioteca Universitaria). Anatomy was to become fundamental for the definition of the modern role of the scientist-physician who, starting from anatomical studies, could discover the laws of nature. In 1757 Benedict XIV added the teaching of obstetrics to the Academy, together with a relevant collection of instruments, thus strengthening the didactic and practical side of the Institute.

The scientific challenge started by Luigi Ferdinando Marsili was interrupted by Napoleon. During the French invasion, the Institute of Science was closed and restored some years later under a new identity, closer to the University of Bologna. Nowadays, the Academy of Science continues its life, thanks to the activity of the university professors. Its seat, decorated with splendid 16th-century frescoes, is in the same palace as the seat of the university rector.

The *Commentarii*

The lectures given by the members of the Academy were collected and published in the *Commentarii,* printed in Bologna by Lelio and Petronio Dalla Volpe from 1731 to 1791 (fig. 1). They represented the local answer to the proceedings of the main European societies and scientific academies, such as: *Acta eruditorium Lipsiae, Mémoires de l'Académie des Sciences de Paris, Journal des Savants* and *Philosophical Transactions of the Royal Society of London.* The Bolognese Academy had strong relations and exchanges with these societies, thus acquiring national and international importance. We wish to name just one of its main foreign members: Voltaire.

Examining the volumes of the *Commentarii,* the pattern of nephrological studies at the Institute of Sciences appears quite clearly, together with the physicians involved. Nephrological research followed three main branches: anatomy of the kidney (by means of microscopic analysis), following the method of Marcello Malpighi; renal pathologies, exposing several case histories, and uroscopy, according to classical Greek medicine which acknowledged diagnostic value to the uroscopic practice.

Nephrological interest can also be found in some hydrological papers, concerning the therapeutic qualities of thermal springs in Italy to treat renal pathologies: Recoaro (VI), Porretta (BO) and Bagni di Lucca (LU), recommended for lithiasis and colics. Water analysis was performed by a team made up of chemists and physicians, in the typical interdisciplinary atmosphere of the Academy.

The following short profiles refer to professors of medicine or anatomy at the University of Bologna who were also members of the Academy and presented their nephrological papers in the *Commentarii.*

Lorenzo Antonio Bonazzoli (Bologna, † 1753)

He wrote on an observation concerning a peculiar conformation of the kidney, found in a man who had died from high fever. His kidneys were joined, forming an arched organ with three pelves and two ureters. Another small duct could be considered as a fourth ureter, since it functioned partially in that way. His bladder was slightly oversized, but on the whole his ill-conformed kidney had functioned normally.

Observationes in intestinis, et renibus habitae. De Bon. Comm., II, 1 (1745), pp 138–142.

Vincenzo Menghini (Budrio, near Bologna, † 1686)

Menghini wrote three hydrological papers, concerning the litholytic qualities of some springs. The author states that the different types of stones classified at the time (tufaceous, arenaceous, gypseous and lateritious) need different types of treatments. Another article by Menghini deals with renal pathology. A man suffering from gonorrhea and with kidney pain expelled small blisters with his urine. The urine was emitted with difficulty and contained blood and blisters as big as chickpeas or even beans. Menghini put the blisters into water, inflated them with air and examined them under a microscope. He concluded that since they presented analogies with the blisters in external cystic tumors, they were symptoms of a tumor in the kidney or the urinary tract. Another paper by Menghini deals with 15 cases of dropsy treated with cream of tartar (acid potassium tartrate, obtainable from must fermentation) which is well known for its laxative and diuretic effects.

De vesiculis quibusdam cum urina emissis: De Bon. Comm., II, 1 (1745), pp 142–144.

De vi calculos dissolvendi in quibusdam aquis quaesita. De Bon. Comm., III, pp 71–72.

Experimenta de largo et diuturno cremoris tartari usu ad hydropisim summopere utili. De Bon. Comm., IV (1757), pp 260–285.

Dissertationes binae de aquarum vi in calculis dissolvendis. De Bon. Comm., V, I (1767), pp 261–274.

Pietro Nanni (Camugnano, near Bologna, † 1717)

Nanni was a professor of medicine at the University of Bologna and was held in esteem by Morgagni for his pro-

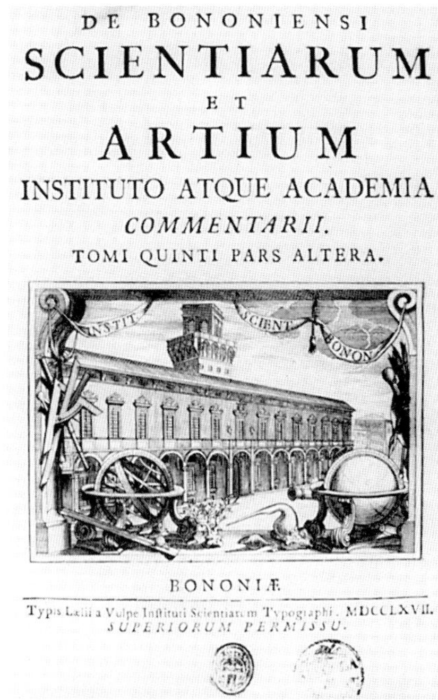

DE BONONIENSI
SCIENTIARUM
ET
ARTIUM
INSTITUTO ATQUE ACADEMIA
COMMENTARII.
TOMI QUINTI PARS ALTERA.

BONONIÆ
Typis Lælii a Vulpe Instituti Scientiarum Typographi. MDCCLXVII.
SUPERIORUM PERMISSU.

Fig. 1. Commentarii of the Institute of Science of Bologna: title page.

found anatomical studies. His lectures showed his vast learning and elegant speech and attracted a large number of students. Nanni published a paper in the *Commentarii,* about the structure of glands (the term used by Morgagni to indicate the kidneys because of their secretory activity). He attempted to classify them, criticizing the subdivision in 'conglobatae' and 'conglomeratae' which had been supported by most of his colleagues. Nanni's analysis, based upon an iatrophysical approach, focused on the distribution and the flow of the blood vessels surrounding the glands. In particular, he wrote that, in order to separate a liquid from the blood, the latter had to be slowed down at a certain point. That point was the one of the maximum ramification of the vessels into capillaries.

De glandulis. De Bon. Comm., I (1731), pp 326–333

Giuseppe Pozzi (Bologna, 1697–1752)

A pupil of Nanni who succeeded the latter to the Chair of Medicine. Pozzi was held in high esteem by Pope Benedict XIV, who appointed him as his Physician Extraordinary. In 1748, he became President of the Academy of Science. Pozzi studied mathematics and geometry, but he achieved fame as an anatomist. He wrote a paper concerning the subcenturiated kidney in the fetus and in

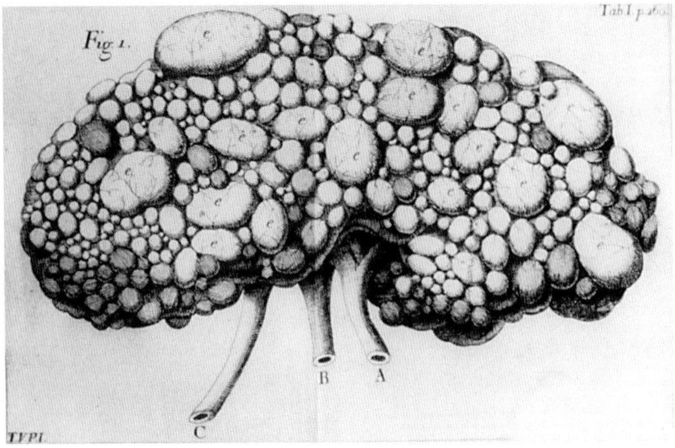

2

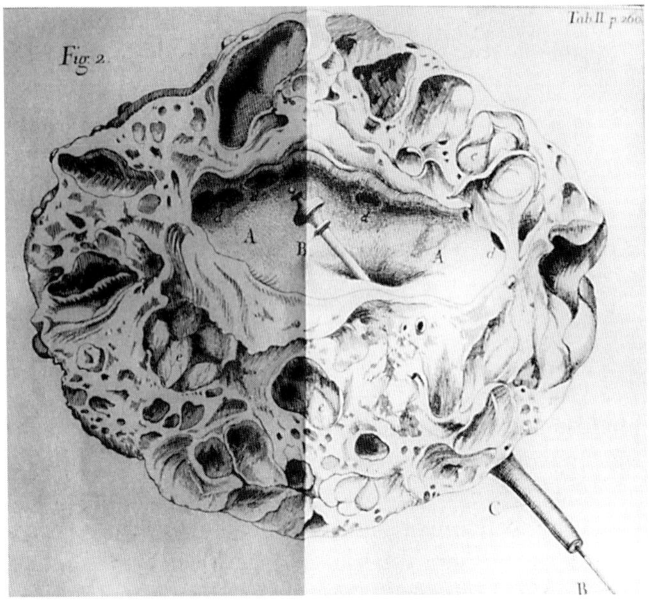

3

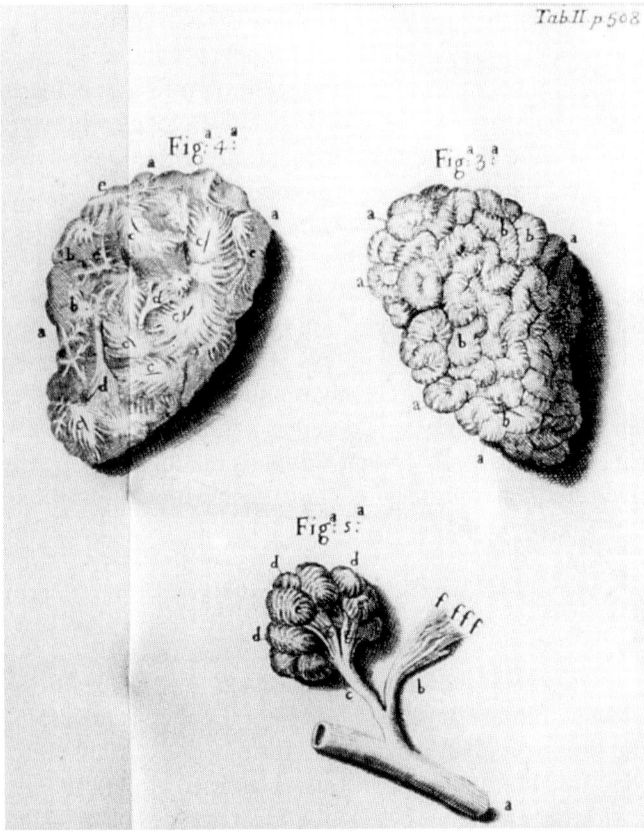

4

Fig. 2. D. Galeazzi: De renum morbis. A polycystic kidney.
Fig. 3. D. Galeazzi: De renum morbis. Drawing of a kidney.
Fig. 4. L. Galvani: De renibus atque ureteribus volatilium. The kidneys of birds.

youngsters. Basing his opinion on direct observation, Pozzi said that the subcenturiated kidneys were diverticula, with the same function as the allantois or pseudoallantois in the fetus.

Observationes anatomicae variae. De Bon. Comm., II, 1 (1745), pp 147–155.

Domenico Maria Gusmano Galeazzi
(Bologna, 1686–1775)

He was a physician of great renown and the father-in-law of Luigi Galvani. Galeazzi was asked to make six public anatomic dissections in front of the Bolognese noblemen, in the anatomical theater, which was considered a great honor. He was called for consultations all over Italy, and in 1734 he was called to the chair of Experimental Physics at the Institute of Science. Galeazzi's method is famous for the importance attributed to prognosis which he considered to be the final aim of case analysis.

The paper, entitled De renum morbis, is introduced by the author's statement that his aim is to investigate the structure of organs and their pathologies through regular observations. He made autopsies of patients of different sexes and ages who had the same symptoms: fever, lumbar region pain and hemorrhages. Autopsy revealed swollen kidneys (particularly the left one) and blisters (some as big as hazelnuts). The blisters were filled with the same serum as that in pelvis and ureter. In the paper a polycystic kidney is shown (fig. 2, 3).

Another paper by Galeazzi concerns stones in the ureter, but we will focus on his third article presented to the Academy. It deals with the case of a young woman with black sweat, weakened by coughing, stomach hemorrhages, fever and vomiting. The woman was treated successfully with water from Brandola (a small town near Modena), known for its antihemorrhagic properties. A few days later the patient fell into a stuporous state and emitted black sweat. Its solid part was examined under a microscope, revealing a fine dust, the grains of which were formed by an aggregation of small particles. Among these particles, some sort of sharp particles could be seen. Her urine became black, too, and was emitted with pain. Galeazzi filtered the urine and examined it under the microscope, observing the same granular structure as in her sweat. He supposed it was made up of saline-sulfurous particles and that the sharp particles were ammoniacal salts. Fogazzi in 1994 (see below) suggested it could have been a case of alcaptonuria.

De renum morbis. De Bon. Comm., V, 1 (1767), pp 249–260.

Historiae duae mirabiles calculorum in ureteribus exsistentium. De Bon. Comm., V, 2 (1767), pp 139–150.

De sudore quodam, atque urina colore nigerrimo infectis. De Bon. Comm., VI (1783), pp 1–12.

Fogazzi GB: The description of polycystic kidney by G.D. Galeazzi. Nephrol Dial Transplant 1988;13:1039–1040.

Fogazzi GB, Cameron JS, Ritz E, Ponticelli C: The history of urinary microscopy to the end of the 19th century. Am J Nephrol 1994; 14:452–457.

Luigi Galvani (Bologna, 1737–1798)

The bicentenary of Galvani's death is being solemnly celebrated this year at the Academy of Science. He published a paper in the *Commentarii* concerning the kidneys of birds. He investigated the structure of their kidneys and ureters. Galvani adopted a technique already used by Galen, typing first the right and then the left ureter, and then both, to verify the tumefaction of the kidney or the ureteral portion above the tying point. He also practiced ureteral incision and saw that the urine flowed between the peritoneum and the intestine. Galvani studied the structure of renal tubules by means of maceration, but, finding this method unsatisfactory, he decided to inject the tubules themselves, thus preceding Hoppe-Seyler and Zaleski by more than a century (fig. 4).

De renibus atque ureteribus volatilium. De Bon. Comm., V, 2, pp 500–508.

Suggested Reading

On the Institute and the Academy of Science

Angelelli G: Notizie dell'origine e progressi dell'Istituto delle Scienze di Bologna e sue Accademie. Bologna 1780.

Angelini A: Anatomie accademiche. Bologna 1993, vol 3.

Bolletti GG: Dell'origine e dei progressi dell'Istituto delle Scienze di Bologna. Bologna 1751.

Cavazza M: La recezione della teoria Halleriana dell'irritabilità nell'Accademia delle Scienze di Bologna. Nuncius 1997;XII:359–377.

Cavazza M: Le Camere dell'Istituto delle Scienze; in: I luoghi del conoscere. Bologna, Università degli Studi di Bologna, 1988, pp 33–43.

Dore P: Origini e funzione dell'Istituto e dell'Accademia delle Scienze di Bologna. Archiginnasio 1940;XXXV:192–214.

Ercolani GB: Accademia delle Scienze dello Istituto di Bologna dalle sue origini a tutto il 1880. Bologna 1881.

Gentili C: Il modello epistemologico dell' «Institutum Scientiarum et Artium» di Bologna; in: I materiali dell'Istituto delle Scienze. Bologna 1979, pp 22–41.

Pallotti V: Per una storia dell'Istituto delle Scienze; in: I materiali dell'Istituto delle Scienze. Bologna 1979, pp 55–62.

Tega W: L'Istituto delle Scienze: L'orizzonte Europeo. Diario scientifico degli accademici bolognesi. Bologna, Università degli Studi di Bologna, 1988, pp 175–184.

Tega W: Anatomie accademiche. Bologna 1986–1987, vol 1–2.

Tega W: L'Istituto e l'Accademia delle Scienze; in: Storia illustrata di Bologna, a cura di W. Tega. Bologna 1989, vol VI, pp 261–280.

On the Scientific Environment of the Time and on the Academy Members

Bernabeo R: La Scuola di Medicina fra XVI e XX secolo; in: L'Università a Bologna: Maestri, studenti e luoghi dal XVI al XX secolo. Bologna 1988, pp 185–194.

Bonomini V, Campieri C, Scolari MP, Zuccoli M: The age-old spirit of nephrology from the oldest university in the world. Am J Nephrol 1994;14:361–364.

De Giovanni A: Lettere e consulti inediti di G.B. Morgagni con introduzione e note del Prof. Luigi Messedaglia. Atti Reale Ist Veneto Sci Lett Arti 1912;71:569–615.

Fantuzzi G: Notizie degli scrittori bolognesi. Bologna 1781–1789.

Gallassi A, Giardina B: L'opera medica di Luigi Galvani; in: Studi e memorie per la storia dell'Università di Bologna, NS. 1985, vol I, pp 461–478.

Jandolo M: Il rene nella visione morgagnana. Pag Storia Med 1957;1:22–29.

Mazzetti S: Repertorio di tutti i professori antichi, e moderni della famosa Università, e del celebre Istituto delle Scienze di Bologna. Bologna 1847.

Thorndyke L: Novità e innovazione nella scienza e nella medicina del Seicento; in: Le radici del pensiero scientifico, a cura di Ph.P. Wiener and A. Noland. Milano 1971, pp 459–473.

Umani Ronchi G: Contributi nel '500 e '600 alla anatomia e fisiologia del rene. Pag Storia Med 1960;4:39–44.

American Journal of Nephrology

Am J Nephrol 1999;19:182–184

Water and Its Effects when Drunk Cold

The Physician's View (1576–1751)

Luciana Bonfante Lorenzo Calò Angela D'Angelo Silvana Favaro
Cataldo Abaterusso Giuseppe Mennella Marcella Normanno
Michela Spinello Augusto Antonello

Institute of Internal Medicine, Division of Nephrology I, University of Padova, Italy

Key Words
Water · Drinking · Health benefit · Mineral water

Abstract
Starting with Baldassare Pisanelli's book *Trattato della natura de' cibi et del bere*, published in Venice in 1586, the controversies that have kept physicians busy over the centuries regarding the relative importance of water in human health are traced. These controversies were of considerable importance as the Latin word for water 'aqua' is derived from the phrase 'a qua vinimus' (from whence we come). However, until the studies of Nicolas Lemery, one of the most important pharmacologists of the 18th century, the controversies were debated using more theoretical, philosophical arguments. Lemery's studies shifted the debates from those based on philosophical arguments to more physiologically and scientifically based arguments.

Ancient physicians (Hippocrates, Erasistratus and Crisippus) described water as a simple body, cold and wet by nature, which surrounds the earth and is itself encircled by air. Although it has no nutritional value, it was considered essential to the diet in that it renders food more digestible.

The ancients also recognized the beneficial effects of spa waters on both humans and animals. It appears to have been the sight of horses afflicted by joint pains rolling in muddy ditches around Abano (now a spa resort) which brought the therapeutic value of mud baths to the attention of early Paduans.

Water obviously has numerous uses in activities related to our daily lives; in agriculture, industry and for domestic chores. What is perhaps less well known is that from the 16th to the 18th century, there was a heated debate between doctors on the subject of cold water. It probably arose because drinking water was frequently chilled either as a result of storage in wells, caves and grottos or by immersion in nitric salts. The custom of mixing mountain ice or snow with water, dating from Roman times was also revived at this time. Those against the imbibing of cold water claimed that it was likely to cause or aggravate conditions such as weakness of the stomach or kidneys, indigestion of the humours, dropsy, gravel and chest pain. A Roman physician, Andrea Bacci [1], contended in a publication of 1576, 'Del Tevere' (The Tiber) (fig. 1) that while cold water should be drunk by those living in the low temperatures of the Northern hemispheres, it could provoke a variety of ailments in the inhabitants of Southern climates, as they had a higher body temperature.

A different view was taken by Baldassare Pisanelli [2], a physician of Bologna, whose practice during the second half of the 16th and early 17th centuries included atten-

KARGER

Fax + 41 61 306 12 34
E-Mail karger@karger.ch
www.karger.com

© 1999 S. Karger AG, Basel
0250–8095/99/0192–0182$17.50/0

Accessible online at:
http://BioMedNet.com/karger

Prof. Augusto Antonello, MD
Division of Nephrology
University of Padova
I–35128 Padova (Italy)
Tel. +39 049 8212155, Fax +39 049 8212151

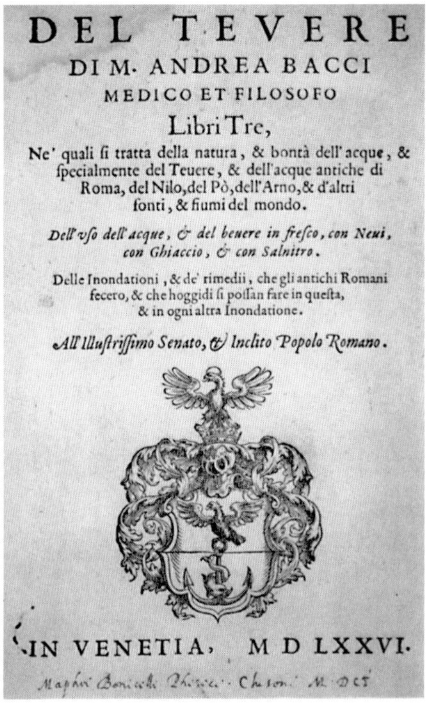
DEL TEVERE
DI M. ANDREA BACCI
MEDICO ET FILOSOFO
Libri Tre,
Ne' quali si tratta della natura, & bontà dell'acque, & specialmente del Teuere, & dell'acque antiche di Roma, del Nilo, del Pò, dell'Arno, & d'altri fonti, & fiumi del mondo.
Dell'vso dell'acque, & del beuere in fresco, con Neui, con Ghiaccio, & con Salnitro.
Delle Inondationi, & de' rimedii, che gli antichi Romani fecero, & che hoggidi si possan fare in questa, & in ogni altra Inondatione.
All'Illustrissimo Senato, & Inclito Popolo Romano.
IN VENETIA, M D LXXVI.

Fig. 1. 'Del Tevere' by Andrea Bacci.

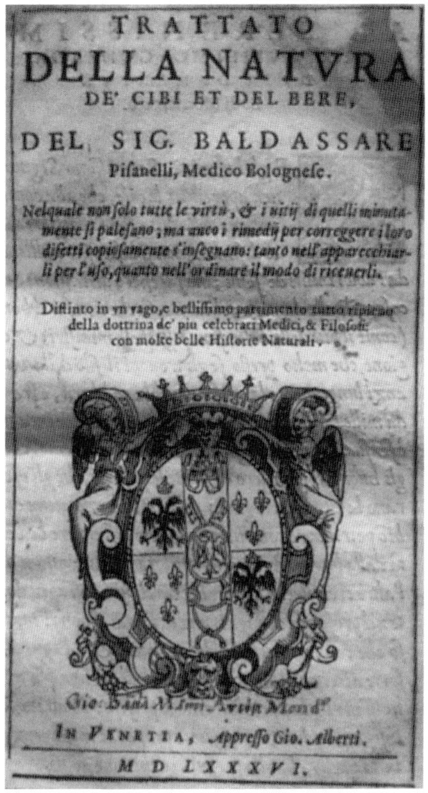
TRATTATO
DELLA NATVRA
DE' CIBI ET DEL BERE,
DEL SIG. BALDASSARE
Pisanelli, Medico Bolognese.
Nelquale non solo tutte le virtù, & i uitij di quelli minutamente si palesano; ma anco i rimedij per correggere i loro difetti copiosamente s'insegnano: tanto nell'apparecchiarli per l'uso, quanto nell'ordinare il modo di riceuerli.
Distinto in vn vago, e bellissimo partimento tutto ripieno della dottrina de' piu celebrati Medici, & Filosofi: con molte belle Historie Naturali.
IN VENETIA, Appresso Gio. Alberti.
M D LXXXVI.

Fig. 2. 'Trattato della natura dei cibi e del bere' by Andrea Pisanelli.

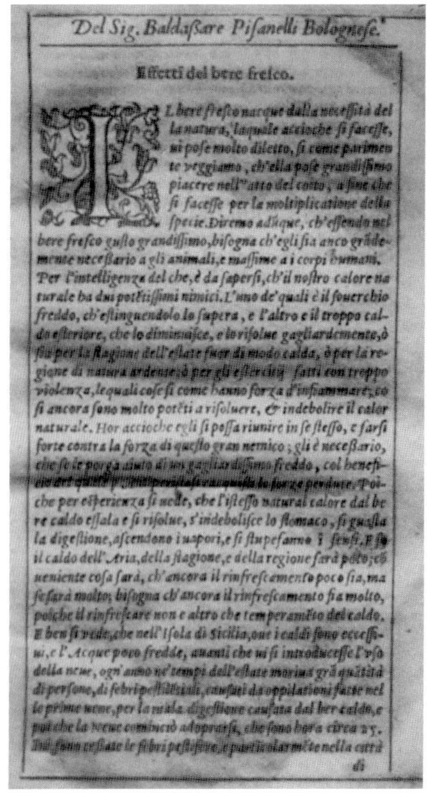
Del Sig. Baldassare Pisanelli Bolognese.
Effetti del bere fresco.

Fig. 3. From 'Del bere fresco' by Baldassare Pisanelli.

dance on the Gonzaga family (rulers of Mantua). His 'Trattato della natura de' cibi et del bere' (Treatise on the nature of food and drink – Venice 1586) (fig. 2) discusses the beneficial and noxious effects of many foods and their use. Water types and the properties necessary for it to be healthy and digestible are also described, together with an explanation of the methods of determining water quality. Pisanelli [2] was a firm believer in the health-giving powers of cold water (fig. 3), stating that it was both thirst quenching and invigorating. Proof of its potency was given in a description of how the use of snow for drinking water had significantly lowered the incidence of plague in Sicily in the mid-1400s. There had been a dramatic reduction in the number of deaths, particularly in the Messina area.

Pisanelli gave a curious explanation for the efficacy of chilled drinking water. He had observed how a glass containing cold water or ice becomes clouded 'as if it were coated by expelled noxious humours' and deduced from this that when ingested, cold water would have the same ability to facilitate excretion of toxic substances from the body.

The debate continued into the 17th century when Antonio Vallisneri [3] lent further support to the use of cold water for therapeutic purposes in 'Dell'uso e dell' abuso delle bevande e bagnature' (The use and abuse of beverages and baths – Naples, 1727). He asserted that cold water could not only break fevers, bringing the body temperature to within normal limits, but was also a remedy for colic. A case was cited in which a patient suffering from violent colicky pains had been treated unsuccessfully with fluids and hot poultices. Vallisneri was called into consultation and prescribed water with a little ice, which brought rapid relief.

The nature and properties of water are thoroughly described in the 'Trattato universale delle droghe semplici' (Universal tract on the simple drugs – Venice, 1751) [4] (fig. 4). The author was Nicolas Lemery, a French pharmacologist famous for his work at the Royal Academy of Science in Paris during the 17th and early 18th centuries. He maintained that the characteristics of water differ according to the type of land through which it flows. In his view, rainwater is the most penetrating and cleansing

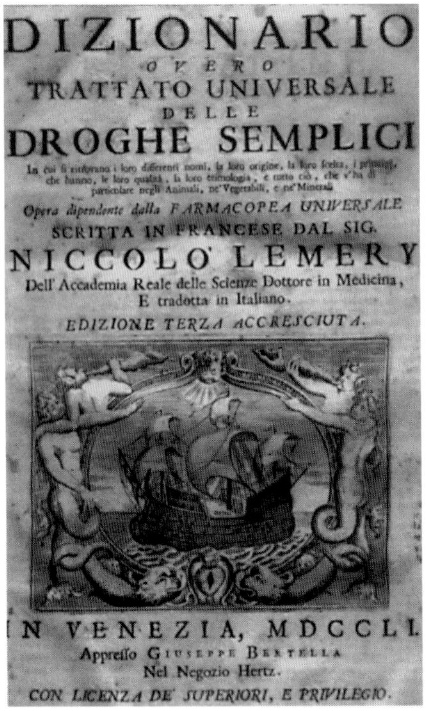

Fig. 4. 'Trattato universale delle droghe semplici' by Nicolò Lemery.

'ordinary' water, as it is enriched by acid salts present in the atmosphere. Spring water was considered the clearest and purest, having been filtered through the earth. If, however, filtration occurs through stone, water becomes heavy and difficult to digest, which may lead to 'coagulation of the humours', a common cause of a number of conditions such as scurvy, renal stones, catarrh, colics and indigestions. These complaints also frequently occur as a result of drinking well water.

River water was said to be the healthiest of all waters because it is warmed by exposure to the sun's rays which also correct any imbalance in its composition. Furthermore, the low salt content makes river water easy to digest. Although this water may often be turbid, it becomes clear if left to settle and can then be filtered. Lemery advised that two to three glasses be taken on an empty stomach in the morning to sweeten acrid humours, moisten the chest, relax the stomach and stimulate diuresis.

In contrast to river water, that of marshland and lagoons was considered stagnant and impure. Well water was considerd to be better for harsh processes involving strong dyes, such as when cotton, corduroy and other soft materials are dyed red. It was not thought suitable for turquoise, yellow and green dyes.

Lemery then turned his attention to mineral waters, which he described as rich in salts derived from mineral or metal deposits. A distinction was drawn between hot and cold mineral waters, the former being heated by subterranean fires with the result that sulphur particles can be seen in still water. Calcium-rich minerals may also colour these waters during their passage through the bowels of the earth. In Lemery's view, the sulphur and volatile salt content of hot mineral waters made them effective in the treatment of many ailments, particularly catarrh, paralysis, sciatica, apoplexy, lethargy and cold humours. Their volatility necessitated, however, that they be drunk at the spring head as they would deteriorate during transportation.

Different qualities were ascribed to cold mineral waters. Lemery considered that their salt and iron content would have the effect of aiding digestion and also made it possible for water to be stored for many years without any loss of its properties, providing that the minerals were present in sufficient quantities and bottles were tightly sealed.

The discussion ends with a description of sea water. Sour, salty and full of purgative mineral salts, this type of water was noted for its ability to relieve pruritus. Lemery also contended that it was an effective safeguard against rabies although it upset stomachs when ingested.

There was occasional interest in water over the following years, stimulated by the findings of illustrious academics who investigated not only its chemical and therapeutic properties, but also its philosophical significance. The etymology of water was even explored, it being suggested that its Latin name derived from the expression 'A qua vinimus' (from where we originate), in that water evaporates into the sky, then returns to earth, making it fertile and so creating life in what would otherwise be sterile, inhospitable terrain [2].

References

1 Andrea Bacci: Del Tevere, Roma, 1576.
2 Baldassarre Pisanelli: Trattato della natura de' cibi et del bere. Venezia, 1586.
3 Antonio Vallisneri: Dell'uso e dell'abuso delle bevande e bagnature. Napoli, 1727.
4 Nicolas Lemery: Trattato universale delle droghe semplici. Venezia, 1751.

Origins of Nephrology – Middle Ages, Renaissance

American Journal of Nephrology

Am J Nephrol 1999;19:185–188

Observations on the *Liber medicine orinalibus* by Hermogenes

Luigi Iorio Faustino Avagliano

Division of Nephrology and Dialysis 'G. De Bosis' Hospital and Montecassino Archive Library, Cassino, Italy

Key Words
Hermogenes · *Liber medicine orinalibus* · Wine examination

Abstract
Our report is based on a text of the philosopher Hermogenes entitled *Liber medicine orinalibus* now conserved in Cod. Casin. 69 (10th century), pp 545–551, of the Montecassino Archive. This text was written in Beneventano-Cassinese characters. The *Liber medicine orinalibus* presents an articulate description of urines, which is interesting because of the information it provides regarding the knowledge of medicine in the 2nd century AD. This text allows us to appreciate the level reached in urine diagnostics that were performed in the medical laboratory annexed to the 'Ospitium'.

Introduction

The text, entitled *Liber medicine orinalibus*, is attributed to the philosopher Hermogenes [1], of whom there is no further mention in the manuscript. Of the various Hermogenes living during antiquity, the most likely author of the *Liber medicine orinalibus* was born in Smirne, son of Charidemus, pupil of Erasistratus, and a follower of Hippocrates [2]. He lived in the 2nd century AD for about 77 years, and wrote many books on medicine. Of many of these only the title is known, yet it has not been possible to find any reference in the *Liber medicine orinalibus*.

Before analyzing the book it is important to make one or two observations: in the then prevailing medical doctrine, which dates back to Hippocrates (4th to 5th century BC) [3], and was later modified by Galen (2nd century AD), each of the four main organic body fluids (blood, phlegm, yellow bile and black bile, also called melancholy or ill humor) regulated man's organism: their equilibrium produced health and their various relationships produced temperament (sanguine, phlegmatic, choleric and melancholic), while the excessive prevalence of one over the other brought about a state of illness. It is also important to remember that in accordance with the knowledge at the time metabolism was supposed to be based on three digestions: the first took place in the stomach, the residues of which made up the excrement, the second digestion occurred in the liver and its residues formed the urine, while the third digestion took place inside the tissues and its residues (content) were also eliminated in the urine.

The text is divided into two parts: the first reports information based on 'empiria', that is to say on the observations of urine, and the second reports a list of the characteristics of urine with their respective prognosis of the disease.

KARGER
Fax + 41 61 306 12 34
E-Mail karger@karger.ch
www.karger.com

© 1999 S. Karger AG, Basel
0250–8095/99/0192–0185$17.50/0

Accessible online at:
http://BioMedNet.com/karger

L. Iorio, MD
'G. De Bosis' Hospital
Via Casilina Nord
I–03043 Cassino (Italy)
Tel. +39 0776 303243, Fax +39 0776 302232

Liber medicine orinalibus

(by Hemogenes, Cod. Cas. 69, pag. 545–551) (fig. 1)

(In the name of Jesus Christ, Our Lord. Here begins the Medical Book on Urine by the philosopher Hermogenes).

To carry out a careful analysis of urine it is necessary to perform many divisions whence to identify its various types.

The first division is to analyze them into two parts: 'Chima' and 'Hypostasin'. There may be further distinct subjects who emit types of urine that are transformed by the emission of others, whose urines undergo a transformation with time. The first eventuality we shall define as transformation of the chima. The second transformation of the hypostasin with the urine that becomes thin or cloudy. In the second in fact, many observations may be made, which we shall analyze on its becoming thin and cloudy, two hours after emission when it loses its heat. After cooling the urines may remain thin and clear, and may neither undergo transformations nor cloudings. Some subjects emit a thin urine which becomes cloudy after cooling. Still others emit a cloudy urine from the very start which does not change after cooling. Yet others emit a urine that is already cloudy, which becomes more cloudy when it cools. Others emit clear urine, which remains such without changing.

In subjects where the last eventuality comes about, it is to be attributed to the stomach, in fact it does not digest food because heating is reduced, that is to say it behaves like a pan that no longer cooks food when there is no fire underneath it.

One of the four humours is reinforced at the expense of the other three, and the body does not have sufficient strength to react, being incapable of carrying out its own functions. When clear urine humours are emitted which become cloudy, the fact certainly denotes a disorder of the upper digestive apparatus. In fact in this case the digestion starts off normal, but then worsens. The emission of cloudy urines which remain as such denote aerophagy, in fact the four humours mix together in a non-equilibrated way because of the infirmity. We now communicate the urinary signs and every type of disturbance provoked by the four humours.

Since the urinary signs are numerous we have divided them up into six colours in order to study them better, as follows: first, white urine; second, orange urine; third, blond urine; fourth, red urine; fifth, flame-coloured urine; sixth, black urine.

White coloured types of urine are indicative of many diseases:

In the aged, since strength is reduced, urine becomes white. White urines are also indicative of fasting and circulation disorders. They are also emitted by those who make excessive use of wine. White and fatty urines denote the prevalence of one humour over the others. When the urines are orange-tinted they are indicative of red melancholy. Blond urine is indicative of the prevalence of one humour over the other three. It may be indicative of a defect in the circulation in the stomach, for the patient who has been unable to sleep. These signs originate from disease from the upper part of the body, where tertian fever is produced.

Flame-coloured urine indicates considerable dehydration if, in addition to its flame colour it is also fatty and cloudy, then it is produced by melancholy. Should you see red urine then this is produced by the blood, since a thickening of the blood (ispissatio sanguinis) is brought about. In other cases this happens because blood flows from a wound. If the urine is black it indicates an abundance of nigra cholera, that must come out with the urine to purify the body. The urine is black because of the blood at the time when it is cooked and is tinted black because of the black melancholy. These signs are indicative of the prevalence of one humour over the others, and are mentioned so that you may recognise healthy urine.

Urine will be healthy when it is neither clear, nor fatty nor cloudy. It will be healthy when the deposits are neither blond, red nor flame-like. And hypostasin will be white, equal and correct not equal, impure and non-cloudy.

To ensure that the sediment corresponds to that described for healthy urine it is necessary that the vessel containing the urine is set on the floor and the deposit on the bottom and at half-way is analyzed.

Here are the signs that are obtained from the first viewing:

At first sight the urine may appear equal because it is immobile. But we must keep account of four signs for a correct examination of the sediment:

The first is water.
The second vision.
The third position (locus).
The fourth time.

According to its consistency water may be strong, soft or hard, and it is necessary to see whether it is white, or changes colour or whether it is tinted, which means that one humour prevails over the others.

It is necessary to take account of the position (regiones) that the residues occupy, and we may distinguish three types:

The first, lower (in the text it is erroneously called 'superiorem'). The second, middle. The third, upper. The latter is found at the top in the urine and is called 'cloud'. The second, middle is called 'procidentes'. The third from the cloud is called 'splanatione'. The cloud that appears at the top in the urine is indication of flatulence, and usually precedes progression towards recovery. The second which is near the 'cloud' indicates sufference of the body's strength because of the prevalence of one humour over the other three, and involves the middle: it is a serious (dura) infirmity, which recovers with some difficulty.

The third is 'splanatione' and appears at the bottom of the urine:

It indicates that the stomach's strength is able to break up and destroy the humour which is cause of the infirmity. It indicates that the same humours which had weakened the body, are beginning to return to normal and to produce full and perfect health. This is the observation of the 'splanatione', the third cloud of urine. The observation of the three regions must be carried out until recovery.

Those who teach that the interpretation of these three signs based on the 'clouds' is to be considered misguided practice and think that there are other signs, base their science on fantasy. We therefore confirm that: If you see that the cloud remains only at the top and stays white, it is an indication that the body is growing stronger, the disease is beginning to cease, and recovery is expected. If you see the cloud in the central part of the urine and you see it curved, it is on the way to recovery, and the middle part of the disease has passed. If you see the third cloud of low part, called 'splanazione' it means that the disease has been overcome.

1

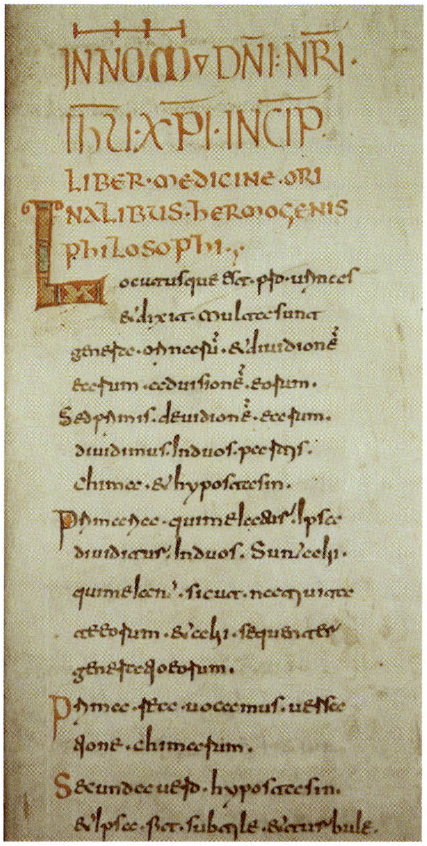

2

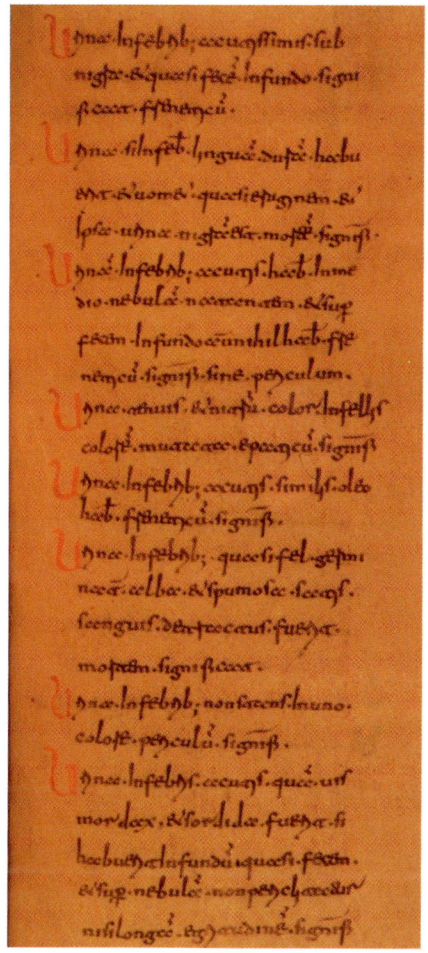

Fig. 1. Beginning of Codex Casinensis 69, p. 545.
Fig. 2. End of Codex Casinensis 69, p. 551.

To be able to show that the infirmity descends from the upper part of the body to the lower part it is expedient to know the three clouds described.

We now inform you what the urinary signs indicative of serious diseases are:

First is orange urine. Second thin. Third black. Fourth similar to the blood of a wound. Fifth thick. Sixth red, which through poor observation appears orange. Seventh crude and hard. Eighth thin and minute. Ninth when there is no sediment. Tenth when there is no middle cloud. Eleventh putrid and bad-smelling. Twelfth if it is similar to olive oil. Thirteenth when the cloud has dispersed and black, cold, orange and phlegmatic.

Signa urinae quae cognoscitur cum nocte in calice miseris et ad lucem videris (Signs of urine placed in a chalice and observed in the light of day)

Pure urine with a fog-like supranatant cloudiness signifies death is near. Cloudy urine or mixed with a murky supranatant cloudiness signifies very long agony. White urine, if it has a faeces-like sediment on the bottom and is mixed with blood, signifies death. Pink mixed urine is not dangerous. Urine if clear, with a bile-like colour and pungent belongs to someone who has fasted. Wine-coloured urine and a faeces-like sediment on the bottom signifies disease. Red-coloured urine accompanied by headaches signifies that a fever is coming on. Very clear urine and frequent urination leads to calculi. Urine that does not change appearance for many hours, or if accompanied by heaviness at kidney level means renal calculosis. Urine which in the middle area has slight heat is indicative of an agitated person who has lost consciousness (fig. 2). Urine which during fever becomes like oil means agitation. Urine which during very severe fever has no deposit and has a foamy cloudiness and is bile-coloured in the middle stratum is a bad sign. Urine which during very severe fevers is very black (subnigra) and there is a faeces-like deposit on the bottom signifies agitation. Black urine with fever that is accompanied by a hard tongue and rust-like vomiting signifies death. Thin black urine which changes in the colour of the bile, signifies sufferance of the liver. Urine which during fever becomes oil-like signifies agitation. Urine which comes out white and frothy during fever and which derives from blood signifies death. Urine that does not remain the same colour during fever is a dangerous sign. Urine which during fever becomes pungent and dirty and has a faeces-like deposit at the bottom and there is a cloudiness above is not a dangerous sign, but is an indication of slow recovery.

Discussion

This urine examination attributed to Hermogenes is comparable to that described in the Hippocratic *Aphorisms* which is a fairly accurate classification of the various species of urine. The different colours of urine are analyzed with greater precision, which was a concept that had already been expressed by Assyro-Babylonian physicians. However, with Hermogenes the examination of urine takes on still greater semiological relevance and paves the way for the more scientific advances several centuries later.

Compared to the Hippocratic text *On the Prognostics*, the urine examination developed by Hermogenes fails to distinguish between pathological urine due to systemic diseases and that due to a pathology of the urinary tract. Prognosis is limited as in the texts of Hippocrates to simply describing the duration and outcome of the disease, but avoids establishing a relationship between the urine characteristics of the urine and a certain disease. The *Liber medicine orinalibus* makes reference to the theory of the humours of Hippocrates and also to his theory of the 'cozione' (cooking). There is no reference whatsoever to the modifications of these theories as introduced by Galen.

To conclude, the text can definitely be attributed to the Hippocratic school, and undoubtedly presents certain semiological shortcomings and reveals an incompleteness in the important differential diagnosis with regard to the texts ascribed to the great Master, yet at the same time it anticipates the considerable importance given to urine examination in the field of semiotics during antiquity and the Middle Ages.

Author's Note

The English translation has been deliberately left in a quasi archaic form, as close and hence as faithful to the original Latin as possible. A rendering in modern scientific English would, it is felt, sacrifice much of the charm of the original document.

References

1 Paulis: Realenciclopädie der classischen Altertumswissenschaft. München, Alfred Druckenmüller Verlag, 1912, VIII, 1, pp 877–878.
2 Corpus Iscritionum Graecorum 3311; Kaibel Epig. Gr. 305.
3 Pezzi G: L'esame delle urine nell'antico a medio Evo. Ministero della Difesa-Marina: pagine di storia della scienza e della tecnica, 1938, vol 10, ser 1.

Origins of Nephrology – Middle Ages, Renaissance

American Journal of Nephrology

Am J Nephrol 1999;19:189–192

Gentile da Foligno, a Pioneer of Cardionephrology: Commentary on *Carmina de urinarum iudiciis* and *De pulsibus*

Mario Timio

Department of Internal Medicine and Nephrology, Hospital San Giovanni Battista, Foligno, Italy

Key Words
Gentile da Foligno · Pulse rate · Urine formation · Urine output

Abstract
Gentile da Foligno was an influential professor and teacher of medicine at the Universities of Bologna, Padua, Siena and Perugia in the first part of the 14th century. He was one of the first physicians to perform human dissection. He authored many important texts and commentaries, among which is the *Consilla,* a collection of therapeutic advices for many diseases. He made a commentary on *Carmina de urinarum iudiciis* (Songs of urinary judgements) and to *De pulsibus* (About pulses) composed by Egidius Corbaliensis. This work is more than a commentary: it is a text attempting to conceptualise the physiology of urine formation. According to his writing, urine associated to the blood passes 'per poros euritides' (through the porous tubules) of the kidney and is then delivered to the bladder. Commenting and explaining the writing on *De pulsibus,* he stressed the importance of heart disease on modulating the colour and output of urine and the relationship between fast pulse rate and urine output. For the originality of his thought and for the conceptualization of the relationship between pulse rate and urine characteristic, Gentile da Foligno could be indicated as the 'first' cardionephrologist in the history of medicine.

Introduction

Foligno is an Umbrian town now mainly devoted to trade. It was founded by the Roman consul C. Flaminius and destroyed by Liutprand who was a Lombard king in the 8th century. Devasted in the Middle Ages by the Saracens and Hungarians, it became a free town at the time of Frederick Barbarossa and was unfortunately strongly damaged by the earthquake of 1997. One of its most eminent citizens was the physician Gentile da Foligno (1272?–1348). There is evidence enough to tell us that Gentile da Foligno was one of the great Italian physicians of his time and surely the greatest among the many physicians born in Umbria. The varied nicknames are no more than a reflection of his fame while he lived: 'the prince of physicians', 'a second Galeno', 'the divine physician', 'the soul of Avicenna', and many Latin variations of his name that usually referred to Foligno as his birthplace.

He was professor in the University of Bologna, Padua, Siena and Perugia and was one of the first physicians to perform human dissection in Italy. This practice allowed him to achieve a great knowledge of the human body mainly of the heart, kidney, and liver.

The knowledge of body organs and the possibility of translating Arabic, Greek and Latin medicine texts, allowed him to write many works and commentaries [1].

Among his writings let me mention the *Commentary of Carmina de urinarum iudiciis* (Songs of urinary judgements) and *De pulsibus* (About pulses) composed by Aegidius Corboliensis [2].

KARGER

Fax + 41 61 306 12 34
E-Mail karger@karger.ch
www.karger.com

© 1999 S. Karger AG, Basel
0250–8095/99/0192–0189$17.50/0

Accessible online at:
http://BioMedNet.com/karger

Dr. Mario Timio
Department of Internal Medicine and Nephrology
Hospital San Giovanni Battista
I-06034 Foligno (Italy)

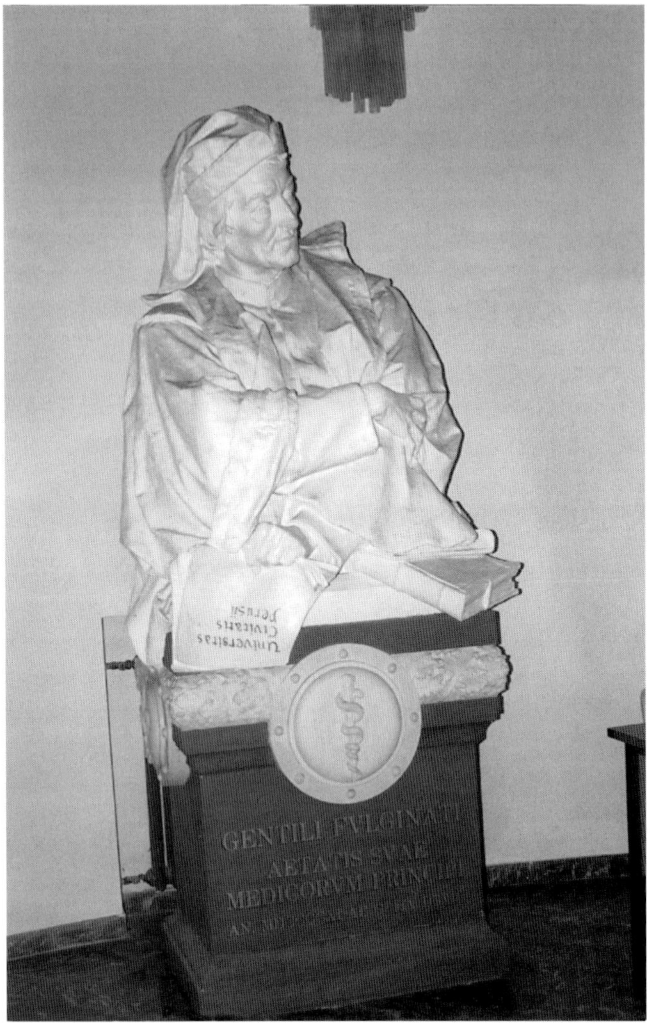

Fig. 1. Bust of Gentile da Foligno (1911), University Library, Perugia (with permission).

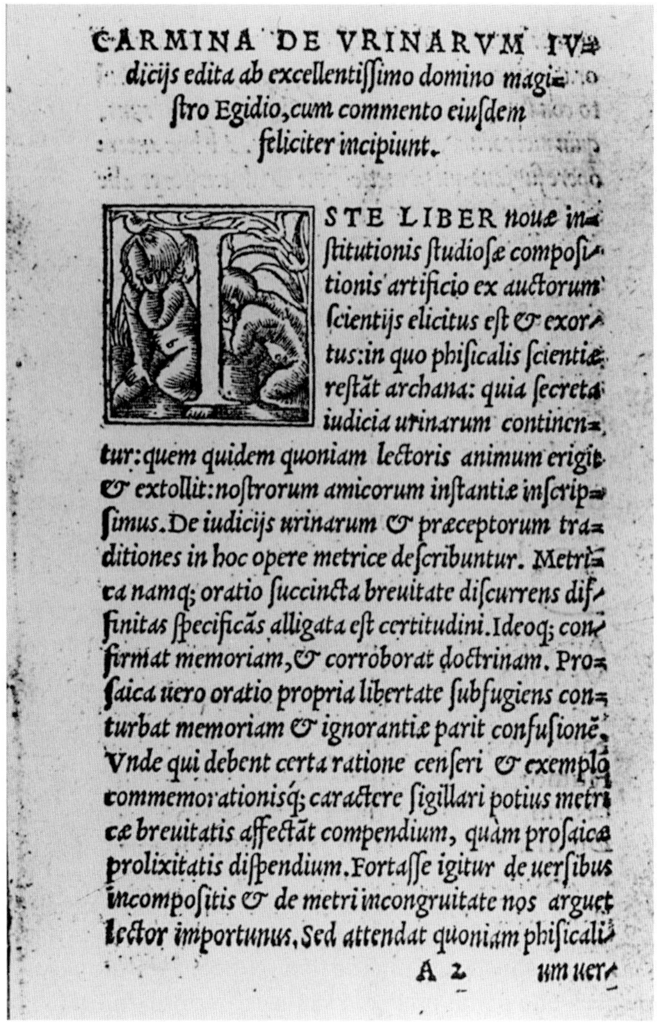

CARMINA DE VRINARVM IV-
dicijs edita ab excellentissimo domino magi-
stro Egidio, cum commento eiusdem
feliciter incipiunt.

ISTE LIBER nouae in-
stitutionis studiosae composi-
tionis artificio ex auctorum
scientijs elicitus est & exor-
tus: in quo phisicalis scientiae
restāt archana: quia secreta
iudicia urinarum continen-
tur: quem quidem quoniam lectoris animum erigit
& extollit: nostrorum amicorum instantiae inscrip-
simus. De iudicijs urinarum & praeceptorum tra-
ditiones in hoc opere metrice describuntur. Metri-
ca namq; oratio succincta breuitate discurrens dif-
finitas specificās alligata est certitudini. Ideoq; con-
firmat memoriam, & corroborat doctrinam. Pro-
saica uero oratio propria libertate subfugiens con-
turbat memoriam & ignorantiae parit confusionē.
Vnde qui debent certa ratione censeri & exemplo
commemorationisq; caractere sigillari potius metri-
cae breuitatis affectāt compendium, quàm prosaicae
prolixitatis dispendium. Fortasse igitur de uersibus
incompositis & de metri incongruitate nos arguet
lector importunus. Sed attendat quoniam phisicali-
A 2 um uer-

Fig. 2. Frontespiece of the *Carmina de urinarum iudiciis.* Town Library, Foligno.

The work of Gentile da Foligno on urine is more than a commentary; it is a text attempting to conceptualise the physiology of urine formation. In addition, this writing is a fascinating and up-to-date description of the different types of urine related to nephropathies, renal stones, and extrarenal diseases. His commentary was famous in Europe until the 17th century.

New Thoughts on Urine Formation, Quality and Volume

The writing of Gentile da Foligno is related to an age when physicians widely resorted to uroscopy, an ancient art whose practitioners focused on the state of many parts of the body, to gain knowledge of the patient's illness [3]. Practitioners usually examined urine in a bladder-shaped glass called a matula, in which they generally distinguished four regions, each of which was supposed to represent a part of the patient's anatomy: the uppermost region stood for the patient's head, the one below for the chest, the third down for the abdomen and the lowest for the urogenital system. Thus, changes occurring in urine at the different levels in the matula indicated the seat of the illness and its nature [4]. This made a large number of variations possible, and suggested many different diagnosis from the visible character of the urine.

The originally of Gentile da Foligno's thought consists in the arrangement of the diagnostic value of urine observation and pulse examination, in a synthesis of Salernitan medicine, which sustained the preeminent value of urine examination and of the classic Greek and Roman medi-

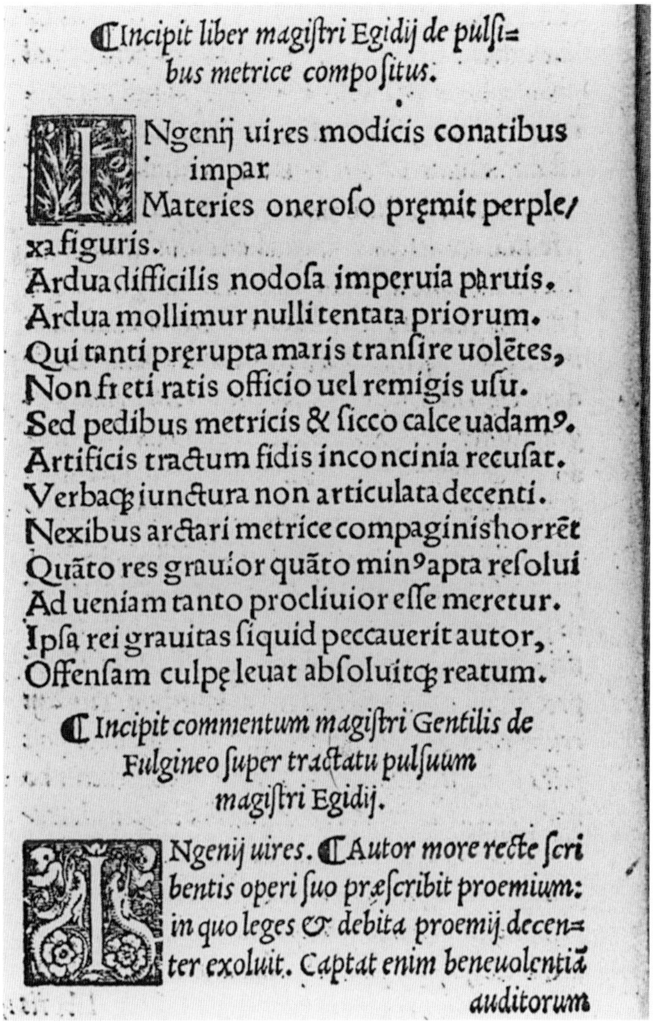
Incipit liber magistri Egidij de pulsibus metrice compositus.

Ingenij uires modicis conatibus impar
Materies onerosa premit perplexa figuris.
Ardua difficilis nodosa imperuia paruis.
Ardua mollimur nulli tentata priorum.
Qui tanti prerupta maris transire uolentes,
Non freti ratis officio uel remigis usu.
Sed pedibus metricis & sicco calce uadamus.
Artificis tractum fidis inconcinnia recusat.
Verbaque iunctura non articulata decenti.
Nexibus arctari metrice compaginis horret
Quanto res grauior quanto minus apta resolui
Ad ueniam tanto procliuior esse meretur.
Ipsa rei grauitas siquid peccauerit autor,
Offensam culpe leuat absoluitque reatum.

Incipit commentum magistri Gentilis de Fulgineo super tractatu pulsuum magistri Egidij.

Ingenij uires. Autor more recte scribentis operi suo praescribit proemium: in quo leges & debita proemij decenter exoluit. Captat enim beneuolentiam auditorum

Fig. 3. The 1st page of the *De pulsibus*. Town Library, Foligno.

cine, which focused on the importance of pulse characteristics.

Gentile da Foligno followed the Theophilus theory of urine formation only partially. According to this theory, urine is the result of processes of 'digestion', where the word 'digestion' indicates a separation between the 'pure' and the 'impure' part of a biological fluid [5]. Gentile da Foligno stated that 'urine is the blood's filtration' *(urina de massa sanguinis eliquatur)*.

According to his writing, the urine associated to the blood is brought to the kidney and then 'per poros euritides' (through the porous tubules) delivered to the bladder. In other words, in Gentile da Foligno's statement, the urine crosses a filtration-like barrier, a hypothesis close to our up-to-date knowledge of the renal physiology. It is worth noting that he explained, on his hypothetical basis, the different kinds of urine in physiological and pathological conditions [6]. In addition, he tried to correct some deceiving statements based on classic uroscopic information [7]. After Theophilus's *De urinis*, he stressed the importance of the characteristics of urine, as a sign of renal and systemic disease.

According to the classic preeminent semeiologic value, urine was especially indicative of two things: either suffering of the liver and veins, or of the kidney and bladder. Gentile da Foligno added a third thing: heart disease. The poverty of medieval doctrine on the subject of heart disease is well known. In congestive heart failure individual parts of the syndrome were regarded as individual clinical entities and were described and classified accordingly [8]. Thus, the expectoration, whether watery or mucoid or foamy, was likely to be characterised as catarrh, and described as a disease of the nose or throat. Similarly, hydrothorax was regarded as a separate disease, called dropsy of the chest. Dyspnea was apt to be described under asthma.

During the middle ages, oliguria as a concept of heart disease was not only described as a kidney disease but was not considered at all by the physicians. Gentile da Foligno stated that small volume urine in the course of acute fever could indicate heart disease; when urine is scanty and black it indicates death. Oliguria and signs of swellings sometimes signify a bad *(humoral)* mixture in the heart, and weakness and wasting of strength are additional signs of abnormal humors [8].

We realise that Gentile da Foligno even if following the old concept of diseases, modulated by humors and body qualities (heat, cold, dryness and humidity), offered ground for new interpretations.

After reciting the character of urine in many diseases, he added an important cause: urinary suppression produced by obstruction above the kidney. In this condition urine is transmitted by veins and is attracted by the lungs. If much urine collects there, the patients suffocate.

In the excerpts from Gentile da Foligno which deal with clinical subjects and which represent the condition of clinical medicine at the first half of the 14th century, we may see the imprint of the new physiology and pathology [9].

Relationship between Pulse Rate and Urine Output

With Gentile da Foligno we come to an original thinker and a new entity; disturbances of urine output and heart disease. Commenting and explaining the writing on *De pulsibus* he stressed the importance of heart disease on modulating the color and output of urine. Perhaps for the first time in the History of Medicine, he underlined the relationship between fast pulse rate (veloci pulsu) and urine output. Even though works on urine and the pulse were included in some manuscripts of the Salerno-Cassino School [11], Gentile da Foligno tried to explain the relationship between pulse variations, heart disorders and urinary abnormalities. This is a relevant observation, considering the era of Gentile da Foligno which was well before the discovery of the Harvean system of circulation of blood and of heart anatomy and physiology. Most of his statements on pulse and heart disorders are in almost similar terms to a recent description of relationship between heart disease and renal derangement.

On the heart anatomy *(De complexione cordis forma)* and physiology *(De motu cordis)*, there is little that cannot be traced to an ancient predecessor or a medieval codifica. Gentile da Foligno's doctrine is a description based for the most part on Galenic physiology, on ratiocination and on analogy. To a lesser extent, in an additional passage it rests on clinical and anatomical observations (based on dissection) and these are partly interpreted according to Pergamena dicta [10] and partially to his personal arrangements.

Gentile da Foligno admitted a very wide variety of causes on palpitation of the heart, which appear to be a conglomeration of ancient doctrine, folklore, simple observation and personal hypothesis. The wide range of causes is paralleled by a much wider range of treatment. Our author attributed great importance to palpitation, which he defines as a trembling movement that befalls the heart. The exposition of the characteristics of the pulse is clear, precise and sometimes innovative, coining some medical words never used in the classic semeiology (i.e. *de pulsu caprizante, martellino, ramoso, flutuante*; i.e. the capricious, hammer-like, branch-like, fluttering pulse). Each new word corresponds to a particular disease. In addition, Gentile da Foligno reminded us how to take the pulse properly: *quomodo tangens pulsum debet tenere manum* (every time you take the pulse, you have to hold the hand).

Gentile da Foligno's Originality and 'Cardionephrology'

On the other hand, Gentile da Foligno placed great emphasis on distinction between pulse derangements that are primary or inherent in the heart pericardium and disease or disturbance that originates in other parts of the body and affects the heart or pericardium secondarily as described by Avicenna and Galen. Among the conditions that could affect heart rate and pulse characteristics, Gentile da Foligno included bladder disease, kidney stones, and urine disorders. All these causes attack the heart removing, consuming or displacing its spirits.

For his originality on urine and pulse relationship, the 'prince of physicians' could be named as the first 'cardionephrologist', this name reflects his fame and his greatness.

Throughout his writing, Gentile da Foligno emphasised therapeutics. In keeping with the prevalent medieval raditionalism, the treatment was mainly humoralistic, even though he introduced the concept that drinking could increase urine output in dropsy patient *(potus diuretico multiplicatur urine)*. In this contest he first used the word *diuretic*.

The wisdom of such a man as Gentile da Foligno is the keynote to newer knowledge, the cause of out-of-dateness of the very knowledge that made such a man great in many fields of medicine, namely of nephrology and cardiology. That doctrine suggests Gentile da Foligno was some centuries ahead of his time.

References

1 Carboliensis E: Carmina de Urinarum Iudiciis. De Pulsibus et commento Gentilis de Fulginea. Basileae, 1529. Biblioteca Communale di Foligno.
2 Bonora F, Kern G: Does anyone really know the life of Gentile da Foligno? Med Secoli 1972; 9:29–53.
3 Reiser SJ: Medicine and the Reign of Technology. Cambridge, Cambridge University Press, 1978, pp 122–143.
4 Dal Canton A, Castellano M: Theory of urine formation and uroscopic diagnosis. Kidney Int 1988;34:273–277.
5 Ideler IL (ed): Theophili De Urinis in Physici et Medici Graeci Minores. Amsterdam, Adolf M. Hackert, 1963, pp 261–283.
6 Baptista de Tortis: Gentilis fulginatis viri eminentissimi in tertium Canonem Avicenna expositio. Venetiis, 1492. Ref. H. 2210/3; Pell 1667/3 GKW 3124/3. Biblioteca Communale di Terni.
7 Hieronimus de Durantibus: Consilia peregregia et toto medici celebratissimi Gentilis de Fulginea. Paduae, 1492. Ref. H. 7574. Biblioteca Communale di Terni.
8 Jarcho S: The Concept of Heart Failure from Avicenna to Albertini. Cambridge, Harvard University Press, 1980, pp 365–373.
9 Thorndike L: 'Consilia' and more works in manuscript by Gentile da Foligno. Med Hist 1959;3:1–10.
10 Kuhn CG: Claudii Galeni opera omnia. Leipzig, Cnoblock, 1821–1833.
11 Pasca M: The Salerno School of Medicine. Am J Nephrol 1994;14:478–482.

Contributions of Padua to Nephrology
(Dedicated to Arturo Borsatti)

American Journal of Nephrology

Am J Nephrol 1999;19:193–198

Bartolomeo Eustachio: A Pioneer in Morphological Studies of the Kidney

A. Mezzogiorno V. Mezzogiorno

Institute of Normal Human Anatomy, Medical School, II University of Naples, Italy

Key Words
Eustachio · Kidney morphology · Anatomy · 16th century medicine

Abstract
The morphological structure of the kidney only started being seriously investigated and truly understood in the 16th century, thanks mainly to Bartolomeo Eustachio. In his *De Renibus*, in fact, he painstakingly described the size, consistency, location and variations of the kidney, to which modern understanding can add very little. In describing the renal parenchyma he stated that it is made up of an external and an internal substance, and recognized the central role of the renal arteries in the excretory function of the kidneys. He made observations regarding the presence of extremely fine arteries that filter urine, the nature and function of the renal tubules and the columns of external substance that protrude between the papillae. There can be no doubt that Eustachio's remarkable achievements made him a pioneer in morphological studies of the kidney.

Historians normally tend to consider the 16th century as medicine's renaissance period, the time when medical culture finally awoke from the empiricism and dogmatism that had dominated it for many centuries. The same century brought fundamental and innovative advances in the morphological understanding of the kidney. If in fact it is true that in the *De Uso Partium* Galen was already clearly aware that the kidneys served to separate urine from blood, it has to be said that the foundation for this statement was just the (incorrect) vitalistic concept of the organ's drawing power [1–4]. The same error was eventually repeated many centuries later by Vesalius. Galen's ideas are, nonetheless, remarkably important for the originality and quantitative experimental reasoning with which they were developed. Quite rightly, Eknoyan [5] aknowledges Galen as 'the founding father of experimental renal physiology'.

Throughout the period of classical and medieval medicine Galen's ideas were forgotten, resulting in a very vague understanding of both the kidney's structure and function. Doctors would make philosophical pronouncements based on theological suppositions and empirical conjecture, and were satisfied with knowing that the kidney separated excess, dangerous serosity from the blood. They focused on examining the urine itself rather than the organ that produced it, thus giving birth to the practise of 'uroscopy', a branch of medicine where illnesses were

KARGER

Fax + 41 61 306 12 34
E-Mail karger@karger.ch
www.karger.com

© 1999 S. Karger AG, Basel
0250–8095/99/0192–0193$17.50/0

Accessible online at:
http://BioMedNet.com/karger

Dr. Antonio Mezzogiorno
Institute of Normal Human Anatomy
Medical School, II University of Naples
Via L. Armanni, 5, I–80138 Naples (Italy)
Tel./Fax + 39 081 5666009

diagnosed through the examination of the urine. Medieval doctors even believed that urine could be used to make predictions. In the German courts, for example, a prince's urine would be inspected by a doctor each morning.

It was not until the 16th century that important Italian anatomists such as Berengario da Carpi (1470–1530), Gabriele Falloppia (1523–1562) and Bartolomeo Eustachio (1510?–1574) first came close to discovering the true structure of the organ of urine formation [6, 7]. The concepts developed by these pioneer scientists were generally accepted and confirmed by their contemporaries and successors, like Caspar Bauhin (1560–1624), André Du Laurens (1567–1609), Johan Vesling (1598–1649) and Thomas Bartholin (1616–1680).

In the *Commentarii super Anathomia Mundini*, Berengario da Carpi agreed with the Pavian professor Gian Matteo Ferrari in denying the presence in the kidney of the Galen-derived 'colatorium', and was also the first to demonstrate the progressive subdivision of the renal veins in the renal substance, as well as to identify the renal papillae. He also described the renal calices surrounding the fleshy corpuscle he termed 'operculum', from the extremity of which the urine would come [8].

Bartolomeo Eustachio is recognized as a main figure in the 16h century. He was a passionate, studious and critical examiner of human forms, and he had dissected a large number of corpses of people who had died from acute and chronic diseases, and had vivisected animals from different species. With Eustachio, detailed investigation became vital to anatomical studies. He mostly committed himself to the study of normal and comparative (pathological) anatomy, and utilized dissection as an investigating tool with which to discover the cause of illnesses. Eustachio and Antonio Benivieni, a Florentine doctor, were the first to make observations regarding pathological anatomy, a new discipline which Giovanni Battista Morgagni (1682–1771) later triumphantly integrated into medicine.

Eustachio was never satisfied with his own work. He would investigate the structure of the human body and of animals with his bare eyes, and with the help of specially arranged lenses for a closer inspection of an organ's intimate structure. Should he not consider this enough, he would then either soak the anatomical pieces in various liquid solutions, or dry them at different temperatures and then inject them with colored solutions through the blood vessels. He pushed scientific investigation to the very limits of his time, in his own way forcing nature to unveil itself and reveal the truth [9, 10].

Marcello Malpighi paid Eustachio special tribute when, confiding in Giovanni Maria Lancisi, he said: '... Should Eustachio have been given the opportunity to combine his anatomical skills with the use of the microscope, he would undoubtedly have reaped such copious fruits that nothing would have been left to his descendants to discover'. No less flattering is Haller's description of Eustachio as 'a man of vigorous mind and one of the brightest anatomists of the 16th century' [11].

Knowledge of Eustachio's life history is rather incomplete and 'patchy', for his birth date is unknown, though it is thought to be between 1500 and 1510; his place of birth is likewise disputed, although it could be either the town of San Severino Marche, or San Severino in Salerno, or Santa Severina in Calabria. Evidence exists, though, in favor of San Severino Marche as the most likely birth place among the three.

Bartolomeo Eustachio's education took place in Rome. Once he had a degree in medicine, he moved from Rome to Urbino, where he offered his services to the 'della Rovere' dukes. When Cardinal Giulio della Rovere moved to Rome, he took Eustachio with him. During his time in Rome, Eustachio was made a professor at the 'Collegio Romano della Sapienza', where he taught anatomy as part of the practical medicine course in accordance with the customs of the time. Anatomy was the discipline to which he was most dedicated.

Eustachio only published one work, the *Opuscola Anatomica*, which consists of six monographs: *De Renibus Structura, De Dentibus, De Auditis Ogano, Ossium Examen, De Motu Capitis* and *De Vena Azygos*. Two of these describe structures which in current anatomy textbooks are named after Eustachio – the Eustachian tube and Eustachian valve. Even for organs that had in fact been investigated by others, his works provide the detailed and remarkable imprint of his hard work and brilliance. Just a few examples worth mentioning are his discovery of the adrenal glands; his incredibly detailed description of the teeth of primary and secondary dentition; his accurate observations on the male and female genital organs (which he referred to as the 'seminal organs'!); his descriptions of the cranial nerves and sympathetic trunk; the accurate description of the branches of aorta and vena cava, and the magisterial description of the azygos system, which previously was virtually unknown. His only inaccuracy lay in the belief that blood flows from the center to the extremities in both the arteries and the veins: this is understandable, since William Harvey was yet to publish the *De Motu Cordis et Sanguinis*.

Eustachio also discovered and described with admirable accuracy the origin, path and outlet of the thoracic duct, which he defined as '... a duct full of white and acqueous humour'. In the preface to the *Opuscola Anatomica*, he stated that he would soon publish another book, the *De Dissensionibus controversii Anatomicis*, and forty-six anatomical plates which would provide a fairly comprehensive anatomical iconography. But, as a matter of fact, by what many medical historians consider inconceivable bad luck (or what we believe were, in fact, nothing but financial limitations), Eustachio published neither the manuscript nor the aforementioned anatomic plates. These manuscripts were found about 150 years later by relatives of Eustachio's ever-faithful collaborator Pier Matteo Pini. On Morgagni's suggestion the plates were published in an elegant volume in 1714 by Giovanni Maria Lancisi, thus providing research and study material for the great 17th century anatomists like Morgagni, Valsalva, Boerhaave, Albino and Haller. This edition of the plates was later followed by one edited and commentated by Andrea Maximino in 1783 (fig. 1).

About Eustachio's anatomical plates, it has to be said that, apart from their incredible precision, he had made them even more interesting by the use of what he called 'geometricus gnomon', an absolutely fascinating system which he used to describe each plate. Rather than just mark the drawings with letters or numbers, Eustachio in fact used a combination of frames and graded reference points, so that every part of the drawing would correspond to the clearly marked longitude and latitude coordinates that framed his drawings. It is important to underline that works published before Eustachio's plates were not nearly as accurate, leading the medical historian Salvatore De Renzi to affirm that 'should Eustachio himself have been able to publish his anatomical plates, Anatomy would then have already been as advanced at his time as it had instead to be about two centuries later'.

Seven of the plates clearly illustrate the morphology of the kidneys and demonstrate the remarkable extent of Eustachio's knowledge by the time *De Renibus Structura* had been published. In this erudite monograph, Eustachio begins with an extremely detailed description of the size, consistency, color and location of the kidneys, to which only very little can be added by modern knowledge. First Eustachio compared the shape of the kidney to a large bean, and specifies that its upper (or cranial) extremity is more rounded than the lower one (or caudal). He then went on to describe the right kidney as generally being slightly more caudal than the left, but also took care to state that the position of the caudal extremity of the organ primarily depends on the kidney's volume, regardless of whether it is the right or the left kidney, as illustrated in the first three plates (fig. 2, 3).

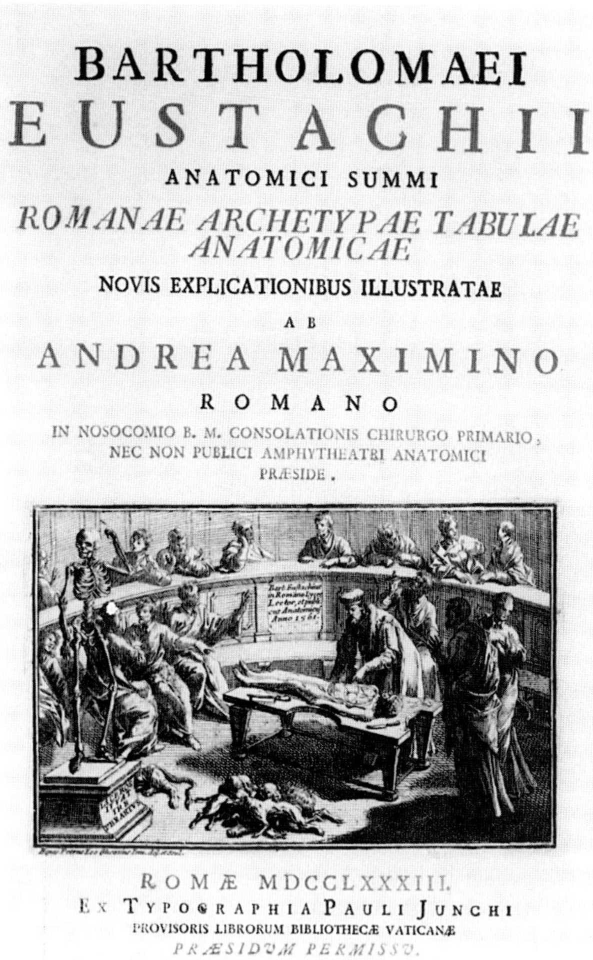

BARTHOLOMAEI
EUSTACHII
ANATOMICI SUMMI
ROMANAE ARCHETYPAE TABULAE ANATOMICAE
NOVIS EXPLICATIONIBUS ILLUSTRATAE
AB
ANDREA MAXIMINO
ROMANO
IN NOSOCOMIO B. M. CONSOLATIONIS CHIRURGO PRIMARIO, NEC NON PUBLICI AMPHYTHEATRI ANATOMICI PRÆSIDE.

ROMÆ MDCCLXXXIII.
EX TYPOGRAPHIA PAULI JUNCHI
PROVISORIS LIBRORUM BIBLIOTHECÆ VATICANÆ
PRÆSIDUM PERMISSU.

Fig. 1. Anatomical demonstration by Bartolomeo Eustachio, on the frontispiece of the *Tabulae Anatomicae*, published by Andrea Maximino (Rome, 1783).

'The consistency of the kidney', said Eustachio, 'is compact and solid, and its color is normally red-brown, occasionally darker, and sometimes pale or whitish, depending on various pathological conditions'. Eustachio also observes that a newborn baby's kidney is lobulated like that of an ox or numerous other animals, whereas in the adult it is always smooth and uniform. He eventually criticized Aristotle for describing the adult human kidney as lobulated.

Eustachio put forth meticulous observations regarding all possible variations in number, origin and caliber of the

2

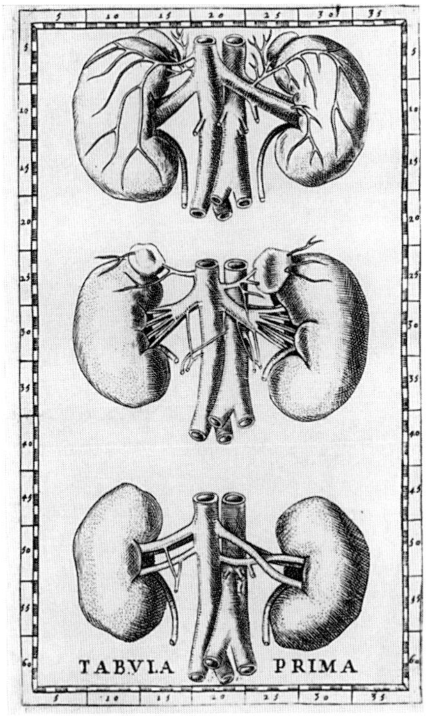

3

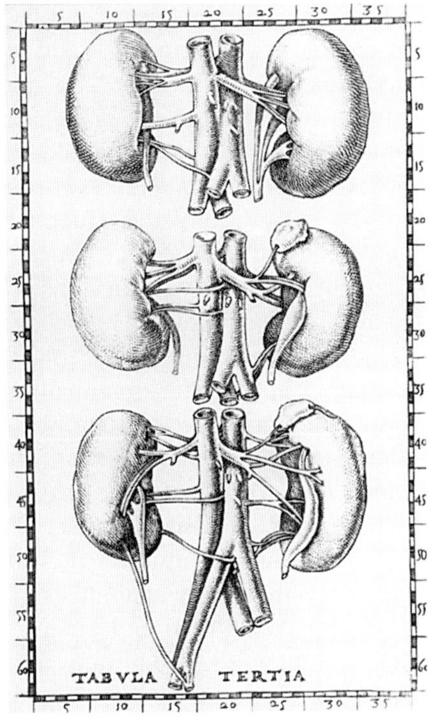

Fig. 2. *Tabula Prima* from Eustachio's *De Renibus Structura.* It clearly shows the position of the caudal extremity of the kidneys in relation to their size. To be noted, here, is that the suprarenal glands are graphically represented perhaps for the very first time.

Fig. 3. *Tabula Tertia* from Eustachio's *De Renibus Structura.* The top illustration shows three renal vessels on the right and a variation in the renal pelvis on the left. The central illustration represents the left ureter in the shape of an oblong bladder, and an artery, originating in the common iliac artery, going into the kidney. The bottom drawing shows some variations of both renal veins and arteries.

blood vessels, which are described to pass into the kidney through a cavity formed by the medial margin facing the spinal column. They are, needless to say, accurately illustrated in the first, third and fourth plate (fig. 2–4). In contrast to his predecessors' belief, Eustachio was more than convinced that various nerves from the celiac plexus penetrate the kidney together with the blood vessels.

He also dwelt at length on the possible anatomical variations of the kidney, affirming the possibility of different shapes or positions, or even numerical differences. He eventually noted that some kidneys can be found much lower than normal, between the fourth lumbar vertebra and the top of the sacrum, in which case the vessels would originate from the division of the vena cava and the aorta and penetrate the back of the kidney, giving us the first description known in medical literature of the congenital condition termed ectopic renal location, which he skillfully illustrated in the fourth plate (fig. 4). He completed this meticulous morphological description by stating that the kidneys are enveloped in two resistant membranes, the inner one being a fibrous tunic which forms a firm, smooth covering which, in some points, continues around the vessels, and an external membrane which is prevented from adhering to the kidney by the presence between the two membranes of a layer of adipose tissue. Lastly, Eustachio set out a complete, accurate description of stones found in the kidneys, ureters and the bladder, concluding that they can begin to form in the kidneys without compromising its structure or its organization.

While describing his study of the renal parenchyma, he confirmed Berengario da Carpi's belief that the renal vein branches out in the renal substance, but in addition stated that it is from the arterial vessels (fig. 5) that urine is secreted. Of even greater importance than this is the identification within the kidney's parenchyma, of three different substances, a statement that definitively abolished the old belief of the kidneys being composed of a single, homogeneous matter. He defined an external substance, reddish-colored, compact and fleshy-looking, which contains minute formations of extremely fine arteries which filter urine. Next, he described a waxy substance, engraved with tiny lines as fine as hairs, each one made up by a bundle of channels (fig. 6), which gather in small papilla-shaped protuberances thus forming a third substance. Among the papillae are small 'glands' which he described as being derived from the external substance: 'instar papillae incumbunt glandulae parvae a substantia renum'. Each papilla is held in a cup-shaped tube which joins others to form two or three short tubes. These in turn link up to form a funnel-shaped sack which extends into the ureter. An enormous number of vessels peregrinate within the three substances. Between the inner and outer-

4

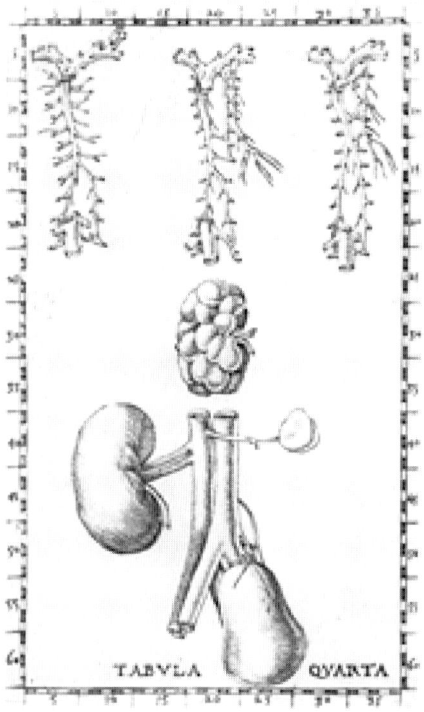

5

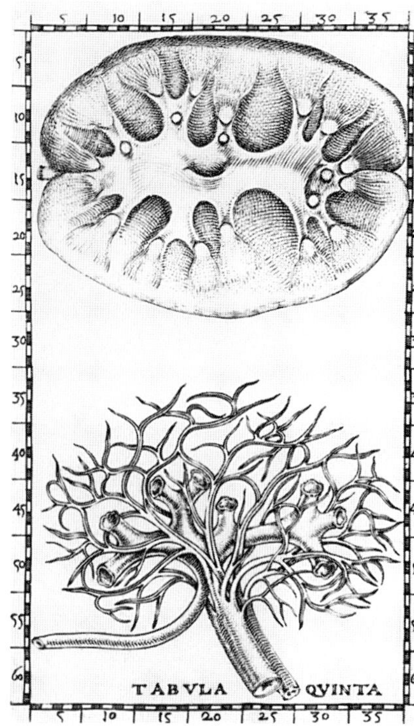

Fig. 4. *Tabula Quarta* from Eustachio's *De Renibus Structura.* The top illustration shows the azygos vein and its variations. The middle illustration depicts a bear's kidney, made up of cherry-sized lobules. The lower illustration shows a kidney which Eustachio described as 'praeter naturam': it is the graphic representation of an ectopic kidney, though its adrenal gland is in the normal position.

Fig. 5. *Tabula Quinta* from Eustachio's *De Renibus Structura.* Top illustration shows the human kidney halved at the hilum. The pyramids through which the ducts pass before converging in the renal papillae are very clear, as is the projection of the cortical substance between them. The bottom drawing shows the subdivision of the renal vessels, and the renal pelvis with the calyces.

most substances, veins connect with veins and arteries with arteries forming well-defined arches which spread out into fine branches that are too small to be seen with the naked eye.

Eustachio's research into the structure of the renal parenchyma represents a fundamental and vital contribution to the advancement of anatomy. His remarkable descriptions include the renal glomeruli, which Malpighi, helped by the use of the microscope, later described with greater accuracy and are therefore known today as 'malpighian bodies'; the nature and function of the renal tubules, which were later described by Bellini and are therefore referred to as the 'ducts of Bellini'; and the external substances which protrude between the papillae and are known today as the 'renal columns of Bertin'. Moreover, he recognized the central role of the arteries in the excretory function of the kidney.

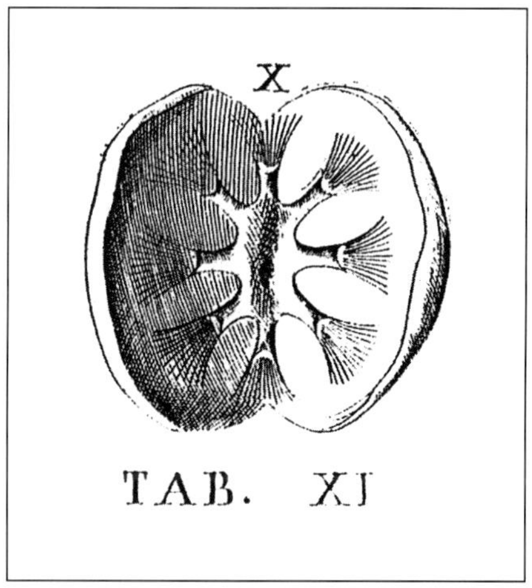

Fig. 6. *Tabula XI* from Eustachio's *De Renibus Structura.* It shows the kidney halved from its convex edge. The filament-like tubules which converge on the papillae in bundles are clearly illustrated.

Eustachio's death is in some ways similar to that of his great predecessor, Vesalius, who died in 1564 during his return from a pilgrimage in the Holy Land. Eustachio died in 1574 during a journey from Rome to Fossombrone, while taking his medical expertise to the bedside of an ill friend, Cardinal Giulio della Rovere. He left Rome as soon as he received a letter from the Cardinal asking him to come, regardless of his own weak physical state, the outcome of a serious episode of gout. His health dramatically deteriorated during the trip, to the extent that he had to stop on several occasions: firstly in Foligno, then in Nocera and finally, in Fossato di Vico, where, on August 27, 1574, he passed away in severe pain and almost destitute.

The death of Eustachio, one of the greatest anatomists of the Renaissance, is fundamentally the death of a doctor who neglected himself and his own health to do all he could for his patients. During his lifetime Eustachio did not seek glory, but only wished, this from his own words, that his work would be recognized by his successors. He would not be disappointed: Joseph Hyrtl (1810), in fact, whose opinion is considerable, defined him as an 'anatomical genius'.

In the light of this noble and exemplary figure of a doctor and scientist, who dedicated every day of his life to the ceaseless quest for truth, we can but bow our heads and learn from his enlightened teachings.

References

1 Belloni L: Per la Storia della Medicina. Sala Bolognese, Forni, 1990.
2 Cosmacini G: La Medicina e la sua storia. Milano, Rizzoli Libri, 1989.
3 Del Gaizo M: Della pratica dell'Anatomia in Italia sino al 1500. Atti R Accad Med Chir 1892;46:194–233.
4 Triolo VA: An interpretative analysis of Galenic renal physiology. Clio Med 1966;1:113–128.
5 Eknoyan G: The origins of nephrology: Galen, the founding father of experimental renal physiology. Am J Nephrol 1989;9:66–82.
6 Portal M: Histoire de l'anatòmie et de la chirùrgie. Paris, Didot, 1770.
7 Sprengel C: Storia Prammatica della Medicina. Napoli, 1826.
8 Mezzogiorno V, Mezzogiorno A, Passiatore C: A contribution to the history of renal structure knowledge (from Galen to Malpighi). Ann Anat 1993;175:391–401.
9 De Renzi S: Storia della Medicina. Napoli, Tipografia del Filiatre-Sebezio, 1846.
10 Grmek MD: Il Calderone di Medea. Bari, Laterza e Figli, 1996.
11 Mezzogiorno A, Mezzogiorno V: Marcello Malpighi. Am J Nephrol 1997;17:269–273.
12 Eustachio B: Tabulae Anatomicae, illustrate da A. Maximino, Roma, 1783.

Contributions of Padua to Nephrology
(Dedicated to Arturo Borsatti)

American Journal of Nephrology

Am J Nephrol 1999;19:199–212

Berengario da Carpi

Natale Gaspare De Santo Carmela Bisaccia Luca Salvatore De Santo Rosa Maria De Santo Vito A. Di Leo Teresa Papalia Massimo Cirillo Alain Touwaide

Chair of Nephrology, Second University of Naples, Italy, and Consejo Superior de Investigaciones Científicas, Instituto de Filología, Madrid, Spain

Key Words
Anatomy · University of Bologna · Commentary in teaching · Kidney structure · Berengario da Carpi · *Commentaria* · Pre-Vesalian anatomy · Renaissance

Abstract
Berengario da Carpi was magister of anatomy and surgery at the University of Bologna from 1502 to 1527. Eustachio and Falloppia defined him as 'the restaurator of anatomy'. He was a great surgeon, anatomist and physician of illustrious patients including Lorenzo II dei Medici, Giovanni dalle Bande Nere, Galeazzo Pallavicini, Cardinal Colonna, and Alessandro Soderini. He had strong links to the intellectuals of his time (Forni, Bonamici, Manuzio, Pomponazzi) as well as with the Medici family. He was respected by the Popes Julius II, Leo X and Clement VII. His main contributions are the *Isogogae Breves, De Fractura calvae sive cranei,* and the illustrated *Commentaria* on the Anatomy of Mondino de Liucci, a textbook utilized for more than 200 years, which Berengario aimed to restore to its initial text. The *Commentaria* constitutes the material for the last part of this paper which concludes with a personal translation of some passages on 'The kidney', where the author gives poignant examples of experimental ingenuity.

Historical Outline

After the great changes occurring in the 14th and 15th centuries that marked the end of the two universal powers of Empire and Papacy, nations were formed as modern states. This occurred first in France and England just after enduring the gruelling trial of the Hundred Years War and the events following thereto. This passage also took place in other parts of Europe but less completely, while in the Balkan Peninsula, quite the opposite occurred, namely the end of independent states and the setting up of the Ottoman Empire.

In Italy, a single state with national identity failed to develop, but instead various states grew, the most important of which succeeded in limiting, but not overcoming traditional Italic particularism. Here the beginning of the modern state coincided with the rise of the city's rule of 'signoria', which evolved from the 'comune'. The greatest of these extended their domain over the surrounding countryside and over the smaller cities, so as to become regional states (the few exceptions to the transformation from 'comune' to 'signoria' regime include: in Venice, for example, the rise and consolidation of an oligarchical rule). The social and civil upheavals and the war between individual states played a considerably important part in bringing about the rise of the signoria and its territorial

KARGER
Fax + 41 61 306 12 34
E-Mail karger@karger.ch
www.karger.com

© 1999 S. Karger AG, Basel
0250–8095/99/0192–0199$17.50/0

Accessible online at:
http://BioMedNet.com/karger

Natale G. De Santo, MD
Chair of Nephrology, Second University of Naples
Via Pansini 5, Pad 17
I–80131 Naples (Italy)
Tel./Fax +39 081 566 6655

Table 1. Historical events between 1450 and 1540

Year	Event
1453	Fall of Constantinople which is conquered by the Turks. Insanity of Henry VI of England. The War of the Roses begins between the Houses of Lancaster and York. Mid-15th century Enclosure Movement in England. Development of sheep farming, transformation of agriculture, rise of large commercial classes.
1455	The War of the Roses begins.
1457	Invention of the Printing Press (Gutenberg).
1460	Henry V, organizer of the Portugese navy, dies. Henry the Navigator withdraws to Cabo de Sagres to coordinate Portugal's discovery enterprises.
1461	Louis XI, King of France. The Turks occupy the Venetian and Genoan possessions on the Black Sea and in the Peloponnese.
1462	The beginning of Ivan III's rule in Russia.
1466	Eastern Prussia is annexed to Poland.
1467	Charles the Bold becomes Duke of Burgundy.
1468	Liège revolts against Charles the Bold.
1469	Marriage between Isabella, Queen of Castile and Ferdinand, heir to the Crown of Aragon.
1473	Birth of Mikolaj Kopernik (Nicolaus Copernicus).
1475	France gains national unity after the 100 Years' War.
1476	The Swiss defeat Charles the Bold at Grandson and Morat.
1477	Maximilian of Hapsburg marries Maria, daughter of Charles the Bold.
1479	Unification of Spain with Ferdinand of Aragon and Isabella of Castile.
1481	John II, King of Portugal.
1482	Peace of Arras between Louis XI and Maximilian of Hapsburg.
1485	Richard III (of York) dies in the Battle of Bosworth Field. The War of the Roses concludes with Henry VI's ascent to the throne.
1487	Bartholomew Diaz reaches the Cape of Good Hope.
1493	Fall of the Kingdom of Granada and end of Muslim rule in Spain. Christoper Columbus discovers the new continent.
1493	In Germany Maximilian I on the imperial throne. Birth of Philippus Theophrast Bombast von Hohenheim (Paracelsus).
1494	Treaty of Tordesillas between France and Portugal.
1496	Marriage between Philip of Hapsburg and Giovanna the Insane.
1503	The Casa de Contratatiòn founded at Seville to watch over the traffic between colonies and the home country with the task of collecting taxes on colonial trade and to receive on behalf of the Crown precious metal from the American mines. The first shipment of negro slaves arrives in America.
1507	M. Waldseemuller, German geographer, proposes baptizing the new world with the name of America.
1509	Creation of the Council of the Indies in Spain. Alfonso de Albuquerque Portuguese governor in India.
1510	The Portuguese conquer Goa.
1511	The Portuguese occupy Macao. Erasmus of Rotterdam publishes *Praise of Folly*.
1513	Portuguese conquest of Ormuz. The conquistador Vasco Nuñez de Balboa crosses the isthmus of Panama and reaches the Pacific.
1514	Birth of Andreas Vesalius.
1515	Francis I King of France.
1516	Treaty of Noyon (regulates the peace between France – Francis I – and Austria, Helvetic Confederation, Pontifical State. Naples to Spain, Milan and Genoa to France). Ottoman conquest of Syria.
1517	The Spanish in the Yucatan. The Portuguese at Canton. The Ottoman conquest of Egypt. Luther's 95 theses against indulgences.
1519	Frankfurt Diet: Charles V becomes Emperor. Magellan's voyage. Hernàn Cortés begins the destruction of the Aztec civilization.
1520	Luther publishes *To the Christian Nobility of the German Nation* (Lutheran doctrine: universal priesthood, free examination of the sacred texts, justification by faith alone, criticism of the sacraments). Papal bulletin *Exsurge domini*.
1521	Papal bulletin *Decet romanum pontificem*; Luther's excommunication. Diet of Worms, Luther's re-excommunication (solemn anathema). Death of Magellan.
1522	The Turks conquer Rhodes.
1523	Gustav I King of Sweden begins the Vasa Dynasty.
1524	Peasants' revolt in Germany. Battle of Frankenhauser and death of T. Müntzer.
1526	Treaty of Madrid between Francis I and Charles V. League of Cognac. Victory of Soliman in the battle of Mohàcs. The Muslim Babour, Signor of Afghanistan founds the Moghul dynasty in India.
1527	The struggle between Huascar Inca and Atahualpa begins for the Inca throne.
1530	Diet of August. *Confessio Augustana* programmatic foundation of the Lutherans.
1534	England, *Act of Supremacy* (Anglicanism, Henry VIII proclaims himself supreme head of the Church of England). First voyage of Jacques Cartier to Canada.
1536	The Turks conquer Mesopotamia.
1540	In Geneva Calvin begins preaching. Ignazio Loyola founds the Society of Jesus.

extension. Later in various cities the signoria received further official recognition by the Empire and the Church, and developed into a principate.

In Poland from 1385, Wladyslaw II Jagiellone became king and the Jagiellonian Dynasty lasted until 1572. In Hungary in 1458, Matthias Corvinus, son of John Hunyadi Regent of Hungary became King, whereas in Bohemia in 1458, George of Podiebrad was elected King. On the death of George of Podiebrad Wladyslaw I of the Jagiellonians was made King of Bohemia, and was also elected King of Hungary. The Jagiellonian Dynasty continued until 1526, when Bohemia and Hungary passed under the Hapsburgs.

In Russia, dominated by the Tarters (Mongols), the Moscow princes grew in strength, brought Ivan I to power (1320–1340) and defeated the Tarters in 1380, but the real founder of the Moscovite power was Ivan III (1462–1505) who, on subjecting the city of Novgorod and numerous Russian principalities, fought against the Tarters and against Poland.

In the Balkans and in Danubian Europe from the 14th century onwards, strong pressure was felt from the Ottoman Turks who defeated the Serbs, occupied Bulgaria, part of Bosnia and of Valacchia and threatened Hungary.

In 1453, Mohammed II conquered Constantinople. The Turks established themselves on the whole of the Balkan Peninsula (1480), Venice lost her possessions in

Table 2. Historical events in Italy during the years 1450–1545

1450	Francesco Sforza, Prince of Milan.
1452	Birth of Leonardo da Vinci.
1454	Peace of Lodi (diplomacy for equilibrium between the Italian States).
1458	Death of Alfonso of Aragon, King of Aragon, Sicily, Sardinia and Naples.
1463	Birth of Pico della Mirandola.
1464	Death of Cosimo de' Medici. Succeeded by his son Piero, who dies in 1469. Francesco Sforza, Duke of Milan since 1450, conquers Genoa.
1466	Death of Francesco Sforza. Succeeded by his son Galeazzo.
1469	Lorenzo de' Medici becomes Signore of Florence.
1471	Borso d'Este is nominated Duke of Ferrara by the Pope.
1476	Murder of Galeazzo Maria Sforza.
1478	Conspiracy of the Mad in Florence. The system of equilibrium between the Italian States in jeopardy.
1480	Ludovico il Moro takes on the protection of the Gian Galeazzo Sforza and usurps the power at Milan. Peace between Lorenzo the Magnificent and Sixtus VI. The Turks disembark at Otranto.
1482	War of Ferrara (The Pope and Venice against Florence, Naples, Milan, Bologna and Mantua).
1484	Peace of Bagnolo. Conspiracy by the Neapolitan barons against the king Ferrante.
1492	Death of Lorenzo de' Medici. Birth of Vittoria Colonna.
1494	Charles VIII conquers the Kingdom of Naples. At Florence the Republic is instituted. Girolamo Savonarola preaches in Florence. Conflict between Milan and Naples. Ludovico il Moro appeals to France.
1494	War for the conquest of Italy, that for its final objective hegemony in Europe.
1495	Battle of Fornovo.
1498	Girolamo Savonarola burnt at the stake.
1499	Louis XII conquers the Dukedom of Milan.
1500	Birth of Benvenuto Cellini.
1501	Birth of Gerolomo Cardano.
1503	Julius II is elected Pope. Spain takes possession of the Kingdom of Naples.
1504	Treaty of Lyon. Spanish dominion in the Kingdom of Naples.
1506	Leonardo paints the 'Gioconda' and begins the construction of St. Peter's Basilica (Bramante).
1508	Michelangelo begins the frescoes in the Sistine Chapel. The League of the Cambrai: Pope (Julius II). France (Louis XII), Spain (Ferdinand the Catholic) against Venice. Birth of Bernadino Telesio.
1509	Venetians beaten at Agnadello.
1510	Holy League: Pope, Venice, Sapin and England against France.
1511	Birth of Vasari.
1512	Battle of Ravenna (the French win, but abandon Milan and Lombardy).
1515	Francis I conquers Milan. Death of Aldus Manutius in Venice.
1516	Machiavelli writes 'The Prince', Thomas Moore 'Utopia', Ariosto 'Orlando Furioso'. Anti-Spanish revolt in Sicily. Birth of Realdo Colombo.
1527	The imperial troups sack Rome. The Florentine Republic is restored.
1529	Peace of Cambrai (between Luisa of Savoy and Margherita of Austria). French renunciation in Naples.
1529	Congress of Bologna. Charles V is crowned Emperor by Pope Clement VII. Italy passes under Spanish influence.
1530	The Medici are restored at Florence. Birth of Giulio Cesare Aranzio, first Ordinary Professor of Anatomy in Italy at Bologna.
1535	Death of Francesco II Sforza. Milan passes to Spain.
1537	War between Venice and the Ottoman Empire.
1543	Birth of Fabrizio d'Acquapendente.
1545	Pope Paul III Farnese creates the dukedom of Parma and Piacenza for his son Pier Luigi. Council of Trent.

Morea, while Genoa lost those on the Black Sea. The Byzantine Empire was destroyed with the fall of the Trebizond Empire. Bayazid succeeded Mohammed II on his death and continued to put Hungary under pressure together with the Hapsburg dominions, Styria, Carinzia and Carniola.

In Germany in 1417 Brandeburg passed the nucleus of Prussia to the Hohenzollerns. During the 14th century and the first decades of the 15th century the imperial crown went to the Luxemberg-Bohemia family and then to the Hapsburgs.

At the beginning of the 16th century the most important political problem was strengthening the state and the unification of power in the countries of the great monarchies that managed to carve out territories. In France, England and Spain, the changes of the state institutions were sharp and profound. As for the politically divided countries, in Germany (which also had a unifying factor in its imperial power) and in Italy, the influence of the medieval institutions resisted.

Events in the Years 1450–1550

Here we focus on Berengario da Carpi, professor of anatomy and surgery at Bologna in the years 1502–1527. Before providing information on his life, his achievements and on his *Commentary* on Mondino's *Anathomy*, it seems appropriate to have a look at his time through a historical outline on the years 1450–1550. Therefore, we have taken the liberty to select some historical events in World history (table 1), paying particular attention to Italy (table 2), as well as to Italian dynasties (table 3). Table 4 lists the popes. The last two tables are most appropriate since the life of Berengario was certainly affected by some Italian dynasties (Medici Family, Pio Family, Gonzaga Family, d'Este Family), and was under the protection of Julius II, Leo X (Giovanni dei Medici), and Clement VII (Giuliano dei Medici). Julius, Leo and Clement (fig. 1) had a great influence on him. They had great admiration for Berengario and helped him as needed. All of them asked him specific professional consultations for their relatives.

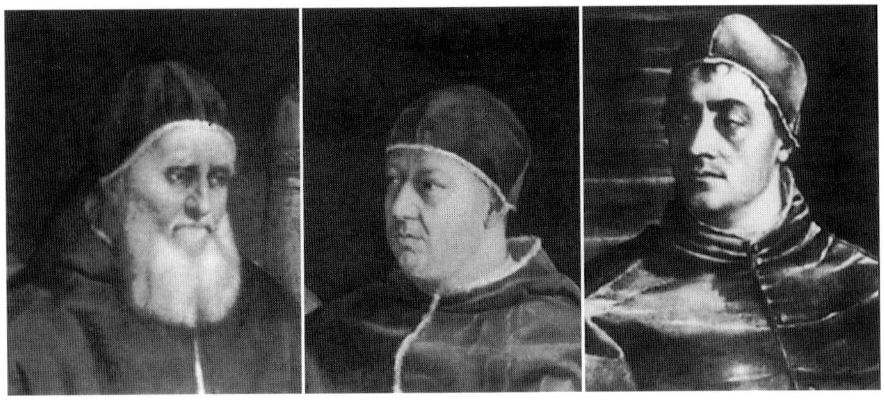

Fig. 1. Popes who supported Berengario. From left Julius II, Leo X, and Clement VII.

Table 3. Some Italian dynasties between the years 1440 and 1550

Appiani (Piombino and the Isle of Elba)
Baglioni (Perugia)
Bentivoglio (Bologna)
d'Este (Reggio, Modena and Ferrara)
Gonzaga (Mantua)
Malaspina (Massa Carrara)
Malatesta (Rimini)
Savoy (Piedmont)
Sforza (Milan)

Table 4. Popes between the years 1455 and 1549

Paul II (Pietro Barbo)
Sixtus IV (Francesco della Rovere)
Innocent VII (Giovanni Battista Cybo)
Alexander VI (Rodrigo Borgia)
Julius II (Giuliano della Rovere)
Leo X (Giovanni de' Medici)
Adrian VI (Adriaan Florisz Boeyens)
Clement VII (Giuliano dei Medici)
Paul II (Alessandro Farnese)

Table 5. Some of Berengario's biographers

Josephus Ferdinandus Gulielminus	1735
M. Portal	1770
Giovanni A. Brambilla	1781
Alessandro Gelati	1844
Salvatore De Renzi	1845
Michele Medici	1857
Paolo Gaitoli	1880
Vittoria Putti	1937
L.R. Lind	1959
R.K. French	1985

Berengario marks pre-Vesalian anatomy and as pointed out by Burggraeve [1], 'it is difficult to keep the balance in this time of great people, in a time during which every hour gives birth to new facts. There is no place for surprise if claims for some discoveries were made by several scientists. At that time there were no journals, no societies, no congresses to give a date to a scientific discovery.'

Digne prédécesseur de Vésale, Berengario est considéré à juste titre par Falloppia et Eustachi comme 'le restaurateur de l'anatomie' [1]. Berengario has a place in every history of medicine; however, there is a group of biographers (table 5) who are worthy of special mention [2–11]. The most famous among them is Mr. Vittorio Putti (fig. 2), born Bologna March 1, 1880 and died in the same city on November 1, 1940. Putti graduated from medical school cum laude at the age of 23 discussing a thesis on formalin's action on the kidney. He studied in Berlin, Dresden, Cologne, Heidelberg, and Bologna (under Codivilla) and became Professor of Orthopedics in Rome at age of 31 (1911) and in Bologna from 1912 to 1940. He touched upon all aspects of his discipline with great skill and class and was a worldwide requested speaker. He was a great surgeon and instructor at Rizzoli Hospital which he brought to great fame. In 1937 he published the biography *Berengario da Carpi*, L. Cappelli Editore, in Bologna which included the Italian translation of *De fractura calvae sive cranei.*

There has been considerable long-lasting discussion about the true name of Jacopo Berengario da Carpi, who is also identified as Iacopo Berengario, Iacopo da Carpi, Il Carpi, Giacomo Barigazzi, Iacopo de Barigatiis, de Baringariis, de Barigariis, Berigariis, Birigariis, de Berengariis, de Barringariis, de Barringatiis, Beringario, Beringerio, Carpus, de Carpo (Rolls of the University of Bologna), da Carpi (from the city where he was born) 'huius nominis defensor et meae patriae'. Only in his testament is it clear that Jacobus de Barigatiis from Carpi was the son of Faustinus the surgeon from Carpi as shown by Policarpo Guaitoli [6] '(Testamentum Domini Magistri Jacobi de Barigatiis. In Christi nomine amen. Anno a Nativitate ejusdem 1528. Indictione prima, die 24 Mensis Martii. Egregius

Excellens Artium ac Medicine Doctor Dominus Jacobus filius quondam Magistri Faustini de Barigatiis de Carpo sanus per gratium Jesu Christi corpore, mente, sensu, visuet intellectu, timens periculum mortis...)'.

Berengario was born in the years 1460–1470. The exact date remains unknown. In *De fractura cranei* he points out that at the time of the Battle of Molinella on July 23, 1467 he was 'satis puer'. He learned a lot from his father, the surgeon Faustino de Barigatiis. He learned practical surgery, care of fractures, everyday gynecology, bedside mannerism. He also learned how to ask for his high professional fees. He was grateful to his father and therefore he stresses that 'nemo enim est peritus chirurgus qui a pueritia non vacavit huic arte' (*De Fractura*, Folio 30a).

Berengario learned humanities (mansuetorum musarum rudimentis) in Carpi with Alberto Pio (who also used to sign Albertus Carpi), son of Lionello, Signore di Carpi, and his wife Caterina Pico della Mirandola under the guide of Aldo Manuzio (sub felici memoria Aldi Manucii romani praeceptoris nostri). However, his latin was poor and Haller stressed that it was 'qualem non expectes ab Aldii Manutii discipulus'. Singer in turn points out that 'He is the worst Latinist. Probably his language prevented his works from being widely read' [12].

The link of Berengario with the Pio Family, Signori di Carpi, was a stable one based on fond friendship and gratitude. To defend those friends on one occasion he used 'mala verba' (nasty words) against the Duke of Ferrara. For this reason Berengario underwent a trial and was fined either to pay 100 ducats or undergo a section of his nose (eidem apsidetur nasus seu nares a vultu). His father, the surgeon, gave the money, the nose was saved, but the time of Berengario in Carpi was over, and he had to go.

Medical Studies

He attended medical school at the university of Bologna (Bononia mea altrice). The list of his teachers includes Gerolamo Manfredi, Chair of General Medicine; Alessandro Achillini (Magnus Achillinus – Great Achillinus) Chair of Logic and Philosophy; Gabriele Zerbi, Chair of Medicine and Philosophy, who gave his last course in Bologna in 1484. He completed his medical studies in 1489. 'Die 3 Augusti 1489 - Aprobatus fuit in artibus et medicina magister Jacobus de Carpo presentatus per Magistrum Cabridem, rectorem. Promotores fuerunt M.r. Johannes de Garzonibus, M.r. Nicolaus de Sabiis qui dedit insigna et M.r. Rufinus de Tuzzi. Nemine discrepante (unanimously).* There is an annotation on the roll: 'hic evasit magnum anatomicum' (this was the beginning of a great anatomist).

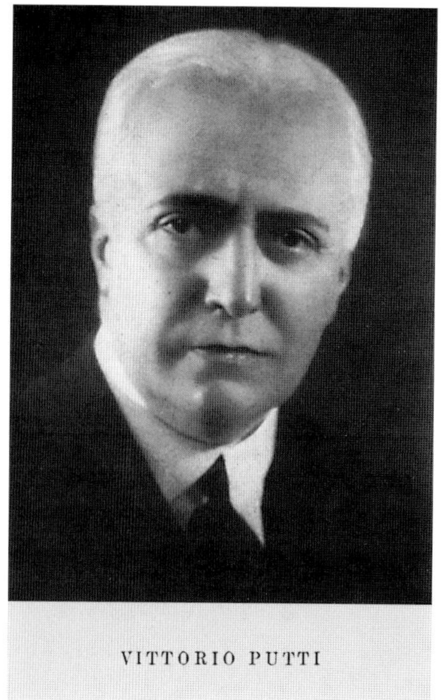

Fig. 2. Vittorio Putti, the most important biographer of Berengario.

Berengario's Intellectual Circle

Berengario had excellent relations with exemplary intellectuals of his time. First of all with Aldo Manuzio (fig. 3), preceptor of Alberto Pio and Berengario da Carpi by advice of Pico della Mirandola and Printer of humanities in Venice. Pietro Pomponazzi, nickname 'il Peretto' for his small frame, was a respected teacher of Philosophy in Bologna. The group also included Lazzaro Bonamici da Bassano, great latinist pupil of Pietro Pomponazzi – a very much sought-after intellectual by the various dynasties – who was preceptor of Ercole Gonzaga. Gianfrancesco Forni taught Logic at the universities of Bologna and Pisa, was with Ercole Gonzaga to whom he taught Arabic. Ercole Gonzaga was second-born to Ercole Gonzaga and Isabella d'Este. Bishop at 16 years of age, cardinal at 21, studied in Bologna with Lazzaro Bonamici who became his preceptor at the suggestion of Pietro Pomponazzi.

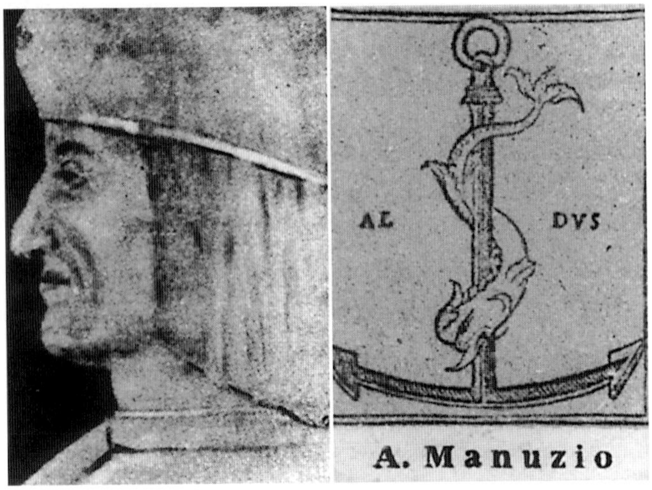

Fig. 3. Aldo Manuzio and the logo of Aldinae Editions of classics.

Teaching at the University of Bologna

At the time of Berengario, lecturers came mainly from Bologna; however, there was place for foreigners, possibly people with teaching experience, people of great name and reputation and only if strictly necessary (excellentes et multi nominis et famae, in casu bene necessario). Berengario had political support and was a man of great reputation. In those days there was no chair of anatomy in Bologna, which was introduced (the first chair of anatomy in Italy) in 1570 with Aranzio.

What did Berengario learn at the University of Bologna in those days? What did he teach subsequently? Raffaele Bernabeo and Giuseppe D'Antuono nicely described the 4-year course [13] in those days, the location of the university, the constitutions, the duties of the professors, how their presence was checked, the fines they paid for unapproved absences, etc., the timing of the lectures which were stressed by the Bell of San Petronio (called Scholara). In this book Stefano Arietti has prepared 2 tables concerning medical instruction in the 14th–15th and 16th–18th centuries, in Bologna (tables 6, 7).

Lectures for Medical Students in Bologna

There were different types of lectures: (1) ordinary (general topics for each fundamental course); (2) extraordinary (defined topics), in the afternoon; (3) advanced courses (usually with experts from abroad); (4) repetitions, usually given by the best students for mandatory courses, or taken as private lessons. Bernabeo and D'Antuono [13] stress the fact that in those days there was the Italian tradition of sending teenagers to university independently of their future activities. University training was not seen as professional training but as an occasion to grow culturally. In fact, there is discrepancy between the number of students registered and those obtaining the medical degree which was a costly procedure and there was no need to obtain it for those who were at the university just to learn and not practice a profession.

Mandatory courses were theoretical medicine, clinical medicine and surgery and there was the duty to learn anatomy from cadavers. The student was obliged to participate in at least two public dissections, but the students participated in many more. Dissections took place at the homes of the teachers, and the cadavers were procured by the students, and later on by the university. There were fixed rules about the number of attendants during practical anatomy. Mondino requested the help of a dissector and also of an ostensor to show anatomical preparations to the students.

Some Discoveries of Berengario da Carpi

According to Singer [12], Carpi 'is the first to describe the vermiform appendix, the first to see arytenoids as separate cartilages, the first to recognize the larger proportional size of the chest in the male and of the pelvis in the female, the first to give a clear account of the thymus gland. He knows something of the cardiac valves. His description of the brain is an advance on Mondino, recognizes the general form of the ventricles, the composition of the choroid plexus out of the arteries and veins, the pineal gland, and the fourth ventricle.'

The First Anatomies Printed with Figures, 1490–1545

The commentary on Mondino is the earliest anatomical treatise that can properly be described as having figures illustrating the text. These figures [12] vary in excellence. Some are not devoid of beauty, and are prepared for the use of artists rather than anatomists.

Table 6. Chairs and textbooks [13] at the Bologna Medical Faculty (13th to 15th centuries)

First year

First morning lecture: Avicenna: Canon (1st book, 1st fen, at exclusion of anatomy; 2nd fen, at exclusion of chapters on necessity of death, diseases of childhood, on diet, on regimen with water and wine, on sleeping and waking)

Second morning lecture: Galen: *On differences of fevers, On complexions, On bad complexion, On simple medicine* (at exclusion of the 6th book), *On critical days* (1st book)

Afternoon lecture: Avicenna: *Canon* (4th book, 2nd fen, 2nd book); Galen: *On internal parts, On critical days* (2nd book); Hippocrates: *Aphorisms* (at exclusion of section 7); Maimonides: *On regimen*

Second year

First morning lecture: Galen: *Book Tegni* (i.e. techniques of medicine); Hippocrates: *On regimen in acute diseases, Prognostics;* Avicenna: *On faculties of the heart*

Second morning lecture: Avicenna: *On accident and disease, On crisis;* Galen: *Method of medicine, On critical days* (3rd book), *Method of medicine, On usefulness of breathing, On putrefaction*

First afternoon lecture: as in the morning

Second afternoon lecture: as in the morning

Third year

First morning lecture: Hippocrates: *Aphorisms* (at exclusion of the 7th section); Galen: *Method of medicine*

Second morning lecture: Hippocrates: *Therapeutics (chapters 6–12); Averroès: Colliget;* Galen: *On natural faculties, On critical days* (2nd book)

First afternoon lecture: texts discussed in the 1st morning lecture during the 2nd year

Second afternoon lecture: texts discussed in the 2nd morning lecture during the 2nd year

Fourth year

First morning lecture: Avicenna: *Canon* (topics discussed in the 1st morning lecture during the 1st year)

Second morning lecture: topics discussed in the afternoon lecture; Hippocrates: *On nature*

First afternoon lecture: texts discussed in the 1st morning lecture during the 3rd year

Second afternoon lecture: texts discussed in the 2nd morning lecture during the 3rd year

Note: In the old constitution lecture is synonymous of chair.

Table 7. Chairs and textbooks [13] at the Bologna medical faculties

Propaedeutic Philosophy Courses for Medicine

1st year: Aristotle: *Physics, On generation and corruption* (1st and 2nd book), *On sleep and wakening, Physionomy.*

2nd year: Aristotle: *On heaven and world, Book Mathaurorum, Book on perception and perceived things, On memory and recording, On breathing, On life and death, On inspiration, On earth's substance.*

3rd year: Aristotle: *On soul* (at exception of part of 1st book), *Methaphysics* (introduction of book 1, second book, part of book 4, books 5–10, book 12), *On length and brevity of life, On cause of animals' movement.*

Medical Course

1st year: Lectures on theoretical medicine: Avicenna: *Canon* (1st book, 1st fen, at exclusion of anatomy; 2nd fen, chapter on nature of seasons; 3rd fen, chapters on necessity of death, on diseases of childhood, on diets, on the regimen with water and wine, on sleep and wakening); Galen: *On differences of fevers, On complexions, On bad complexion, On simple medicine* (at exclusion of chapter 6), *On internal parts* (at exclusion of the 4th book, *On critical days* (1st and 2nd book); Avicenna: *Canon* (4th book, 2nd fen; 2nd book); Hippocrates: *Aphorisms* (at exclusion of section 7); Maimonides: *On regimen.*

Courses on practical medicine: Avicenna: *Canon* (3rd book: *On special disease).*

2nd year: Lectures on theoretical medicine: Galen: *Small art, On critical days* (3rd book), *On differences of fevers, On putrefaction, On usefulness of breathing;* Hippocrates: *Prognostico, On regimen in acute diseases;* Avicenna: *On faculties of the heart, On crisis.*
Lectures on practical medicine: as in the 1st year.

3rd year: Lectures on theoretical medicine, all the texts discussed in the previous 2 years: Galen: *Method of medicine* (books 7–12), *On natural faculties;* Averroès: *Colliget.*
Lectures on practical medicine: as in the 1st year.

4th year: Lectures on theoretical medicine: the texts of the previous years: Hippocrates: *On nature.*
Lectures on practical medicine: as in the 1st year.
The medical course also included:
Lecture on surgery: Galen: *On tumors contrary to nature, On ulcers, On wounds, On bone luxations and fractures* (from 1737 on). Lecture on anatomy (from 1570 on).
Lecture *On simples* (from 1534 on), subsequently on fossils, plants and animals (from 1561 on). Chemical lecture (from 1737 on). Lecture *On surgical intervention.*
Note: In the old constitution lecture is synonymous of chair. Lectures on theoretical medicine and lectures on practical medicine were divided into ordinary lectures, extraordinary lectures and advanced course mainly presented by outside experts.

Relations to Zerbi

Berengario hated Zerbi, and has left us with many testimonies. He hated him without reason. Zerbi was a respected scientist of his time and in fact was professor in Bologna, Padua, and Rome. However, Zerbi had written that Carpus derives from the Latin carpere (to steal).

The Years 1502–1527

He was nominated Magister of Surgery in 1502 and, later on, also Magister of Anatomy. His role was confirmed up to 1527. His retirement from the university

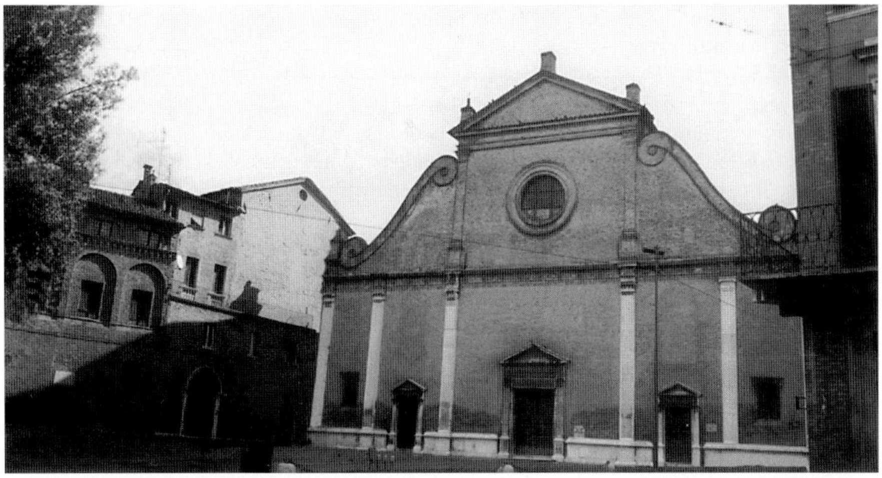

Fig. 4. The church of St. Francis in Ferrara.

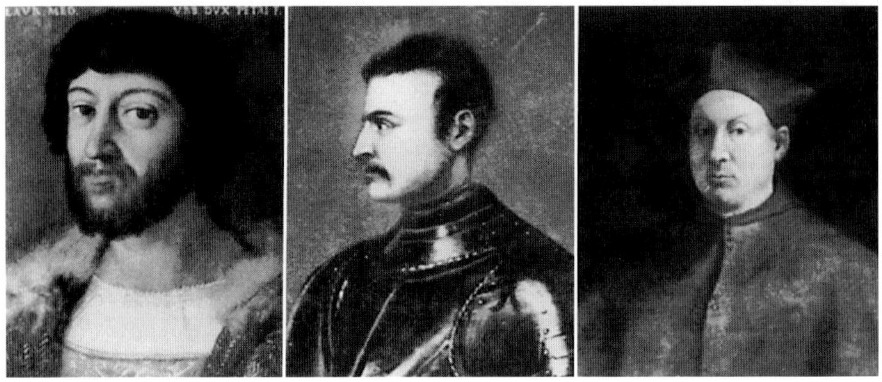

Fig. 5. Renowned patients of Berengario. From the left to right Lorenzo dei Medici, Duke of Urbino (Lorenzo II), Giovanni dalle Bande Nere (middle) and Cardinal Pompeo Colonna (on the right).

post remains unexplained. The charge of vivisection and difficulties with the Holy Inquisition have been invoked, but never proved. After retirement from his post in Bologna he worked for his friend Ercole Gonzaga who granted him a nominal salary of 25 ducats. Nothing is known about the death of Berengario and about his place of burial. He had expressed the will to be buried in the Church of St. Francis in Ferrara (fig. 4) and many historians of medicine say that this was the case, but a clear-cut demonstration is still lacking. Berengario was a great teacher, very much admired by students, to whom he performed great services. In a roll of the university of Bologna in those days we read: 'ad lecturam chirurgiae D.M. Iacobus de Carpo habet sat scholarium, D.M. Dominicus de Lana nihil valet vel parum'. In addition, a note points out that 'D.M. Dominicus de Lana vix habet tres scholares et parum valet. M. Iacobus de Carpo. Iste habet X vel XII scholares et illis satisfecit.' Indeed, many students from countries North of the Alps were attracted to Bologna by Berengario's reputation.

Driven by his professional capabilities, the fame of Berengario grew. On July 4, 1506 Berengario was made a citizen of Bologna. This honor was given by Pope Julius II by means of a *breve* to 'Dilecto filio Jacopo Barigatiis de Carpo Civis Civitatis Bononiensi in artibus et medicinae magistro'. In these years, he also edited interesting books (table 8).

Renowned Patients of Berengario

Leo X in 1513 asked the Senate of Bologna to allow Berengario to go to Florence to take care of Alessandro Soderini, relative of Cardinal Soderini and of the Medici Family, without a reduction of salary and granting substitution with another expert lecturer for the time needed to heal the patient.

In 1517, Berengario took care of Lorenzo dei Medici, Duke of Urbino (fig. 5, left) who underwent cranial trephination for a skull fracture received in battle. The patient healed. This was an impetus to the preparation, within

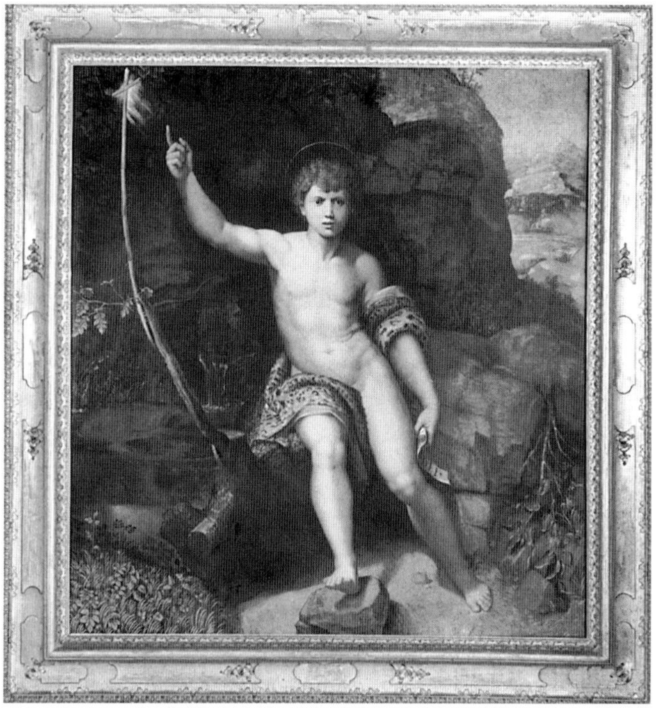

6

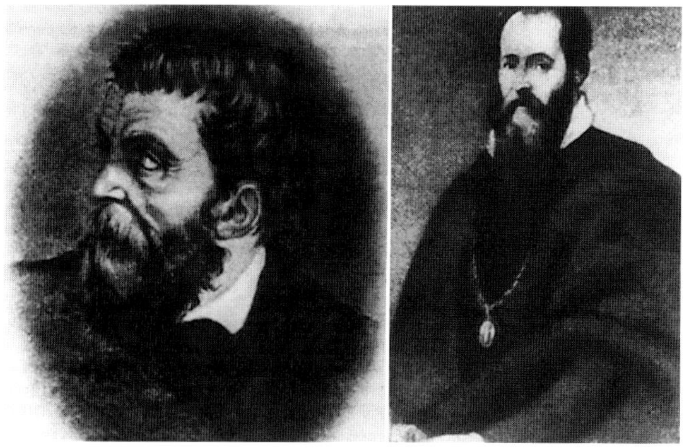

7

Fig. 6. St. John in the desert. Art Gallery at Bologna.
Fig. 7. Benvenuto Cellini and Giorgio Vasari (left to right).

2 months, of the *De Fractura calvae sive cranei* which, of course, was dedicated to the illustrious patient: 'please accept this small book which deals with skull fractures which I have elaborated at the maximum of my capabilities and is dedicated to you to fulfil a promise to your request at the time I took care of the wounds of your head'.

In 1520, Berengario took care of Marchese Galeazzo Pallavicini, a gouty man with kidney disease and generalized edema (qui ab urinali aquositate in venis totius aggregata suffucatus est, et haec aquositas induxit squinantian, pro qua applicavimus ventosam sine scarificatione divertendi causa et ventose per poros cutis implebantur pura aquositate).

In 1525, Clemente VII asked Berengario to go to Piacenza to cure Giovanni dalle Bande Nere (fig. 5, middle) wounded in battle on February 18 of that year. The patient was grateful to Berengario for consultation, but selected another surgeon for the operation!

Giorgio Vasari and Benvenuto Cellini on Berengario

After Berengario successfully cured Cardinal Colonna (fig. 5, right side) he asked in payment a painting on wood by Rafael. The painting (fig. 6) represents St. John in the Desert (166 × 150.5 cm), which according to Putti is presently in the Art Gallery of Bologna. According to Vasari (fig. 7, right side) 'Rafael had painted a Saint John in the Desert for Cardinal Colonna who having been severely ill had been assisted by Jacopo Berengario da Carpi a physician who healed him. Berengario asked for Rafael's painting as honorarium. The painting is now in the possession of Francesco Benintendi' [14]. However, on this painting, which in 1720 was given to the city of Bologna by Francesco Mastri, there is still no agreement about the authorship.

Now let's move to Cellini (fig. 7, right) who in his *Vita* written in the years 1558–1566 [15] reports: 'Capitò a Roma un grandissimo cerusico il quale si chiamava Jacopo da Carpi. Questo valente uomo infra gli altri medicamenti prese certe cure disperate di mali francesi ... fattosi cognoscere questo valente uomo mostrava di sanare meravigliosamente queste cotai infermità, ma voleva far patto prima che cominciassi a curare; è quali patti erano a centinaia e non a decine. ... era molto litterato, meravigliosamente parlava di medicina. Il papa volse che lui restassi al suo servizio, e quest'uomo disse che non voleva restare al servizio di persona al mondo.' (In those days a great physician named Berengario da Carpi arrived in Rome. This skillful man adopted desperate cures for French disease. He was successful in handling such dis-

Table 8. List of publications

1	*Anothomia Mundini noiuter Impressa ac per Carpum castigata* Anno Domini 1514, Die XII Augustii, Impressa per Istiniuanu Ruberie Quarto volume, Roman Characters, 2 columns, 42 lines, 26 folios
2	*Tractatus De Fractura Calve sive Cranei* cm 20.4 × 14 (quarto volume), round characters, 1 column, 39 lines Impressum Bononiae per Hyeronimum de Benedictis, Anno MDXVIII
3	*Carpi Commentaria cum amplissimis additionibus super anatomia Mundini una cum textu eiusde in pristinu & verum nitore redacto* Impressum Bononiae per Hyeronimum de Benedictis, Anno MDXXI The volume, a quarto edition, sums up a total of 528 folios numbered with Roman numerals and is printed with Roman types, 1 column per folio, each consisting of 39 lines. The last folio is the registrum and points out that all are quaternions, before concluding 'Laus Deo. God be praised!'
4	*Isagoge Breves perlucide ac uberrime in Anatomia humani Corporis* Impressum Bononiae p. Benedictu Hectoris, Anno MDXXII sub die XXX Decebris 72 folios, 20 figures (second edition per Hyeronimum de Benedictis 1523)
5	*Galeni Pergamneni Libri Anatomici* Bononiae in Aedibus Ioannis Baptistae Phaelli, Mense Septebri, MDXXIX, 152 folios, 20 × 14.5 cm (quarto volume). Roman Characters, 1 column, 38 lines

eases; however, before starting therapy, he used to make pacts, such pacts were not by tens, but by hundreds of ducats. He was a humanist and a good public speaker of medicine. The Pope asked him to be archiater, but he refused.)

Cellini continues: 'Passando un giorno casa dalla mia bottega vide a sorta certi disegni infra i quali erano parecchi bizzari vasetti. Volse il dicto maestro che gnene facessi d'argento. Con tutto quello che il detto valente uomo bene me gli pagassi fu l'un cento maggiore l'onore che mi apportorno'. (One day he entered my workshop and saw some drawings among which some bizarre small jugs and asked me to make them in silver. The money I received was adequate; however, the honor I received for this work was hundreds of percent greater.)

Commentaria on Mondino

According to Guy de Chauliac, le père de la chirurgie française [16], 'Mundinus Bononiensis qui super anatomiam scripsit, et eam fecit multoties, et magister meus Bertuccius per hunc modum: situato corpore in banco faciebat de ipso quatuor lectiones, in primis tractabantur membra nutritiva, quia cito putrebilia; in secunda membra spiritualia, in tertia membra animata, in quarta extremitates tractabantur.'

Burggraeve [1] in turn stresses that the 'principal merit of Mondino is that he is among those who used cadavers to teach anatomy in public courses'. During the Renaissance the first anatomist who deserves mention is Mondino who published a treatise of anatomy. This was used for nearly two centuries as a manual for the students and as a foundation for the lectures of professors who were obliged by law to read and to comment on it. The *Commentaria* were illustrated with a total of 21 figures. Indeed, Berengario probably had the privilege of working with Ugo da Carpi, the famous xylographer born in Carpi (ca. 1480) and died in Bologna in 1532. Ugo da Carpi studied the works of Albrecht Dürer (Nürnberg 1471–1528) as well as those of H. Burgknair (Augusta 1473–1531) in Venice and developed a new technique [17–19] which utilized a series of boxwood blocks laid one upon the other, and obtained unsurpassed *effects of chiaroscuro* [17, 18]. The primacy of Ugo da Carpi in xylography was attested by Vasari.

The graphic approach of the *Commentaria* on Mondino (fig. 8) is not different from that used by Gerolamo Benedetti for *De immortalitate animae digressio* of Giovanni Francesco Pico della Mirandola (fig. 9). In the *Commentaria* there is a difference concerning the name of the pope, the coat-of-arms, and the vignette describing the teaching of anatomy. Within the frame, the pope of the time is recalled (Leo X), and the center holds the symbol of the Medici Family. At the base of the column on the left appears the coat-of-arms of the Pio Family, Signori di Carpi. In the vignette, the teacher is depicted on the left in a sitting position addressing the students. Standing in the middle is the dissector while the students stand on the right. The book was dedicated to Giulio dei Medici, Cardinal and Vice Chancellor of the Vatican in Bologna, to whom in the preface Iacopo Berengarius wishes good health and happiness (salutem felicitatem dicit) and has the goal to spread the glory of Mondino. The book was put under the patronage of Giulio dei Medici and of his Family (the descendants of Cosimo de Medici) from whom also Pope Leo X, the reigning pope, originated. The author declares that he had initially thought to dedicate the book

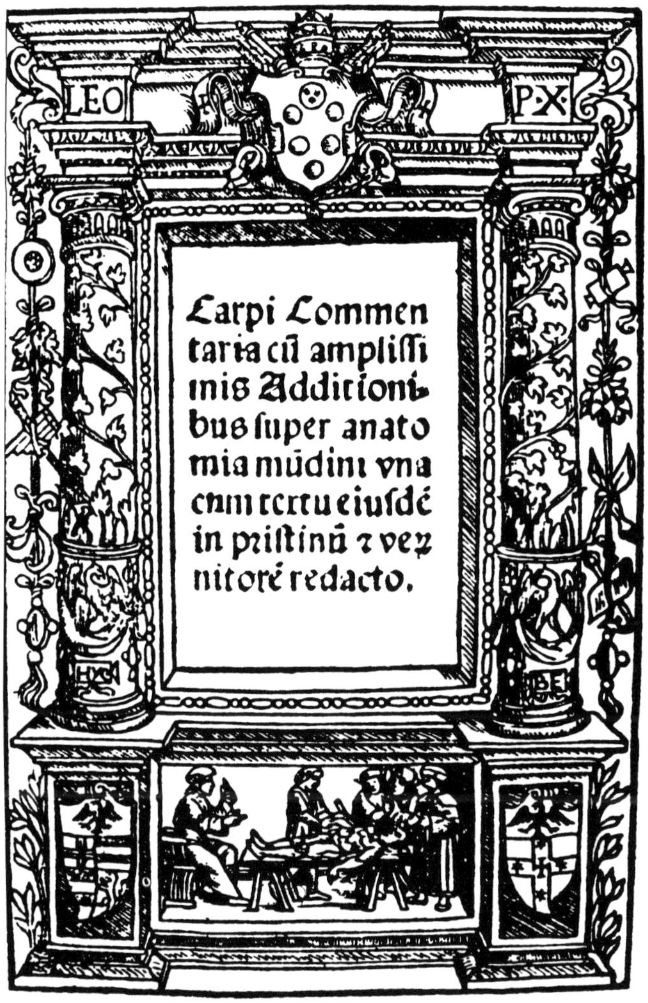

Fig. 8. Frontispiece of Carpi Commentaria on Mondino (Biblioteca Nazionale, Naples).

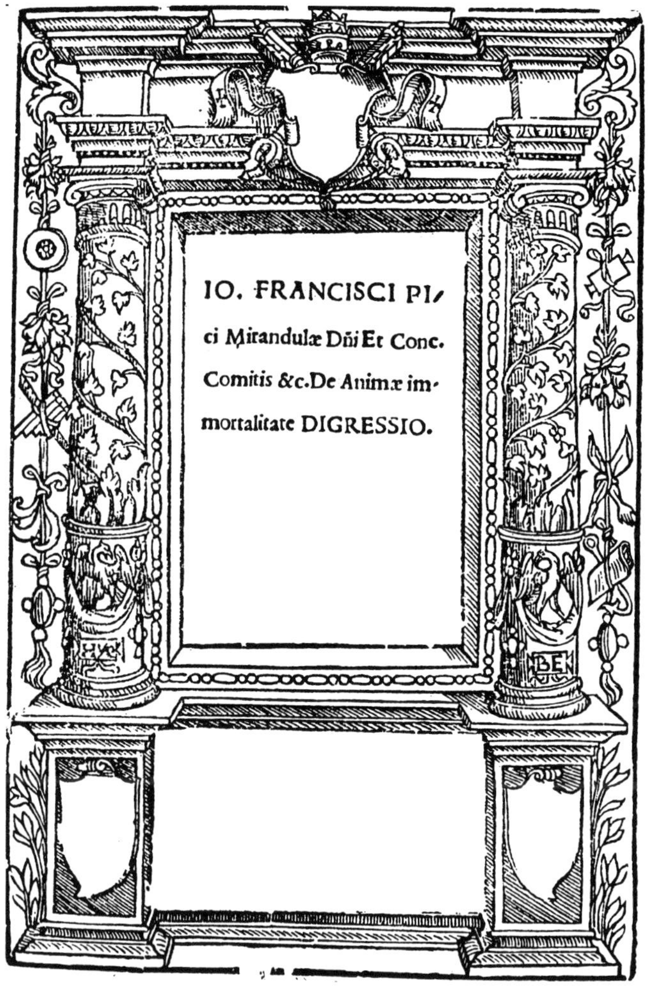

Fig. 9. Frontispiece of 'De anima immortalitate' of Francesco Pico della Mirandola.

to Lorenzo dei Medici (Duke of Urbino) to whom Machiavelli five years earlier had dedicated *Il Principe – The Prince* and finally concludes hoping that Giulio might accept his offer.

The Use of Commentary in Anatomical Teaching

In a paper on Berengario's technique of commentary, French [11] writes: 'The commentary had been the vehicle of medical education for some two and a half centuries when Berengario produced this in 1521... which was unique among his predecessors and contemporaries in producing a dissection-based anatomy in commentary form'. Berengario does not fragment the text of Mondino which is presented in chapters. The goal is that of restoring the text to pristinum sensum by adding the parts which might have been lost, by cutting those which have been spuriously added during the years. There is also the need to restore the initial order of sequence. Subsequently, he provides, as was usual in those days, an expositio which enucleates the difficult points of the text and discusses them. Following French [11], one easily learns about the personal technique of Berengario in the *Commentaria* on Mondino, which is derived from that mastered by Gentile da Foligno. The technique may be summarized as follows: the reader is introduced into the general problems of the whole topic (digressiones), then, if needed, Berengario would discuss the opinions of other

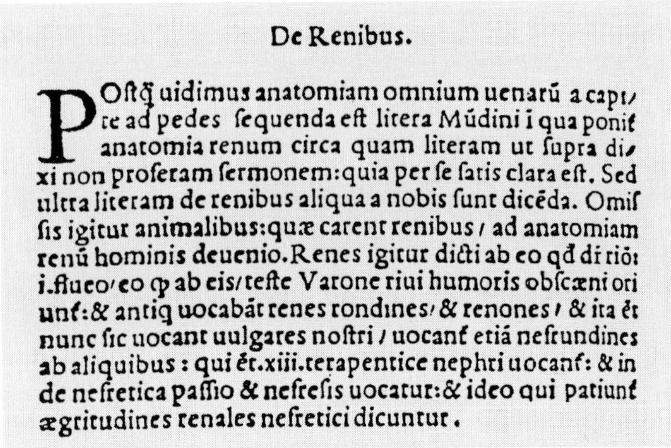
De Renibus.

Postq̃ uidimus anatomiam omnium uenarũ a capite ad pedes sequenda est litera Mũdini i qua ponit anatomia renum circa quam literam ut supra dixi non proferam sermonem: quia per se satis clara est. Sed ultra literam de renibus aliqua a nobis sunt dicẽda. Omissis igitur animalibus: quæ carent renibus, ad anatomiam renũ hominis deuenio. Renes igitur dicti ab eo qđ ri riõ: i. fluo, eo q ab eis, teste Varone riui humoris obscæni oriunt: & antiq uocabãt renes rondines, & renones, & ita ẽt nunc sic uocant uulgares nostri, uocant etiã nefrundines ab aliquibus: qui ẽt. xiii. terapentice nephri uocant: & in de nefretica passio & nefresis uocatur: & ideo qui patiunt ægritudines renales nefretici dicuntur.

Fig. 10. Anastatic copy from the original of some passages on the kidneys (Folio CLXXVIIverso) from *De renibus* in Carpi *Commentaria*, with translation in the right column.

On kidneys

CLXXCVIIverso

After we have seen the anatomy of all the veins from the head to the feet, we have to follow Mondino's text, where the anatomy of kidneys appears. We shall not discuss this chapter, as we have said above, because it is clear enough in itself. But, we have to add some data to his chapter on kidneys. Living thus aside the animals, which have no kidneys, we come to the anatomy of kidney in man.

Now, they are called kidneys *(renes)* from what is called river *(rion)*, i.e. *flow,* for the reason that, according to Varro, the flows of dirty humour arise from them. And the Ancients called the kidneys *(renes) rondines* and *renones*, like people do also nowadays. They are called also nefrundines by some, and they are also called *nephri* in 13th book of *terapentik*; in the *Treatise on nephretic disease* it is called *nephrisis*; for this reason, people who suffer of diseases of kidneys are called *nefretici*.

authorities. He subsequently introduces his anatomical findings as 'propositions' and gives proof for them (demonstratio) in the form of sensory experience (ad sensum). Demonstrations lacking the test of the sense are left sub judice.

The Kidney

In the *Commentaria*, the kidneys are thoroughly discussed in folios CLXXVIIverso – CLXXXrecto. We provide (fig. 10) a copy of lines 1–13 in folio CLXXVIIverso (the introduction to the topic). We also provide a copy (fig. 11) of lines 27–37 in folio CLXXVIIIverso and of lines 1–34 (folio CLXXIXrecto) which report on personal experiments of Berengario and provides his opinion about the existence of a sieve (colatorium) in the kidneys. Our personal translations of the passages in figures 10 and 11 are added to the figures.

A Comment on the Previous Passages

Berengario stresses immediately that Mondino's text on 'De Renibus' is clear enough, therefore he wants to add his own observation. Then he says that there are no kidneys in the animals and makes a philological approach on the origin of the words 'kidney and kidney diseases'. At this point he erronously quotes the *terapentike** which does not exist, instead of the *Therapeutike**.

Berengario experiments on the kidney. His experiment consists of injecting warm water in the emulgens vein to see whether it penetrates the urinary channel. This did not happen since the kidney was swollen and full of water. Therefore, he goes on by cutting the kidney surface and by repeating the injection of warm water in the vena emulgens and under these experimental conditions the water disappears. At this point he decides to open the renal channel (ureter) at the kidney extremity along the longer axis of the kidney. Part of the water penetrates the tissues, part of it finally enters the urinary channel through structures which resemble glandular tissue found in women's breasts. But Berengario looks for exact answers for his experiment (highest precision) devoted to finding a connection of the emulgens vein with the parenchyma, which is achieved by thin ramifications stretched on the breast-like glandular tissues. In a series of experiments he demonstrates that urine is not formed through a milk-like exudation process. Finally, he has a negative opinion about the existence of a sieve (colatorium), and has no difficulty in admitting the need for further experiments. At this time, however, he does not have enough data and appropriately waits to study additional kidneys.

Perhaps it should be stressed here that Berengario in the *Isagogae Breves* will soon be able to perform experiments on the site of urine's origin in the human fetus, and to underline the weakness of the kidney in diabetes, and their weakness in edema.

Accepi renes & poſui
ſiringam aqua calida plenam in uena emulgente:& uolui
uidere an ex uena emulgente penetraret ad porrum uriti/
dem aqua/ fortiter eam impellendo:& inueni ꝙ non:ueri
tas eſt ꝙ ren implebatur aqua & in magnũ eleuabatur tu/
morem/hoc uiſo ſuperficialiter:uulneraui renem:& dein/
de iterum cum ſiringa per uenam emulgẽtem in tali:rene
impoſui aquam etiam calidam ut melius aperirentur por/
ri & uenæ renum:&,tunc pẽr plagam prædictam ſuperfi/
cialem renis/exibat aqua a me per ſiringam itromiſſa:hac
experientia uiſa aperui porrum uritidem uſq; ad concauũ
renis:& per longitudinem renis inueni in ſubſtantia renis
media porrum uritidem eſſe in concauitate renis dilatatũ

CLXXIX

ad inſtar lacunæ:in qua lacuna iudicio meo generantur la
pides renum & tunc facta tali aparitione & inciſione ĩ por
ro uritide impoſui iterum ſiringa in uena emulgente eiuſ/
dem renis aperti & inciſi:& impellẽdo aquam cum ſirin/
ga per uenam emulgentem exibat talis aqua a ſubſtantia
renum inciſa circa porrum uritidem/& etiam exibat p par
tem interiorem porri uritidis aqua:ueritas eſt ꝙ maior q̃ti
tas exibat per concauitatem.i.per illam lacunam:quam fa
cit porrus uritides in renem q̃ per partem carneam renis:
& in illa lacuna ſiue in illo uacuo qđ facit porrus uritides
ſunt certæ carnes:quæ aſſimilantur papillis mamillarum
mulierum:ſunt tamen minores:& circa illas carnes exibat
aqua illa per me prius in rene intromiſſa cum ſiringa in ue
na emulgente.Et ego diligentiſſime uolui uidere qua uia
talis aqua exibat a uena emulgente ad porrum uritidem:
& uidi uenam emulgentem terminari de magna uena in
minores uenas/deinde ĩ minores:& uidi illas minimas ue
nas tẽdere uſq; ad extremas partes renum/ & uidi aliquas
ex prædictis uenis paruis tendere uerſus porum uritidem
ad illas carnes prædictas ſimiles papillis mamillarum/ &
circa eas uidi terminari tales uenas paruas portãtes aquã
urinalem ad lacunã porri uritidis prædictam : & prædictæ
carnes papillares habẽt baſim uerſus partem in qua termi
nantur rami uenæ emulgentis & cuſpidem uerſus lacunã
porri uritidis.Et porrus uritides nerueus eſt:perforatus fo
ramine notabili ubi ẽ cuſpis talis carnis papillaris/ forte ut
tale foramẽ nõ claudat . Et alias ego cogitabam ꝙ a carne
tali papillari reſudaret urina in cõcauitatem porri uritidis
eo modo quo reſudat lac a carne papillæ : & hoc nõ potui
uidere.Hæc ſupra ſcripta ſunt a me/tanq mihi impfecte co
gnita uſq; in hodiernũ diẽ/forte ꝙ ſuccedentibus pluribus
ſubiectis pro anatomia renũ(ut ſpero)certificabor de ma/
iori reſolutione talis colatorii an ſit in natura uel ne . Et ſic
pro nunc hæc ſufficiant pro opinionibus colatorii.

Fig. 11. Anastatic copy from the original of some passages on the kidneys (Folio CLXXVIIIverso and CLXXIXrecto) of the text in Carpi *Commentaria* on Mondino, with translation in the right column.

CLXXVIIIverso

I received kidneys and I put a syringe full of warm water in the emulgens vein; I wanted to see, pushing strongly the water, whether it would penetrate from the emulgens vein to the urinary channel. And I have found that not. The truth is that the kidney was full of water and was swollen, forming a big tumor. Once I saw that, I lacerated superficially the kidney; and, furtherly, with the syringe, I introduced again into this kidney water which was also warm, through the emulgens vein, so that the channels and veins of the kidneys became more open. And then, through the superficial incision of the kidney said above, the water introduced by myself with the syringe went away. Once I saw this experience, I opened the urinary channel till the cavity of kidney; and, on the whole length of the kidney, I found, in the middle of the substance of the kidney, that the urinal channel is dilated in the concave part of the kidney like a cavity; and, in this cavity, stones arise, in my opinion.

CLXXIXrecto

Once seen that and cut the urinary channel, I put once again the syringe in the draining vein of the same kidney, open and cut. And, while I pushed water with the syringe through the draining vein, this water went out of the substance of the kidneys cut around the urinary channel; and water went also out through the lower part of the urinary channel; the truth is that a higher quantity of water went out through the concave part of the kidney, i.e. through the cavity which the urinary channel produces within the kidney, than through the fleshy parts of the kidney; and, in this cavity, it is to say: in this void which the urinal channel produces, there are some fleshes, which are similar to the extremity of women's breast; they are smaller, however; and the water introduced by me into the draining vein by means of the syringe went out around these fleshes.
I wanted to see with the highest precision through which way this water went out of the draining vein into the urinary channel. And I saw that the draining vein is a large one which ends in veins smaller and smaller. And I saw that the very small veins are extended till the end of the kidney. And I saw that some of the small veins described above are stretched in the direction of the urinary channel through the fleshes we said to be similar to the extremities of women's breast. And, around these fleshes, I saw that these little veins which carry the urinary water we said, end near the cavity of the urinary channel we have described above. And the glandular fleshes we have said, have their bottom oriented towards the part in which the branches of the draining vein end, and their top oriented towards the cavity of the urinary channel. And the urinary channel is of nervous matter: it is perforated with a visible perforation where there is the top of this flesh like breasts extremities, probably to avoid that the perforation could be obturated.
Other times, I thought that urine could exude from this flesh similar to breasts extremities into the cavity of the urinary channel, in the way in which milk is exuded from the flesh of breasts extremities. But, I haven't been able to see that.
All this has been described by me as still imperfectly known by me till now. Maybe, if more cases of anatomy of kidneys happen (as I hope), I shall confirm, about the higher permeability of this *colatorium,* whether it is in nature or not. Now, this is enough on the opinions dealing with the *colatorium.*

Acknowledgements

Supported by funds made available at the Second University of Naples.

The authors are pleased to acknowledge the support received from many sources. In particular they wish to thank the Bibliothèque Nationale de France, Paris, France; Biblioteca Comunale, Carpi; Biblioteca Nazionale, Naples; Biblioteca Istituto Mazzini, Naples; The Archiginnasio of Bologna; The Pinacoteca of Bologna; Studio Canonab, Naples, and Doctor's University Service, Naples. The following individuals provided extraordinary help: Dr. Giulia Colussi, Naples, Dr. Leonardo Gallo, Naples; Dr. Marina Zuccoli, Bologna; Dr. Marisa Ursano, Naples; Dr. Daniela Gragnaniello, Ferrara; Dr. Gianfranco Arietti and Dr. Gaetano La Manna, University of Bologna, and Dr. Joseph Sepe, Maryland.

References

1 Dr. Burggraeve: Œuvres Médico-Chirurgicales. Paris, Ballière, 1862, vol 1, pp 26–30.
2 Portal M: Historie de 'Anatomie et de la Chirurgie. Paris, 1770, pp 271–281.
3 Guglielmini JF: De claris Bononiae anatomicis. Oration in theatro anatomico recitata (1735). Typographia S. Thomae Aquinatis, Bononiae, 1735.
4 Gelati A: Iacopo Berengario da Carpi; in: Memorie storiche e documenti sulla città e sull'antico principato di Carpi. Carpi, Pederzoli e Rossi, 1879–1880, (1840), pp 179–200.
5 Medici M: Compendio Storico della Scuola Anatomica di Bologna. Dal rinascimento delle scienze e delle lettere a tutto il secolo XVIII. Bologna, Tipografia Governativa della Volpe e del Sassi, 1857.
6 Guaitoli P: Appendice sulla precedente memoria; in: Memorie storiche e documenti sulla città e sull'antico Principato di Carpi. Carpi, Pederzoli e Rossi, 1879–1880, pp 203–242.
7 Putti V: Berengario da Carpi. Saggio biografico et bibliografico seguito dalla traduzione del *'De Fractura calvae sive cranei'.* Bologna, Cappelli Editore, 1937.
8 Brambilla GA: Storia delle Scoperte Fisico-Medico-Anatomico-Chirurgiche fatte dagli Uomini Illustri Italiani. Milano, Imperial Monistero di San Ambrogio Maggiore, 1781, Tomo II, Parte I, pp 127–140.
9 De Renzi S: Storia della Medicina in Italia. Napoli, Tipografia del Filiatre-Sebezio, 1845, vol III.
10 Lind LR: Jacopo Berengario da Carpi. A short introduction to anatomy (Isagogae Breves). Chicago, University of Chicago Press, 1959.
11 French RK: Berengario da Carpi and the use of commentary in anatomical teaching; in Wear A, French RR, Lonnie IM (eds): The Medical Renaissance of the Sixteenth Century. Cambridge, Cambridge University Press, 1985, pp 42–74.
12 Singer C: A short history of anatomy and physiology from the Greeks to Harvey (the evolution of anatomy). New York, Dover, 1957.
13 Bernabeo AR, D'Antuono G: La scuola medica di Bologna, settecento anni di storia. Bologna, Firma Libri, 1988.
14 Vasari G: Le Vite Dé più Eccellenti Pittori, Scultori et Architetti. Bologna, Heredi di Evangelista Dozza, 1647.
15 Cellini B: Vita di Benvenuto Cellini orefice e scultore fiorentino da lui medesimo scritta. Milano, Società Italiana dei Classici Italiani, 1806.
16 Guy de Chauliac: Anatom. 1363, Cap I, Doctr I, 136 3.
17 da Carpi Ugo: Enciclopedia Zanichelli a cura di Edigeo. Bologna, 1995.
18 da Carpi Ugo: Enciclopedia Treccani, 1951, vol IX, p 142.
19 da Carpi Ugo: Thesauro de scrittori. Venetia, Ludovicus, 1525.

Contributions of Padua to Nephrology
(Dedicated to Arturo Borsatti)

American Journal of Nephrology

Am J Nephrol 1999;19:213–221

Jewish Medicine and the University of Padua: Contribution of the Padua Graduate Toviah Cohen to Nephrology

Shaul G. Massry[a] Miroslaw Smogorzewski[a] Elizur Hazani[b]
Shaul M. Shasha[b]

[a]Division of Nephrology and Department of Medicine, University of Southern California, School of Medicine, Los Angeles, Calif., USA; [b]Division of Nephrology, Western Galilee Hospital, Nahairya, Israel

Key Words
Jewish medicine · University of Padua · Cohen, Toviah · Nephrology, 17th century

Abstract
During the period of the 11th to 17th century, the access of Jews to European universities was restricted and even those who were fortunate enough to be admitted to a university were not awarded a degree at the end of their studies. An exception to this situation was the University of Padua that allowed Jewish students to study and awarded them degrees; indeed 229 physicians graduated from this university between 1409 and 1721. Among these physicians there were many luminaries such as Joseph Del Medigo, Salmon Congeliano and Toviah Cohen. The latter made many contributions to the field of nephrology. In this treatise *Maaseh Toviah* he discussed uroscopy, kidney function, body fluid homeostasis and obstructive uropathy.

In order to understand the relationship between Jews, Jewish medicine and the University of Padua, one must be familiar with Jewish medicine in the medieval period and the situation of medicine and its practice as well as with the process of medical education in Europe during the 12th century and onward. Therefore, a short background is in order.

Jewish Medicine before the 12th Century

As indicated in previous publications [1, 2], the medical knowledge among Jews up to the 5th century was derived from three sources. First, the Bible which provided extensive principles for maintaining hygiene and prevention of diseases as well as explicit codes for dietary regimens. Second, anatomical observations obtained during the dissection of animals for the sake of determining their suitability for eating (kosher) which provided a pathological basis for the understanding of the disease process. Third, clinical observations made by rabbis and scholars on the presentation of various ailments. None of this information was codified in medical books, but rather it was incorporated into religious books (the Bible, the Mishna and the Talmud).

KARGER
Fax + 41 61 306 12 34
E-Mail karger@karger.ch
www.karger.com

© 1999 S. Karger AG, Basel
0250–8095/99/0192–0213$17.50/0

Accessible online at:
http://BioMedNet.com/karger

Shaul G. Massry, MD
Chief Division of Nephrology, University of Southern California School of Medicine
2025 Zonal Avenue
Los Angeles, CA 90033 (USA)
Tel. +1 323 226 7337, Fax +1 323 226 5390

The first Jewish medical book is *Safer Harfuoth* of Asaph Judaeus (Asaph Harufeh) who lived either in the 3rd or the 6th century [2]. This was followed by the books of Isaac Judaeus (Isaac Israeli, 850–950 AD) and included books on fever, on urine, on remedies and on guidelines for physicians [2]. Then came the medical writings and books of the great Jewish physician of the 12th century, Maimonides who lived between 1135 and 1205 [1]. There were other less significant Jewish books. Most of these were written in Arabic which was the prevailing language during the glorious times of the Islamic culture. Some of these books were written in Hebrew.

In the 12th century, rigid Islamic orthodoxy, which did not encourage scientific endeavors, was on the rise. As a result, the hub for the intellectual and scientific progress began to shift from the Islamic centers to the more scientifically receptive Christian Europe. Also, the emergence of Islamic fundamentalism and of sects like Almohades in North Africa and Spain forced Jews and Jewish Scholars to drift to other European countries. These events created at least two significant challenges for Jews and Jewish medicine.

First, the universities of Europe did not admit Jews and even those universities which did accept Jewish students did not permit them to take the final examination for the degree.[1] This situation almost precluded Jews from studying medicine at the universities of Europe. However, Jews were interested in being doctors for several reasons. First, this profession provided a great status in the community. Second, the Jewish religion and the great rabbis gave great support to the physician by stating: 'One cannot live in a city which does not have a doctor within its boundaries.' Third, the discrimination against the Jews by the authorities of Europe at the time made it extremely difficult for Jews to engage in other professions.

Despite these conditions, Jews continued to study medicine by utilizing the common and accepted practice of the time that one can gain medical knowledge and become a physician by working with a noted practicing physician. This process, however, was costly since the student was required to pay a substantial amount of money to the physician-teacher. Therefore, this approach was common among families of physicians where fathers taught sons without cost. Also, students sought to marry daughters of famous physicians with the stipulation that the dowry would be a commitment of the father of the bride to teach the groom the art and the practice of medicine. This phenomenon is probably the reason behind the finding of dynasties of Jewish physicians among the Jewish families of the time. Also, the practice of private teaching of medicine among the Jews may explain the large number of Jewish physicians in European towns and cities despite their small Jewish population and despite the inability of Jews to enter universities [3].

Second, the prevailing language of medical books in Europe was Latin with which Jews were not familiar. The scholars of the Jewish community solved this problem by translating Arabic and Latin books into Hebrew making the medical knowledge of the time available to the Jewish students of medicine. This translation fervor was so widespread that by the 16th century there were about 15,000 medical Hebrew manuscripts available in various libraries [4]. This phenomenon led the Rector of the University of Leipzig to lament the following in 1518 [4]:

> 'In the libraries of the Jews, a treasure of medical science lies hidden, a treasure as scarce as is to be found in other language. Nobody ... will be able to get access to this treasure without intimate knowledge of the Hebrew grammar.'

Jewish scholars also translated Arabic and Jewish medical writings into Latin, a process which facilitated the infusion of significant and important medical knowledge into Europe.

Thus, due to the hostile attitude of the European universities to Jews during the period between the 12th and 16th century, the study of medicine by Jews was difficult and the writing of medical books by Jews was hampered. Indeed, there is no known noted Jewish medical book during this period of time. However, Jewish scholars contributed greatly to medicine of that time through their translation effort.

University of Padua

One of the great universities of Italy is the University of Padua which essentially emerged from the student body of the University of Bologna [5–8]. In 1222, a group of students had a quarrel with the city of Bologna, and they decided to migrate to Padua. They were accompanied by some of their teachers and laid the foundation for the University of Padua. It must be mentioned that, at the time, universities were in reality a group of students who selected their teachers and formed their educational organization. The University of Padua flourished in the 14th century under the rule of the Carrara family. However,

[1] The reasons for this attitude are complicated and multifactorial and require extensive discussion. Therefore, they could not be included in this article.

the greatest time and prosperity of the University of Padua began when Venice gained control of Padua in 1405.

The University of Padua was tolerant to others and accepted protestants and Jews. This was possible since the University of Padua was outside the papal control. This tolerance and liberal approach attracted students from many countries, and they were organized according to their nationalities (Naciones). Indeed, even in the early days of the university (1228 AD), there were already four groups of nations including French and Romans, Spaniards and Catalans, Germans, and Italians. The study of medicine at the University of Padua began in 1250 and in the beginning of the 14th century a faculty was established that taught medicine, physics and natural sciences.

Jews, Jewish Medicine and the University of Padua

In the hostile environment toward the Jewish students by the European universities, there was a bright light shining from Padua and its university which exercised considerable tolerance toward the Jews [5–11]. This was evident from the beginning of the 14th century and reached its peak between the 16th and the 18th century. This favorable attitude led Jews to migrate to Padua, and in the early part of the 17th century (1616 AD) there were about 700 Jews living in Padua.

The first Medical Doctorate was bestowed on a Jew by the University of Padua in 1409. Between 1517 and 1619, 80 Jews graduated from the Medical School of Padua, and this number increased significantly, thereafter. Indeed, 149 Jews received the degree of Doctor of Medicine from the University of Padua between 1619 and 1721, and the number increased to 325 by 1816. Some of these physicians achieved fame and distinguished themselves by their scholarly contributions. Among these were Joseph Del Medigo, Salmon Congeliano and Toviah Cohen. A list of the Jewish physicians who graduated from Padua has been published by Modena and Morpurgo [11].

Many of the Jewish graduates of Padua returned to their original countries and cities where they practiced medicine. A case in point is Poland which had many families of physicians who studied in Padua (about 50 physicians). These include the De Jonases in Lemberg (Lvov), the Montaltos in Lublin, the De Limas and Wincklers in Posen (Poznan), the Gordons in Vilna and Marpurgos in Cracow. Del Medigo practiced in Vilna, Frankfurt and Prague [10]. As we will discuss later, Toviah Cohen practiced in Cracow, Adrianopole and Constantinople. Thus, the medical teaching in Padua exerted a far-reaching influence on Jewish medicine and its practice in many countries and cities.

The University of Padua was sensitive to its Jewish students in other ways as well. The Jews were allowed to wear the black beret, similar to that of non-Jewish students, rather than the yellow beret required of Jewish students in other institutions. This sensitivity was also manifested in the diploma of the Doctorate of Medicine granted to Jewish graduates [10]. Figure 1 provides a picture of the diploma of Copilius Pictor whose Jewish name was Koppel (or Jacob) Maler. The diploma starts with the inscription 'In Dei Aeterni Nomine Amen', i.e., in the name of eternal God. This in contrast to 'In Christi Nomine, Amen', i.e., in the name of Christ, in the diploma for Christian graduates. The date of the diploma of the Jewish graduates also differed from that in the diploma of Christians. For example, the date in Pictor's diploma was 'Currente Anno MDCLXXXXV' while in a Christian diploma the dates were linked to the birth of Christ such as 'Anno a partu Virginis' or 'Anno a Christi Nativitate'. In addition, the diplomas were signed by witnesses and the university sought Jewish witnesses to sign the diploma of Jewish graduates. The diploma of Pictor was signed by Sabbatheus Marini, a Paduan Hebrew doctor of philosophy and medicine and by the Venetian Jewish doctor Simon Mischita. Finally, the ceremony of the presentation of the diplomas for the Catholic graduates was held in the church and was presided by the bishop while that of Jewish graduates took place in a location in the university and was presided by an nonclerical official. Similar consideration was made for non-Catholic Christians during the presentation of their diploma. Later the University of Padua created the Collegium Venetum (Venetian College) to organize the ceremonies for the presentation of the diplomas to Jews and non-Catholic Christians. The first head of the Collegium Venetum was Santorio Sanctorius.

Another manifestation of the Jewish influence on Padua medicine and of the respect of Padua scholars for the Hebrew language is found in the book of Andreas Vesalius *De Humani Corporis Fabrica.* Vesalius gave Hebrew names together with Latin and Greek names of anatomical structures (fig. 2). The Hebrew terms were provided to Vesalius by the Paduan Jewish Scholar Lazaro de Frigis who obtained them from the Talmud and from the Canon of Avicenna which was translated into Hebrew.

Although the tolerance of the University of Padua to Jews was a unique phenomenon, it was not without some biases and adverse attitude towards Jewish students. For example the tuition for Jews was double of that for non-

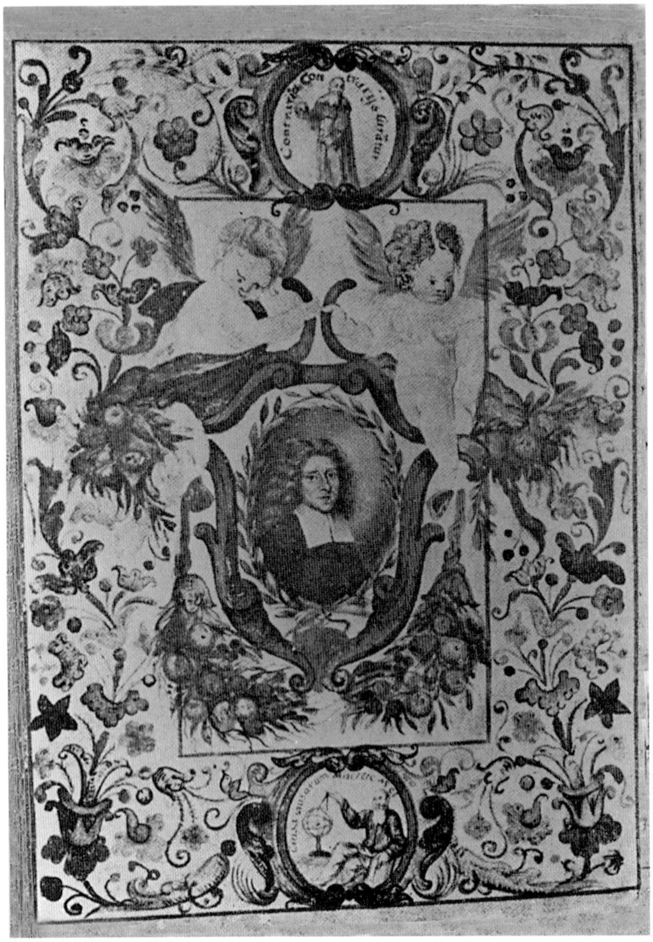

Contra vim Con ... nulla ... herbis

a

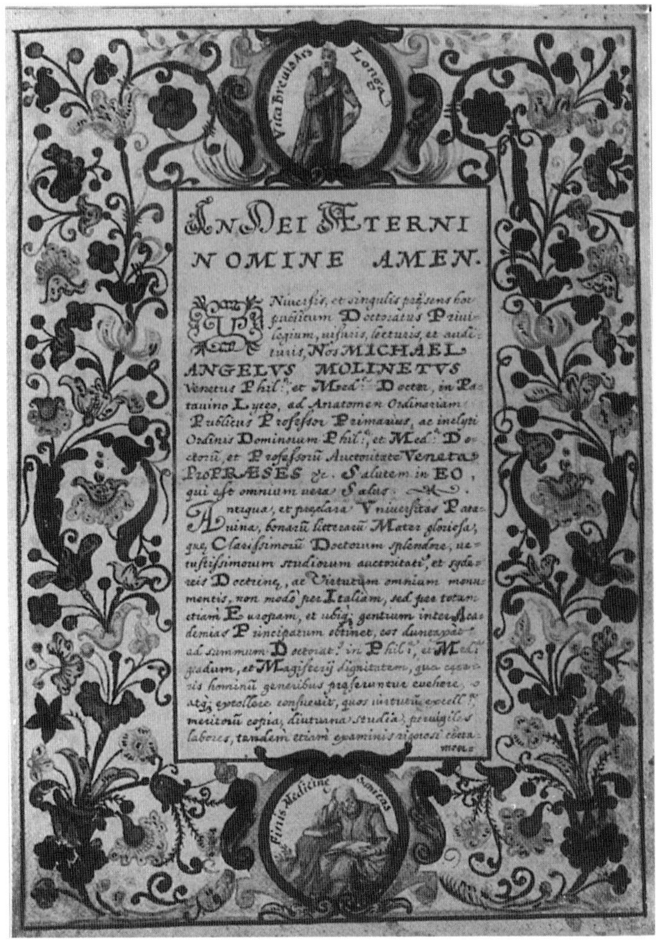

Vita Brevis Ars Longa
IN DEI ÆTERNI
NOMINE AMEN.

b

Fig. 1a, b. Diploma of Capillus Pictor, a medical graduate of Padua. For the difference between the Jewish diploma and the Catholic diploma granted by the University of Padua, the readers are referred to the text of the article.

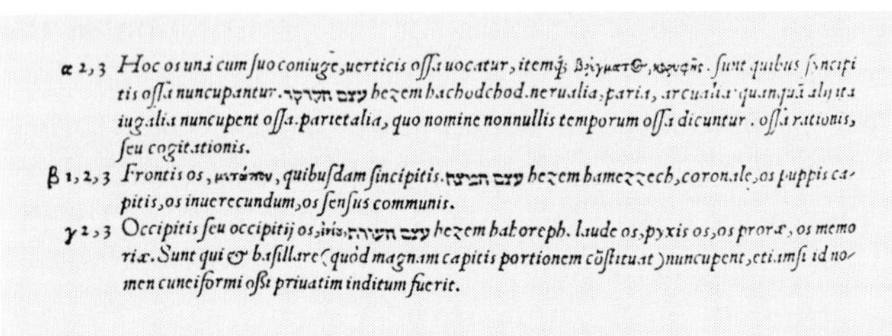

α 2, 3 Hoc os unà cum suo coniuge, uerticis ossa uocatur, itemq́; βρέγματος, κορυφῆς. sunt quibus sincipitis ossa nuncupantur. עצם הקדקד bezem bachodchod. neruealia, paria, arcualia quanquā alij ita iugalia nuncupent ossa. parietalia, quo nomine nonnullis temporum ossa dicuntur. ossa rationis, seu cogitationis.
β 1, 2, 3 Frontis os, μετώπου, quibusdam sincipitis. עצם המצח bezem bamezzech, coronale, os puppis capitis, os inuerecundum, os sensus communis.
γ 2, 3 Occipitis seu occipitij os, ἰνίου, עצם העורף bezem baboreph. laude os, pyxis os, os proræ, os memoriæ. Sunt qui & basillare (quòd magnam capitis portionem cōstituat) nuncupent, etiamsi id nomen cuneiformi ossi priuatim inditum fuerit.

Fig. 2. A photograph of a text from the anatomy book of Andreas Vesalius *De Humani Corporis Fabrica* which shows the Hebrew names of various bones.

Jews. Jewish students were also subjected to special taxes such as the requirement to provide after their graduation 170 pounds of sweets and meat to Christian students. These inconveniences were outweighed by the exceptional scholarly and intellectual opportunities provided to Jews by the University of Padua.

Toviah Cohen (1652–1729)

Biography

Toviah Cohen, also known Tobias Kohn or Katz or Tobiasz Kohn, is a graduate of the University of Padua (fig. 3) [12–14]. He was the last physician of a family of many physicians. His grandfather (Eleazer Cohen) who came to Crakow from Safed, Palestine was a physician.

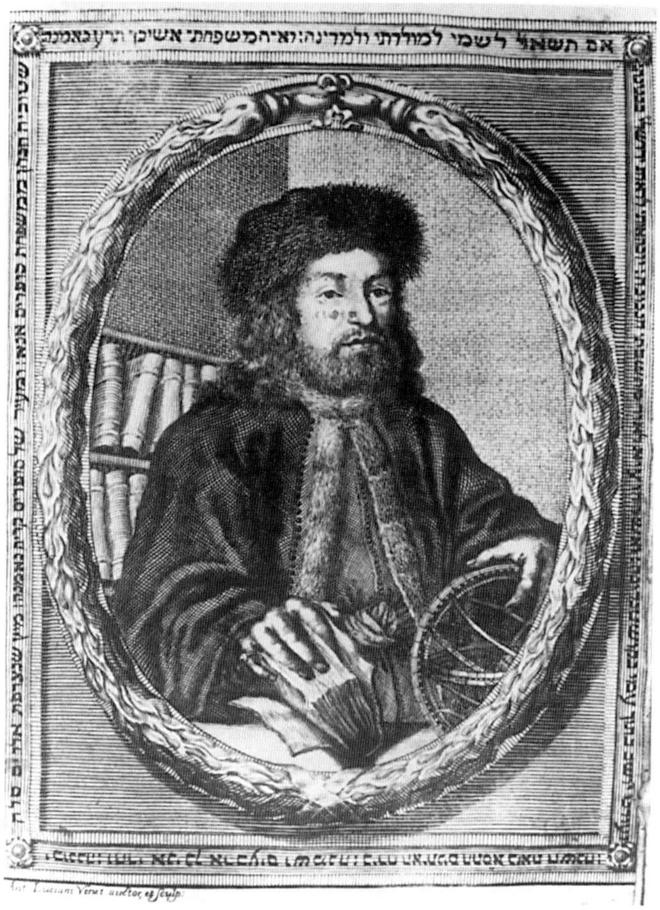

Fig. 3. A portrait of Toviah Cohen. Note the Hebrew writing that frames the picture. It translates as follows (clockwise from left upper corner): 'If you ask for my name, my ancestry and my country I shall answer: know ye that I am Toviah the Cohen. I come from a learned family and from a city of learned people, Metz the faithful city that is in France, may God guard it forever. I will be forty-eight in September this year, 1701, and I live with my people in Constantinople. And may (God) who published my thoughts grant me the chance to see the rebuilding of Jersualem.' The statement reflects his deep religious belief and his yearning to live in Jerusalem which he fulfilled later in his life.

His father Moses Kohn practiced medicine in Noral, Poland but he was forced to leave in 1649 to Metz, France because of the atrocities of the Cossacks against the Jews. He had two children; one of them was Toviah who was born in 1652. Eight years after the birth of Toviah, his father died. Toviah and his brother were raised by their uncle since their mother remarried and left Metz. The uncle sent the two children to Cracow for Jewish education. Toviah entered a Jewish school (Yeshivah) in Cracow.

Toviah was very enthusiastic to continue his education and to study medicine since this profession was a family tradition. There are some indications that he engaged in medicine before his formal medical studies suggesting that he gained medical knowledge by working under the tutelage of a practicing physician. He soon realized that he needs a formal education in the medical field which could only be provided by a university. However, it was extremely difficult at that itme for Jews to be admitted to a German University. Therefore, he and his friend Gabriel Felix sought, and after great difficulties, obtained permission from Frederick Wilhelm I, the Grand Elector of Brandenburg, to enroll in the University of Frankfurt an der Oder. The Grand Elector supported them financially during their studies. Indeed, Toviah and his friend Felix entered the university on June 17, 1678. They felt indebted to the Grand Elector and as a gesture of their appreciation they gave him a scroll containing tables of Hebrew grammar. However, there was one caveat in this arrangement; they were not allowed to take the examination for a degree from the university.

Toviah left Frankfurt for Padua to obtain his degree in medicine. He enrolled in the University of Padua in 1681 and 2 years later (June 25, 1683), he received the title of Doctor of Medicine. Toviah was always attracted by Padua which was tolerant to Jews, provided an excellent intellectual atmosphere, and was a ferment for new ideas in medicine such as the chemical philosophy of Paracelsus for the basis of health and disease compared with the humoral theory of Galen.

After his graduation from the University of Padua, he went back to Cracow and practiced medicine there. Several years later he went to Adrianopole and then to Constantinople. With the support of Prince Maurocordata and the great Vazir Rumi Pasha he rose to be the Court Physician of Sultan Ahmad III.

His success in Adrianopole and Constantinople permitted him to accumulate great wealth and quietness of mind that allowed him to devote time to scholarly endeavors. These efforts resulted in his famous Hebrew book מעשה טוביה, *Ma'aseh Toviah*, i.e. the work and story of Toviah, which he wrote in Adrianopole. In order to publish his book, he enticed the publisher Jacob Aboab of the publishing house Stamparia Bragadina to print the book which appeared in 1708 (fig. 4). The preface to the book was written by Salmon Conegliano (1642–1719 AD) a noted and famous physician and teacher of the time, who also was a graduate of the University of Padua. The book of Toviah was immediately accepted by Italian and German physicians of the time; it was published in five

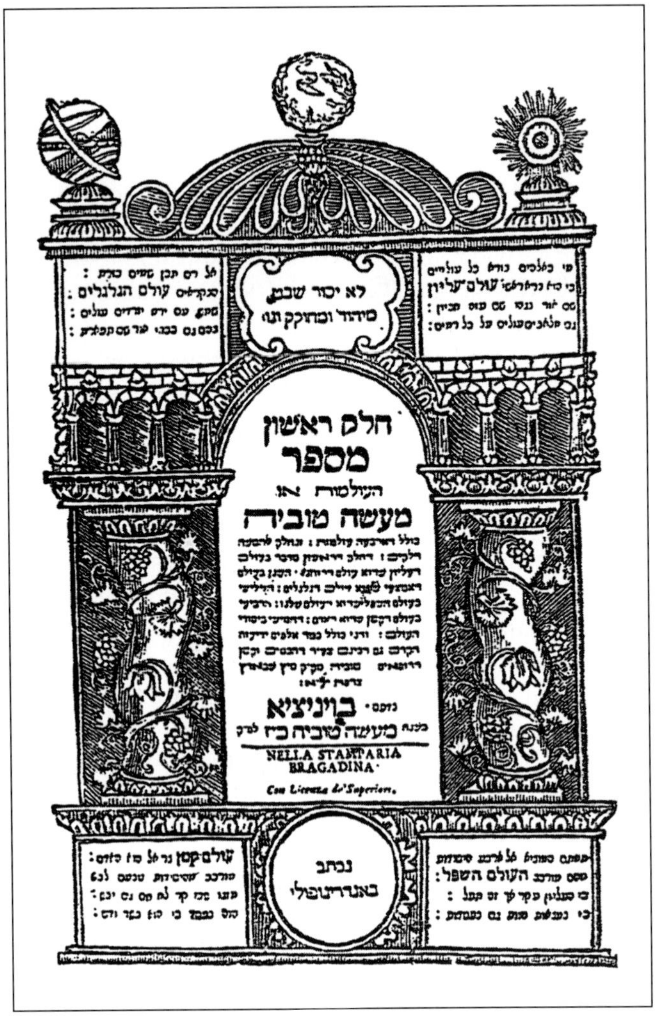

Fig. 4. Title page of the first edition of *Ma'aseh Toviah*. It indicates that it was written in Adrianopole and published in Venice by the publishing house Stamparia Bragadina.

additional editions, the last of which appeared in 1907. The first is the most accurate and ornate of the five editions.

In recognition of his success and fame, he was asked back to Padua to provide a lecture during the meeting of the Faculty of Padua. This event was a source of great pride for him.

After a short visit to Poland to meet friends and family, he returned to Constantinople. In 1724, he decided to settle in Jerusalem to concentrate on the study of religion and religious writings. This is not surprising since his father was a rabbinical scholar and his grandfather came from Palestine. In fact, he expressed his wish to go to Jerusalem in the writings which frame his portrait which was published in his book (fig. 3). Toviah died in 1729 at the age of 77 and is buried in Jerusalem. He seems to have come to the City of David rich and wealthy but died poor. He states: 'All I had was stolen and taken from me.'

Medical Writings of Toviah

Toviah lived in a transitional period of medicine. The influence of Hippocratic and Galenic concepts still existed but new challenges to these ideas were put forward as a result of new trends in medicine. Dissection of the human body had advanced greatly and provided detailed information about the structure of the various organs. These aspects of medicine were championed by Andreas Vesalius (1514–1564 AD) and Realdo Colombo (1516–1559 AD) in the University of Padua [15, 16]. The microscope was invented at the end of the 16th century and permitted new discoveries. William Harvey (1578–1657 AD) discovered the circulation and Malphighi (1628–1694 AD) described the renal corpuscle. Therefore, the medical writings of Toviah were influenced by both the old and new trends of medicine.

One must emphasize that the fame of Toviah is not due to special discoveries, originality or creativeness but it is due to the vast knowledge he presented in his book *Ma'aseh Toviah*, and the fact that he wrote it in Hebrew and made his knowledge available to his Jewish brethren. Thus, he is a famous physician for the Jews but little is mentioned about him in the historical accounts of medicine and not even in the Turkish medical sources.

The book is an encyclopedic treatise of 138 pages. It has two parts. The first encompasses five sections that deal with theology, astronomy and natural sciences. The second part which constitutes about a third of the book deals with medicine, hygiene, medical botany and secret diseases (syphilitic afflictions). One section discusses the diseases of the 'Closed Garden', i.e. gynecological and obstetrical diseases. Another provides information on the disease of the 'Fruit of the Body', i.e. diseases of children.

One of his interesting concepts is provided in figure 5. Toviah compared the anatomy of the body to the various parts of a house. The hair is the roof, the ears are represented by the corner of the roof, the eyes are the windows of the house and the mouth is its door. The lungs represent the upper level of the house which provides ventilation. The liver and spleen are the middle story where cooking occurs and where the cellar (spleen) is found. The kidney is the water well and the lower intestines are the lavatory. The feet provide the foundation of the house. Again, this notion is not his original concept but he described it in a more detailed and elaborate way than previous similar analogies. Indeed, William Harvey (1578–1657) also compared certain organs of the body to certain parts of a house; the stomach is the kitchen and the lung is the parlor of the house.

One of Toviah's original medical description is that of 'plica polonica' [14]. Although some doubt this fact, he definitely described the etiology, prevention and treatment of plica polonica. This entity was common among Polish indigent people and presented itself by entangling and sticking together of the head hair giving rise to rope formations, irritation of the skin of the scalp and headache. He indicated that the plica polonica is the result of a lack of cleanliness and inappropriate hygiene of the hair. Indeed, the individuals affected with the disease did not wash, clean and comb their hair even once a year. This practice resulted in infection of the root of the hair and thrombosis of the superficial veins. Toviah provided preventive measures as well as remedies for this condition.

Toviah's Contribution to Nephrology

Toviah provided in his book discussions on the urinary tract and on urine. He considered the kidney the well of the urine, the ureters the drainage tubes of the well, and the bladder represented the pool for the storage of the urine. He defined the urine as a juice that is derived from the blood and is generated by the kidney from drinking liquids and eating moist, watery food stuff; this definition implies two principles. First, the urine is either secreted or filtered by the kidney from the blood. These concepts were known at this time and were influenced in part by the work of Galen [17]. Second, water and fluid intake is the source of the urine, an idea that fits our current concept.

He clearly stated that the urinary system is required for the maintenance of the body and this system may be afflicted by many illnesses. This concept embodies the notion that the urinary system is essential for body homeostasis. Similar ideas are found in the aphorisms of Maimonides [1].

Toviah considered that the study of the characteristics of the urine (constitution, appearance, volume, color and odor) provides important clues to various aliments of the body. These concepts have been espoused by Greek, Byzantine and Jewish physicians before him [1, 2]. The significance of urine examination, as Toviah saw it, led him to provide ten cautionary caveats to ensure the accuracy of this procedure (table 1).

His thoughts about urine volume are interesting. A normal urine volume indicates that the amount of urine is in proportion to the amount of fluid intake. A large urine

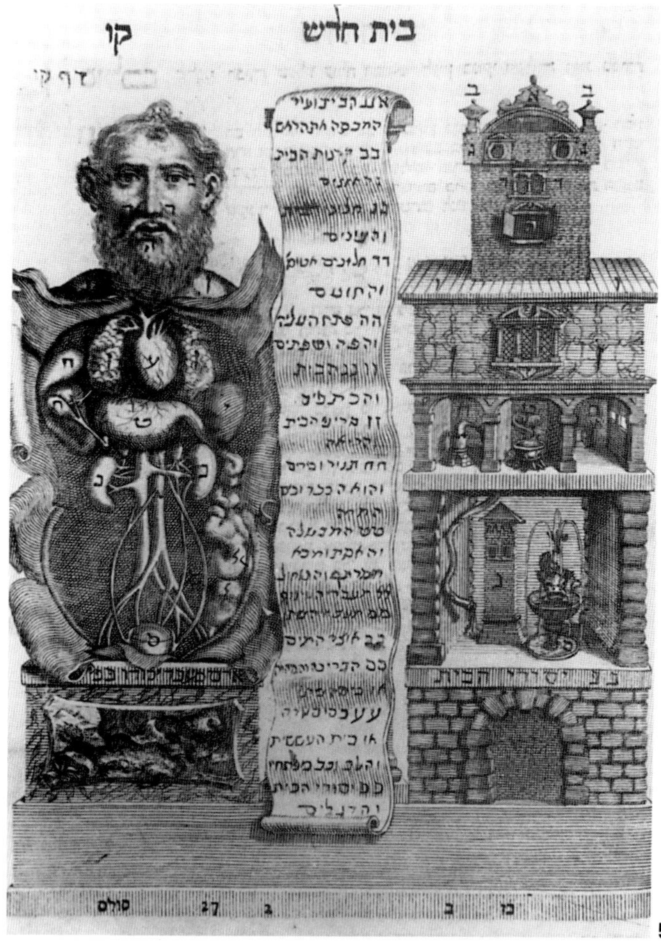

5

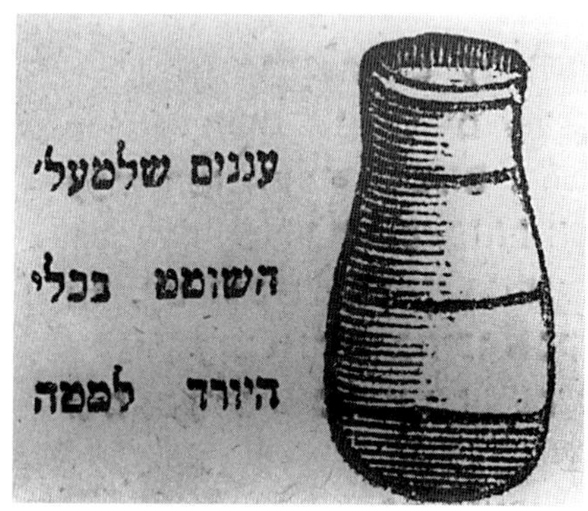

6

Fig. 5. Comparison of the body to a house. See the next for explanation.

Fig. 6. Picture of the flask recommended by Toviah for urine collection. Just as the physicians divide the body into three parts, the head, the chest and the abdomen, so is the urine in the vessel divided into three parts. They are: the top part (the clouds that are above) is associated with the head (diseases?), the second part (wandering in the vessel) is associated with the chest (disease?), and the bottom part (yeast or sediment), where matters of illness and of digestion are observed. The translation of the Hebrew writings are as follows: clouds that are above (upper line), wandering in the vessel (middle line) and sediment (lower line).

volume suggests wetness of the body (overhydration), and small volume denotes dryness of the body or excess perspiration (dehydration). These statements clearly relate urine volume to the state of body fluid and is in concert with modern day notions of fluid homeostasis and the important role of the kidney is this process.

Toviah indicated that the pool of the urine (bladder) is made of two skins (tunica or layers), one with the force which draws and the other with the force that propels the urine into the two tubes from the kidneys to the bladder.[2]

He, of course, did not realize that the urine reaches the bladder through the peristaltic movements of the ureters. On the other hand, he raised, most likely, for the first time, the concept of vesicoureteral reflux through the force of the muscular layer of the bladder to propel urine back into the ureters.

Toviah defined four ailments that may affect the urinary system. First, 'urinary retention' which is due to several causes including blood clots, thick mucus, excess spirit, stone, verruca or polyp. This condition is associated with renal pain (colic) which could be easily differentiated from abdominal colic (affliction of the intestine). 'The kidney pain is stuck like a wedge in one side, right or left, and at times, it will extend from below the navel along the ureters. At all times there may be a delay (oliguria) our shut down (anuria) of urine.' In contrast, abdominal colic spreads from one side to the other almost all over the abdomen and at times with bowel sounds. If urinary retention is due to a lodged stone, Toviah recommended drinking tea made of certain herbs that are capable of promoting diuresis and breaking down stones.

The second ailment of the urinary system is 'hesitancy of urination' which should more appropriately be called burning urine ('dysuria' in Latin and the 'burning disease' in German). This condition may be recognized by three signs: (1) the urine drips like boiling water, drop after drop continuously, (2) pain is experienced during urination, not before and not after, and (3) it is mainly due to fever of the kidneys and bladder (urinary tract infection) and at times stone in the bladder. He proposed the use of drugs that cool and cleanse the bladder (treat infection), and the patient should drink barely water, herbal tea and juices.

The third ailment is 'dripping of the urine' (the 'cold disease' in German). This condition is caused by coldness of the abdomen and at times of sour mucus. It is called dripping since the patient gives one drop and stops, then a second drop, and a third drop, all with pauses between drops. (This ailment may fit enlargement of the prostate or afflictions of the urethra.)

Table 1. Ten mandatory caveats for the observation of urine

1	The urine must be sampled once and not many times[a]
2	This must be in the morning on an empty stomach, when the food is already digested[b]
3	The urine should be taken in a clear, transparent pumpkin-shaped glass vessel[c]
4	The container should be covered and kept in a warm place in order to protect it from cold and heat, and from direct sunlight
5	The urine must not be observed less than 1 h after sampling[d]
6	And no later than 6 h, which is the time limit for observing the cloudiness and other components of the urine[e]
7	If during this time the urine is altered due to an external or internal cause, the container should be immersed in a cup of water so that the urine may resume its original form
8	Observation of the urine must be performed in a well-lighted place, but not in direct sunlight
9	Urine must not be sampled after the drinking of wine, nor after eating saffron or taking medication like rhubarb, which easily alter the urine[f]
10	The physician who fears that the urine may be altered by exposure to air or to sunlight should place his hand on the side of the container facing the sun to serve as a barrier between the sun and the container

[a] This is most likely to ensure that one would obtain the whole volume of the urine which is in the bladder at the time of urination.
[b] This ensures that the urine characteristics are not influenced by products of food taken by the patients.
[c] Toviah thought that various layers of the urine as displayed in a pumpkin-shaped flask (fig. 6) reflect diseases of various parts of the body. The top part is associated with the head, the second part is associated with the chest and the bottom part reflects ailment of digestion.
[d] To ensure that sediments had already settled.
[e] To ensure that urine characteristics were not altered by external or internal (bacteria) conditions.
[f] Toviah had recognized that alcohol and drugs may alter the characteristics of the urine.

The four ailments is 'polyuria' which denotes 'continuous urination with no ability to stop and it is called diabetes in Latin'. This illness has two characteristics. (1) The urine is exactly like clear water without any change (dilute urine), and (2) the urine is very white and clear.

Thus, it is apparent that the writings of Toviah about the urinary system described the relationship between

[2] This notion is most likely derived from other information available at the time. Although Masaria of Padua claimed that the bladder has one coat, Jean DeWigo of Genoa in 1503 described that the bladder has two coats. This was later confirmed by anatomical studies conducted at the University of Padua by Vesalius and others.

fluid intake and urinary output, body fluid homeostasis and the effect of overhydration and dehydration on urine volume, the role of the kidney in this fluid homeostasis, and four ailments that afflict the urinary system which include urinary tract obstruction, urinary hesitancy (infection) dribbling, and polyuria. He provided an interesting clinical differential diagnosis between renal and abdominal colic. He also raised the possibility that the bladder may participate in the genesis of vesicoureteral reflux.

References

1 Massry SG: Maimonides: Physician and nephrologist. Am J Nephrol 1994;14:307–312.
2 Massry SG, Smogorzewski M, Hazani E, Shasha SM: Influence of Judaism and Jewish physicians on Greek and Byzantine medicine and their contribution to nephrology. Am J Nephrol 1997;17:233–240.
3 Shatzmiller J: Jews, Medicine and Medieval Society. Berkeley, University of California Press, 1994, pp 1–35.
4 Berger N: Why medicine?; in Berger N (ed): Jews and Medicine: Religion, Culture, Science. Beth Hatefusoth, 1995, pp 13–32.
5 Bylebyl JJ: The school of Padua, humanistic medicine in the sixteenth century; in Health, Medicine and Morality in the Sixteenth Century. Cambridge, Cambridge University Press, 1979, pp 335–370.
6 Major RH: A History of Medicine. Springfield, Thomas, 1954, pp 327–333.
7 Ruderman DB: Jewish Thoughts and Scientific Discovery in Early Modern Europe. New Haven, Yale University Press, 1995, pp 100–117.
8 Castiglioni A: The Medical School of Padua. Ann Med Hist 1935;7:214–227.
9 Nevins M: The Jewish Doctor: A Narrative History. London, Arnson, 1996, pp 43–49.
10 Fredenwald H: The Jews and Medicine. KTAV Publishing House, 1994, pp 253–256.
11 Modena A, Morpurgo E: Medici Churghli Ebrei Dottorate e Licenziate nell' Università di Padova dal 1617 al 1816. Bologna, Forni Editori, 1617 pp.
12 Allan N: A Jewish physician in the seventeenth century. Med Hist 1984;28:324–328.
13 Cohen T: Ma'aseh Toviah.
14 Bershon M: Tobiasz Kohn: Lekarz Polaski w XVII wieku, Drukarnia Czao, Krakow, 1872.
15 De Broe ME, Sacre D, Snelders ED, De Weert DL: The Flemish anatomist Andreas Vesalius (1514–1564) and the kidney. Am J Nephrol 1997;17:252–260.
16 Eknoyan G, De Santo NG: Realdo Colombo (1516–1559). A reappraisal. Am J Nephrol 1997;17:261–268.
17 Eknoyan G: The origins of nephrology: Galen, the founding father of experimental renal physiology. Am J Nephrol 1989;6:66–82.

Contributions of Padua to Nephrology
(Dedicated to Arturo Borsatti)

American Journal of Nephrology

Am J Nephrol 1999;19:222–225

Giovan Battista Morgagni, a Pioneer of Clinical Nephrology

Augusto Antonello Lorenzo Calò Luciana Bonfante Giuseppe Mennella
Cataldo Abaterusso Michela Spinello Silvana Favaro Angela D'Angelo

Institute of Internal Medicine, Division of Nephrology, University of Padova, Italy

Key Words
Morgagni · Autopsy · Uremia · Rokitansky · Virchow

Abstract
In the 18th century, Giovanni Battista Morgagni was the first to propose that specific signs and symptoms are linked to particular anatomical changes at autopsy and that these changes were the cause of the disease. This paper describes the report by Morgagni wherein he linked the anatomic findings at autopsy, specifically atrophied kidneys, with the signs and symptoms of a disease now known as uremia. From these findings, Morgagni felt that he had identified the factors responsible for the disease as well as its clinical course.

Today, thanks to the great progress made in the fields of histology, immunology and molecular biology, diseases involving the nephron are well known. In past centuries, little if anything was known about its pathology. Fundamental strides in clinical methodology were made by Giovan Battista Morgagni (1682–1771; fig. 1) in his renowned work *De Sedibus et Causis Morborum per Anatomen Indagitis,* published in Venice in 1761 (fig. 2).

Morgagni is rightly considered to be the discoverer of organic pathology in that, thanks to his enormous capacity for critical speculation, he was able to establish very clear criteria in his anatomical and clinical studies. He demonstrated how local kidney damage could be recognized, and showed how it indicated functional alterations in the organ, with related phenomenological and clinical expressions.

After studying medicine at Bologna under the guidance of Valsalva, Morgagni came to the University of Padua and, at the age of only 29, was first professor of theoretical medicine and then anatomy. His treatise *De Sedibus* is an admirable collection of the clinical cases he studied over a period of almost 50 years, many of which were accompanied later by autopsy findings. In this particular field, Morgagni was a follower of that cultural tradition which had already made itself felt in Europe during the preceding century, best personified by Théophile Bonet (1620–1689).

The great novelty introduced by Morgagni, a concept which lay at the basis of his anatomoclinical thinking, was that if the signs and symptoms most frequently observed in vivo in many patients corresponded regularly to common alterations in the organs in question, then such alterations could be considered the cause of disease, and the hypothesis of mere coincidence could be excluded [1].

Following the tradition of his times, Morgagni gave a topographic classification of diseases, from the head to

KARGER
Fax + 41 61 306 12 34
E-Mail karger@karger.ch
www.karger.com

© 1999 S. Karger AG, Basel
0250–8095/99/0192–0222$17.50/0

Accessible online at:
http://BioMedNet.com/karger

Prof. Augusto Antonello, MD
Division of Nephrology
University of Padova
I–35128 Padova (Italy)
Tel. +39 049 8212155, Fax +39 049 8212151

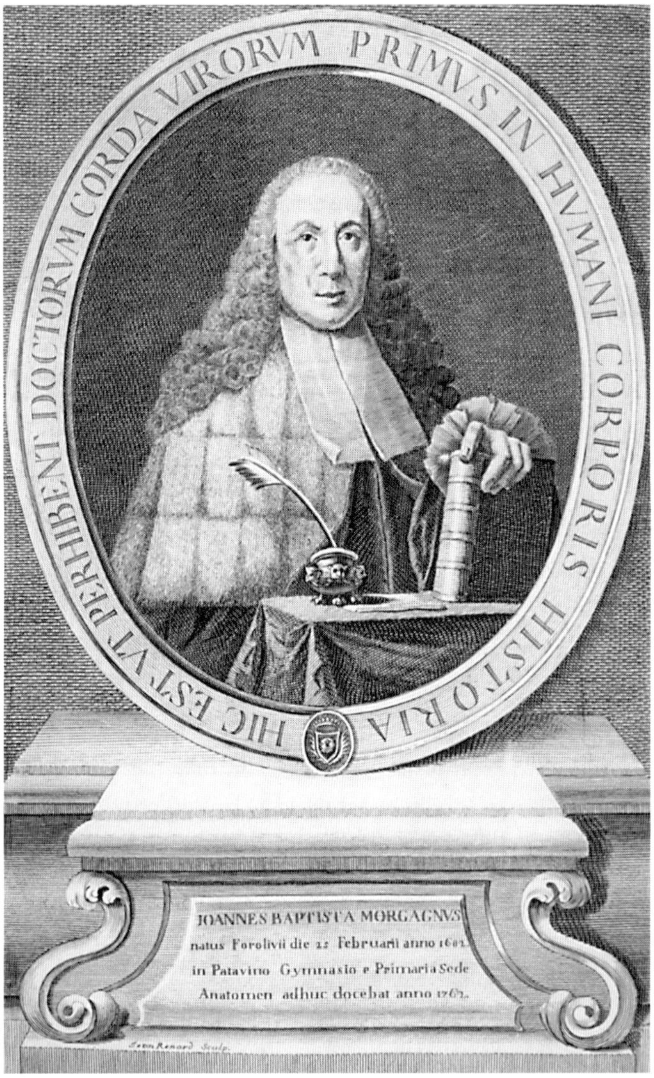
HIC EST VT PERHIBENT DOCTORVM CORDA VIRORVM PRIMVS IN HVMANI CORPORIS HISTORIA
JOANNES BAPTISTA MORGAGNVS
natus Forolivii die 25 Februarii anno 1682
in Patavino Gymnasio e Primaria Sede
Anatomen adhuc docebat anno 1762.

Fig. 1. Portrait of Morgagni.

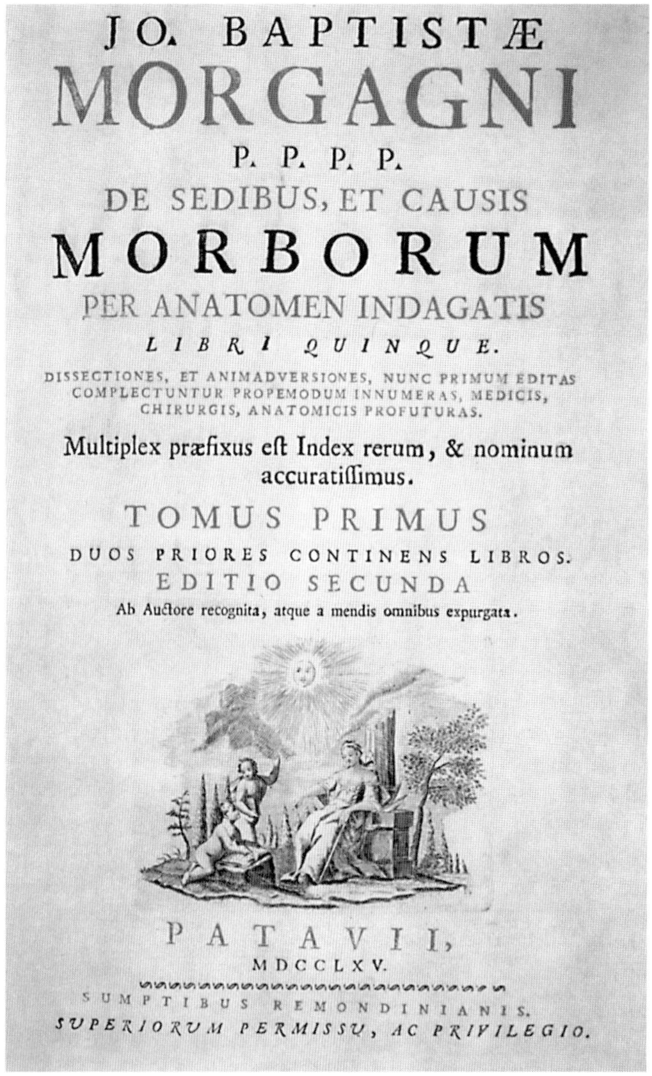

JO. BAPTISTÆ
MORGAGNI
P. P. P. P.
DE SEDIBUS, ET CAUSIS
MORBORUM
PER ANATOMEN INDAGATIS
LIBRI QUINQUE.
DISSECTIONES, ET ANIMADVERSIONES, NUNC PRIMUM EDITAS COMPLECTUNTUR PROPEMODUM INNUMERAS, MEDICIS, CHIRURGIS, ANATOMICIS PROFUTURAS.
Multiplex præfixus eſt Index rerum, & nominum accuratiſſimus.
TOMUS PRIMUS
DUOS PRIORES CONTINENS LIBROS.
EDITIO SECUNDA
Ab Auctore recognita, atque a mendis omnibus expurgata.
PATAVII,
MDCCLXV.
SUMPTIBUS REMONDINIANIS.
SUPERIORUM PERMISSU, AC PRIVILEGIO.

Fig. 2. *De sedibus et causis morborum per anatom indagatis.*

the lower limbs. It must, however, be recognized that, in *De Sedibus*, Morgagni made no attempt to interprete the etiopathogenesis of the various diseases he studied.

Morgagni described a whole series of nephropathies, most of which were cases of kidney stones. In this regard, he was an upholder of the theory that bladder and urethral forms were of renal origin. He described numerous anatomical anomalies, such as double pelvis and arterial and venous vessels, monolateral renal agenesis, ectopic kidneys, and the more frequent occurrence of renal cysts in the elderly. He also noted the association of liver and kidney cysts, and that between the presence of large renal cavities and hemoptysis.

If we continue our reading of *De Sedibus*, letter XXX is of great interest. It describes a patient who, in the last few months of his life, presented symptoms of nausea, vomiting, and headache associated with episodes of loss of consciousness. The most interesting autopsy finding in this case was the description of two greatly shrunken, hard, irregularly shaped, greyish kidneys.

Morgagni commented on his observations by stating that he had treated other patients with the same symptoms and that, on autopsy, they showed the same morphological picture. He therefore concluded that this renal pathology was the cause of the symptoms described.

3

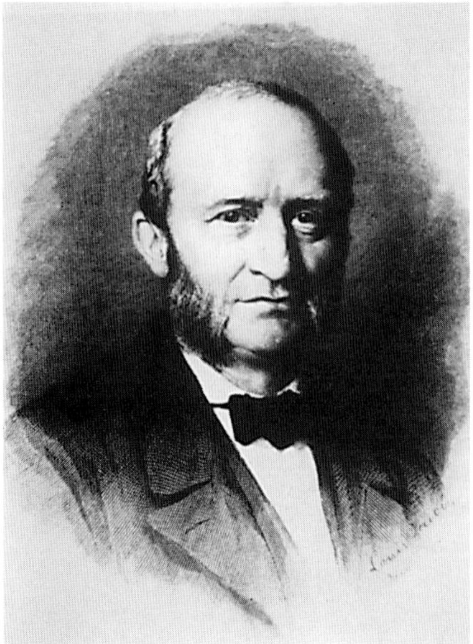

4

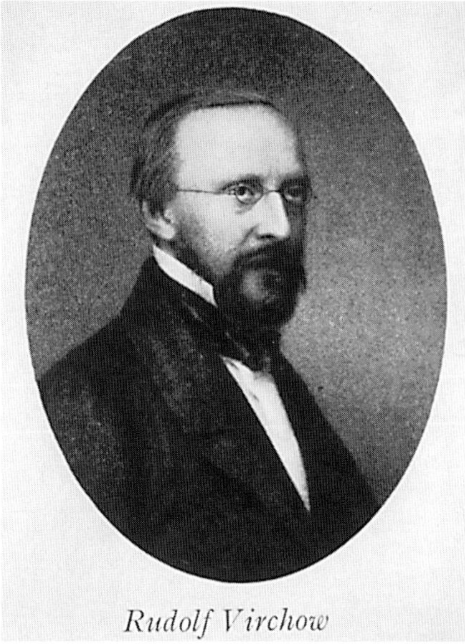

Fig. 3. Portrait of Rokitansky.
Fig. 4. Portrait of Virchow.

It should be noted here that this was one of the first, if not the very first description of what we now call uremia, although of course at that time Morgagni was not aware of the physiopathological features of this condition, which are now common knowledge.

Morgagni's work was based exclusively on macroscopic observation of the various organs of the human body. Although the microscope was already in existence, it was still a rather unmanageable instrument and often defective, in view of the still imperfect characteristics of its lenses. In the following years, continual technical improvements led to the production of more precise and reliable microscopes, so that, during the 19th century, macroscopic anatomy became associated with microscopic study of various tissues.

It was in this field that the figure of Carl Rokitansky (1804–1878; fig. 3) emerged. Rokitansky upheld the humoral theory of diseases, according to which they were caused by alterations in the components of the blood, mainly fibrins and proteins. According to Rokitansky, every altered protein was the cause of a specific disease. He also conducted important histological studies, mainly regarding phlogosis, and applied them to kidney diseases. He distinguished an acute form which, in his opinion, affected the renal cortex, was diffuse or had many points of phlogosis, and later also involved the tubules, from a chronic form with the same histological characteristics but with less tissue damage, which more easily led to atrophy.

However, like Morgagni, Rokitansky did not classify diseases in general and kidney diseases in particular, in common with another great anatomical pathologist of those times, Rudolf Virchow (1821–1902; fig. 4). Virchow, who may be called the first modern pathologist, identified cellular pathogenesis as the origin of disease. He believed that diseases were manifestations of cellular reactions to pathogenic factors which, in turn, modified the chemical and physical structures of the cells themselves. Virchow studied renal phlogosis with particular attention. In his opinion, it developed from an increase in the volume of epithelial cells in which granular material of protein origin was deposited. This led to the disappearance of the nucleus, the death of the cell and hence to the appearance of sclerotic tissue. In Virchow's view, therefore, the organism was not much more than the simple sum of the cells composing it, and disease was essentially the sum of cellular alterations [2]. From the early 19th century and until the middle of the 20th, the general classification of renal diseases, still very uncertain and based mainly on clinical data, was that proposed by Ellis [3]. It involved two phases: (a) acute onset, and (b) a quiescent phase. The former could result in the death of the patient, either directly or after a transitory edematous phase. The latter either led to death due to chronic kidney failure, or to recovery.

These were, however, the years in which great improvements in optical microscopy were being made and new scientific knowledge, as a result of the development of immunohistochemistry, revealed the pathogenetic mechanisms of kidney diseases in an increasingly more complete and accurate manner, so that they could be included in classifications made precisely as a result of histological studies.

Important contributions in this field were made by Ellis [3] and Volhard and Farr [4], although it should be noted that the main differences between the works of these authors lie in the nomenclature they adopted rather than in deeper conceptual divergences.

Today, renal biopsy has become an essential aid for the correct diagnosis of nephropathy. For example, histological correlations between post-streptococcal glomerulonephritis and proliferation of glomerular cells provide increasingly clear pictures.

Immunofluorescence, electronic microscopy, and experimental models have revealed the existence of diseases of the immune complex.

Thus, thanks to new discoveries partly favored by technological advance, renal pathologies are steadily easier to identify and treat. But we should remember that these great strides are the result, over the centuries, of the admirable intuition and of the formidable anatomical and clinical speculative capacities of Giovan Battista Morgagni.

References

1 Zanobio B, Armocida G: Storia della Medicina. Milan, Masson, 1997.
2 Grmek MD: Il concetto di malattia. In Storia del Pensiero Medico Occidentale. Bari, Laterza, 1996, vol 2, pp 254–289.
3 Ellis A: Natural history of Bright's disease: Clinical histological and experimental observations. Lancet 1942;i:1.
4 Volhard F, Fahr T: Die Bright'sche Nierenkrankheit. Berlin, Springer, 1914.

Contributions of Padua to Nephrology (Dedicated to Arturo Borsatti)

American Journal of Nephrology

Am J Nephrol 1999;19:226–233

Santorio Sanctorius (1561–1636) – Founding Father of Metabolic Balance Studies

Garabed Eknoyan

Renal Section, Department of Medicine, Baylor College of Medicine, Houston, Tex., USA

Key Words
Renaissance · Sanctorius · Metabolic balance · Insensible perspiration · Instrumentation

Abstract
The intellectual renaissance of the closing decades of the sixteenth century provided the fertile ground in which the budding spirit of scientific inquiry emerged in the seventeenth century. Direct observation, soon augmented by instrumentation that allowed for quantification and, therefore, verification, became the revelatory medium for the progress of the sciences. In medicine, progress depended on the application of the exact sciences of chemistry, mathematics and physics to the study of function. One of the medical luminaries of this early scientific revolution was Santorio Sanctorius (1561–1636), whose principal contributions were his studies on insensible perspiration and his instrumental inventions. To study insensible perspiration, he designed a movable platform attached to a steelyard scale that allowed for the quantification of changes in body weight of subjects who partook in their daily activities on the platform. After years of self-experimentation, he applied his device to the study of patients. Unfortunately, his records are lost. What survives is a summary of his observations in a series of aphorisms published under the title of *Ars de statica medicina,* in 1614; 3 years after he was appointed Ordinary Professor of Theoretical Medicine in Padua. To enhance the bedside evaluation of patients, he also designed instruments to quantify the pulse, temperature, and environmental humidity. For his pioneering and detailed balance studies, Sanctorius clearly deserves the title of founding father of metabolic balance studies.

The challenges to ancient orthodoxy and scholasticism, increasingly voiced by Renaissance humanists during the closing decades of the sixteenth century, culminated in the seventeenth century in a fundamental, and although dispersed but nevertheless a large scale, attempt to change the view of the whole of the natural world. One of the more perplexing and astonishing moments in scientific thought, the seventeenth century has been appropriately dubbed 'The Insurgent Century' [1]. It was then that the explanation of the natural world advanced by Aristotle (384–322 BC), and accepted as dogma for centuries past, came under scrutiny and considered to be no longer adequate. Once the rationale for direct, rather than textual, observation of nature became the rule, it quickly became evident that there were just too many contradictions between the recorded, often theoretical, descriptions of the ancients and those that were being actually observed.

KARGER

Fax + 41 61 306 12 34
E-Mail karger@karger.ch
www.karger.com

© 1999 S. Karger AG, Basel
0250–8095/99/0192–0226$17.50/0

Accessible online at:
http://BioMedNet.com/karger

Garabed Eknoyan, MD
Department of Medicine
Baylor College of Medicine
One Baylor Plaza, Houston, TX 77030-3498 (USA)
Tel. +1 713 798 4748, Fax +1 713 790 0681

The problem became all the more critical when the power of observation began to be magnified by the growing use of instrumentation. The resultant intellectual revolution, began by the philosophers (Bacon, Descartes) and astronomers (Copernicus, Kepler), provided the very foundations of scientific research and the roots of modern science that was to flourish in the centuries to come [2, 3]. As subjective description was replaced by objective measurements (mathematics, physics), scientific experiments in the form of repeatable and reproducible phenomena became possible. In astronomy, what Copernicus (1473–1543) had demonstrated mathematically, Galileo (1564–1642) confirmed by repeated, reproducible and quantifiable observation, using instruments to extend the senses. It was then that experimental tradition became well established, and perception, augmented by new instrumentation, became a constant revelatory medium for the progress of the sciences.

This new and revolutionary spirit of scientific inquiry also affected the biological sciences [4]. In medicine, revolt was channelled against the authority of Galen (130–200), whose voluminous writings formed the bulk of the medical texts that were becoming widely available in their original version following the advent of the printing press (1454). The rebellion began in anatomy. Andreas Vesalius (1514–1564), the more famous and better known of the advocates of the direct observational method in anatomy, vigorously argued that those who sought medical truth should put aside medical texts and directly study the human body [5]. It is ironical that none other than the principal victim of these attacks, Galen, had advocated that the path 'to become expert in all matters of plants, animals, and metals ... was by personally inspecting them, not once or twice, but often' [6]. The difference was that the method which Galen had professed now became accepted and vigorously applied. It is also ironical that it was the very rediscovery of direct observation that determined the limitations of the anatomical approach that Vesalius and his contemporaries had advocated. Accurate knowledge of structure did not provide an understanding of function, and the dead bodies that were being examined meticulously did not yield the secrets of life. Indeed, even when dissection was performed on live bodies, the secrets of nature remained elusive. Vesalius, who did resort to vivisection, could not advance the understanding of renal function beyond that of Galen [6, 7]. This is what Vesalius had to say about renal function: 'the office of purgation is most fitly performed by the kidneys ... they quickly draw the greater part of the serous humor of the liver toward themselves and strain it from the blood. In order that they may accomplish this more handily, a notable vein and likewise an artery are extended to the kidney; the kidney receives the serous humor into a membranous sinus ... covered by a double tunic ... and expels the urine off into another sinus which is prolonged as the urinary passage and constructed like a vein ...'. The recurrent reference to veins is a central tenet of the teaching of Vesalius who believed that 'nature gave straight fibers to the veins, by means of these it draws blood into its cavity' [8]. Thus, while anatomists gradually evolved a concern for function, and therefore physiology, their explanations were structural and remained descriptive but did provide the fertile grounds on which the new science of physiology would thrive and prosper.

Progress occurred only when the exact sciences of chemistry, mathematics and physics began to be applied to medicine. Explanation of function on a chemical basis started with Paracelsus (1493–1541), who was in fact one of the first to attack the ancients and challenge the teachings of Galen [9]. He is considered the founder of the Iatrochemical School, that was to reach its height in the work of Jean Baptist van Helmont (1577–1644) and Franciscus Sylvius (1614–1672). Physics and mathematics were the two other growing exact sciences to be used in order to provide an explanation of function [10, 11]. René Descartes (1596–1650), who did much to encourage the practice of experimentation, brought the human body, the 'earthen machine' as he called it, into the sphere of physics (iatrophysics) [12]. The language of iatrophysical medicine became that of mechanics (iatromechanics) or mathematics (iatromathematics). Giovanni Borelli (1608–1679) brought to the study of action and movements a knowledge of physics and is considered the founder of the iatromechanical school. While Santorio Sanctorius (1561–1636) applied mathematics to the study of medicine and is considered a founder of the iatromathematical school [13, 14].

This pace in the effort to understand and explain function, which emerged gradually in the sixteenth century, increased in the seventeenth century, but remained remarkably restricted to islands of learning. Interestingly, by and large most of the scientists who led the scientific revolution in the seventeenth century were trained or worked in Padua. Padua, which had emerged from its medievalism and achieved some degree of fame in the fourteenth century, came under the protection of Venice in 1440, an event that would ultimately provide it with the intellectual freedom which was instrumental in making it the most distinguished center of learning in Europe during the second half of the sixteenth and most of the

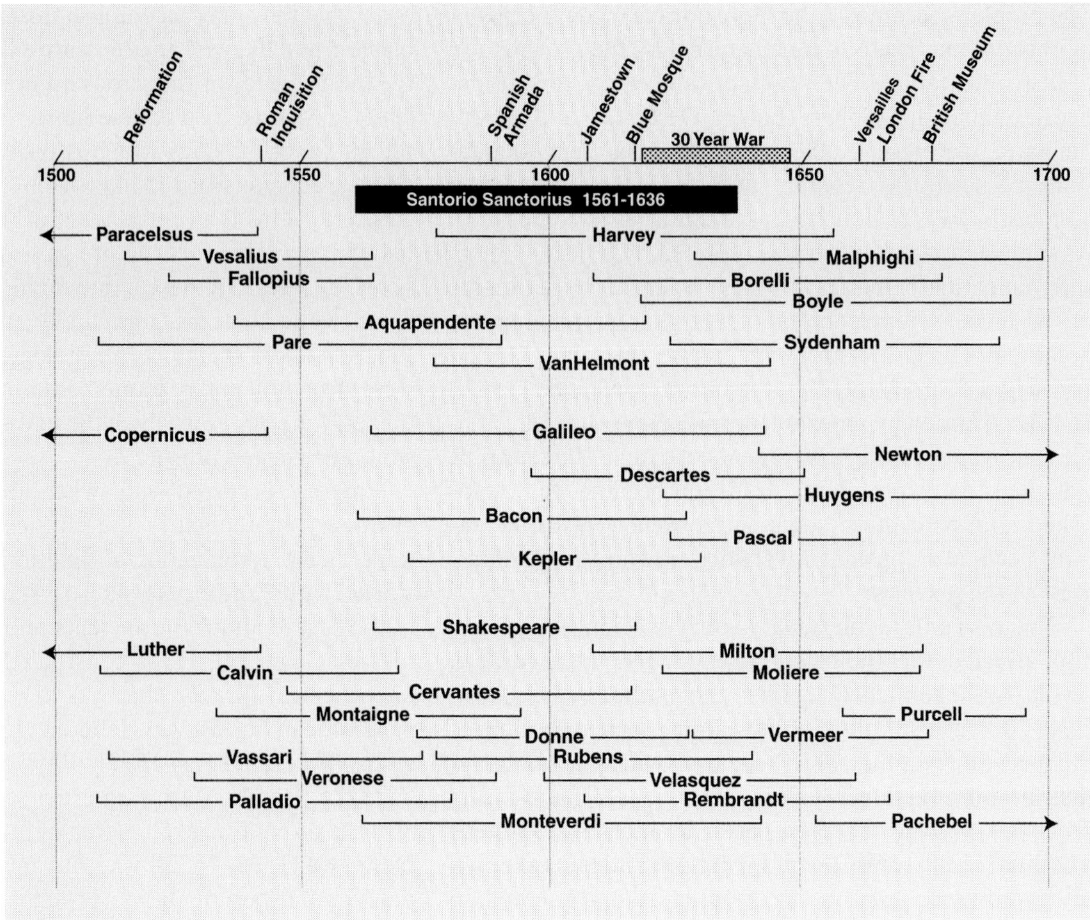

Fig. 1. Time line showing some of the prominent contemporaries of Santorio Sanctorius in medicine, the sciences and liberal arts.

seventeenth century. This was perhaps truest of its medical faculty which was founded in 1250 [15]. The era of medical science in seventeenth century Padua was an interlude which exhibits a surprising flash that was fundamental to the development of the modern methods of medical research. It was in this atmosphere that Galileo and Harvey, the two most celebrated Paduan figures, were trained to think and solve the problems of the new sciences. Eminent amongst the early scientific experimenters and a figure whose work spans the transition from the 16th to the 17th century is Santorio Sanctorius, a contemporary of Galileo and a predecessor of Harvey in Padua (fig. 1).

Santorio Sanctorius (1561–1636)

Santorio Sanctorius was born on March 29, 1561, in Capodistria, the capital of Istria, then under the rule of Venice and still known by its Roman name of Justinopolis (fig. 2). Of patrician descent, and the oldest of four children, his father, Antonio, was a Friulian nobleman who had been appointed Chief of Ordnance of the city and his mother, Elisabetta Cordonia, was of a prosperous and noble Istrian family. His connections to nobility were to come to good stead, both during his childhood education and subsequent career appointments. His schooling which began in Capodistria, continued in Venice where he received private education in the home of family friends, the powerful Morosinis. In 1575, at the age of 14, he began his studies at the University of Padua, first in philosophy and later in medicine (table 1). In 1582, he

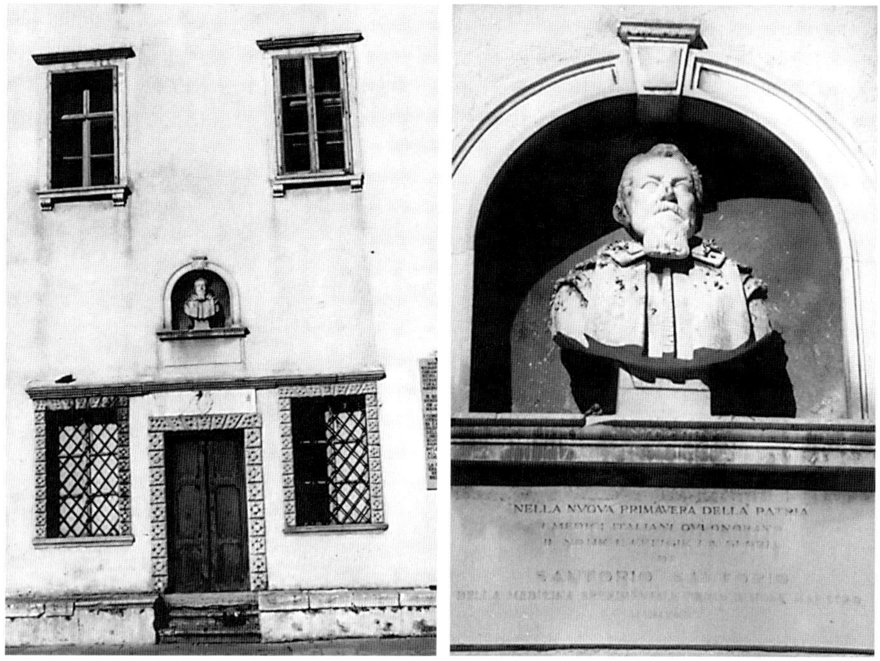

Fig. 2. The house of Santorio Sanctorius in Justinopolis (now Koper), marked with a commemorative bust placed in his honor by Italian physicians characterizing him as 'First Eminent Teacher of Experimental Medicine'.

received his degree in medicine at the age of 21, one year younger than Vesalius had received his in 1537, and three years younger than Harvey would receive his in 1602, both from the same school [16–18].

Five years after graduation he seems to have been recruited to practice medicine in the various courts of eastern Europe. After some 12 years, he returned to Venice in 1599 to continue his practice of medicine. In Venice, he became part of the intellectual circle which gathered at the home of his childhood friend and classmate, Andrea Morosini, and included such luminaries as Galileo, Fabrizzio de Aquapendente (1537–1619) and Fra Paolo Sarpi. Shortly after his return to Venice, he published in 1602 his first book: *Method of Combating All the Errors which Occur in the Art of Medicine* (table 2). It was this book on differential diagnosis that established his fame and coupled with the strength of his social connections led to the invitation to serve as Professor of Theoretical Medicine in Padua in 1611. Galileo, who had served as Professor of Mathematics (1593–1610) had just left, Fabrizzio de Aquapendente was then Professor of Anatomy and teaching in the amphitheater he had built in 1595, and Harvey who had completed his studies in Padua (1593–1602) had long left.

The position of First Ordinary Professor of Theoria had been vacant since 1603. In Santorio, the chair acquired an experienced practitioner, an investigator of

Table 1. Santorio Sanctorius (1561–1636)

1561	Born March 29, Capodistria (Justinopolis, Koper)
	Begins studies in Venice (Morosinis)
1575	Begins university studies in Padua
1582	Receives medical degree
1582	Begins medical practice and research studies
1611	Professor of Theoretical Medicine, Padua
1616	President, Collegio Venetio, Padua
1624	Returns to medical practice, Venice
1630	President, Venetian College of Physicians
	Chief Health Officer, Venice
1636	Dies on February 22, Venice

Table 2. Bibliography of Santorio Sanctorius

1602	*Methodus vitandorum errorum omnium qui in arte medica contigunt*
1612	*Commentaria in artem medicinalem Galeni*
1614	*De Statica medicina*
1625	*Commenteria in primam Fen primi Canonis Avicennae*
1629	*Commenteria in primam sectionem Aphorismorum Hypocratis*
1629	*De remediorum inventione*
1638	*De lithotomia seu calculi vesicae consultatio* co-authored with L. Batarourum (posthumous)
	De instrumentis medicis (unpublished)

some consequence, and a creative spirit whose influence extended well beyond the borders of Padua. As Professor of the Theory of Medicine, his responsibilities were to interpret and teach the Aphorisms of Hippocrates, the Art of Medicine of Galen, and the first part of the Canon of Avicenna. Over the years he would publish his lectures as commentaries on the work of all three (table 2). Commentaries which had started as student aids for learning had evolved into scholastic endeavors of some merit in the modernization of teaching [19], at least until the first half of the seventeenth century. Amongst the more than 60 extant copies of the Commentaries on Avicenna, the one by Sanctorius is deservedly famous because it was so uncharacteristic in its genre for the inclusion of scientific instruments designed by the author to quantify (pulse, temperature, humidity) the study of patients. Their inclusion indicates that Sanctorius used them in the teaching of medicine [18, 20]. However, the book that was actually to establish his position in posterity as a scientist was a relatively short text on insensible perspiration, titled *Ars de statica medicina* and published in Venice in 1614.

During the term of his tenure as Professor of Theoretical Medicine, he was appointed President of a new college (Collegio Veneto) in 1616, a position he held for 8 years until 1624, when at the age of 63 he resigned to return to the practice of medicine in Venice. In recognition of his contributions, the Venetian Senate granted him the title of professor and an accompanying salary for life. The fact that he had several powerful connections in the Venetian Senate, including his schoolmate Morosini, no doubt facilitated this well deserved, but rarely granted honor. In 1630, he was appointed President of the Venetian College of Physicians and Chief Health Officer to control the plague that was then ravaging Venice. He died, at the age of 75, on February 22, 1636, from what is said to be complications of urinary tract disease from which he had suffered for several years. Buried in the Church dei Servi in Venice, his bones were disinterred during the looting of Venice on Napoleon's orders, following the Treaty of Milan. His bones, entrusted to the Professor of Anatomy of Padua, were ultimately buried in his home town of Capodistria, while his presumed skull is preserved in the Anatomical Museum of Padua.

A man of small stature, with a trim beard, Sanctorius never married, dedicating all his time to his work. A tireless investigator, inspired by the exact sciences, he focused on selected issues that he studied exhaustively. In his work he demonstrated unprecedented patience and perseverance. His studies on insensible perspiration, at which he worked so assiduously, were superior in approach, design and meticulousness to any others of his time. A man ahead of his times, who preceded the other luminaries of the century (fig. 1), Sanctorius was recognized by his contemporaries as one of the major figures of the seventeenth century and considered the equal of Harvey. The *Ars de Statica medicina* underwent 28 editions and remained in demand well into the end of the eighteenth century and was translated into Italian, English, German and French [15, 21].

Scientific Contributions

The principal contributions of Sanctorius were his studies on insensible perspiration and his instrumental inventions. The latter is at the very core of his metabolic studies on insensible perspiration. The instrument he developed for its study consisted of a movable platform, attached to a steelyard scale, on which the subject would partake in daily activities, that allowed for the measurement of changes in body weight (fig. 3). His work began as one of the first self experimentation studies in which he would partake a meal set on the table before him until his weight reached a predetermined quantity. If he then remained on the balance for a while, he could observe his weight becoming gradually lighter. He recognized that this decline in weight represented a loss of matter, the loss of which he called insensible perspiration. During the course of the experiment, he would weigh the stool and urine excreted and subtract them from the final change in weight to verify the loss attributed to insensible perspiration.

After years of self-experimentation, he applied the instrument to the study of other subjects. In the letter presenting a copy of *De Statica* to Galileo, he claims to have studied more than 10,000 subjects in the span of 25 years [15]. That would entail the daily study of at least one subject literally on every single day of the 25 years! It is unfortunate that the data he collected is not preserved and that he elected to summarize his findings in a series of aphorisms. While criticized for this shortcoming, it should be kept in mind that at the time of his studies, he was in constant movement in Eastern Europe and that data books, as we conceive them today, were not in fashion. Additionally, the text is not a mere listing of aphorisms, such as the forerunner of them all the Hippocratic Aphorisms. Rather, each aphorism is followed by an explanation, which, in paragraphs of varying lengths, provides the rationale of the information distilled in the aphorisms.

The notion of insensible perspiration was not new [22, 23]. Galen had identified it quite clearly as: 'mouths placed on the skin pass out whatever is redundant of vapors and smoke ... and the other excretion, which has no name because it is not commonly known, since it escapes observation ... is insensible perspiration (adelos diapnoe)', and was cognizant of its overall metabolic consequences '... the amount of urine passed everyday shows clearly that it is the whole of the fluid drunk which becomes urine, except that which comes away with the dejections, or passes off as sweat, or as insensible perspiration'. This was the basis of the central role of bathing and lustrations in Greek and Roman medicine.

What Sanctorius accomplished was to bring to bear the scientific method in documenting these earlier observations by quantifying them by instrumentation, verifying them by repeated examination, and extending them to the study of the determinants of its variation. The importance he attached to the role of insensible perspiration is stated in Section I, Aphorism II: 'If a physician, who has the care of another's health, is acquainted only with sensible supplies and evacuations, and knows nothing of the waste that is daily made by insensible perspiration, he will only deceive his patient, and never cure him'. A general notion of his concepts can be gleaned from the following quotes. Section III, Aphorism LXXVI: 'In the first hours after eating a great many perspire a pound or near; and after that to the ninth two pounds; and from the ninth to the sixteenth scarce a pound.' Section I, Aphorism VI: 'If eight pounds of meat and drink are taken in one day, the quantity that usually goes off by insensible perspiration in that time, is five pounds.' Section 1, Aphorism XIV: 'Sixteen ounces of urine is generally evacuated in the space of one night; four ounces by stool, and forty ounces upwards by perspiration.' Section I, Aphorism LXXXIX: 'Vomiting diverts urine and perspiration.' Section I Aphorism XCIV: 'Those who piss more than they drink, little or nothing perspire.' Section III Aphorism XIV: 'Robust persons discharge their food for the most part by perspiration. Those not so strong by urine, and the weak chiefly by an indigested chyle.'

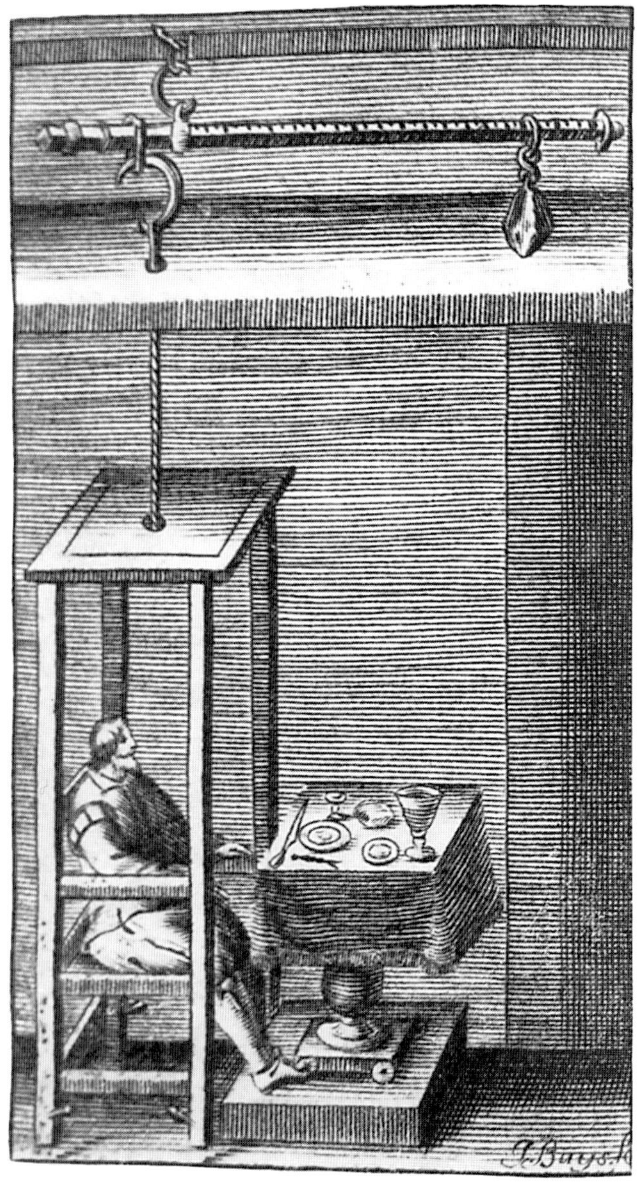

Fig. 3. The metabolic balance devised by Santorio Sanctorius for the study of insensible perspiration. From *De Statica medicina,* 1690.

This is well beyond what Galen and all his successors had said about insensible perspiration. It is a first effort to obtain physiological data and provide a quantitative basis to pathophysiology by meticulous study and precise instrumentation [24, 25]. Not only did he study insensible perspiration, but documented its fluctuations under the influence of such variables as air, food, age, movement, repose, sexual activity and drink. Published in 1612, and by his admission having taken 30 years to complete, *De Statica medicina* is the result of studies that must have been initiated at or about 1582 when the rudiments of the scientific revolution were just beginning to gel. As such, they were not only innovative, but advanced for their time and laid the basis of all future metabolic studies. In our balance experiments today, we handle intakes and outputs of the body essentially as Sanctorius did, except for the addition of chemical analysis to what he only characterized in terms of weight and volume.

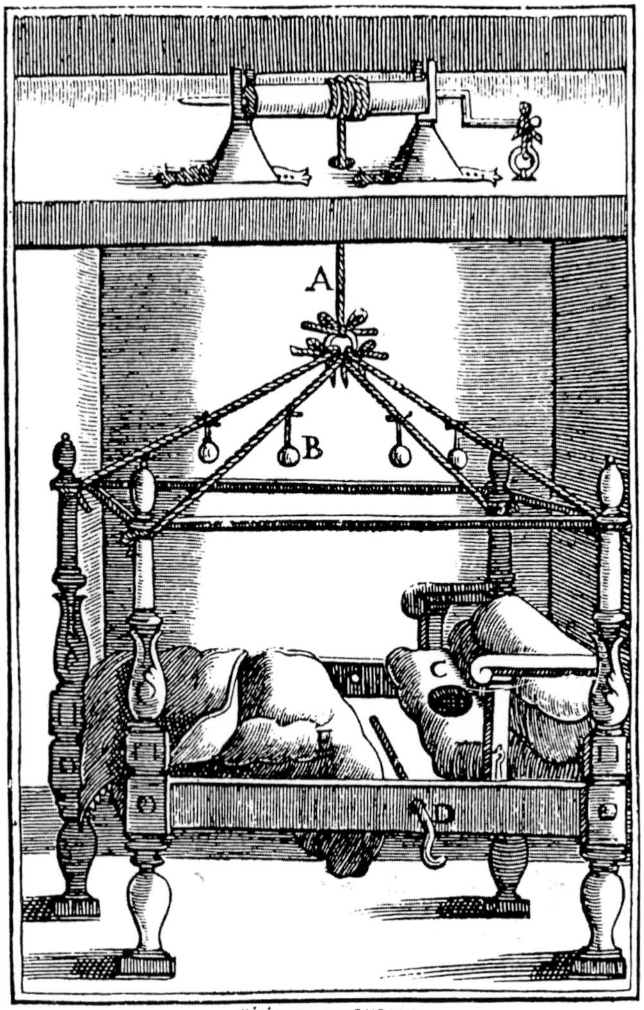

Héliogravure DURAND.

FIG. 11. — Lit mécanique.

Fig. 4. 'Lectus artificiosus' – a mechanical bed for the care of invalids – whose advantages Sanctorius characterizes as especially meritorious because the patient can remain comfortably seated in bed; can defecate in bed through a special foramen; can move the bed position by the four metal balls suspended from the top; and can be moved while seated allowing for transportation and change of linen.

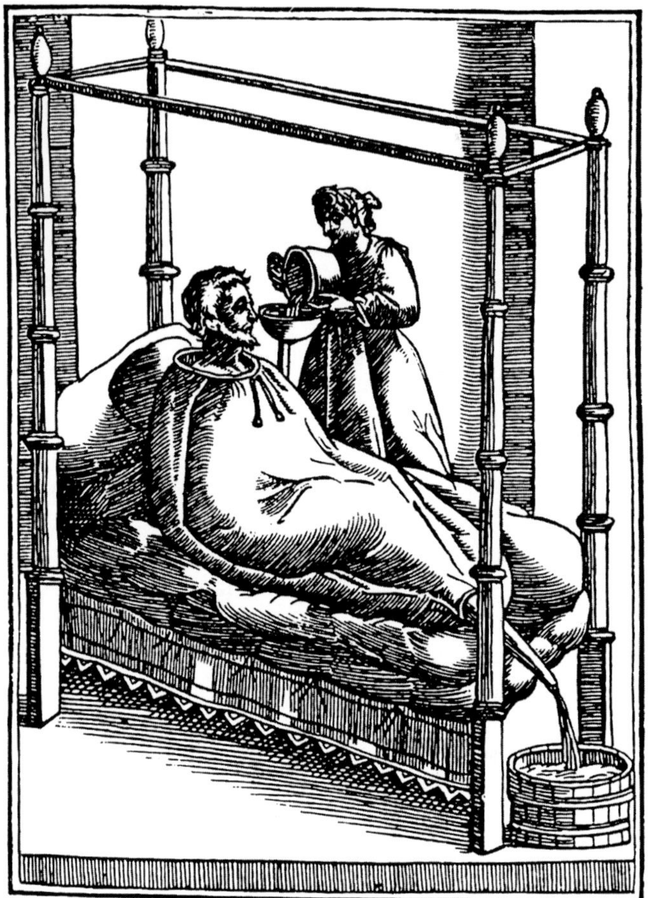

Héliogravure DURAND.

FIG. 7. — Appareil pour prendre un bain dans le lit.

Fig. 5. 'Balneatorium' – a leather bag that allows bathing or hydrotherapy of the patient in bed. After placing the patient in the bag, the neck of the sack is drawn together with a string, then cold or hot water can be poured through a tube at the upper and drained through another at the lower end of the bag.

To evaluate him by current criteria, his work was clearly novel, acknowledged by his contemporaries, and provided the stimulus for research by others not only in the 17th century, but well into the 20th century. In fact, his studies did not reach full fruition until the beginnings of the 20th century when they were resuscitated by the use of the matter of perspiration for calculating basal and total metabolism [26].

Conclusion

Although best remembered for his metabolic studies, Sanctorius made equally important and original contributions to instrumental precision in medicine [25]. The balance he used in his studies was but a forerunner of other instruments to come. Among others, these included a thermometer to measure temperature, a hygrometer to record moisture, a pulsilogium to quantitate the pulse, a mechanical bed for the care of incapacitated patients (fig. 4), and a device to bathe the sick in bed (fig. 5). He alluded to these instruments in his early publications, and had intended to publish their detail in a volume that remained only a manuscript, now lost, *De instrumentis medicis.* Ultimately, he incorporated them into his *Commentary on Avicenna* published in 1625 (table 2).

For all his innovative approach and contributions, Sanctorius clearly deserves not only the title of founding father of metabolic studies, but also that of clinical experimentation, objective physiological measurement and medical instrumentation.

References

1 Singer C: The Insurgent Century. Downfall of Aristotle (1600–1700): New Attempts at Synthesis; in Singer C (ed): A History of Scientific Ideas. New York, Dorset Press, 1959, pp 218–287.
2 Boas-Hall M: The Scientific Renaissance 1450–1630. New York, Dover, 1994.
3 Shapin S: The Scientific Revolution. Chicago, University of Chicago Press, 1996.
4 Barry J Jr: Measures of Science. Theological and Technological Impulses in Early Modern Thought. Evanston, Northwestern University Press, 1996.
5 Eknoyan G, De Santo NG: Realdo Colombo (1516–1559). A reappraisal. Am J Nephrol 1997;17:261–268.
6 Eknoyan G: The origins of nephrology – Galen, the founding father of experimental renal physiology. Am J Nephrol 1989;9:66–82.
7 DeBroe ME, Sacré D, Snelders ED, De Weerdt DL: The Flemish anatomist Andreas Vesalius (1514–1564) and the kidney. Am J Nephrol 1997;17:252–260.
8 The Epitome of Andreas Vesalius. Translated by L.R. Lind. New York, Macmillan, 1949.
9 Eknoyan G: On the contributions of Paracelsus to nephrology. Nephrol Dial Transplant 1996; 11:1388–1394.
10 Brown TM: The College of Physicians and the acceptance of iatromechanism in England. Bull Hist Med 1970;44:12–30.
11 Brown TM: Physiology and the mechanical philosophy in mid-seventeenth century England. Bull Hist Med 1977;51:25–54.
12 Carter RB: Descartes' Medical Philosophy. The Organic Solution to the Mind-Body Problem. Baltimore, Johns Hopkins University Press, 1983.
13 Boas M: The establishment of the mechanical philosophy. Osiris 1952;10:412–541.
14 Osler W: The Evolution of Medicine. Birmingham, Classics of Medicine Library, 1982, pp 126–182.
15 O'Malley CD: The lure of Padua. Med Hist 1970;14:1–9.
16 Castiglioni A: Life and work of Sanctorius. Med Life 1931;38:727–786.
17 Sigerist HE: The Great Doctors. A Biographical History of Medicine. New York, Norton, 1933, pp 150–156.
18 Grmeck MD: Santorio Sanctorius, DSB 1975; 12:101–104.
19 Sarton G: Was any attempt made by the editors of the late Latin editions of Avicenna's Canon to modernize it? Isis 1952;43:54.
20 Siraisi NG: Avicenna in Renaissance Italy. The Canon and Medical Teaching in Italian Universities after 1500. Princeton, Princeton University Press, 1987.
21 Quincy J: Being the Aphorisms of Sanctorius. Newton, London, 1712.
22 Benedict FG, Root HF: Insensible perspiration: Its relation to human physiology and pathology. Arch Intern Med 1926;38:1–35.
23 Renbourn ET: The natural history of insensible perspiration: A forgotten doctrine of health and disease. Med Hist 1960;4:135–152.
24 Bing FC: The history of the word 'metabolism'. J Hist Med All Sci 1971;26:158–180.
25 Mitchell SW: The Early History of Instrumental Precision in Medicine. 1892. New York, Lenox Hill (Bart Franklin), reprinted 1971.
26 Newburgh LH, Wiley FH, Lashmet FH: A method for the determination of heat production over long periods of time. J Clin Invest 1931;10:703–732.

American Journal of Nephrology

Am J Nephrol 1999;19:234

Section dedicated to: Carl William Gottschalk

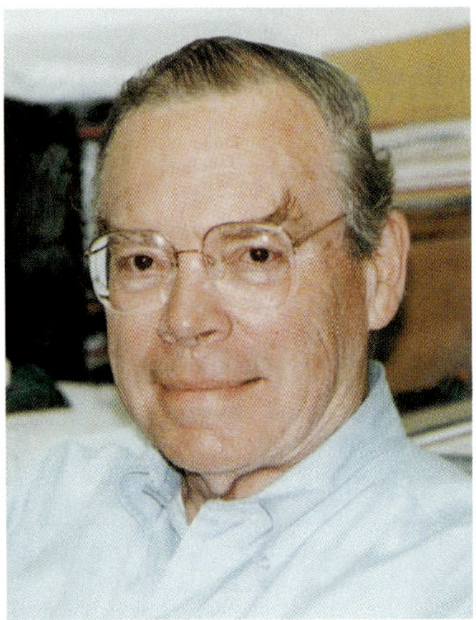

1922–1997

KARGER

Fax + 41 61 306 12 34
E-Mail karger@karger.ch
www.karger.com

© 1999 S. Karger AG, Basel

Accessible online at:
http://BioMedNet.com/karger

Origins of Renal Physiology
(Dedicated to Carl Gottschalk)

American Journal of Nephrology

Am J Nephrol 1999;19:235–242

Carl Gottschalk – Physiologist, Bibliophile and Historian of Nephrology

J. Stewart Cameron

Renal Unit, Guy's Hospital, King's College, London, UK

Key Words
Carl Gottschalk, childhood, education, history of nephrology contributions, scientific contributions, teaching career

Carl Gottschalk was scholar, scientist and gentleman; and a gentle man. Few could escape being captivated by his combined ability and modesty, or fail to retain fond memories of his kindness together with admiration for the high standards he set for himself. We miss him and regret his absence at this meeting, which he would so much have enjoyed, and to which he would have contributed as always, with grace and perception. We honour him today with this symposium, both as a scientist and as a historian of Physiology and Nephrology.

Carl William Gottschalk was born on April 28th 1922, in the small town of Salem, Virginia, into a family of German origin. His father, also named Carl, was born in 1884 in Treffurt an der Werra, a small town in the landschaft of Hessen, and emigrated from Germany to South Africa in 1909. There he farmed ostriches, but the fashion for ostrich plumes waned, and after unsuccessful attempts at gold mining in what was then the British colony of Rhodesia (now Zimbabwe), he designed and repaired cigarette-making machines in Port Elizabeth in Natal. In 1914, now aged 30, he again became restless and emigrated to New York, moving on to Lynchburg, Virginia, but lived the rest of his life in Salem, near Roanoake, where he owned a cinema, an automobile repair shop and other property. There he married Lula Helbig (b. 1879), also of German origin, and had two sons, Walter (b. 1918) who trained as a mathematician at Roanoake College and the University of Virginia, and Carl. Carl senior died of a stroke in 1969, whilst Lula had died of acute glomerulonephritis in 1946, during Carl's internship (fig. 1).

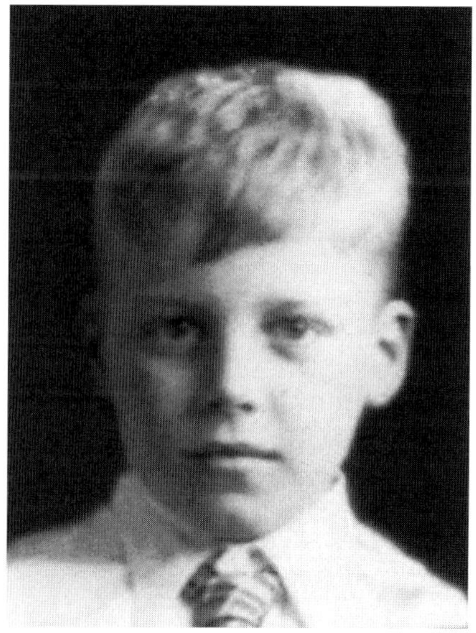

Fig. 1. Carl at about the age of 9 years, taken from a family snapshot around 1931.

As a child, Carl William was studious, quiet, and even then had two characteristics which would mark his subsequent career: he was a collector, and an acute observer. As well as the more usual stamps and coins, Carl also col-

KARGER
Fax + 41 61 306 12 34
E-Mail karger@karger.ch
www.karger.com

© 1999 S. Karger AG, Basel
0250–8095/99/0192–0235$17.50/0

Accessible online at:
http://BioMedNet.com/karger

Emeritus Professor J.S. Cameron
Elm Bank, Melmerby, Penrith
Cumbria CA10 1HB (UK)
Tel. +44 1768 881804, Fax +44 1768 881105, E-Mail jstewart-cameron@email.msn.com

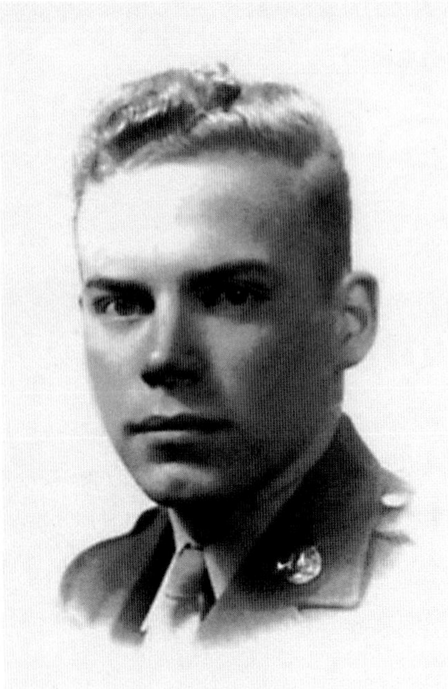

Fig. 2. Carl in 1947/8 in the Army. During this time he spent time researching the effect of cold on the performance of Army personnel, and also amassing the most complete collection of subarctic butterflies available, now in the Peabody Museum, New Haven, Conn.

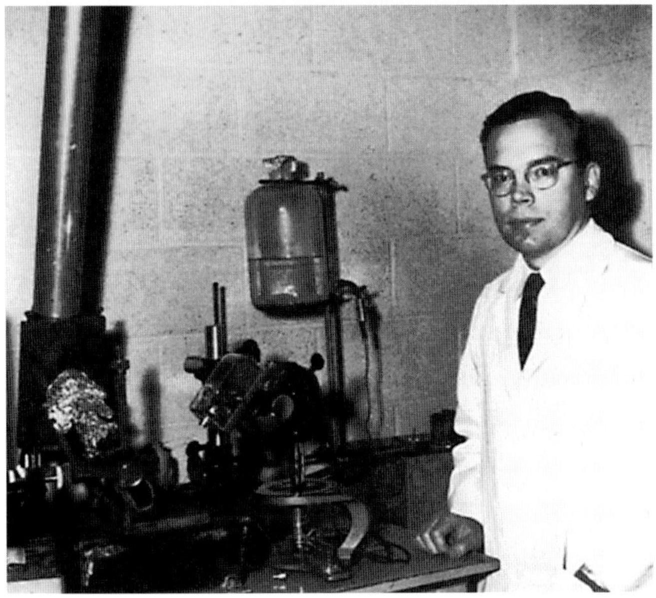

Fig. 3. Carl in his laboratory in the late 1950s or early 1960s. He began using micropuncture of the mammalian kidney in 1955, and was responsible for this technique becoming a central tool in the investigation of renal physiology throughout the 1960s and 1970s.

lected butterflies, and his collection came to include when he was only 15 years old one butterfly hitherto unknown, which eventually was named after him – *Stryman cecrops gottschalkii*. There is little doubt that his character of careful observation was shaped by these early experiences in entomology. Leaving high school he graduated BS from Roanoke College, Virginia, in 1942 and took his MD in the University of Virginia only 3 years later as part of an accelerated course in Medicine running during the war (fig. 2).

During his time as an intern at the Massachussetts General Hospital, he met and married in 1947 a nursing student, Helen Scott, who was his wife for over 40 years; they had 3 children. After this he entered the Army, and encountered medical research for the first time when based at Fort Knox, Kentucky, studying the physiological effects of cold exposure on army personnel, which work led to five reports and scientific papers [1–5]. However, these did not, as one might expect, include his first publication: this had appeared when he was only 20 years old, in *Entomological News* [6], describing his work on the butterflies of his locality in Roanoke and Montgomery Counties, Virginia. His love of butterflies went with him to St James' Bay and Labrador in the Canadian Arctic, when his military service took him there to study the effects of cold, and he made the most complete collection of subarctic butterflies yet assembled, which was donated to the Peabody Museum of Yale University, and still graces their collection.

Leaving the Army, he returned to Boston for 2 years (1948–50) in the physiology laboratory at Harvard of Eugene Landis, followed by a further 2 years as resident in Medicine, during which he trained, not in Nephrology – which did not exist as an independent specialty at that time – but in Cardiology. It was in Landis' laboratory that he first studied the physiology of the kidney, examining the effect of the then novel adrenal cortical hormones [7] and interstitial pressure [8], in an attempt to better understand congestive heart failure and hypertension.

Then in 1952 he moved to the University of North Carolina at Chapel Hill to become a Clinical Cardiologist and (at first Assistant) Professor of Medicine and Physiology. He used to say it was the only offer he had, but the idea of returning to the South must have long been close to his heart. Although initially appointed to a clinical post, he realized his first love was not clinical but investigative medicine, and thereafter devoted himself to bench research. He lived and worked in Chapel Hill for the rest of his life, and had a deep love of and loyalty to this place and its people, which was reciprocated in full. The only cloud during these long and happy years in Chapel Hill was when his wife Helen died in 1988 of amyloidosis, bereaving him and their 3 children, 1 of whom had herself become a physician.

In 1995, Carl went to the meeting in Bar Harbor, Maine, to commemorate the centenary of Homer Smith's birth. At that meeting he met Dr Susan Fellner; they became inseparable and were married the following year. Carl knew he had coronary heart disease but this was not a major problem. However, they were cruelly separated after only a brief period of happiness together when Carl died unexpectedly on October 15th 1997 during an exercise stress test. All of us lost something precious that day.

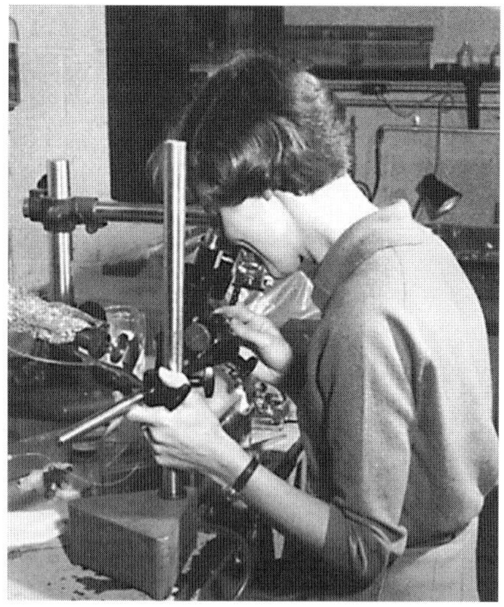

Fig. 4. Margaret (Peggy) Mylle (b. 1927), Carl's associate in the classic studies on the concentrating mechanisms of the kidney, and many other papers throughout the 1960s. Like Carl himself, she was self-taught in techniques of micropuncture, but her skills were legendary; she taught the technique to many other renal physiologists.

Carl Gottschalk: The Scientist

In Chapel Hill, Carl set up what was to become one of the leading physiology laboratories of subsequent decades. The beginnings were modest: a single small laboratory, and only some less than modest local funding (USD 2,000). He continued his interests in renal tubular interstitial and peritubular capillary pressures, using the techniques pioneered in Landis' laboratory [9, 10], including attempts at micropuncture, despite initial discouragement from Richards himself. Shortly after he was joined by Margaret (Peggy) Mylle (b. 1927 in Harrogate, England), for whose technical expertise in micropuncture Carl remained grateful, almost in awe, all his life (fig. 4). She came to Chapel Hill in 1956 after graduating BS and MA in 1952 and 1954 at the University of Western Ontario and Holyoake College, Canada, following the suggestion of a friend who was already in Chapel Hill. She was largely self-taught so far as micropuncture was concerned, having worked with Murray Barr on chromatin previously. Her skills were crucial in the success of the research that Carl conducted in the 1950s and 60s, until she left for family reasons in 1967.

Carl had become interested in one of the major unresolved dilemmas in the study of renal function at that time: how urine more concentrated than plasma was formed [11]. The role of vasopressin in permitting dilute urine was already clear, but how concentrated urine could be elaborated remained a mystery. Carl recalled [11]: 'During a visit of Homer Smith ... I had the opportunity to discuss the counter-current hypothesis with him. Smith believed that the loop of Henle played no part in the concentrating mechanism, and that the osmotic concentration of urine occurred as a result of active water transport out of the collecting ducts.'

This view Smith elaborated in his classic books of the 1950s. In contrast, the Swiss physiologist Heinrich Wirtz (1914–1993) (who spent a year in Smith's laboratory in 1950) proposed in 1951 on the basis of work by the physical chemist Werner Kuhn (1899–1963) going as far back as 1942, that the vasae rectae and Henle's loop together could function as a counter-current exchanger to build up a medullary osmotic gradient, with *passive* absorption of water [12], together with regulation of collecting duct permeability to water to obtain variation in urinary concentration. In 1951, Wirtz and his colleagues had made the crucial observation of the presence of a corticomedullary osmotic gradient, using freezing-point depression studies on slices of cortex and medulla [13].

However, even though Smith had rejected Wirtz and Kuhn's model, Carl was intrigued [14]: 'The smart boys don't believe in it,' Smith said. 'On the other hand, having no formal training in renal physiology and not burdened by establishment biases, I found the hypothesis very appealing.'

These last laconic comments are typical of Carl. He and Mylle applied the hitherto neglected technique of

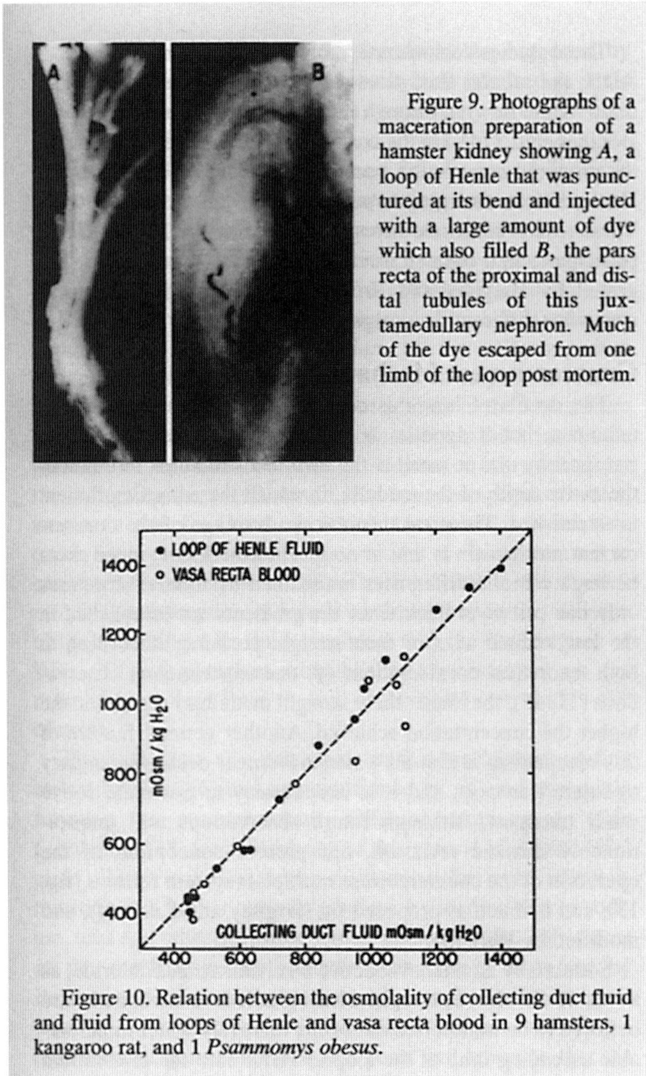

Fig. 5. Two crucial figures in one of the two classic papers on the concentrating mechanism from Gottschalk and Mylle in 1959 (see text). [Reproduced with permission from reference 22].

micropuncture to the problem in a novel way. As is well known [15], Arthur Newton Richards (1876–1966) and Joseph T. Wearn (1893–1984) had pioneered micropuncture of the amphibian tubule in their classic paper of 1922 [16]. Thereafter it was little practised outside of Richards' laboratory, and indeed Richards himself was doubtful if others could produce useful results using the technique, and discouraged its use. Micropuncture of the mammalian kidney had been carried out successfully only by Arthur Walker, Phyllis Bott and Muriel MacDowell in 1941 in Richards' laboratory [17], after which there were no more studies in the area for more than a decade.

Wirtz was aware that micropuncture studies would be necessary to test their hypothesis, but was able only to puncture the vasae rectae in the papilla, finding, as predicted, a high osmolality [18]. Then Gottschalk and Mylle conceived and carried out a similar series of micropuncture experiments, using a nanoliter method for freezing-point depression which had just been published in 1955 [19]. As so often happens, a technical advance was required to permit the testing of a new hypothesis. First [20] they confirmed Walker's surprising finding that the fluid within the distal tubule – in their case of the rat – was as or more dilute than plasma, even when the urine was ten times as concentrated as plasma; they were able also to identify distal tubules unequivocally for the first time. Wirtz [21] then obtained similar data. Clearly, there had to be a diluting segment between the concentrated papilla and the distal tubule. Then Gottschalk and Mylle managed the hitherto impossible task of identifying and puncturing the loop of Henle in the hamster, chosen because of its elongated papilla, which anatomical feature had long been known to be present in species with the ability to elaborate of highly concentrated urine [22]: the crucial observations showed that the tubular fluid was as concentrated as the urine and the blood in the vasae rectae, proving the existence of a diluting segment between the medullary tubule and the distal tubule. Their results, which provided overwhelming support for the countercurrent hypothesis, were a landmark in renal physiology and were so treated in a recent issue of the *Journal of the American Society of Nephrology* launching a series of such articles on the recent history of our specialty (fig. 5). In his commentary on this re-publication of their 1959 paper in the *American Journal of Physiology,* Carl wrote [11]: 'Nothing I had ever done before or have done subsequently was as thrilling as obtaining these data.'

They postulated the differences which must exist between the descending limb, where passive removal of water must take place down an osmotic gradient, and the ascending limb, with active lumen-to-basal transport of solute. At first Homer Smith remained sceptical, despite the unequivocal nature of the data, and did not mention the countercurrent theory at all in his second book on the kidney published in 1956 [23] although before he died in 1962 came to accept it in the light of Carl's data [24], albeit with continued reluctance – which is surprising, given the elegance of the concept and its operation. Only after publication of his own papers did Carl finally meet Wirtz face to face, as Klaus Thurau recalled [25].

The small Chapel Hill laboratory rapidly became a place of pilgrimage to learn micropuncture, which as a result of Carl's work became a dominant technique in renal physiological research for two decades. In 1958, Bill Lassiter joined the team, and a series of seminal papers bearing the names of Gottschalk, Lassiter and Mylle poured out during the 1960s, dealing with urinary acidification and solute exchange along the nephron [26–30]. Mylle herself made the quinhydrone microelectrodes which enabled the pH of the minute tubular fluid samples to be determined [26]. Then came work with François Morel, on sabbatical leave from France, which led to a new technique of tracer injection, to follow water transport [31, 32].

Although at first interested in the function of the normal mammalian kidney, in the late 1960s and early 1970s Carl pioneered the study of micropuncture in a number of disease states: potassium depletion (in collaboration with Lou Welt) [33, 34], acute renal damage induced by obstruction, sodium dichromate and ischaemic damage (with Bill Arendshorst and Bill Finn) [35–38], and (together with Marjorie Allison of Glasgow and Elvira Arrizurieta of Buenos Aires) reduction of renal mass and immune-induced glomerulonephritis [39–41]. These various methods of renal reduction allowed examination of glomerulotubular balance in disease, which Carl termed the 'adaptive nephron' [39, 41]. In several papers he reported the use of the technique of nephron microdissection popularized by Jean Oliver in a co-ordinated fashion, correlated with the functional studies, co-authoring papers with the master of microdissection [38, 42, 43]. He studied also the still vexed question of the complex handling of urate by the nephron [44, 45].

During all these years he produced a number of scholarly and beautifully-written summaries of knowledge of various aspects of renal physiology, many the results of invited lectures.

Studies later in the 1970s and early 1980s involved the role of the renal nerves in determining sodium and water excretion [46–48], showing that the water diuresis in the denervated kidney was accompanied by decrease in sodium reabsorption without any detectable change in glomerular filtration rate (GFR), whilst renal nerve stimulation induced an increase in sodium reabsorption, again without any change in GFR.

Although Carl Gottschalk's administrative and personal talents generally flowered in the local setting of Chapel Hill, where with great skill and success he took on many burdens in local committees, at two points he had a decisive influence on national affairs. The first occurred when he was asked to chair the Special Committee on Renal Disease, to examine the pressing problem of long-term treatment of patients in renal failure. This was recognition of his absolute integrity and fairness which he applied to his own and everyone else's affairs. He was thus the ideal chairman in dealing with disputed issues. His committee's report [49] recommended that dialysis treatment be available to all who needed it, without denial for financial reasons – a proposal not viewed with favour by the Bureau of Budget who commissioned the report! However, it paved the way for the famous public law 92–603 of 1972 guaranteeing treatment for renal failure to US citizens. The influence of the Gottschalk report – as it came to be known – was not confined to the United States. I remember reading it avidly in 1967, and using it in our (less successful) arguments with government officials in the United Kingdom about our nascent chronic renal failure program. The second was when he became President of the American Society of Nephrology in 1975, serving on its national executive for 3 years.

In addition in 1979, together with Robert Schrier, he took over editing the 3rd edition of Strauss and Welt's *Diseases of the Kidney*. This fruitful collaboration continued through until the 6th edition, published in 1997. This book was and still is the standard American text on Nephrology against which all other similarly comprehensive efforts must be judged.

Carl Gottschalk: Bibliophile and Historian of Nephrology

Most, if not all major contributors to medical science like Carl have a keen sense of how the study of the past can illuminate the present, and help shape the future. Carl, however, carried this awareness into the public domain, with a series of studies of the history of Nephrology, especially renal physiology, published over 30 years from 1969 to 1997 [50–62], and was working actively on projects in the history of Nephrology when he was lost to us. His contributions culminated for most of us, I suppose, in the volume published by the American Physiological Society in 1987, which he helped assemble and edit: *Renal Physiology: Men and Ideas* [63]. It was, and 10 years later still is, the key work in the field.

Also, on behalf of the International Society of Nephrology, we must thank Carl for two successful endeavours: the Historical Archive series appearing in *Kidney International*, which he founded, contributed to and edited for more than 15 years, and the Commission for the History of Nephrology, which he started and chaired for a similar period. That both are active and expanding today, although he stepped down from these duties a few years ago, is a tribute to his success in launching them.

We do not know when Carl began collecting books. I suspect it was very early – probably whilst still a child. One of his mentors, Jean Oliver, had no children, regarding Carl more as a son than a colleague, and fuelled this quest by bequeathing him his own collection of books, reprints and manuscripts to do with the kidney, in the knowledge I am sure of Carl's already developed passion. For more than 40 years, Carl shrewdly, patiently and persistently amassed a collection of works on the history of medicine, particularly those relating to the study of Nephrology. Much of this collecting was done during summer visits to London over the years, where he became known to all the many antiquarian and medical booksellers in the city.

First the house had to be enlarged, then enlarged again to accommodate the collection. It was fortunate that by the time the garage succumbed under the tide of books there was almost no works bearing on the field of renal physiology and renal disease that Carl did not already possess. In addition, he had a substantial collection of rare or first editions of general literature, in keeping with his wide range of intellectual interests.

I think Carl loved the process of collecting almost as much as the possession and reading of the works. Leon Fine, a fellow collector of fine books, wrote to me: 'Whenever we met, we would exchange battle stories about books won, and books lost ...'

As his collection became more and more complete, the hunt for rare volumes in the excellent condition he always required became ever more difficult – and therefore ever more exciting. Many of us were able to share with Carl and Leon their excitement when they produced a unique exhibit of original material relating to the history of renal physiology and medicine at the International Society of Nephrology meeting in Los Angeles in 1984 [64] – which in addition resulted in there being an event relating to the history of our subject at all subsequent Congresses of the ISN.

Books truly were Carl's lifelong passion. If this word 'passion' seems a little too strong in this context, we should remember that Ralph Waldo Emerson said once [65]: 'a man's library is a sort of harem ...'

We cannot know if Carl thought of his collection in this way, but his delight in the look and feel of books, the hand-made paper, the exquisite type, the leather binding, their smell – and even their sound as some creaked open – was evident to all, and illustrates the passion of the bibliophile. Never was he happier than when delighting appreciative fellow bibliophiles with his collection.

Carl's collection of books and reprints is unique: nowhere is the archive of primary sources for our specialty assembled so completely, especially his collection of original reprints of key papers in the history of Nephrology, many with original autographs. I believe that to get close to Carl's spirit, one needs only to sit down at his library desk, pick up, open and browse through one of his volumes, knowing that he had done the same many times. It is good to know that his collection – and his exquisite kidney-shaped desk, another gift from Jean Oliver – will rest in the Wilson library at the University of North Carolina in Chapel Hill, available to scholars of medical history, a suitable memorial to a remarkable and loveable man.

Acknowledgements

I would like to thank particularly Susan Fellner Gottschalk for her help in the preparation of the biographical part of this paper. Also Mabel Purkerson for allowing me sight of material on Margaret (Peggy) Mylle Richardson prior to publication, Peggy Richardson herself and Leon Fine for their memories of Carl, Bob Berliner for sight of his unpublished appraisal of Carl's contribution to renal physiology, and Bill Blythe and Bill Arendshorst for background material.

References

1 Blair EA, Gottschalk CW: Efficiency of Signal Corps operators in extreme cold. Armored Medical Research Laboratories. Project No 57, 22nd January 1947.
2 Molnar GW, Blair JR, Gottschalk CW, Layton WM, Osgood LE, Zimmerman WJ, Johnson CA: Energy expenditure and endurance of men in an arctic bivouac. Medical Departmental Field Research Laboratory, Report No 6-64-12-02(13), 1st April 1950.
3 Talbott JH, Gottschalk CW, Henry CB, Blair JR, Kolovis RE: Report of cold injury research team, Medical Research and Development Board, Office of the Surgeon General, Department of the Army, 20th March 1951.
4 Gottschalk CW, Riggs DS: Protein-bound iodine in the serum of soldiers and of Eskimos in the Arctic. J Clin Endocrinol Metab 1952;12: 235–243.
5 Gottschalk CW: Frostbite. Mod Concepts Cardiovasc Dis 1953;2:202–205.
6 Wood CE, Gottschalk CW: The butterflies of Roanoke and Montgomery Counties, Virginia. Entomol News 1942;53:143–146, 159–164, 191–197.
7 Tosteson DC, deFriez AIC, Abrams M, Gottschalk CW, Landis EM: Effects of adrenalectomy, desoxycorticosterone acetate and increased fluid intake of on intake of sodium chloride and bicarbonate by hypertensive and normal rats. Am J Physiol 1951;164:369–379.
8 Gottschalk CW: A comparative study of renal interstitial pressure. Am J Physiol 1952;169: 180–187.
9 Gottschalk CW, Mylle M: A micropuncture study of the pressures in the proximal tubules and peritubular capillaries of the rat kidney and their relation to ureteral and renal venous pressures. Am J Physiol 1956;185:430–439.
10 Gottschalk CW, Mylle M: A micropuncture study of the pressures in the proximal and distal tubules of the rat during osmotic diuresis. Am J Physiol 1957;189: 323–328.
11 Blythe WB: In memoriam Carl William Gottschalk (1922–1997). Kidney Int 1998;53:1–2.
12 Wirtz H, Hargitay B, Kuhn W: Das Multiplikationsprinzip als Grundlage der Harnkonzentrierung in der Niere. Z Elektrochem 1951;555: 539–558.
13 Wirtz H, Hargitay B, Kuhn W: Lokalisation des Konzentrierungsprozesses in der Niere durch direkte Kryoscopie. Helv Physiol Pharmacol Acata 1951;9:196–207.
14 Milestones in Nephrology: Micropuncture study of the mammalian urinary concentrating mechanisms: Evidence for the countercurrent hypothesis. CW Gottschalk and Margaret Mylle, with comments by CW Gottschalk and MA Knepper. J Am Soc Nephrol 1997;8:153–164.
15 Peitzman S: Micropuncture and the mechanistic kidney; a new look at a classic experiment. Bull Med Hist 1991;65:366–375.
16 Wearn JT, Richards AN: Observations on the composition of glomerular urine, with particular reference to the problem of reabsorption in the renal tubules. Am J Physiol 1922;71:209–227.
17 Walker AM, Bott PA, Oliver J, MacDowell MC: The collection and analysis of fluid from single nephrons of the mammalian kidney. Am J Physiol 1941;134:580–595.
18 Wirtz H: Der osmotische Druck des Blutes in der Nierenepapille. Helv Physiol Pharmacol Acta 1953;11:20–29.
19 Ramsay JA, Brown RHJ: Simplified apparatus and procedure for freezing-point determinations upon small volumes of fluid. J Sci Instrum 1955;32:372–375.
20 Gottschalk CW, Mylle M: Evidence that the mammalian nephron functions as a countercurrent multiplier system. Science 1958;128: 594.
21 Wirtz H: Der osmotische Druck des Blutes in den corticalen Tubuli der Rattenniere. Helv Physiol Pharmacol Acta 1956;14:353–362.
22 Gottschalk CW, Mylle M: Micropuncture study of the mammalian urinary concentrating mechanism: Evidence for the counter-current hypothesis. Am J Physiol 1959;196:927–936.
23 Smith HW: Principles of Renal Physiology. London, Oxford University Press, 1956.
24 Smith HW: The fate of sodium and water in the renal tubules. The Sixth Harlow Brooks Memorial Lecture. Proc NY Acad Sci 1959;35:293–316.
25 Thurau K: In memoriam: Carl William Gottschalk, MD 1922–1997. Am J Kidney Dis 1998;31:xlvi–xlvii.
26 Gottschalk CW, Lassiter WE, Mylle M: Localization of urinary acidification in the mammalian kidney. Am J Physiol 1960;198:581–585.
27 Lassiter WE, Gottschalk CW, Mylle M: Micropuncture study of net transtubular movement of water and urea in nondiuretic mammalian kidney. Am J Physiol 1961;200:1139–1147.
28 Lassiter WE, Gottschalk CW, Mylle M: Micropuncture study of renal tubular reabsorption of calcium in normal rodents. Am J Physiol 1963; 204:771–775.
29 Lassiter WE, Mylle M, Gottschalk CW: Net transtubular movement of water and urea in saline diuresis. Am J Physiol 1964;206:669–673.
30 Lassiter WE, Mylle M, Gottschalk CW: Micropuncture study of urea transport in rat renal medulla. Am J Physiol 1966;210:965–970.
31 Gottschalk CW, Morel F, Mylle M: Tracer microinjection studies of renal tubular permeability. Am J Physiol 1965;209:173–178.
32 Morel F, Mylle M, Gottschalk CW: Tracer microinjection studies of the effect of ADH on renal tubular diffusion of water. Am J Physiol 1965;209:179–187.
33 Gottschalk CW, Mylle M, Jones NF, Winters RW, Welt LG: Osmolality of renal tubular fluids in potassium-depleted rodents. Clin Sci 1965;29:249–250.
34 Jones NF, Mylle M, Gottschalk CW: Renal tubular microinjection studies in normal and potassium-depleted rats. Clin Sci 1965;29: 261–275.
35 Arendshorst WJ, Finn WF, Gottschalk CW: Nephron stop-flow pressure response to obstruction for 24 hours in the rat kidney. J Clin Invest 1974;53:1497–1500.
36 Finn WF, Arendshorst WJ, Gottschalk CW: Pathogenesis of oliguria in acute renal failure. Circ Res 1975;36:675–681.
37 Arendshorst WJ, Finn WF, Gottschalk CW: Pathogenesis of acute renal failure following temporary renal ischemia in the rat. Circ Res 1975;37:558–568.
38 Biber TUL, Mylle M, Baines AD, Gottschalk CW, Oliver J, MacDowell A: A study by micropuncture and microdissection of acute renal damage in rats. Am J Med 1968;44:664–705.
39 Arrizurieta de Michnik EE, Lassiter WE, Lipham EM, Gottschalk CW: Micropuncture study of glomerulotubular balance in the rat kidney. Nephron 1969;6:418–436.
40 Allison MEM, Lipham EM, Lassiter WE, Gottschalk CW: The acutely reduced kidney. Kidney Int 1973;3:354–363.
41 Allison MEM, Wilson CB, Gottschalk CW: Pathophysiology of experimental glomerulonephritis in rats. J Clin Invest 1974;53:1402–1423.
42 Kramp RA, MacDowell M, Gottschalk CW, Oliver JR: A study by microdissection and micropuncture of the structure and function of the kidneys and nephrons of rats with chronic renal damage. Kidney Int 1974;30:136–144.
43 Fetterman GH, Allison MEM, Wilson CB, Gottschalk CW: Structural changes of experimental glomerulonephritis in rats as revealed by microdissetion. Pathol Annu 1978;13:55–79.
44 Kramp RA, Lassiter WE, Gottschalk CW: Urate-2-14-C transport in the rat nephron. J Clin Invest 1971;50:35–48.
45 Cook MA, Adkinson JT, Lassiter WE, Gottschalk CW: Uric acid excretion by the rat kidney. Am J Physiol 1975;229:586–591.
46 Colindres RE, Gottschalk CW: Neural control of renal tubular sodium reabsorption in the rat. Single nephron analysis. Fed Proc 1978;37: 1218–1221.
47 Colindres RE, Spielman WS, Moss NG, Harrington WW, Gottschalk CW: Functional evidence for renorenal reflexes in the rat. Am J Physiol 1980;239:F265–F270.
48 Szalay L, Colidres RE, Jackson R, Gottschalk CW: Effects of chronic renal denervation on conscious unrestrained rats. Urol Nephrol 1986;18:3–18.
49 The 'Gottschalk report': Report of the special commission on chronic renal failure to the bureau of budget. Department of State, Washington, D.C., 1967.
50 Gottschalk CW: Dr AN Richards and kidney micropuncture. Ann Intern Med 1969; 71(suppl 8):28–37.

51 Gottschalk CW: Introduction. Jean Redman Oliver Festschrift. Kidney Int 1974;5:75–76.
52 Gottschalk CW: Bright's disease – An historical perspective; in Controversies in Nephrology 1979. Proceedings of the first conference, January 18–19, 1979. Washington, Georgetown Nephrology Division, 1979, pp 1–21.
53 Gottschalk CW: Odyssey of the glomerular filtration coefficient. Proc Int Union Physiol Sci 1983;15:237.
54 Arendshrost WJ, Gottschalk CW: Glomerular filtration dynamics: Historical perspective. Am J Physiol 1985;248:F163–F174.
55 Gottschalk CW: History of the urinary concentrating mechanism. Kidney Int 1987;31:507–511.
56 Gottschalk CW: The application of micropuncture techniques to analysis of renal function: A personal view. Am J Kidney Dis 1990;16:536–540.
57 Gottschalk CW: A history of renal physiology to 1950; in Seldin D, Giebisch G (eds): The Kidney: Physiology and Pathophysiology, ed 2. New York, Raven Press, 1992, pp 1–29.
58 Gottschalk CW: Elucidation of kidney function by micropuncture: An historical perspective. Bull Acad Med Belg 1992;147:162–169.
59 Gottschalk CW, Berliner RW, Schreiner GW: The American Society of Nephrology and its beginnings; in Tannen RL, Fine LG, Gottschalk CW, Schreiner GW (eds): A Quarter Century of Nephrology. Commemorating American Society of Nephrology's 25th Anniversary, American Society of Nephrology, 1992, pp 1–8.
60 Gottschalk CW: Alexander Schumlansky's De structura renum. Am J Nephrol 1994;14: 32–324.
61 Gottschalk CW: Homer William Smith: A remembrance. J Am Soc Nephrol 1995;5:1984–1987.
62 Gottschalk CW, Fellner SK: History of the science of dialysis. Am J Nephrol 1997;17: 289–298.
63 Gottschalk CW, Berliner RW, Giebisch G (eds): Renal Physiology: People and Ideas. Bethesda, American Society of Physiology, 1987.
64 Fine LG, Gottschalk CW: Photostat facsimile. Available in the Wellcome Library of the History of Medicine, London.
65 Emerson RW: In praise of books; in The Conduct of Life. Leipzig, Bernhard Tauchnitz, 1860, pp 64.

Origins of Renal Physiology
(Dedicated to Carl Gottschalk)

American Journal of Nephrology

Am J Nephrol 1999;19:243–256

History of Renal Physiology in Germany during the 19th Century

Klaus Hierholzer[a] Karl Julius Ullrich[b]

[a]Department of Clinical Physiology, Free University of Berlin, and [b]Max Planck Institute of Biophysics, Frankfurt/Main, Germany

Key Words

Renal physiology · Henle · Ludwig · Heidenhain · Fick · Helmholtz · du Bois-Reymond

Abstract

The roots of renal physiology in Germany in the last century have been traced. Vitalistic concepts became replaced by physical, chemical and mechanistic laws which govern biological processes. First, the main exponents of renal physiology, J. Henle, C. Ludwig and R.P.H. Heidenhain, are discussed, then the (indirect) contributions of A. Fick, K. Peter, H. Helmholtz, E. du Bois-Reymond, J.L. Schönlein and A. Dohrn are evaluated. The original literature bearing on renal physiology in the 19th century is screened by a survey of publications in *Pflügers Archiv* and *Archiv der experimentellen Pathologie und Pharmakologie*. We point to the international cooperation in the field. At the turn of the century, renal function was adequately described by a theory of glomerular filtration, tubular secretion and tubular reabsorption.

Introduction

In the present paper we attempt to delineate the early development of renal physiology in our country. We concentrate mainly on the 19th century. Before that there was no systematic research in renal physiology, as there was none elsewhere in the world. From the beginning of this discussion we have to stress that the gradual development of a reliable theory of urine formation was the achievement of many groups inside and outside of Germany. It is impressive to realize how even in the 19th century, scientists (J. Müller, W. Bowman, C. Bernard, C. Ludwig, R.P.H. Heidenhain, E.H. Starling, A. Fick, A.R. Cushny and others), their departments, and concepts interacted across national borders. Table 1 depicts the historical context of some of the relevant scholar who participated. Modern renal physiology with its many ramifications is a tree with many roots in numerous laboratories. We like to trace some relevant ones in our country.

In his *Textbook of Physiology*, Hildebrandt [8] summarized the then available knowledge of renal physiology: 'The human body, like all other living beings, is gifted with a vital force (vis vitalis), which causes the particular state of the living body, i.e. life (vita)' (§57). Urine is watery and contains the same substances as blood but in different concentrations. 'Excretion of this juice (urine) occurs in both kidneys (renes) by transfer within the renal cortex of water and certain other substances into tubules (tubuli uriniferi) of the inner area (substantia tubulosa) ...' (§460). This vitalistic concept was challenged, when Wöhler [58] in 1828 succeeded in synthesizing urea in vitro '... without the need of an animal ...', and it finally became replaced by mechanistic, physical and chemical laws which provided a scientific and reliable basis for the

KARGER

Fax + 41 61 306 12 34
E-Mail karger@karger.ch
www.karger.com

© 1999 S. Karger AG, Basel
0250–8095/99/0192–0243$17.50/0

Accessible online at:
http://BioMedNet.com/karger

Prof. Klaus Hierholzer
Schlappengasse 12
D–78476 Allensbach (Germany)
Tel./Fax +49 7533 3619

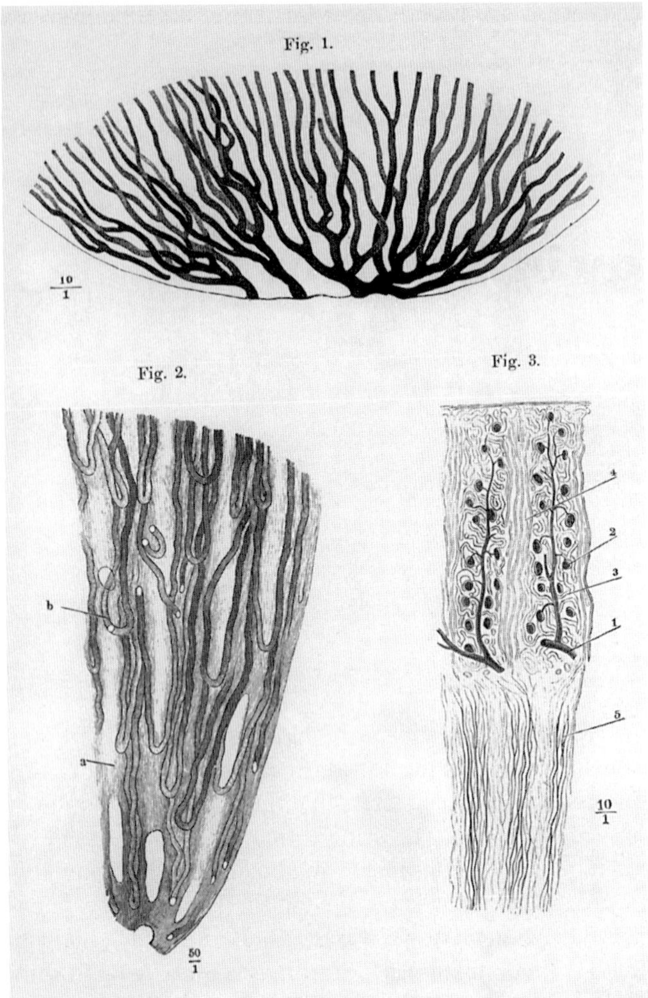

Fig. 1. Section through the papilla of a kidney, injected from the ureter. From Henle's 'Grundriss der Anatomie des Menschen' [25]. Cited from Hierholzer [21].

Table 1. Historical context of scholars discussed in the present paper

German Scholars		
1793	Schönlein, Johann Lukas	1864
1800	Wöhler, Friedrich	1882
1801	Müller, Johannes	1858
1803	Liebig, Justus, v.	1873
1809	*Henle, Jacob*	1885
1816	*Ludwig, Carl Friedrich Wilhelm*	1895
1818	du Bois-Reymond, Emil	1896
1821	Helmholtz, Hermann Ludwig Ferdinand v.	1894
1821	Virchow, Rudolf	1902
1829	Fick, Adolf	1901
1834	*Heidenhain, Rudolf Peter H.*	1897
1837	Basch, Ritter v., Siegfried Samuel Karl	1905
1840	Dohrn, Anton	1909
1845	Röntgen, Wilhelm Conrad	1923
Foreign scholars with whom they interacted		
1779	Berzelius, Jöns Jakob	1848
1791	Faraday, Michael	1867
1813	Bernard, Claude	1878
1816	Bowman, William	1892
1849	Mahomed, Frederick	1884
1866	Cushny, Arthur Robertson	1926
1866	Starling, Ernest Henry	1927

explanation of living processes. In Germany this change most dramatically occurred in the Department of Anatomy (and Physiology) of Johannes Müller in Berlin. Müller still considered the possibility of the existence of a special vital force. His assistants, particularly Helmholtz, du Bois-Reymond, Henle, Brücke and others, turned exclusively to physicochemical forces in the attempt to analyze biological processes.

What were the pertinent contributions of German scientists to renal physiology in the 19th century which eventually led to a consistent and more sophisticated theory of renal function? In the following, we would like to discuss this question in some detail.

Contributions to Renal Physiology

The main experimental and conceptual contributions in our country undoubtedly came from Jacob Henle in Berlin, Heidelberg and Göttingen, from Carl Ludwig in Leipzig and From Rudolf Heidenhain in Breslau, with their respective coworkers. Their scientific careers and their work has been discussed and evaluated in many previous articles to which we refer in the bibliography. In the context of the present discusssion it suffices to remember that:

Jakob Henle [21–25], basically an anatomist, discovered the loop arrangement of medullary tubules (tubuli uriniferi) which eventually paved the way for the explanation of urine concentration by the counter current system. Figure 1 is taken from an article by Henle [25]. In a letter to Ludwig he describes his observation and opens a discussion as to the possible functional importance of the peculiar structure. Henle by no means concentrated exclusively on renal structure and function. He has been quoted saying: 'One has only to sweep over a piece of fresh tissue with a razor blade in order to make a pertinent discovery ...' [see 38, p 236 and ref in table 2, IIIb]. He apparently swept over many different tissues. As we have dis-

Table 2. Original papers, relevant for the development of renal physiology published in *Pflügers Archiv* (Archiv für die Gesammte Physiologie der Menschen und Thiere) and in *AePP* (Archiv für Experimentelle Pathologie und Pharmakologie) from the beginning of their appearance to the turn of the 19th century: papers are grouped according to different topics; topics and/or titles are translated and shortened, papers from *AePP* are printed in italics

Author(s), city	Title	Vol–year–page
(Ia) Analytical methods		
Jaffé M, Königsberg	Indican in urine	3–1870–448
Strassburg G, Bremen	Bile acids in urine	4–1871–461
Seegen J, ?	Sugar in urine	5–1872–375
Fokker AP, Goes	New technique for uric acid	10–1875–153
Pflüger E, ?	Quant. analysis of urea	21–1880–248
Habel L, Fernholz J	Quant. analysis of chloride in urine	23–1880–85
Müller W, Christiania	Copper oxide and alcali on uric acid	27–1882–22
Müller W, Christiania	Copper oxide and alcali on creatinine	27–1882–59
Müller W, Christiania	Copper oxide and alcali on urine	27–1882–86
Müller W, Christiania	Analysis of sugar in urine	27–1882–86
Pflüger E, Bohland K, Bonn	Analysis of nitrogen in human urine	36–1885–102
Weyl Th, Meyer A, ?	Nitrates in urine	36–1885–456
Pflüger E, Schenck F, Bonn	Analysis of urea in human urine	38–1886–325
Pflüger E, Schenk F, Bonn	Analysis of urea	38–1886–530
Pflüger E, Bohland K	Analysis of urea	39–1886–1
Pflüger E, Bohland K	Analysis of urea	39–1886–143
Leo H, Berlin	Urinary excretion of trypsin	39–1886–246
Arnold C, Wedemeyer K, ?	Analysis of nitrogen in urine, comparison of techniques	52–1892–592
Schulz H, Greifswald	Determination of sulfur in urine	57–1894–233
Schöndorff B, ?	Determination of urea in tissues and fluids	62–1896–1
Lohnstein Th, ?	Densitometric analysis of glucose in urine	62–1896–82
Salkowski E, ?	Analysis of 'alloxur' bases in urine	69–1898–268
Rösel R, ?	Quant. analysis of iodine in urine	77–1899–22
Heubach H, Bonn	*Quant. analysis of alcohol in urine*	*8–1878–446*
Pohl J, Prag	*Analysis of globulin in urine + serosal fluids*	*20–1886–426*
Schumacher II, ?	*Quant. analysis of mercury in urine*	*28–1891–138*
Jolles A, Wien	*Quant. analysis of mercury in urine*	*44–1900–160*
Farup, Christiania	*Quant. analysis of mercury in urine*	*44–1900–272*
(Ib) Experimental techniques		
Salkowski E, Berlin	Isolated kidney perfusion and microsc. inspection	54–1893–607
Jacobj C, Strassburg	*Apparatus for blood perfusion of isolated organs*	*26–1890–388*
Jacobj C, Strassburg	*Technique of artificial blood perfusion of isolated perfused organs*	*36–1895–330*
(II) Urine composition and urinary excretion		
Pflüger E, Bonn	Gas content of urine, bile, saliva, milk	2–1869–156
Salkowski E, Berlin	Chemical analysis of urine (urea and various organic acids)	2–1869–356
Huizinga D, ?	Glucose in urine	3–1870–496
Seegen J, ?	Glucose in normal urine	5–1872–24
Baumstark F, Greifswald	Two pathologic dyes in urine	9–1874–582
Hoppe-Seyler F, ?	Biliary compounds in urine	10–1875–208
Esoff J, Petersburg	Urobilin in urine	12–1876–50
Baumann E, ?	'Brenzcatechin' in urine	12–1876–63
Baumann E, ?	Paired sulfuric acids in urine	12–1876–69
Munk I, Berlin	Phenol forming compound in urine	12–1876–142
Gergens E, Baumann E, Strassburg	Guanidin, dicyandiamidin, cyanamid in urine	12–1876–205
Külz E, ?	Glucose in normal urine	13–1876–269
Dehn A, ?	Potassium salts excretion	13–1876–353

➤

Table 2 (continued)

Author(s), city	Title	Vol–year–page
Valentin G, ?	Diffraction indices of urine	17–1878–255
Oppenheim H, ?	Human urea excretion, various conditions	23–1880–446
Vetlesen HJ, Christiania	Reducing substance in urine after intake of terpentine	28–1882–?
Gehrig F, ?	Encymes in urine	38–1886–35
Heffter A, Rostock	Sulfur in urine	38–1886–476
Helwes F, Hannover	Rennet in urine	43–1888–384
Hagemann ?, Berlin	Reducing substances in horse urine	43–1888–501
Pott R, ?	Reliability of uric acid analysis in urine	45–1889–389
Salkowski E, ?	Carbohydrates in urine, fermentation	54–1893–607
Meyer F, Bonn	Canine urine composition after meat intake	55–1894–272
Jolles A, Wien	Urobilin in urine	61–1895–623
Rosemann R, ?	Pattern of human nitrogen excretion	65–1897–343
Marcuse G, Breslau	Pattern of phosphorus excretion after intake of casein	67–1897–373
Schöndorff B, ?	Urea content of several body fluids	74–1899–357
Beck A, ?	Excretory pattern in bled and food-depleted frogs	77–1899–290
Gottlieb R, Wien	*Iron excretion in urine*	*26–1890–139*
Heuss E, Bern	*Lactic acid in human urine*	*26–1890–147*
Mosso U, Torino	*Excretion of salicylic acid and derivatives*	*26–1890–267*
Mocatelli R, Roma	*Lactic acid content of human urine*	*27–1890–158*
Schreiber, ? + Waldvogel, Göttingen	*Uric acid excretion under phys. and pathol. conditions*	*28–1891–69*
Starck v, Kiel	*Urobilin in canine urine*	*33–1894–373*
Cloetta M, Strassburg	*'Uroprot' acid in urine*	*40–1898–29*
Stockmann R, ?	*Excretion of tannic acid*	*40–1898–147*
Poduschka R, Prag	*Excretion of allantoin*	*44–1898–59*
(III) Renal physiology and pathophysiology		
(IIIa) Structure/function relationship		
Bial M, Breslau	Function of renal epithelia, storage of compounds	47–1890–116
Kostjurin SD, Charkow	*Importance of renal smooth muscles*	*25–1889–184*
(IIIb) Process of urine formation		
Heidenhain R,	Exp. analysis of urine formation	9–1874–1
Grützner P, Breslau	Blood pressure and urine excretion	11–1875–370
Nussbaum M, ?	Secretion in kidneys	16–1878–139
Nussbaum M, ?	Secretion in kidneys cont.	16–1878–580
Grützner P, Breslau	Physiology of renal secretion	24–1881–441
Schmidt A, ?	Site and mechanism of excretion of carmine	48–1891–34
Liebermann L, ?	Properties of renal parenchyma, pH and different compounds	50–1891–55
Liebermann L, Budapest	Chemical processes connected with secretion of urine	54–1893–585
Pregl F, Graz	Cause of high C/N ratios in human	75–1899–?
Jacobji C, Sobieranski Wv, Strassburg	*Functions of isolated perfused kidneys*	*29–1892–25*
Suter F, Meyer H, ?	*Normal secretion of urine in humans*	*33–1894–241*
Seelig A, Königsberg	*Local sugar excretion in organs*	*37–1896–156*
Seelig A, Königsberg	*Local sugar excretion in organs*	*38–1897–158*
Breul L, Strassburg	*Sugar excretion, influence of diet*	*40–1898–1*
(IIIc) Acid-base excretion		
Sawicki A, ?	Acid excretion and work	5–1872–285
Buchheim R, ?	Renal acid excretion	12–1876–326
Pflüger E, Bonn	Excretion of acids and bases	44–1889–273

Table 2 (continued)

Author(s), city	Title	Vol–year–page
(IIId) Renal circulation (cf. Ib)		
Högyes A, ?	*Experiments on renal circulation*	*1–1873–299*
(IIIe) Extrarenal effects on renal function		
Sachs B, New York	Influence of spinal cord on kidneys	25–1881–299
Bleibtreu L, Bonn	Muscular work on urea excretion	46–1890–601
Müller K, Berlin	*Influence of skin on renal function*	*1–1873–429*
Quincke H, Bern	*Influence of sleep on renal function*	*7–1877–115*
Quincke H, Kiel	*Urine excretion at day and night*	*32–1893–211*
Spiro ?, Strassburg	*Hemoconcentration affects urine and lymph flow, effect of colloids*	*41–1898–148*
(IIIf) Effect of drugs and poisons		
Quincke H, Kiel	*Urine pattern after intake of 'copaibalsam'*	*17–1883–273*
Mürset A, Bern	*Intoxication nephritis from aloin and axalic acid*	*19–1885–310*
Penzoldt F, Erlangen	*Intake of naphthalin on urine pattern*	*21–1886–34*
Albertoni P, Pisenti G, ?	*Renal effects of acetone and aceto-acidic acid*	*23–1887–393*
Werner R, Löhmimgen	*Bile and bile salts on renal function*	*24–1888–31*
Morishima K, Leipzig	*Effect of poisoning with curarin ...*	*28–1891–28*
Nencki M, ?	*Methylmercaptane in urine after intake of asparagus*	*28–1891–206*
Walti L, Strassburg	*Renal effects of atropine*	*36–1895–411*
(IIIg) Diuresis/diuretics		
Filehne W, Breslau	Contributions to diuresis, Introduction	51–1902–565
Filehne W, Biberfeld, Breslau	Introductory experiments	51–1902–569
Ruschhaupt W, ?	Interaction of two salts in diuresis	51–1902–574
Pototzky C, ?	Effect of several diuretics on excretion of salt, including Na-depleted animal	51–1902–595
Ercklentz W, ?	Effect of saline infusion on Cl excretion	51–1902–599
Ruschhaupt W, ?	Effect of surgical maneuvers on salt diuresis	51–1902–619
Schroeder Wv, Strassburg	*Diuretic actions of caffeine*	*22–1887–39*
Schroeder Wv, Strassburg	*Diuretic actions of caffeine*	*24–1888–85*
Hoffmann A, Heidelberg	*Therapeutic use of theobromine deriv.*	*28–1891–1*
Rüdel G, Heidelberg	*Influence of diuresis on urine pH*	*30–1892–41*
Pfaff F, Brnian (Bohemia)	*Diuretic effects of digitalis glycosides (humans and animals)*	*32–1893–1*
Sobieranski Wv, Marburg	*Mechanism of action of diuretics*	*35–1895–144*
Jacobj C, Strassburg	*Experimental renal diabetes*	*35–1895–213*
Rost E, Heidelberg	*Excretion of caffeine + theobromine*	*36–1895–56*
Bondzynski St, Gottlieb R, ?	*Methylxanthin in urine after intake of caffeine and theobromine*	*37–1896–385*
Hellin D, Spiro K, Strassburg	*Effects of caffeine + phloridzin in nephritis*	*38–1897–368*
Schwarz L, Prag	*Physiology and pharmacology of diuresis*	*43–1900–1*
Magnus R, Heidelberg	*Effect of saline infusion on diuresis*	*44–1900–68*
Magnus R, Heidelberg	*Effect of saline infusion on diuresis*	*44–1900–396*
Ach N, Strassburg	*Diuretic action of purine derivatives*	*44–1900–319*
(IIIh) Pathophysiology		
Antweiler X, Breidenbend P, Bonn	Glucose in diabetic urine	28–1882–179
Bohland C, Schurz H, ?	Excretion of uric acid and nitrogen in leukemia	47–1890–469
Liebermann L, ?	Content of phosphoric acid in horse urine under different conditions	50–1891–57
Smith-Jerome WJ, ?	Abnormal excretion of sulfur in a dog	60–1895–233

➤

Table 2 (continued)

Author(s), city	Title	Vol–year–page
Annuschat A, ?	*Excretion of lead in lead poisoning*	*10–1879–261*
Jaarsveld GJ + Stokvis, Amsterdam	*Renal disease and formation of hippuric acid*	*10–1879–268*
Hallervorden ?, ?	*Renal excretion of ammonia under pathologic conditions*	*12–1880–?*
Stadelmann E, ?	*Excretion of ammonia in diabetes mellitus and diabetic coma*	*17–1883–419*
Minkowski O, ?	*Oxybutyric acid in urine of diabetics*	*18–1884–35*
Minkowski O, ?	*Oxybutyric acid in urine of diabetics*	*18–1884–147*
Külz R, Marburg	*Dextra-rotatory oxybutyric acids (diab)*	*18–1884–20*
Schreiber J, Königsberg	*Experimental albuminuria in humans*	*19–1885–237*
Schreiber J, Königsberg	*Experimental albuminuria in humans*	*20–1886–85*
Wolpe H, Königsberg	*Oxybutyric acid in diabetic urine*	*21–1886–138*
Riess L, ?	*Nitrogen excretion under antipyretics*	*22–1887–127*
Török L, Pollak S, ?	*Formation of cylinders in urine*	*25–1889–87*
Livierato E, Genova	*CO_2 excretion in diabetics*	*25–1889–161*
Neuberger J, Leipzig	*Calcareous deposits in kidneys*	*27–1890–39*
Gerhardt D, Schlesinger W, Strassburg	*Excretory pattern (Ca, Mg, acids) in diabetics*	*28–1891–83*
Seelig A, Königsberg	*Renal effects of thoracic compression*	*28–1891–263*
Tillie J, Edinburgh	*Hemoglobinuria after blood pressure oscillations*	*29–1892–170*
Limbeck Rv, Prag	*Uremic intoxication*	*31–1893–180*
Weintraud W, Strassburg	*Excretion of acetone and acids in diabetes mell.*	*34–1894–12*
Bondsynski St, Gottlieb R, Heidelberg	*Xanthin derivatives in leukemic urine*	*36–1895–127*
Riedl A, Kraus R, ?	*Renal excretion of microorganisms*	*37–1896–1*
Klecki Cv, Krakau	*Renal excretion of microorganisms and influence of diuresis*	*39–1897–173*
Scholz W, Graz	*Carbon content of urine in fever*	*40–1898–326*
Ruschhaupt W, Heidelberg	*Acetone glycosuria*	*44–1900–127*
(IV) Ureters and bladder		
Engelmann ThW, Utrecht	Peristalsis in ureters	2–1869–293
Edlefsen G, Kiel	Urine layers in bladder	3–1870–585
Treskin S, Mstislawl	Bladder and kidney function, urea excretion	5–1872–324
Falck FA, Kiel	Physiology of urinary bladder	19–1979–431
Sokoloff O, Luchsinger B, Bern	Physiology of ureters	26–1881–464
Edlefsen G, Kiel	Urine layers in bladder	43–1888–314
Zeissl M v, ?	Innervation of urinary bladder	53–1893–560
Zeissl M v, ?	Innervation of urinary bladder	55–1894–569
Exner S, Wien	Paralysis and distensibility of bladder	55–1894–303
Hauc A, ?	Reflexes in urinary bladder	73–1898–453
Lewin L, Goldschmidt, Berlin	*Reabsorption of foreign compounds from urinary bladder*	*37–1896–60*
Lewin L, Berlin	*Penetration of particles through wall of urinary bladder*	*40–1898–287*
(V) Different additional topics of general importance		
Engelmann ThW, Utrecht	Electromot. forces in frog skin	4–1871–321
Heidenhain R, Breslau	Experiments on salivary glands	9–1874–335
Heidenhain R, Breslau	Secretion in stomach	19–1879–148
Heidenhain R, Breslau	Histology and physiology of small intestine	43–1888–suppl.
Koeppe H, Giessen	Isotonia/osmotic pressure of saline	65–1897–492

cussed at a previously meeting of this Association [21, 22], Henle's contributions include the description of epithelia, the histological analysis of various cell systems (liver cells, retinal and corneal structures, muscle cells, closed (endocrine) and open glands, the description of the origin and nature of germ cells and hair). As a teacher he was enthusiastic and dedicated. In fact he was the first anatomist who in Berlin, in Müller's department, offered a histology course and attracted many students to histological studies. Many of these students would later become important scientists, like Helmholtz, du Bois-Reymond, Haeckel, Schwann and Virchow. In Göttingen, Robert Koch belonged to his coworkers. With him he worked together on 'contagious' diseases and bacterial growth.

Carl Ludwig [26–35], on the basis of histological and injection studies and experimental work with semipermeable membranes, described the renal circulation and formulated a filtration/reabsorption hypothesis of urine formation. As early as 1842/3 [31, 32] in his 'Habilitations' thesis he discussed the question: 'What is the driving force for urine excretion?' One has considered vital, chemical and/or mechanical (physical) forces, which would separate fluid through the membranes of blood and glandular vessels: He dismissed the ('nonexisting') vital force and chemical forces as underlying glomerular fluid separation. Instead he deduced from his meticulous recording of vessel diameters that local hydraulic forces would drive filtration of fluid through the porous vessel walls. Figure 2 represents his view of the arrangement of intrarenal capillaries and the adjacent vessels. As he pointed out, results from technical model experiments supported his hydraulic concept.

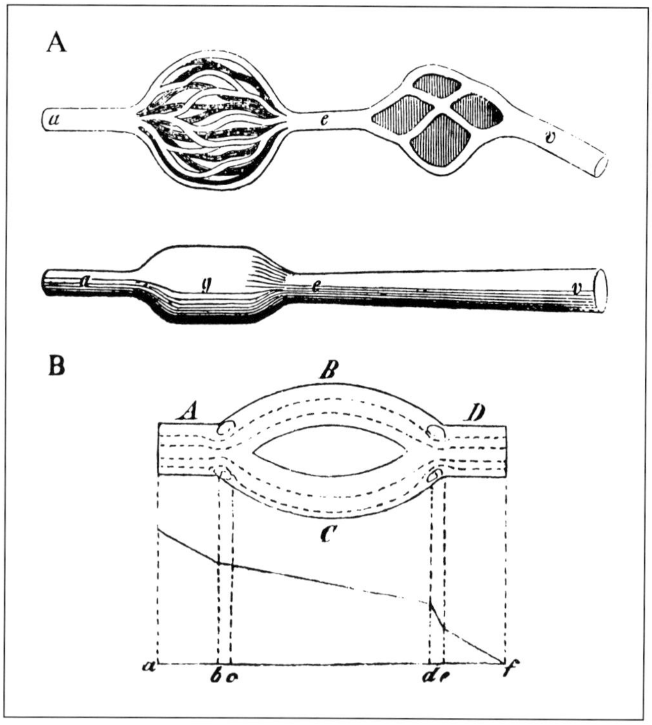

Fig. 2. Ludwig's representation of renal microvasculature (**A**) and of pressure profiles across the capillary bed (**B**). Cited from Thurau et al. [28].

In the context of the discussion of Bowman's and Heidenhain's theories (see below), it is pertinent to note that experimental data supporting Ludwig's filtration concept were also reported by Pautynski [52] and Henschen [48]. Pautynski, working in the Department of Pathology in Heidelberg, injected indigo dye into the jugular vein of rabbits and observed blue glomeruli and unstained convoluted tubules when he killed the animal soon after the injection. Basically, the same approach was used by Henschen, working in Ludwig's department and in Stockholm. He also observed immediately after injection an initial blue staining of glomeruli and concluded: '... the dye present in blood first passes the glomeruli. Under the pertaining high pressure filtration of dye occurs ...'

We mention only briefly that Ludwig opened the door to quantitative experimental physiology when he introduced his kymograph for the continuous recording of living processes (1847) and his 'Stromuhr' for the quantitative registration of organ blood flow (1876). He and his coworkers were among the first to develop an apparatus for the in vitro perfusion of isolated organs, including the kidney (1865/6). Ludwig had an enormous impact on scientific progress not only through his own ingenious work but also through the many coworkers he attracted and trained over the years. Schröer [26] lists not less than some 250 pupils (including names like J. Bernstein, H. Pickering Bowditch, A. Fick. O. Frank, W.H. Gaskell, C.J. Hüfner, I.P. Pawlow, W. Rutherford, and E. Pflüger) from practically all European countries, Egypt, Japan and USA, who came to Ludwig's department in Leipzig. It is therefore understandable that Henle, when he had made his important discovery, contacted Ludwig to inform him and to tempt him to provide a functional interpretation [cf. 21]. This stimulated Ludwig to repeat Henle's study which he was able to confirm [see letter from Ludwig in ref. 21].

Rudolf Peter Heinrich Heidenhain [36–41] also was one of the leading German physiologists of his time. He started his career in du Bois-Reymond's department in Berlin, were he was exposed to modern scientific argu-

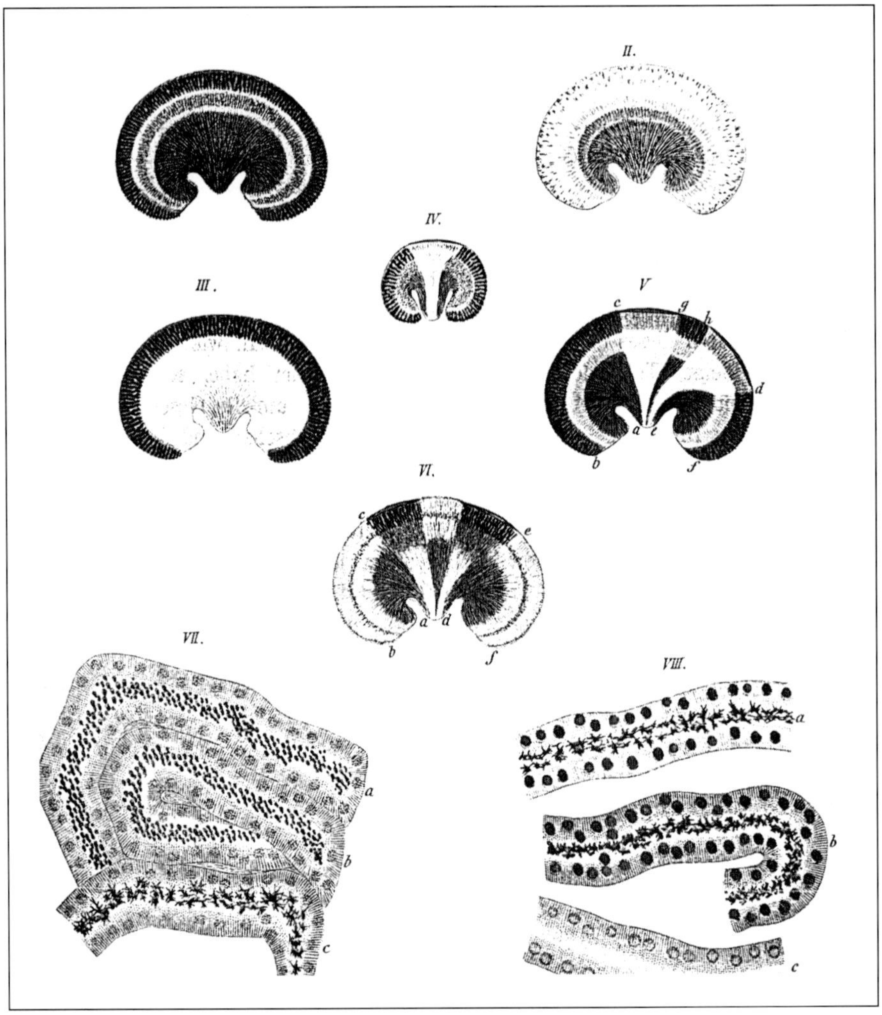

Fig. 3. Experimental results obtained by R.P.H. Heidenhain in 1883 after intravenous injection of indigo dye into a rabbit. From Heidenhain and Neisser [40].

mentation and experimentation and at the same time became immunized against vitalistic concepts. From 1859 on he held the chair of physiology and histology at the university of Breslau. His department was open to many young scientists, as has been listed by Grützner [38] in his very moving and personal obituary shortly after Heidenhain's death.

Heidenhain, on the basis of carefully controlled dye injection studies, provided experimental proof for the existence of proximal tubular secretion as a principal transport process involved in urine formation. If one could demonstrate, he argued, that in the absence of glomerular 'water filtration' certain renal epithelia would continue to excrete solutes, this would be proof of secretion and would therefore support Bowman's theory of urine formation. In figure 3 (PA 1874), we present a summary of his findings which he obtained after injection of an indigo dye (indigoblauschwefelsaures Natron). Indeed, he observed directly proximal secretion; initially, however, he overlooked that his results were not an argument against Ludwig's concept of water *and* solute filtration at the glomerular level but rather an important extension. Heidenhain's studies were repeated and extended by Nussbaum (table 2, IIIb) who injected dyes into the portal circulation of frogs and confirmed cellular dye uptake in the absence of glomerular filtration. He thus confirmed tubular secretion; however, from comparable experiments with urea he concluded that urea too would be excreted by cellular secretion and would in turn drag water along. Grützner [47] from Heidenhain's department performed additional experiments and he also tried to repeat the experimental approach of Henschen [48]. Basically, he confirmed Heidenhain's secretion concept and rejected Henschen's results as 'unphysiological'. In the paper in 1881, he summarized the available data at that time, including the work of Wittich [57].

Heidenhain's interests were not limited to renal physiology [36–38] but extended to general considerations of structure/function relationships, to blood and circulatory physiology, to properties of nerves and muscles, to secretory processes outside the kidneys (salivary, gastric, mammary, parotid and pancreatic glands and bile production), on lymph formation and on intestinal absorption. He also was a devoted teacher, who took great care enriching his lectures with physiologic experiments. Grützner [38] remembered: 'Sometimes he presented too much for a normal student ...'.

Other Contributions to the Progress of (Renal) Physiology

Several scientific developments outside the field exerted important impacts on renal physiology. We can only briefly point to some of them:

Adolf Fick [42–44], formerly one of Ludwig's students and later a prosector in Ludwig's department in Zürich, was appointed professor of physiology in Würzburg (1868). He had studied mathematics and medicine. He made a seemingly indirect but rather profound contribution to renal physiology by presenting the concept that cardiac output and cardiac stroke volume could be calculated from pulmonary oxygen uptake and/or pulmonary carbon dioxide clearance. We quote from the proceedings (Sitzungsberichte) of the 'Physical-Medical Society in Würzburg' (Physikalisch-medicinische Gesellschaft in Würzburg) on July 9, 1870: '... One should measure how much oxygen an animal takes up from the air and how much CO_2 is released. Furthermore, one has to take a sample of arterial and a sample of venous blood during the time of the experiment. In both, one has to measure oxygen content and CO_2 content ...' [42, cf. 44, p 183]. Thus, a flow rate can be calculated by dividing $Q - O_2$ with the a-v oxygen difference: $Q_{bl} = Q_{O_2}/(O_{2_a} - O_{2_v})$. The potential importance of this mathematical expression for renal physiology has apparently first been recognized by Heidenhain [see 38]. He attempted to calculate glomerular filtration rate from the renal excretion of urea, which according to Ludwig's hypothesis was excreted solely by a glomerular process. It is obvious that the 'Fick principle' in essence is the first formulation of the clearance concept which later would become a rather universal tool in the hands of renal physiologists. An interesting coincidence is that in the same sesssion where Fick presented his provocative paper in 1870, another scientist, the young Wilhelm C. Röntgen, was accepted as a member of the Würzbug Medical Society, i.e. a man who later significantly albeit indirectly contributed to progress in the field by providing a new imaging technique applicable also to the kidneys.

Morphological roots of renal physiology are personified by Henle, Heidenhain and Müller, as we have discussed. However, one leading morphologist of his time with predominant renal interests has to be mentioned:

Karl Peter [13], professor in Greifswald, was an extremely successful experimental anatomist, who has not received the proper credit he deserves. Towards the end of the last century he was engaged in maceration studies with renal tissues of man and several animals (sheep, pig, rabbit, cat, mouse). He also used injection of stained lime and reconstructed microscopic images of tubules. In 1909 he published his material on macroscopic and microscopic renal anatomy in a book [13]. He described the tubular system, sizes of tubular segments and their arrangement in renal tissue, the longitudinal heterogeneity of renal epithelia and pertinent species differences, not to mention his intensive studies on renal embryology. From Peter's invaluable work we present a tubular image in figure 4. Peter also noticed that the kidneys of different species contained thin loops of different lengths. He correlated this finding with the normal specific weight of the urine and concluded: 'The order of sequence of water content of the urine equals almost exactly the order of lengths of the thin loops. ... I think that this puzzling parallelism between water content of urine and length of the thin part of loop justifies to assume that this segment is charged with the task to reabsorb partly the fluid of glomerular origin.' It took a long time until this peculiar parallelism met its explanation.

Hermann Helmholtz and *Emil du Bois-Reymond*, both students of Johannes Müller, turned away from vitalistic concepts and became 'physicomechanists', working in close contact with Henle, Ludwig and other nephrologists. Helmholtz was a brilliant physiologist and physicist. His contributions reach from the derivation of the 'law of conservation of energy' to the development of the first ophthalmoscope, from extensive experimental work in physiology of optics, to sound perception and hydro- and electrodynamic problems [see 15, 21]. du Bois-Reymond also became a 'physical physiologist' who concentrated on electrophysiology. He was an ingenious inventor of measuring equipment, described the resting current in nerves and discovered electromotive changes associated with nerve excitation. He also worked in muscle physiology

4

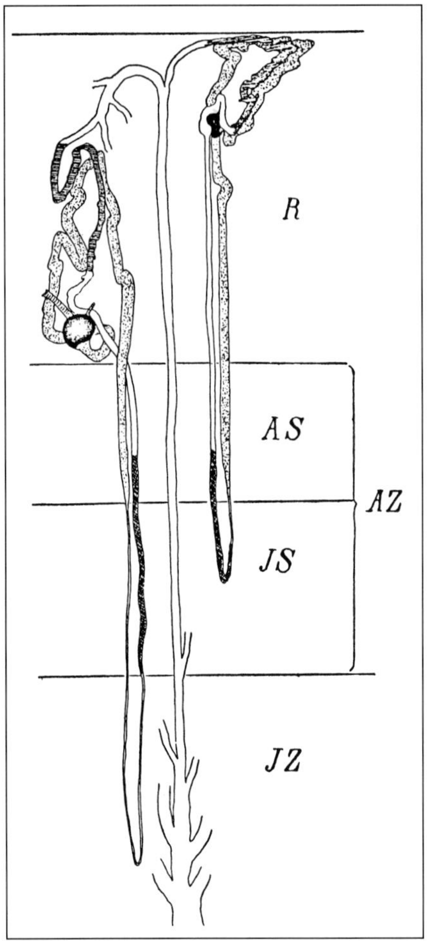

5

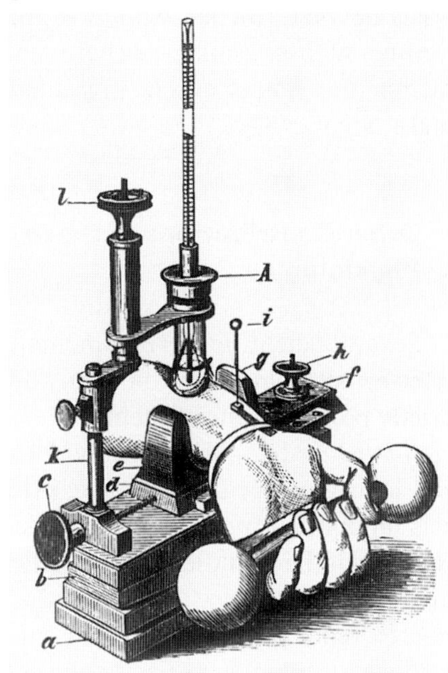

Fig. 4. Schematic presentation of two tubules of mammals. R = Cortex; AS = outer stripe; IS = inner stripe; AZ = outer zone; IZ = inner zone. From Peter [13], text, fig. LVIII.

Fig. 5. Improved sphygmomanometer for the measurement of human blood pressure. From Basch [45], cited from Bleker [2].

[15, 21]. Both, Helmholtz and du Bois-Reymond actively contributed to the antivitalistic physical (and chemical) atmosphere in which all biological disciplines could unfold and prosper.

Concerning physical technology a contribution of *Siegfried Samuel Karl v. Basch* should not be overlooked. He designed a sphygmomanometer for the nonvasive measurement of human blood pressure [2], which under normal conditions he reported to range between 135 and 165 mm Hg. In several cases of Bright's disease he recorded values above 200 mm Hg. The technique is shown in figure 5 [45]. It took several decades until the method was replaced by the technique of Riva Rocci in 1909 [2].

Concerning chemistry which influenced the development of biological sciences in Europe by providing new chemical methods and scientific concepts, free of vitalistic speculations, we have, in figure 1, listed the names of *Wöhler, Liebig* and *Berzelius*, to quote only a few outstanding scientists. Through their basic work in inorganic and organic chemistry they provided a reliable analytical basis for the evaluation of chemical processes in the kidneys and of chemical driving forces which participate in the formation of urine. The impact of chemistry on physiology has been discussed by Rothschuh [15].

A pathophysiological root from which renal physiology could benefit and draw experience is personified by *Johann Lukas Schönlein*, a pathologist and internist, who initially worked in Würzburg, later in Zürich and finally in Berlin. Here he was one of the founders, together with *Johannes Müller*, of the 'Berlin school'. He introduced quantitative physical and chemical methods into clinical medicine and studied relevant topics such as daily variations of urine secretion, pH changes of urine, and the urea concentration of various tissues in various renal diseases [51]. We know this from lecture notes which were collected and published by some of his students [16]. His most important contribution to renal physiology, however, was the description of 'rheumatic purpura rubra' (now 'Schönlein-Henoch syndrome') as a clinical entity with typical renal lesions [16].

Finally, comparative aspects emerged, as we have discussed in connection with Peter. *Anton Dohrn* has to be mentioned here since he was the biologist who most clearly recognized the need for and the advantages of comparative approaches. This is most clearly documented by the 'Stazione Zoologica' which he was able to establish in Napoli, in close connection with and supported by du Bois-Reymond in Berlin [21]. From this department in Napoli many impulses reached biological and physiological institutions all over Europe, who shared laboratory space in the stazione and pursued comparative and marine biological topics. Ludwig, who initially had been reluctant, finally became a convinced supporter of the marine biological institute. This was also true for Heidenhain.

Additional Original Contributions to Renal Physiology

In the following, we attempt to provide some additional information by following the rootlets of nephrological research in two leading German periodicals: Pflüger's *Archiv für die gesammte Physiology des Menschen und der Thiere* (Archives of Total Physiology of Man and Animals) and Klebs, Naunyn and Schmiedeberg's *Archiv für experimentelle Pathologie und Pharmakologie* (Archives of Experimental Pathology and Pharmacology) which were established in the second part of the last century. The titles of these journals indicate the broad field which they intended to cover.

In table 2, we have collected and extracted relevant original articles which were published in the second part of the 19th century. Also included are papers on relevant analytical and methodological aspects. The articles have been grouped under different topics and reflect the different aspects which could be studied with the methodological arsenal available at that time. The code (volume/year/page) included in table 2 permits direct access to the original papers in the 2 respective journals. Obviously, table 2 is not a complete record of all activities in renal physiology in the last century. *Virchow's Archives* and a few other journals as well as Proceedings of several German academies would have to be extracted in addition to the two periodicals listed. However, this is beyond the scope of the present paper.

It is interesting to note the gradual accumulation of quantitative analytical methods which paved the way for new experimental approaches. From today's perspective the initially narrow analytical basis can hardly be imagined. At second thought the statement of Ludwig becomes understandable – that a concise description of intrarenal transport mechanisms, and their driving forces, such as 'endosmosis', had to await chemical methods that would allow a precise comparison of blood and urine composition under different conditions (Ludwig in Wagners Handwörterbuch [33]). As the table reflects, it gradually became possible to measure more and more substances in plasma and urine and to determine quantitatively the renal excretory pattern of many compounds. The developed was so rapid that as early as in 1877 F. Hoppe-Seyler [from 38] expressed the opinion that most physiologists would lack the adequate competence in all natural sciences to perform research in all fields of their disciplines. Therefore, he postulated that chairs for physiology, biophysics and biochemistry should be founded! This was a rather revolutionary proposal – to our knowledge the first time that the terms 'biophysics' and 'biochemistry' were used – and it is not surprising that some contemporary scientists fiercely refused such plans. Pflüger [from 38] reacted with the statement: 'Subdivision of physiology in physiological physics and chemistry, thus, is philosophically inadmissible (!) and practically impossible.'

As to the authors listed in table 2, it is apparent that experimental research was carried out in many different places. The departments of Göttingen, Leipzig, Berlin and Breslau were particularly active centers, but other places like Heidelberg, Strassburg, and Vienna also contributed to progress in the field. All these places attracted young scientists from Germany and abroad. Thus, there existed, already in these early days, a quite impressive international cooperation.

From the papers listed we should like to point to some of special importance: Several groups were interested in a technique for isolated organ perfusion (cf. Ellinger in [1] p 378ff and literature in table 2). Two early attempts had been reported in 1849 by Löbell and in 1862 by von Bidder in their dissertations. Most actively pursued was this approach by Ludwig and his associates. Jacobj, as listed in table 2, had developed a rather sophisticated apparatus for the in vitro perfusion of isolated organs and reported experimental data on the functional properties of isolated kidneys. His rather elaborate technique included two perfusion chambers, one for the in vitro perfusion of an isolated lung for blood oxygenation and a second one for the perfusion of the isolated organ of interest, e.g. a kidney. In figure 6 we present the technical design of Jacobj.

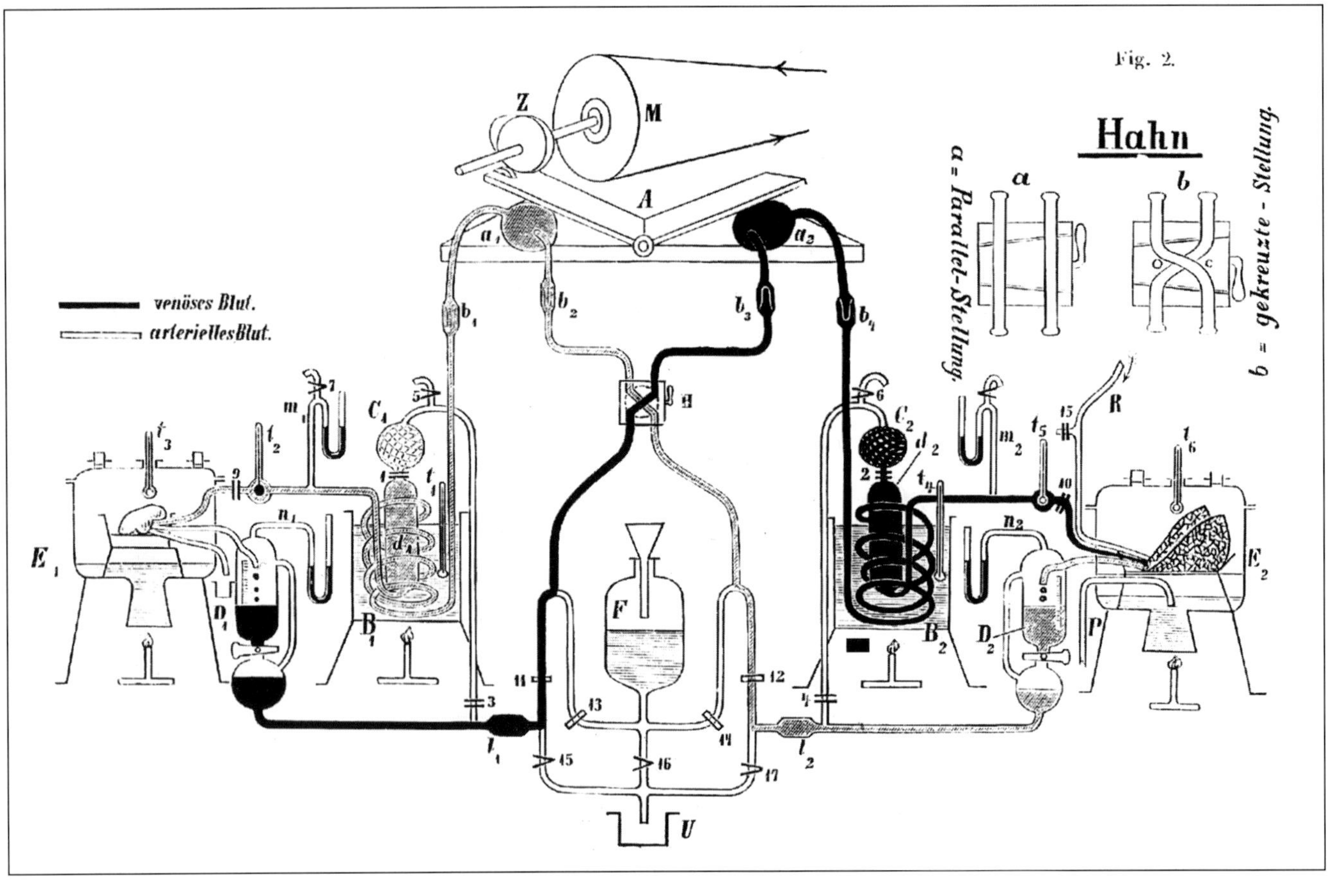

Fig. 6. Apparatus for the artificial in vitro perfusion of isolated organs with oxygenated blood. From Jacobji (Arch Exp Pathol Pharm 1895, cit. in table 2, Ib).

A focus of interest was the change of renal function in diabetics, the question of normal and pathological sugar excretion and the appearance of several acids and compounds in diabetes and diabetic coma. Interest focused also on renal effects of chemical drugs and poisons which were sometimes used as chemical tools, particularly in the attempt to define diuretic mechanisms. Finally, we have included a few articles which indirectly may have influenced progress in renal physiology by providing information on other relevant biological systems such as glands and frog skin.

Conclusion

At the turn of the century a host of experimental data was available and awaited interpretation in the frame of a unified theory of renal function. Controversies in details threatened to obstruct progress. We therefore like to close by citing two scientists who attempted to combine the essence of the various existing hypotheses in a unified theory. Filehne (table 2, IIIg) in the introduction to a remarkable series of original papers on 'diuresis' pointed out that the challenge was not merely to distinguish between Ludwig's and Heidenhain's theory. The essentials of the Ludwig concept had been developed further in the sense of Heidenhain and one should experimentally test the existence of tubular reabsorption as well as tubular secretion. Progress in renal physiology had most carefully been followed and summarized by R. Metzner, a former associate of Ludwig in Leipzig, later working in Basel. At the beginning of this century he discussed the 'production and excretion of urine' in an extensive review article [12]. The paper contains a detailed description of renal anatomy and histology and discusses functional parameters such as renal blood flow, urine production, influences of blood pressure and of chemical compounds. As to the mechanisms involved in urine formation he combined the concepts of Bowman, Ludwig and Heidenhain to a rather consistent logical theory. We quote [pp 209–210]:

'(1) Ludwig's proposal that plasma minus protein flows out of the glomerulus, is a very likely one. ...

(2) The hypothetical assumption of Ludwig that the ultrafiltrate becomes concentrated by water reabsorption on its way through the tubuli uriniferi has been strongly supported by newer experimental evidence. ... (water diffusion and active functions of tubular epithelium must be involved) ...

Uric acid, phosphoric acid and substances normally not contained in blood undergo true secretion in the tubules ... Certain structural 'condensators' may possibly also mediate reabsorption processes. ...'

Metzner rightfully pointed to the fact that a real contradiction between Ludwig's and Bowman-Heidenhain's theory never existed, with the exception of Heidenhain's refusal of glomerular filtration. Thus, at the turn of the century the kidney was quite adequately described by a biological system that included glomerular filtration, tubular secretion and tubular reabsorption.

Acknowledgements

The authors wish to acknowledge the competent help of Prof. Dr. J. Bleker and the librarians Ms. U. Bradis and Ms. B. Klische, and Dr. U. D'Orazio from the Free University Berlin.

References

Textbooks, Monographs and Reviews

1 Bethe A, Bergmann GV, Emden G, Ellinger A (eds): Handbuch der normalen und pathologischen Physiologie, vol 4: Resorption und Exkretion, Berlin, Springer, 1929.

2 Bleker J: Die Geschichte der Nierenkrankheiten. 1972, Mannheim, Boehringer.

3 Boylan JW (ed): Founders of Experimental Physiology. München, Lehmann, 1971.

4 Eknoyan G, De Santo NG, Capaaso G, Massry SG (eds): History of Nephrology. Reports from 1st Int Conf, Naples/Montecassino, 1993, pp 255–502.

5 Gottschalk CW, Berliner RW, Giebisch GH (eds): Renal Physiology, People and Ideas. Bethesda, American Physiology Society, 1987.

6 Gottschalk CW: A history of renal physiology to 1950; in Seldin DW, Giebisch G (eds): The Kidney. New York, Raven Press, 1992, pp 1–29.

7 Groeben C, Hierholzer K: Emil du Bois-Reymond–Anton Dohrn, Briefwechsel (Letters). Berlin, Springer, 1985.

8 Hildebrandt DF: Lehrbuch der Physiologie. Erlangen, Johann Jacob Palm, 1796, §57, chap 20.

9 Kayser H (ed): Schriften Theophrasts von Hohenheim genannt Paracelsus. Leipzig, Insel Verlag, 1924.

10 Ludwig C: Nieren und Harnbereitung; in Wagner R (ed): Handwörterbuch der Physiologie mit Rücksicht auf physiologische Pathologie. Braunschweig, Vieweg & Sons, 1844, pp 628–640.

11 Lyons AS, Petrucelli RJ: Medicine, an Illustrated History. New York, Harry N. Abrams Inc. Publishers, 1978.

12 Metzner R: Die Absonderung und Herausbeförderung des Harnes (The formation and excretion of urine); in Nagel W (ed): Handbuch der Physiologie des Menschen. Braunschweig, Vieweg + Sons, 1907, vol II, pp 207–448.

13 Peter K: Untersuchungen über Bau und Entwicklung der Niere. Jena, Verlag Gustav Fischer, 1909.

14 Pollak K: Wissen und Weisheit der alten Ärzte: Die Heilkunst der frühen Hochkulturen. Eltville, Bechtermünz-Verlag, 1993, Indian medicine, pp 159–244, Chinese medicine, pp 245–287, Ancient American Medicine, pp 289–360.

15 Rothschuh KE: 'Physiologie'. Der Wandel ihrer Konzepte, Probleme und Methoden vom 16. bis 20. Jahrhundert, Orbis Academicus, vol II/15. München, Verlag Karl Alber Freiburg, 1968, pp 231–252.

16 Schönlein JL: 'Allgemeine und spezielle Pathologie und Therapie' nach JL Schönleins Vorlesungen, niedergeschrieben und herausgegeben von einigen seiner Zuhörer, ed 5. St. Gallen, Literatur-Comptoir, 1841.

17 Schrier RW, Gottschalk CW (eds): Diseases of the Kidney, ed 4. Boston, Little, Brown, 1988.

18 Seldin DW, Giebisch G (ed): The Kidney, ed 2. New York, Raven Press, 1992.

19 Spunda F: Das Weltbild des Paracelsus. Wien, W. Andermann Verlag, 1941.

20 Toellner R: Illustrierte Geschichte der Medizin. Salzburg, Verlagsbuchhandel Andreas & Andreas, 1986. German translation of: Histoire de la medicine, de la pharmacie, de l'art dentaire et de l'art vétérinaire. Paris, Societé française d'éditions professionnelles, médicales et scientifiques, 1978.

Selected Literature on/from Prominent German (Renal) Physiologists

Jacob Henle

21 Hierholzer K: Carl Ludwig, Jacob Henle, Hermann Helmholtz, Emil du Bois-Reymond and the scientific development of nephrology in Germany. Am J Nephrol 1994;14:344–354.

22 Kinne-Saffran Evamaria, Kinne RKH: Jacob Henle: The kidney and beyond. Am J Nephrol 1994;14:355–360.

23 Henle J: Handbuch der rationellen Pathologie. Braunschweig, Vieweg, 1847.

24 Henle J: Zur Anatomie der Nieren. Mittheilungen an die Göttinger Gesellschaft der Wissenschaften, Januarheft: 4–12, Bibliothek der Georg-August-Universität, Göttingen, 1862.

25 Henle J: Grundriss der Anatomie des Menschen. Braunschweig, Vieweg, 1883.

Carl Friedrich Wilhelm Ludwig

26 Schröer H: Carl Ludwig, Begründer der messenden Experimentalphysiologie; in Degen H (ed): Grosse Naturforscher. Stuttgart, Wiss. Verlagsges., 1967, Band 33: Extensive Bibliography of Ludwig up to 1967.

27 Schröer H: Carl Ludwig; in Boylan J (ed): Founders of Experimental Physiology. München, Lehmann Verlag, 1971, pp 169–180.

28 Thurau K, Davis JM, Häberle DA: Renal blood flow and dynamics of glomerular filtration: Evolution of a concept from Carl Ludwig to the present day; in Gottschalk CW (ed): Renal Physiology, People and Ideas. Bethesda, American Physiological Society, 1987, pp 31–62.

29 Gottschalk CW: A History of Renal Physiology to 1950, in [7], pp 1–29, 1992.

30 Hierholzer K: Carl Ludwig, Jacob Henle, Hermann Helmholtz, Emil du Bois-Reymond and the scientific development of nephrology in Germany. Am J Nephrol 1994;14:344–354.

31 Ludwig C: De viribus physicis secretionem urinae adjuvantibus, Marburge Cattorum; Habschr, 1842.

32 Ludwig C: Beiträge zur Lehre vom Mechanismus der Harnsecretion. Marburg, Elwert, 1843, pp 1–42.

33 Ludwig C: Nieren und Harnbereitung; in: Rudolph Wagner's Handwörterbuch der Physiologie mit Rücksicht auf physiologische Pathologie. Braunschweig, Vieweg, 1844, Bd II, pp 628–640.

34 Ludwig C: Einige neue Beziehungen zwischen dem Bau und der Funktion der Niere, Sitzungsber. d. Kgl. Akad. d. Wiss., Wien, 1863, Mathem. Nat. Cl. 49B, pp 725–733.
35 Ludwig C: Von der Niere; in Stricker S (ed): Handbuch der Lehre von den Geweben des Menschen und der Thiere. Leipzig, 1871/2, Bd I, p 489.

Rudolf Peter Heinrich Heidenhain

36 Bernstein J: Rudolph Heidenhain. Naturwiss Rundschau 1897;12:606–607.
37 Kruta V: Heidenhain, Rudolf Peter Heinrich; in: Dictionary of Scientific Biographies. New York, Charles Scribner's & Sons, 1970, pp 224–227.
38 Grützner P: Zum Andenken an Rudolf Heidenhain (Obituary). Pflügers Arch Ges Physiol 1898;72:220–265.
39 Gottschalk CW: A History of Renal Physiology to 1950; in ref (7), 1992, pp 1–29.
40 Heidenhain R, Neisser A: Versuche über den Vorgang der Harnabsonderung, Pflügers Arch Ges Physiol 1874;9:1–27.
41 Heidenhain R: Die Absonderung der festen Harnbestandteile; in Hermann L (ed): Handbuch der Physiologie. Leipzig, Vogel, 1883, vol 5, pp 1279–1373.

Adolf Fick

42 Fick A: Über die Messung des Blutquantums in den Herzventrikeln (On the measurement of blood volume in heart ventricles). Report of the XIV. Session of the Physical-Medical Soc, Würzburg, 1870, XVI.
43 Fick A: Gesammelte Schriften in 4 Bänden, Bd II: Physiologische Schriften. Stahel'sche Verlagsanstalt, 1903.
44 Fick A: In Boylan J (ed): Founders of Experimental Physiology. München, Lehmann Verlag, 1971, pp 181–184.

Original Papers (Reports)

45 Basch SS, Ritter V: Einige Ergebnisse der Blutdruckmessung an Gesunden und Kranken. Z Klin Med 1881;3:512.
46 Gottschalk CW: A History of Renal Physiology to 1950, in (7), 1992, pp 1–29.
47 Grützner P: Zur Physiologie der Harnsecretion. Pflügers Arch Ges Physiol 1881;24:441–466.
48 Henschen S: Om indigosvafvelssyradt natrons afsöndering i njurarne. Akademisk afhandling, Stockholm, 1879. (German translation in Hoffmann-Schwalbe 1880, vol 8, p 347.)
49 Hierholzer K, Winau R: Pioneer nephrologists of Berlin. Am J Nephrol 1992;12:442–450.
50 Hierholzer K: Carl Ludwig, Jacob Henle, Hermann Helmholtz, Emil du Bois-Reymond and the scientific development of nephrology in Germany. Am J Nephrol 1994;14:344–354.
51 Hierholzer J, Hierholzer C, Hierholzer K: Johann Lukas Schönlein and his contributions to nephrology and medicine. Am J Nephrol 1994;14:467–472.
52 Pautynski JF: Über die Abscheidung des indigoschwefelsauren Natrons durch die Nieren unter normalen und pathologischen Bedingungen. Virchows Arch 1880;79:393–407.
53 Schipperges H: Vom Wesen der Natur und vom Wesen der Zeit bei Paracelsus; in Keel HJ, Nager F (eds): 500 Jahre Paracelsus. Bern, Hallwag, 1994, pp 11–15.
54 Smith HW: Highlights in the history of renal physiology. The Bulletin, Georgetown University Medical Center 1959;13:4–48.
55 Sperber I: Studies on the mammalian kidney. Zool Bidrag Fran Uppsala 1944;22:249–431.
56 Ullrich KJ, Jarausch KH: Untersuchungen zum Problem der Harnkonzentrierung und Harnverdünnung. Pflügers Arch Ges Physiol 1956;262:537–554.
57 Wittich W.v. Über Harnsekrete. Arch Pathol Anat 1856;X:325–330.
58 Wöhler F: Über die künstliche Bildung des Harnstoffs. Poggendorffs Ann Phys Chem 1828;12:253–256.

Origins of Renal Physiology
(Dedicated to Carl Gottschalk)

American Journal of Nephrology

Am J Nephrol 1999;19:257–265

British Contributions to Renal Physiology: Of Dynasties and Diuresis

Leon G. Fine

Department of Medicine, Royal Free and University College Medical School, University College London, UK

Key Words
Renal physiology · Water homeostasis · Glomerular-filtration rate · Vasopressin · Sodium homeostasis

Abstract
British contributions to renal physiology trace back to the seminal contribution of William Bowman, who defined the structure of mammalian nephron and its blood supply and pointed out its likely mode of function. A series of contributions followed, which stemmed from a distinguished lineage of physiologists based at University College London and which had, as its high point, the establishment by Ernest H. Starling, in 1899, of a method for measuring oncotic pressure and the subsequent demonstration that glomerular filtration requires a hydrostatic pressure in excess of oncotic pressure in the glomerular capillaries. Arthur Cushny published a monograph on renal function in 1917 which had wide influence. The homeostasis of water and sodium chloride were the subjects of important contributions by Verney and De Wardener, respectively. Little contribution was made by British renal physiologists to the understanding of single nephron function with the emphasis being largely on integrative physiology.

Renal Physiology in Britain

In 1785 William Withering described a preparation of digitalis leaf for a woman with dropsy 'which acted very powerfully upon the kidneys, for within the first twenty-four hours she made upwards of eight quarts of urine' [1]. Whilst this experience could be described as one of the earliest serious interventions in the workings of the human kidney in England, its implications in terms of the links between cardiac output and renal excretion of salt and water took two centuries to emerge.

William Bowman (1816–1892)

William Bowman must lay claim to being one of the luminaries of renal physiology [2] even though his principal discovery is generally thought to be anatomical in nature. In 1837, he joined the medical department of King's College London, where he was appointed as junior demonstrator in anatomy and curator of the museum. At the tender age of 25, he was elected to the Fellowship of the Royal Society. One year later, in 1843, he was to publish a paper which has become a classic, *On the structure and use of the Malpighian bodies of the kidney with observation of the circulation through that gland* [3]. No other contribution since that of Malpighi in 1666 [4] had a more

KARGER

Fax + 41 61 306 12 34
E-Mail karger@karger.ch
www.karger.com

© 1999 S. Karger AG, Basel
0250–8095/99/0192–0257$17.50/0

Accessible online at:
http://BioMedNet.com/karger

Prof. Leon G. Fine
Department of Medicine
Royal Free and University College Medical School
University College London, 5 University Street
London WC1E 6JJ (UK)

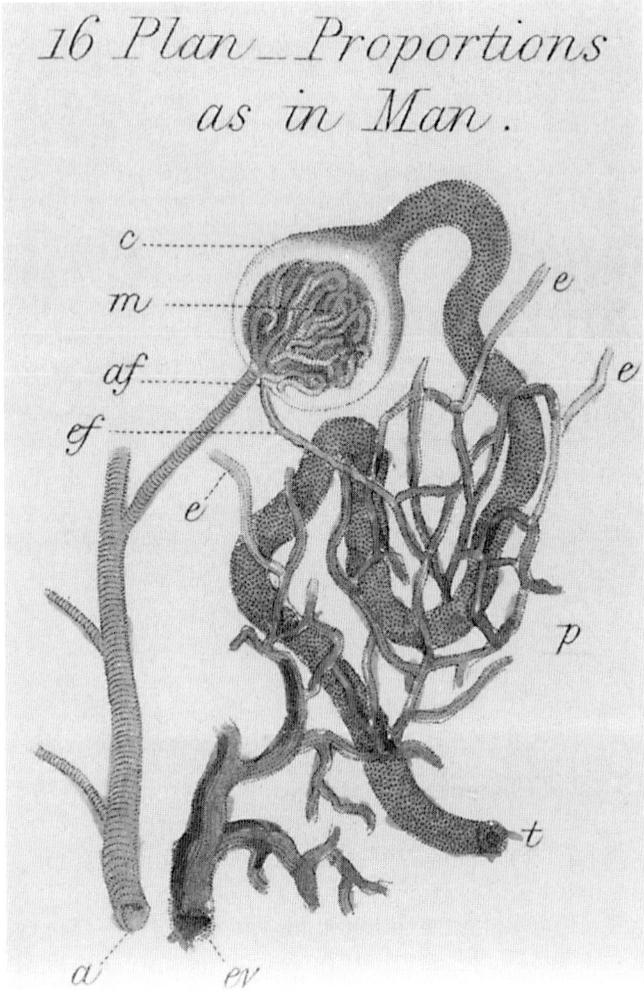

Fig. 1. Bowmans depictions of the human nephron.

profound impact on the understanding of how the kidney functions than Bowman's.

For this single paper on the kidney, Bowman's place was assured in the history of nephrology, but it is sobering to note that his principal interests lay elsewhere. He functioned almost entirely as a 'medical scientist' for much of his career until, in 1848, he turned to the practice of ophthalmic surgery and was elected as first President of the Ophthalmological Society of Great Britain. He was made a baronet in 1884.

Bowman's publication coincided roughly with that of Ludwig in 1842, the latter making crucial observations on the physical forces governing ultrafiltration [5]. Both capitalised on advances in the techniques of microdissection and vascular injection and both elucidated the relationship between glomerular capillaries, arterioles and peritubular capillaries. Yet, there is no evidence to show that these investigators had any communication with each other.

Bowman's investigations on the structure of the kidney ranged over a wide variety of species included horses, rabbits, parrots, frogs, guinea pigs, boa constrictors and humans. In each, he noted a tuft of capillaries fed by one arteriole and drained by another. These 'Malpighian bodies' (glomeruli) he saw to be 'invested by a cyst of capsule of precisely similar appearance to the basement membrane of the tubes'. The single plate, illustrating his paper of 1842, shows the accuracy with which his observations were made (fig. 1). The depiction of the human nephron remains unsurpassed as a precise and correct depiction of the proximal part of the nephron.

The fact that the coloured injected material (lead acetate and potassium dichromate) in many instances burst through the glomerular tuft into the capsule and the proximal tubule allowed Bowman to conclude that these two structures were in continuity. Only the fine details are missing from his observation, i.e. that the glomerular capillaries are invested with a layer of epithelial cells in continuity with those of the capsule and that there is a juxtaglomerular pole with unique features.

Bowmans insights into the physiology of this unique structure are best described in his own words:

> 'It would be difficult to conceive a disposition of parts more calculated to favor the escape of water from the blood than that of the Malpighian body. A large artery breaks up in a very direct manner into a number of minute branches which suddenly open into an assemblage of vessels of far greater aggregate capacity than itself and from which there is but one narrow exit. Hence must arise a very abrupt retardation in the velocity of the current of blood. The vessels in which this occurs are uncovered by any structure. They lie bare in a cell from which there is but one outlet, the orifice of the tube. ... Why is so wondrous an apparatus placed at the extremity of each uriniferous tube if not to furnish water to aid in the separation and solution of the urinous products from the epithelium of the tube. ... The secretion is brought from the tubules of the gland (i.e., glomerular capillaries) in a fluid state and only becomes solid (i.e. the solid urine of some reptiles) by reabsorption of its aqueous portion after it has traversed the tortuous canals (i.e. tubules) wherein it was formed.' (Words in parentheses are the present author's).

He went on to suggest that some constituents of the urine are secreted by the tubules. His findings were rigorously supported by the studies of Ludwig, who proposed the existence of a protein-free, cell-free filtrate of plasma containing all the urinary constituents, which is formed by the glomerulus by the hydrostatic force within the capillaries. Ludwig proposed that part of the filtrate is absorbed by the tubules by a force resulting from the concentration of blood in the peritubular capillaries and negated the idea of tubular secretion [5].

The Physiology Dynasty of University College London and Ernest Starling

It is, perhaps, not exaggerated to refer to a 'dynasty' in physiology at University College London (UCL), established in 1828 as the first liberal, non-denominational university in England for 'effectively and multifariously teaching, examining, exercising and rewarding with honours in the liberal arts and sciences the youth of our middling rich people' [6].

The first Professor of Physiology and Surgery was Charles Bell, who gave the first inaugural lecture of the college in 1828. Bell's description of motor and sensory nerves has been likened to Harvey's description of the blood as one of the most fundamental observations in all of human physiology.

In 1836 William Sharpey was appointed to the Chair of Physiology which he held for nearly 40 years. Although he was an inspiring teacher and introduced the microscope for practical demonstration, it was his students who came to dominate the subject.

Sharpey was succeeded by John Burdon Sanderson and it was with him that William Osler chose to work when he spent 18 months in England learning the scientific underpinnings of medicine [3]. Burdon Sanderson established physiology as a compulsory subject for all medical students and he introduced the experiment as a central feature of the educational process. He convened the first meeting of the Physiological Society in his house. This scientific organisation was to become the cement which bound together physiologists around Briatin. In 1883 Burdon Sanderson was succeeded by Prof. E.A. Schafer who changed his name to Sharpey-Schafer in honour of his teacher. He made important contributions to the understanding of the antidiuretic properties of pituitary extracts on the kidney (see below).

In 1903 a widely reported speech was given to the National Anti-Vivisection Society, accusing a teacher in the Physiology Laboratory of UCL, William Bayliss, of having carried out a cruel experiment on an unanaesthetised dog. In fact, he had given a lecture showing an experiment on a dog already anaesthetised, which was being studied by his brother-in-law, Ernest Starling, the Professor of Physiology. Bayliss brought a libel case against his accusers and won it. He donated the £ 2,000, awarded for damages, to the College. Bayliss later succeeded to the Chair of Physiology.

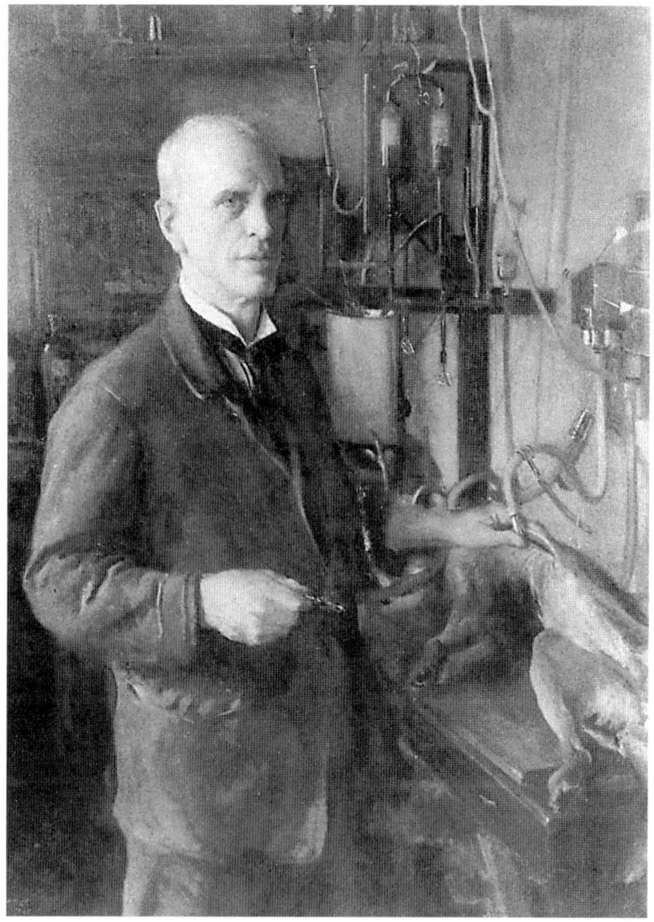

Fig. 2. Ernest Henry Starling (1866–1927).

But it is to Ernest H. Starling (1866–1927, Jodrell Professor of Physiology from 1899 to 1923; fig. 2) that credit must go for the most substantial contribution to renal, and cardiac and hormonal physiology. Starling introduced the word 'hormone'. The forces governing the passage of fluid out of capillaries and the 'law of the heart', named after him, have retained his name in the annals of physiology and medicine. He established the Institute of Physiology in 1909 and expanded it later to include pharmacology. In 1923 he resigned his Chair and remained on at UCL as a Royal Society Professor.

Starling was the first to introduce the concept of oncotic pressure and to appreciate the counterbalancing of hydrostatic and oncotic pressure on transcapillary fluid exchange. In 1899, in his paper on *The Glomerular Functions of the Kidney*, published while working at Guy's

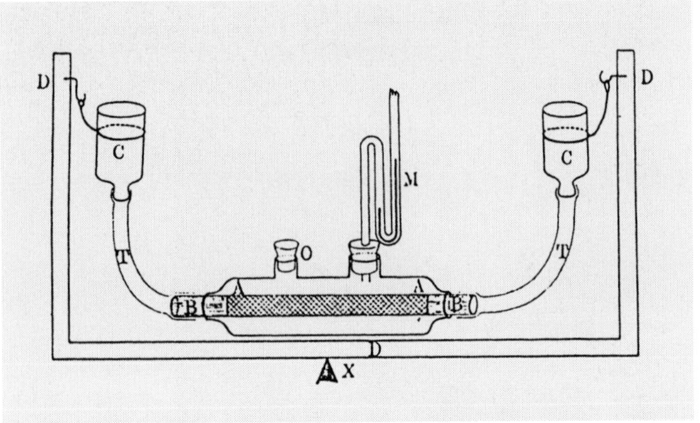

Fig. 3. Starling's osmometer [7]. The tube, BB, is made of silver gauze connected at each end to a tube of solid silver. Round the gauze is wrapped a piece of peritoneal membrane (as in making a cigarette). This is painted all over with a solution of gelatin (10%) and then a second layer of membrane applied. Fine thread is now twisted many times round the tube to prevent any disturbance of the membranes, and the whole tube is soaked for half-an-hour in a warm solution of gelatin. In this way one obtains an even layer of gelatin between two layers of peritoneal membrane, and supported by the wire-gauze. This tube so prepared is placed within a wide tube, AA, which is provided with two tubules at the top. One of these, O, is for filling the outer tube, the other is fitted with a mercurial manometer, M. Two small reservoirs, CC, are connected with the outer ends of BB by means of rubber tubes, TT. The whole apparatus is placed in a wooden cradle, DD, pivoted at X, and provided with a cover, so that it may be filled with fluids at different temperatures if necessary. The colloid solution is placed in AA, and the reservoirs, CC, and inner tube, BB, are filled with a salt solution. The apparatus is then made to rock continuously for days or weeks by means of a water motor. (The two reservoirs, CC, are corked, and connected by means of a tube, in order to avoid evaporation.) In this way the fluid on the two sides of the membrane is continually renewed, and the attainment of an osmotic equilibrium facilitated.

Hospital, he measured plasma protein concentrations and presented measurements of colloid osmotic pressure in dogs [7] using an osmometer which he designed (fig. 3). He derived from these measurements the minimal arterial pressure which could sustain glomerular filtration. He coined the term 'maximum secretory pressure of the urine' by which he meant the difference between the 'arterial pressure and the maximal ureteral pressure' (a surrogate for intratubular pressure). His simple conclusion is a masterpiece of reasoning:

'... The results given in this paper show that, so far as the experimental evidence goes, the glomerular epithelium may be looked upon as a simple filtering membrane resembling, in many particulars, a membrane of gelatin. The osmotic pressure of the proteids of the plasma is about 25–30 mm Hg. When the pressure in the glomerular capillaries rises above this point, filtration takes place through the glomerular epithelium, the filtrate representing simply plasma minus proteid. The higher the pressure in the glomerular capillaries the more rapid would this process go on.'

Starling's paper of 1899 is remarkable in other respects which are not generally appreciated. His ability to deduce from a well-designed experiment that an increase in the colloid content of a solution of 1 g/dl raises the osmotic pressure by about 4 mm Hg was crucial to the determination of ultrafiltration pressure (which Starling termed 'maximum secretory pressure'). The fact that he was able to show that urine formation ceases when the blood pressure in the glomeruli approaches the osmotic pressure of the serum proteids, was interpreted by Starling as affording an 'a priori argument in favour of the view that the process occurring in the glomeruli is one of filtration'.

In the same paper, he studied the phenomenon which we now call 'osmotic diuresis'. He argued that 'if the glomerular function is a mere filtration we should expect that the more rapid the process, the more nearly would the urine, which is turned out into the ureters, resemble in composition, reaction and osmotic pressure, the blood plasma, since the glomerular filtrate hurried through the tubules, would have very little time to undergo any changes resulting in its concentration'. He did the experiment by injecting normal saline and concentrated saline and dextrose solutions into dogs and confirmed his prediction that 'the more rapid the secretion (formation) of urine, the more closely does its osmotic pressure approximate that of the blood plasma'.

He considered those factors which might be concerned in promoting an increased glomerular transudation i.e. '(1) a rise of the pressure in the glomerular capillaries; (2) quicker blood flow through the capillaries and (3) diminished amount of proteids in the blood plasma'. After injection of NaCl or dextrose he observed a diuresis which outlasted the 'hydraemic plethora' and resulted in an increased concentration of the blood and 'therefore a diminution of the volume of circulating fluid'. In another experiment he found that he could obviate the increase in arterial blood pressure and kidney volume caused by the infusion, by removing blood simultaneously from the carotid artery. In this case the diuresis was prevented. He concluded that it is the 'state of the blood vessels and the general blood-pressure' which determine the diuretic response rather than direct effect on the kidney cells. This diuresis may be the result of two factors, i.e. hydraemic plethora and consequent rise in the pressure and velocity of blood in the kidneys (or) a direct dilator effect of the injected substance on the renal blood vessels.

Starling was succeeded at University College London by A.V. Hill who was to receive the Nobel Prize for his work on the energy of muscle contraction. He was followed, in 1926, by Charles Lovatt Evans, a pupil of Starling. In 1966 Andrew Huxley became the Jodrell Professor and, in 1963, he and Bernard Katz, the first Professor of Biophysics, were both awarded the Nobel Prize for their work on nerve conduction [6].

Arthur Cushny

The link to an important step in the understanding of renal function is provided by yet another UCL person, Arthur Cushny, Professor of Pharmacology. Starling had invited him to prepare a monograph on the kidney which he published as *The Secretion of the Urine* in 1917 [8]. His introduction, in the form of a response to Starling, is interesting:

> 'The growth in the literature on the kidney has been extraordinary since the time when you and I began to work on it, and this increase in bulk has not gone along with an improvement of quality, but rather the reverse. No other organ of the body has suffered so much from poor work as the kidney, and in no other region of physiology does so much base coin pass as legal tender. It was therefore necessary to sift thoroughly through this mass of printed matter of over 6,000 pages, and I have read it carefully and, as far as might be, sympathetically, though I must confess that my patience has been sorely tried by some papers in which the depth bore no proportion to the length'.

It is difficult to know how to evaluate Cushny's role in the intellectual debate of the time. On the one hand, there was the view of Ludwig and Bowman that the kidney filters and reabsorbs and on the other hand, that of Rudolf Heidenhain, who maintained that urine formation is dependent entirely on active tubular and glomerular secretion of solutes and fluid [9]. It may be said that Cushny provided no new information which resolved the debate in any way. On the basis of his extensive review of the literature, he called his own view, the 'modern view'. He said: 'I do not flatter myself that this treatise obtains finality in regard to the secretion of the urine; that is impossible at the present time. If it serves as an advance post from which others may issue against the remaining ramparts of vitalism, its purpose will be obtained'.

His reference to vitalism may have been an obtuse reference to Heidenhain's view that the cells of the kidney are endowed with an intrinsic property of secretion and, quite inappropriately, this was considered negatively to represent a 'vitalistic' point of view. In fact Heidenhain was careful to avoid this impression when he said that the words 'life of a cell' are only 'an expression indicating the totality of unknown physical and chemical processes occurring in the cells ...'.

Cushny's 'modern view' rejected the notion of tubular secretion completely. He saw filtration as being a physical process occurring in the glomerulus and reabsorption occurring in the tubules by an undefined intrinsic activity of the epithelium. He believed that Heidenhain had based his rejection of the concept of glomerular filtration on incorrect numbers. Cushny summarised his overview of kidney function as follows:

> 'The function of the kidney may thus be shortly defined as the filtration of the non-colloid constituents through the capsule and the absorption of 'Locke's fluid' through the tubule cells. The capsule furnishes the tubules with the fluid as it exists in the circulation and the tubules return to the blood the fluid best adapted for the tissue and allow the rest to escape in the urine. Thus if the plasma is too rich in sugar or chloride, the filtrate also contains it above the threshold value; the epithelium however returns it at the optimal or threshold concentration and the remainder passes into the ureters. If much water has been ingested and the filtrate is correspondingly dilute, the subtraction of the optimal solution leaves the excess water in the urine along with the urea and other waster products.
>
> The formation of the glomerular filtrate is due to a blind physical force; and the absorption of the tubules is equally independent of any discrimination, for the fluid absorbed is always the same, whatever the needs of the organism at the moment.
>
> The 'modern view' dispenses with the power of the kidney to discriminate between minute changes in the composition of blood, and thus renders it superior to the rival view of specific secretion. It is impossible at present to prove it correct, but this is unnecessary. It is sufficient to show that it is in accordance with a large body of observations. Even if it fails to offer a complete explanation of these, it merely requires further development and not abandonment'.

Cushny's monograph apparently had great influence and it was later revised in a second edition in 1926 which added little that was new. With the wisdom of hindsight it is illuminating to see how a 'powerful figure' who had written one of the most famous of systematic pharmacology textbooks and who had held sway in Berne (1889–1890), Strasbourg (1891–1893), Michigan (1893–1905), London (1905–1918) and Edinburgh (1918–1926), achieved such prominence without having contributed any original data of a substantial nature to the field.

E. Bruce Mayrs

E.B. Mayrs (1891–1963) worked with Cushny in the last period his life in Edinburgh and found that creatinine, sulphate and phosphate were concentrated to the same extent in the urine but that urea did not follow the same pattern. He defined urea as a 'threshold substance' and the others as non-threshold substances. With his colleague [10] he argued that any non-threshold substance could be used to derive 'the proportion of plasma which comes into direct contact with renal cells' and, since tubular secretion for these had been ruled out, it is possible to measure GFR.

His measurement of GFR in 11 anaesthetised rabbits using the formula:

$$GRF = \frac{UV\ (\text{sulphate})}{P\ (\text{sulphate})}$$

is still in current use, but is now applied to substances shown more rigorously to be excreted by filtration only. Mayrs deserves full credit for formulating and applying a suitable clearance method for the measurement of glomerular filtration in an experimental animal for the first time. Prior to his retirement, Mayrs occupied the Chair in Pharmacology at Queens College in Belfast from 1928 to 1957.

From the above it is evident that there was a sound infrastructure in Britain for the study of kidney function until the 1920s and that the English physiologists featured prominently in the scientific advances. What is puzzling is the fact that, for no obvious reason, this momentum was lost and it appears that little of substance was added at the level of single nephron function thereafter. Instead the pendulum swung to the side of whole body homeostasis and the role of the kidney in this process.

Control of Water Homeostasis: Vasopressin

This topic has been reviewed masterfully by Fitzsimons [12]. Around the end of the nineteenth century, textbooks of physiology admitted that absolutely nothing was known about the function of the pituitary gland. But things were to change and British physiologists were to lead the field.

In 1895 Edward Schafer (Sharpey-Schafer) turned his attention to the effects of the injection of glandular extracts on various systemic functions. He and Oliver described the sharp rise in blood pressure which was produced by intravenous injection of pituitary extracts [13]. After it was reported that the pressor substance was derived from the neurohypophysis, Schafer and Vincent confirmed this [14].

In 1901 Schafer, who had moved to Edinburgh as Professor of Physiology, reported that pituitary extracts caused a prolonged diuresis independent of any effect on the renal vessels or blood pressure. He and Percy Theodore Herring, who was Professor of Physiology at Andrews University, concluded that there must be a direct action on the renal epithelium.

In contrast to this observation, Schafer also noted an antidiuretic effect which preceded the diuresis and a rise in blood pressure and suggested that there may be two separate substances in the pituitary acting on the kidney. In his Croonian lecture of 1909, Schafer stated:

> 'It is further noticeable that in a large proportion of experiments a common phenomenon is a temporary diminution or cessation of urine flow, even although the blood-pressure is raised to a considerable extent and the kidney volume markedly increased; conditions which – on the mechanical or filtration theory of urine secretion – should inevitably produce diuresis. There is, in fact, very often at first an inhibition of secretion (followed in the majority of cases by the characteristic secretory activity), even although the vascular conditions are throughout favourable to the occurrence of free secretion. The extract is therefore liable to cause two effects which are antagonistic to one another. The most reasonable explanation of this is afforded by the supposition that the gland contains not only a substance which stimulates the kidney cells to activity but also another substance which depresses their activity, and this to so great an extent in certain cases that the kidney ceases to secrete, although all the vascular conditions for urine excretion are of the most favourable character. Nevertheless, the secretory substance usually ultimately prove the more potent: or it may be that the kidney cells are more susceptible to its influence.'

He also alluded to the polyuria which is often observed in injuries to, and tumours in the base of the brain.

Despite this, Schafer was more focussed on the polyuric effect of posterior pituitary extracts, which he attributed to irritation and/or hypertrophy of the pars intermedia, which causes the syndrome of diabetes insipidus, a conclusion which is now known to be incorrect. His principle contribution, therefore, was to focus attention on an internal secretion rather than on a mechanism including nerves. It was left to others to perform experiments on conscious humans where the antidiuretic effects of pituitary extracts became clear.

It was much later, when the subject was taken up again by a British researcher, Geoffrey Wingfield Harris, Professor of Physiology at the Institute of Psychiatry in London. In his 1955 monograph, *Neural control of the pituitary gland* [15], using a remote control method of stimulating the supraoptico-hypophyseal tract of anaesthetised rabbits, he showed that temporary inhibition of water diuresis occurred. This antidiuresis was associated with the appearance of antidiuretic hormone in the urine. This work formally established the role of the nerve supply to the neurohypophysis in regulation of ADH secretion.

The concept of osmoreceptors, while not strictly residing in the domain of renal physiology, also deserves attention. In the 1920s Ernest Basil Verney collaborated with Starling at UCL. They found that urine produced by an isolated dog kidney perfused by a heart-lung preparation was similar to that produced in diabetes insipidus in both amount and composition. They wrote [16]:

> 'We suggest, therefore, that some substances or substances with an action similar to that of pituitrin are normally present in the intact mammal and serve as the means whereby the kidney is controlled in its important function of regulating the output of water and of chloride. The isolated kidney is divorced from this regulating mechanism – a mechanism which has presumably been produced during phylogenetic development in response to the request for an increasing control over salt-and-water metabolism. It is not surprising, then that without this aid the kidney functionally reverts to the type of gland characteristic of the fish and amphibian classes of the vertebrate phylum. In these classes, so far as we have been able to find urinary analysis in the literature, the chloride percentage in the urine is always below that in the blood plasma.'

They further found that the diuresis could be inhibited by posterior pituitary extracts and that correction of a perfused-head preparation to their heart-lung-kidney preparation returned urine volume and composition to normal. These experiments provided the most definitive evidence that the production of concentrated urine by the kidney depends on the pituitary.

Later, Verney and colleagues administered a large volume of water by stomach tube to dogs and noted a delay of 15 min between peak water load and peak diuresis [12]. They concluded that:

> 'The secretion of water, over and above that required for the solutes in the urine, is conditioned by and dependent upon a fall in the concentration in blood and kidney of the antidiuretic principle of the pituitary body. The secretion of the antidiuretic principle is itself controlled, through the intermediation of the nervous system, by the concentration of water in blood and tissues.'

In 1947 Verney gave the Croonian lecture of the Royal College of Physicians [17]. Fitzsimons notes its landmark quality [13] and the fact that, a half of century later, not one of its conclusions has been invalidated. He described experiments in which urine flows were measured in conscious dogs in response to injection or perfusion of various solutions into the carotid arteries. Verney found that an intracarotid injection of hypertonic NaCl caused a profound inhibition of urine flow in a dog undergoing water diuresis but that a similar injection made into the malleolar vein or an intracarotid injection of isotonic NaCl did not. The character of the inhibition closed parallelled that obtained by intravenous injection of posterior pituitary extracts. Removal of the posterior lobe of the pituitary reduced the inhibitory response to less than 10% of baseline.

Verney then went on to test other substances which increase osmotic pressure in the carotid blood and found that other hyperosmotic solutions have the same effect, e.g. $NaSO_4$ and sucrose. Prolonged infusions decreased urine flow gradually and this could be matched by posterior pituitary extract. He concluded that an increase of only 1% in the osmotic pressure of aortic blood was adequate to reduce water diuresis. Recovery of urine flow after cessation of the infusion was associated with a fall in antidiuretic hormone (fig. 4). Verney's insightful overview was as follows:

> 'Water diuresis, then, is fitly and accurately described as a condition of physiological diabetes insipidus, and there can be little doubt that the antidiuretic secretion of the neurohyophysis is a hormone in the physiological sense that its liberation is mainly and continually governed by the contemporary concentration of sodium chloride in the carotid arterial plasma. The physiological fitness of this control is emphasised by its quantitative aspects, in that changes within the range and of the order of 1% in the osmotic pressure of the arterial blood lead, through the intermediation of the antidiuretic hormone, to changes in the rate of water excretion within the range and of the order of 1000%; the maintenance of near constancy in the osmotic pressure of the internal environment is thereby achieved.'

Control of Sodium and Extracellular Volume Homeostasis

Whereas the generally held view of regulation of sodium homeostasis until the 1950s was that this was achieved by alterations in GFR, mediated by changes in blood pressure, renal nerve activity and plasma oncotic pressure, it slowly became apparent that regulatory activity resided in the renal tubules.

In 1961 a seminal experiment was performed in Sharpey-Schafer's Department of Medicine at St Thomas's Hospital by De Wardener, Mills, Clapham and Hayter who showed that, in normal dogs receiving large amounts of salt-retaining steroids and vasopressin and in which GFR had been substantially reduced by mechanical means, an infusion of saline caused a rise in urinary sodium excretion [11]. Hugh De Wardener and Ivor Mills were working as lecturers in the department and Mills had recently returned from the National Institutes of Health where he had worked with Fred Bartter on aldosterone. In

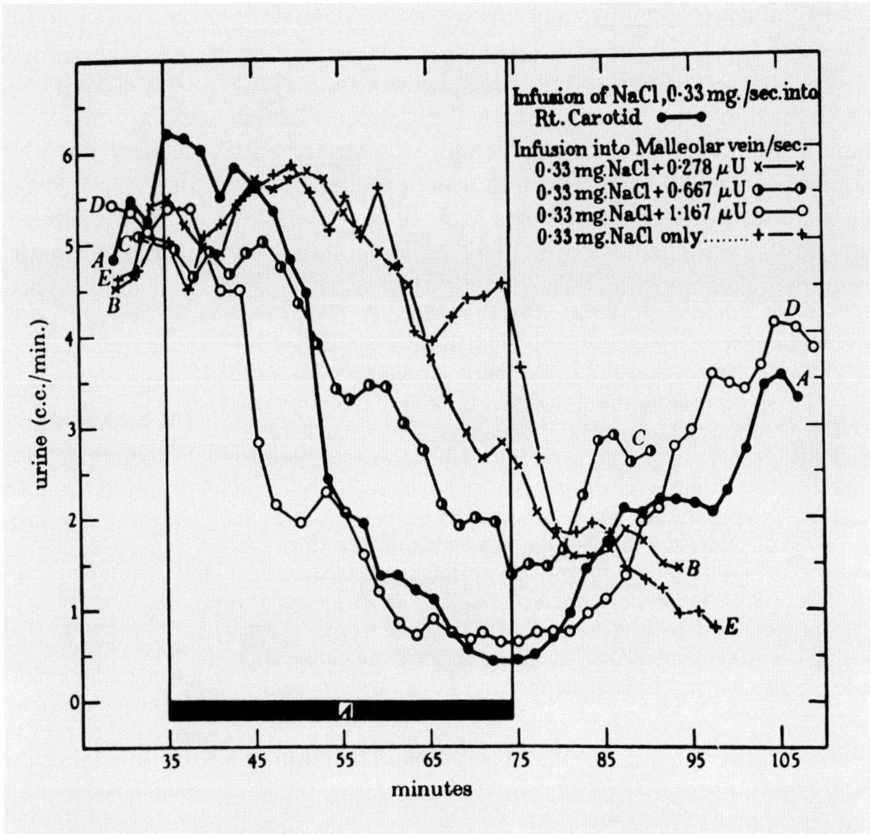

Fig. 4. Assay of release of postpituitary antidiuretic substance during prolonged intracarotid infusion (39.5 min, rectangle A) or 1.243 *M* NaCl at 0.2725 ml/min in the bitch 'Nicky'. Calculated local increase in osmotic pressure is 1.80%. Curve A, intracarotid infusion; Curve E, intravenous infusion of NaCl at same rate; Curves B, C and D show responses to intravenous infusion with postpituitary extract 0.28, 0.67 and 1.17 μU/s, respectively. Abscissa: Approximate time after test dose of water. From Verney [17].

part it was to demonstrate that this hormone did not play an important regulatory role, that the experiment was done in the first place.

Subsequent experiments by the same group controlled for dilutional effect, haematocrit, sodium concentration, plasma protein, arterial and venous pressure, renal blood flow and GFR and under all circumstances, the saline infusion caused a natriuresis. The release of a circulating natriuretic substance was postulated.

Despite decades of work the elusive natriuretic factor(s) was slow in surfacing. The atrial natriuretic family of peptides emerged in the 1980s as clearly defined entities whereas other putative 'hormones' remained elusive.

As in many areas of science it was the initial experiment rather than the emergences of a defined outcome that was important. De Wardener's approach had opened the door to wider thinking about a process that was thought to be rather simple. It is hardly surprising that a process as fundamental to the maintenance of tissue perfusion, as sodium and volume homeostasis, is backed up by multiple fail-safe devices, yet this was not generally appreciated prior to the spate of experiments which followed the work of Hugh De Wardener and colleagues and which elucidated a variety of mechanisms of regulation of tubular handling of salt and water.

Conclusions

British physiologists appear to have contributed more to the understanding of integrated kidney function and how it is regulated, than to the detail of the precise glomerular and tubular mechanisms of filtration, reabsorption and secretions. The lineage of renal physiologists starting with William Bowman and Ernest Starling constituted a major force in the field, at least until the middle of the twentieth century.

References

1 Withering W: An Account of the Foxglove and Some of Its Medical Uses: With Practical Remarks on Dropsy and Other Diseases. Birmingham, Swinney, 1785.
2 Fine LG: William Bowman's description of the microscopic anatomy of the kidney. Nephrol Dial Transplant 1995;10:2147–2149.
3 Bowman W: On the structure and use of the Malpighian bodies of the kidney with observations on the circulation through that gland. Phil Trans R Soc Lond 1842 (part 1):57–60.
4 Malpighi M: De Viscerum Structura: De Renibus; in: Opera Omnia. London, Scott, 1666, pp 87–100.
5 Ludwig C: De Viribus physicis secretionem urinal adjuvantibus. Marburg, Elwert, 1842.
6 Harte N, North J: The World of UCL, 1828–1990. London, University College London, 1991.
7 Starling EH: The glomerular functions of the kidney. J Physiol (Lond) 1899;24:317–330.
8 Cushny A: The Secretion of the Urine. London, Longmans, Green, 1917.
9 Heidenhain R: Versuch über den Vorgang der Harnabsonderung. Pflügers Arch Ges Physiol Menschen Tiere 1874;9:1–27.
10 Mayrs EB, Watt JM: Renal blood flow and glomerular filtration. J Physiol (Lond) 1922;56: 58–68.
11 De Wardener H: Control of sodium excretion; in Renal Physiology: People and Ideas. Bethesda, American Physiology Society, 1987, pp 217–246.
12 Fitzsimons JT: Control of vasopressin release; in Renal Physiology: People and Ideas. Bethesda, American Physiology Society, 1987, pp 277–308.
13 Olivier G, Schafer EA: On the physiological action of extracts of pituitary body and certain other glandular organs. J Physiol (Lond) 1895; 18:277–279.
14 Schafer EA, Vincent S: The physiological effects of extracts of the pituitary body. J Physiol (Lond) 1899;25:87–97.
15 Harris GW: Neural control of the pituitary gland. Physiol Soc Monogr 3, 1955.
16 Verney EB, Starling EH: On secretion by the isolated kidney. J Physiol (Lond) 1922;56:353–358.
17 Verney EB: The antidiuretic hormone and the factors which determine its release. Proc R Soc Lond B Biol Sci 1947;135:26–106.

American Journal of Nephrology

Am J Nephrol 1999;19:266–273

Origins of Renal Physiology in the USA

Gerhard Giebisch Robert W. Berliner

Department of Cellular and Molecular Physiology, Yale University School of Medicine, New Haven, Conn., USA

Key Words

Renal physiology · National Institutes of Health · Comparative physiology · Clearance · Micropuncture

Abstract

Research in renal physiology began later in the USA than in Europe. Initial studies in the early 1900s dealt with the pathophysiology of renal failure. Micropuncture study of single nephron function was initiated in the laboratory of A.N. Richards in the early 1920s and with the later addition of microperfusion provided important insights into the site and mechanisms of solute transport. In parallel, with the leadership of Homer Smith, the development of noninvasive clearance methods to measure glomerular filtration rate and renal blood flow initiated a fruitful period of quantification of renal hemodynamics and of transport by the tubules. The steady progress of renal physiology in the USA owes much to the generous support of basic reasearch by the National Institutes of Health. It is also worthy of mention that progress in renal physiology in the US owes much to work carried out in clinical departments and to the type of comparative studies exemplified by work at the Mt. Desert Island Biological Laboratory.

Dr. R.W. Berliner holds a joint appointment in the Department of Medicine.

Introduction

Development of research in renal physiology in the USA is of relatively recent origin compared with the much earlier pursuit of similar activities in continental Europe. It was only in the early part of this century that significant advances in nephrology occurred in the USA. That early work was largely limited to pathophysiological studies in which the excretion of urea, electrolytes and of organic dyes during the progression of renal failure was explored. Major increases in physiological work occurred in the early twenties of the present century and especially after World War II. Several important influences stimulated basic research in the USA including physiological investigations of kidney function. These are summarized in table 1.

First, the Flexner report [1], published in 1910, led to a profound change in the structure of American medical schools. Establishment of a full-time faculty in both basic science and clinical departments, emphasis on scholarship and the application of scientific theory to medical problems encouraged the inclusion of basic research into the activities of clinical departments of American medical schools. As a consequence of such developments, some of the best research in renal physiology over the last 50 years was not confined to basic science departments but has emerged from departments of internal medicine, pediatrics, and pathology.

KARGER

Fax + 41 61 306 12 34
E-Mail karger@karger.ch
www.karger.com

© 1999 S. Karger AG, Basel
0250–8095/99/0192–0266$17.50/0

Accessible online at:
http://BioMedNet.com/karger

Gerhard Giebisch, MD
Department of Cellular and Molecular Physiology
Yale University School of Medicine
333 Cedar Street, New Haven CT 06520-8026 (USA)
Tel. +1 203 785 4076, Fax +1 203 785 4951, E-Mail gerhard.giebisch@yale.edu

Table 1. Contributions to renal physiology: important influences

Flexner Report
National Institutes of Health
Intramural research and training (Shannon, Berliner)
Extramural research and training (grant and fellowship programs)
Research in both basic science and clinical departments
Activities of American Society of Nephrology

Another important influence in the flowering of renal physiology and indeed of all of biomedical research in the United States in the last half century has been the acceptance by the federal government of the need to support both basic and applied research and the phenomenal growth of that support through the National Institutes of Health. It is notable that in that movement two men who were themselves important contributors to renal physiology played key roles in making the federal government the major supporter of medical research in general.

A.N. Richards was, during World War II, the chairman of the Committee on Medical Research of the Office of Scientific Research and Development (OSRD). The progress of the research supported by that organization during the war suggested that a continuation of such support would be appropriate, and through Richards' efforts the medical research projects that had been supported by OSRD were transferred to the National Institutes of Health (NIH) for support. The NIH had, at that time, been in existence for over 50 yers but had been relatively small and almost all of its research had been carried out in its own intramural laboratories. Acceptance of responsibility for research on a national scale had not previously been in its purview.

The NIH program of support for medical research more widely had a rather modest beginning and grew relatively slowly during its earlier years. Its later exponential expansion was largely the result of the effective leadership and political skills of James A. Shannon.

Shannon had originally established himself as a leading renal physiologist in Homer Smith's department in the 1930s. During the war he had a leading role in the search for new antimalarial drugs. His career at the NIH began in the late 1940s when he was recruited to be director of intramural research for the newly established National Heart Institute. Over the next few years he organized a group of intramural laboratories and recruited to their leadership a number of scientists who became leading figures in their fields.

Among the Heart Institute laboratories was the Laboratory of Kidney and Electrolyte Metabolism which became a major center of renal physiology. Under the leadership successively of Robert Berliner, Jack Orloff and Maurice Burg, the laboratory has not only made important research contributions to renal physiology, but also provided a training ground for many who have become major contributors to the field.

After a few years in the Heart Institute, Shannon moved into the office of the Director of NIH, succeeding to that position in 1955 and continuing as leader of NIH until 1968. Through his vision of the potential for research to revolutionize medicine and his ability to convince the leaders of Congress of the soundness of his views, he was able to provide for the support of medical research at a level previously unthinkable. During the period of his directorship the funds for extramural grants grew by a factor of more than 15!

It was, in fact, this growth of funds for medical research that made possible the development of the academic medicine visualized in the Flexner report by making possible significant research efforts in clinical departments of schools of medicine as well as in the basic sciences. Whereas previously a full time position in a clinical department was often a luxury that could be afforded only by an individual with an independent income or with a busy private clinical practice, it became possible to create new positions with support from funds supporting the research of the incumbent. Along with many other areas of biomedicine, renal physiology has prospered, not only in basic science but also in clinical departments.

Pathophysiology and Biochemistry

The advances in renal physiology in the USA can be traced back to several roots, listed in tables 2 and 3. First among these was pathophysiological research, especially biochemical studies, in several clinical departments. Common to most of them is that the physiological questions frequently evolved from clinical problems.

The activities of T. Addis [2], F. McLean [3], O. Folin [4] and D.D. Van Slyke [5] may serve as examples (fig. 1). These investigators were interested in urea excretion, especially the complex relationship between plasma urea concentration, urine flow rate and urea excretion. Many of their efforts were directed at finding a useful index of kidney function during progression of renal failure. That

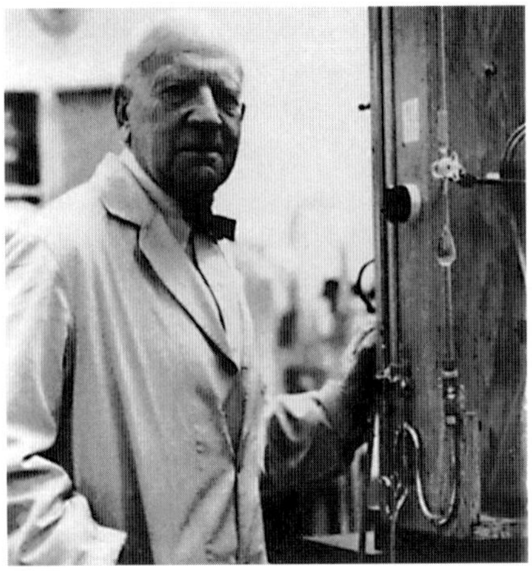

Fig. 1. D.D. Van Slyke (1883–1971). (1) Analytical methods: amino acids, urea, volumetric and manometric analysis of total CO_2 (HCO_3^-), 'buffer value', titration curve of oxy- and reduced hemoglobin. (2) Clinical chemical studies: blood gas and electrolyte measurements in clinical disorders, series of papers entitled Factors Controlling the Electrolyte and Water Distribution in the Blood. (3) Monographs (with J.P. Peters): *Quantitative and Clinical Chemistry* (two volumes); chapter on hemoglobin and oxygen, and carbonic acid and acid-base balance were landmark contributions.

Table 2. Contributions to renal physiology: pathophysiology, biochemistry and comparative physiology

Pathophysiology	Biochemistry	Comparative physiology (MDIBL)
Addis	Van Slyke	Marshall
Rowntree	Henderson	Smith
Peters	Folin	Chambers
Loeb	McLean	Kempton
Goldring-Chasis	Hastings	Forster
Gamble	Nash-Benedict	
Elkinton-Danowski		
Seldin		

Table 3. Contributions to renal physiology: clearance and single tubules (micropuncture and microperfusion)

Clearance	Single tubules: micropuncture and microperfusion
Van Slyke	Richards, Wearn
Smith	Walker, Oliver
Pitts	McDowell, Bott
Berliner	Gottschalk, Burg, Grantham, Orloff

measuring changes in the kinetics of urea excretion would be useful was initially suggested by Ambard [6]. The constant that he proposed to describe the relationship, however, proved not to be reproducible. A major step was the development of improved analytical methods for the measurement of urea in blood urine [5, 7] and an analysis of the relationship of urine flow to urea excretion [3, 5]. Work by Van Slyke and his associates [5] finally led to the conclusion that at high rates of urine flow, a constant volume of blood referred to as the 'maximal urea clearance' is cleared of urea [5]. This concept served as a useful background for subsequent clearance studies. Foremost among these was the work of H. Smith and his associates that led to the development of the inulin clearance and the noninvasive measurements of the glomerular filtration rate. Also included in table 2 are several investigators who made significant biochemical achievements. Most of them were associated with D.D. Van Slyke's laboratory at the Rockefeller Institute and participated in studies dealing with urea and acid-base excretion by the kidney [5, 8].

Another important advance in renal physiology, preceded by clinical studies, was the discovery that the excretion of phenol red (phenolsulfonphthalein, PSP) could serve as a useful measure of renal function. Phenol red was extensively used in evaluating the progression of renal disease after it had been shown by L. Rowntree and T. Geraghty to be rapidly and almost completely excreted by the kidneys following intravenous administration of a small dose [9]. This observation led E.K. Marshall and J. Vickers [10] and later Marshall and M. Crane [11] to use phenol red to demonstrate that the renal tubules had the capacity for secretion by a specific saturable transport mechanism. At the time of these investigations, secretion of solutes by the kidney was not a popular concept but became firmly established after these incisive studies by Marshall and his collaborators [10–12]. These studies also paved the way for acceptance of subsequent evidence that, in the case of both urate and potassium, certain solutes may be both reabsorbed and secreted. It is now, of course, generally accepted that filtration, reabsorption and secretion participate in urine formation.

The activities in the laboratory of J. Peters at Yale are another example of the application of physiological concepts of water and electrolyte transport to the study of human disease mechanisms (fig. 2). For many years Peters' laboratory was a center for careful balance and renal function studies which dealt with a variety of metabolic disorders, including diabetic coma, heart failure, infections, thyroid disorders and toxemias of pregnancy. Significant as were such studies, Peters' most imporant contributions were probably (1) his part in producing with Van Slyke that bible of mid-century clinical chemistry [13] and (2) the many young investigators he inspired to continue in scientific research [14–17]. Peters was also involved in the introduction into clinical departments of the flame photometer, invented during the later years of World War II. The development of accurate and rapid methods for measuring sodium and potassium in small samples of body fluids was a major methodological breakthrough, because previous methods were time-consuming and difficult. The flame photometer quickly became an essential tool for renal function and balance studies [18].

Robert Loeb [19] at Columbia and James Gamble at Harvard were also physiologically oriented clinicians whose interest in abnormal fluid and acid-base metabolism included many investigations. Gamble especially focused on the relations between plasma electrolyte patterns, shifts of fluid and ions between fluid compartments, and especially distortions of the cation and anion composition. Gamble also developed a novel way of presenting the distribution of electrolytes in body fluids by juxtaposition of anion and cation columns ('Gamblegrams'). This provided a useful didactic way of describing body fluid abnormalities. Gamble's work [20, 21] also advanced the design of optimal replacement solutions for the treatment of a wide variety of electrolyte disorders.

Further examples of pathophysiological investigations involving the use of physiological approaches include the work of Goldring and Chasis [22], with H. Smith at the New York University, and of Elkinton and Danowski who were strongly influenced by Peters at Yale. Don Seldin provides another example of a successful investigator with a broad range of research interests and with a strong focus on physiological approaches to the study of electrolyte and renal disorders. As stated by himself, many research questions evolved from the practice of internal medicine [23, 24].

2

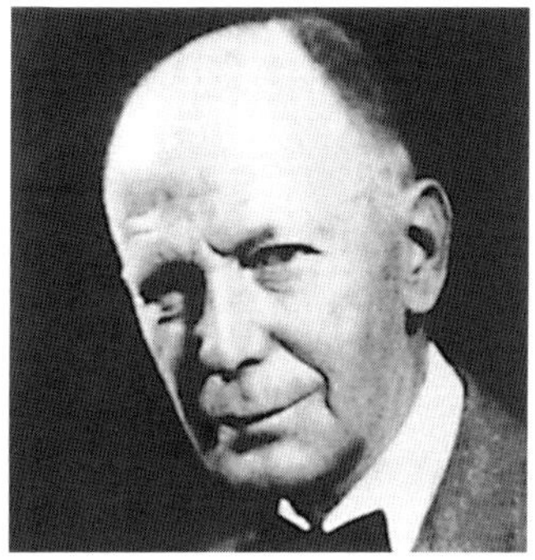

3

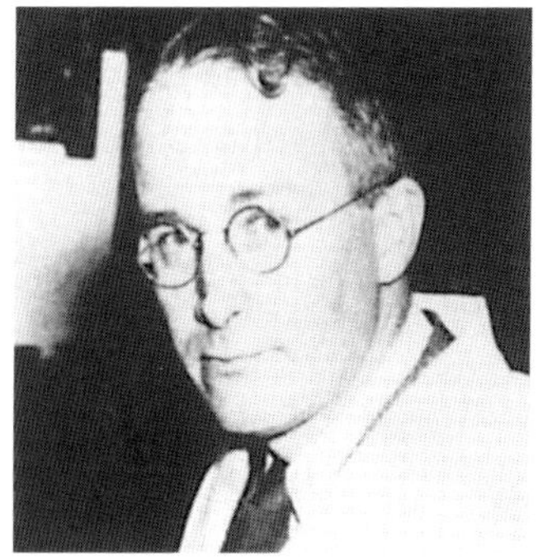

Fig. 2. John P. Peters (1887–1955). (1) Application of physiological principles to study disease mechanisms. (2) Introduction of flame photometer into clinical medicine (American Cyanamid, Perkin-Elmer). (3) Extensive application of balance techniques (urea, nitrogen, ions, water, calories). (4) Studies on renal mechanisms underlying acid-base and endocrine disorders, diabetes, heart failure, and edema, shock, dehydration, acute and chronic renal failure, toxemias of pregnancy and thyroid disorders. (5) Monographs: *Body Water, The Exchange of Fluids in Man. Quantitative Clinical Chemistry* (two volumes, with D.D. Van Slyke).

Fig. 3. E.K. Marshall (1889–1966). (1) Demonstration of tubule secretion of phenol red (measurement of free and bound dye) (with J.L. Vickers), 1923. (2) Description of saturation of the secretory mechanism of organic acids (with M.M. Crane). (3) Described aglomerular kidneys (with A.L. Grafflin), 1928–1929 (goose fish, toadfish); absence of sugars in urine.

Comparative Physiology

The comparative physiology of the kidney has been a focus of a number of studies, especially at Mount Desert Island Biological laboratory (MDIBL). That institution which just celebrated its centennial [25, 26] has contributed in a major way to the advancement of renal physiology. Two men, E.K. Marshall (fig. 3) and Homer Smith laid the foundation for the studies of kidney function for which the laboratory has become distinguished. Marshall had, with Vickers and with Crane, shown that the amount of phenol red excreted in the urine far exceeded the amount that could be filtered at the glomeruli because a large fraction of the phenol red in the plasma was bound to the plasma protein. What we now consider to have been a clear demonstration of secretion by the renal tubules failed to convince some of the leading figures, notably Cushny and A.N. Richards. Marshall became aware of the aglomerular status of the goosefish and its availability at Salsbury Cove, Me., the site of the MDIBL. So he joined the laboratory to study the excretion of phenol red in the goosefish, finding, of course, that it was rapidly excreted in the urine. Secretion of solutes by the renal tubules has, since then, never been in doubt.

Among the findings of Marshall's study of the goosefish was that glucose did not appear in the urine, even after the administration of phlorizin. This is said to have suggested to Smith that a nonmetabolized sugar might be a suitable substance with which to measure glomerular filtration. Of course, although suggesting that sugars were not secreted, their absence from goosefish urine did not prove that they might not be reabsorbed by the tubules. Indeed the first sugar proposed by Smith's laboratory for measuring glomerular filtration, xylose, turned out to be partially reabsorbed. It was only later that Smith's group and, simultaneously, Richards' laboratory came up with inulin as the marker neither secreted nor reabsorbed [27–30].

Marshall and Smith had a long history of interaction. Smith had worked under Marshall during World War I and it was through the influence of Marshall that Smith subsequently went on to earn his doctoral degree. Although Smith had been interested in the study of body fluids, he had not undertaken to study the function of the kidney until he was approached by Goldring and Chasis, two young clinicians with a problem concerning urea excretion in febrile patients. It is not clear what if any light they were able to throw on that particular problem but it launched a highly successful collaboration and led to the flowering of American renal physiology under the influence of Homer Smith.

Several other developments at the MDIBL had a significant impact on renal physiology in providing model systems for the study of the mechanisms of fluid and ion transport. Among these were the discovery of the shark rectal gland by Wendell Burger [31], the nasal salt gland of marine birds by Knut Schmidt-Nielsen [32] and the development of the teased flounder tubule preparation by Roy Forster [33]. A detailed account of the wide range of comparative physiological activities at the MDIBL has recently been published [25].

R. Chambers and R.T. Kempton [34] also deserve mention for their investigations showing that fragments of chick mesonephros cultured in vitro formed small cysts that secrete anionic dyes such as phenol red into the lumen. These studies provided an important early stimulus for subsequent work demonstrating secretion of phenol red into the lumen of teased flounder tubules and its accumulation into cortical renal tissue [35, 36].

The work of R. Chambers was also important for suggesting the possibility of kidney micropuncture. A.N. Richards refers to his having observed R. Chambers in 1921 puncturing erythrocytes. He discussed these experiments with his associate, J.T. Wearn, who thought of the possibility of puncturing single amphibian glomeruli to obtain fluid from Bowman's capsule for chemical analysis [27].

Clearance and Homer Smith

The introduction of inulin as a reliable substance for the accurate measurement of the glomerular filtate had a major impact on renal physiology because the inulin clearance made possible quantitative measurements by noninvasive techniques of reabsorption and secretion by the tubules. The term 'clearance' had been introduced by D. Van Slyke as an index of renal function (see above) but the idea of using the clearance of a substance to measure glomerular filtrate originated with the Danish physiologist P.B. Rehberg [37; see also E.B. Mayrs, 38]. Rehberg suggested that the clearance of creatinine might be suitable because of the many substances excreted in the urine it was the most highly concentrated. If urine were formed only by filtration and reabsorption, the clearance of the most highly concentrated solute would have to be a measure of filtration rate. As was shown subsequently [39, 40]. however, creatinine is secreted in the human kidney but its clearance has remained a useful index of glomerular function in the diseased kidney. The search for a substance whose clearance could be used for the accurate measurement of the glomerular filtrate led H. Smith (fig. 4) and his associates and simultaneously the laboratory of A.N. Richards to inulin [41].

The use of inulin as a reliable substance for measuring glomerular filtration rate was the beginning of quantitative renal physiology and this development owes very much to Smith [42–48]. Reabsorption and secretion could now be measured in a variety of experimental conditions and the renal effects of hormones, diuretics and changes in electrolyte and acid-base could be characterized. The observation that iodine-containing urologic contrast media such as Diodrast and Hippuran had exceedingly high renal clearances suggested not only that these substances were secreted into the urine but that these clearances must approach the renal plasma flow. Smith and his associates developed the Diodrast clearance for measuring renal blood flow, and later replacing Diodrast with the more easily measured *p*-aminohippuric acid (PAH) [46]. Clearance studies by Smith, Pitts and Berliner, to mention those most eminent in the USA, laid the foundation for the impressive body of knowledge of renal excretion of fluid, titratable acid, sodium, chloride, bicarbonate, potassium and many other solutes. The application of clearance methods also provided insight into the mechanisms underlying renal disease processes and Smith and his associates deserve credit for having played a major role in bringing quantitative clearance concepts into clinical medicine. It is fair to state that Smith dominated the field of nephrology in the USA for many years [27, 48].

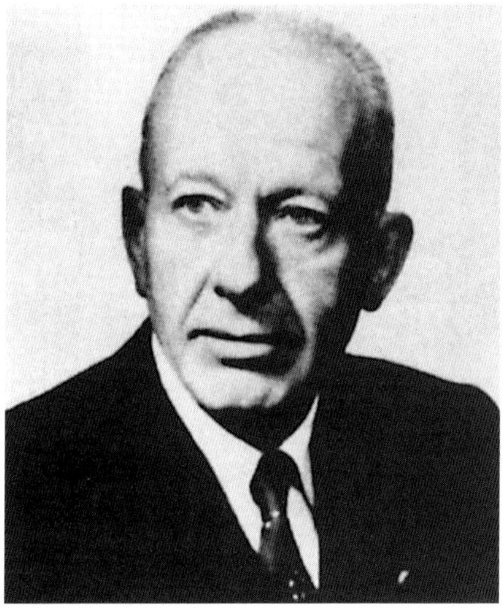

Fig. 4. H.W. Smith (1895–1962). (1) Comparative physiology of fluid and electrolyte metabolism; evolution of the kidney. (2) Renal clearance concept: glomerular filtration rate, effective renal blood flow, tubular transport capacity (Tm), excretion of water and excretion of sodium. (3) Monographs: *The Physiology of the Kidney* (1937), *Lectures on the Kidney (Porter Lectures)* (1943) and *The Kidney: Structure and Function in Health and Disease* (1951).

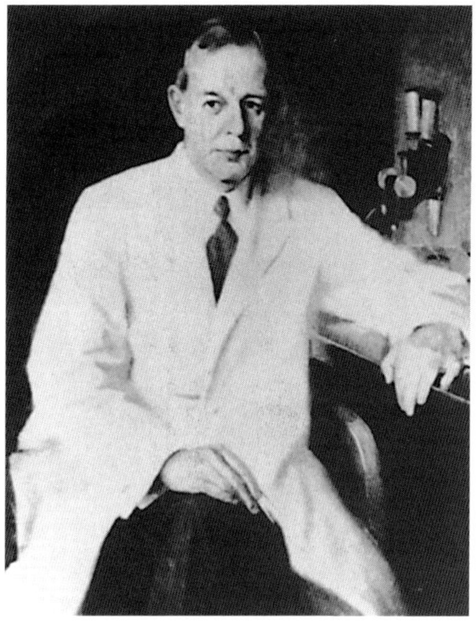

Fig. 5. A.N. Richards (1876–1966). (1) Introduction of kidney micropuncture (with J.T. Wearn, 1893–1984 and A.M. Walker, 1896–1955). (2) Validation of filtration-reabsorption theory of urine formation (1924). (3) Direct localization of specific nephron transport sites (puncture, perfusion of amphibian tubule, 1937). (4) Puncture of mammalian tubules (1941; in A.N. Richards' laboratory; A.M. Walker, P.A. Bott, J.R. Oliver and M.C. McDowell).

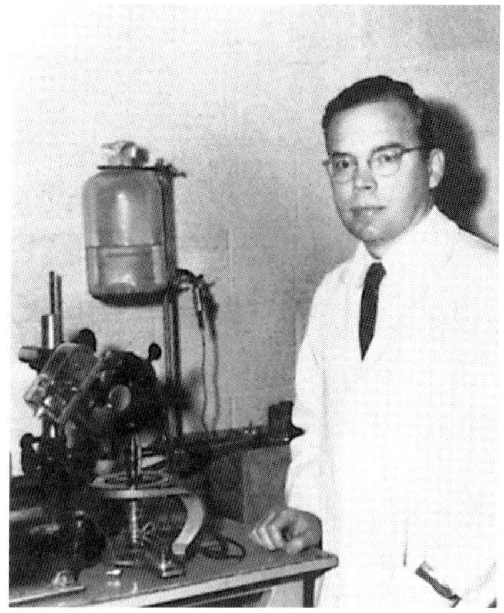

Fig. 6. C.W. Gottschalk (1922–1997). (1) Revived micropuncture studies. (2) Hydrostatic pressure measurements along the mammalian tubule. (3) Validation of countercurrent mechanism of urine concentration. (4) Micropuncture studies of ion and water movement in the mammalian kidney (osmolality, urea, pH). (5) Studies on the effects of sympathetic nervous system on renal electrolyte transport.

Single Tubules: Micropuncture and Microperfusion

Studies on the function of single nephrons in the USA can be broadly divided into two periods: the first, starting in the 1920s and lasting to the beginning of World War II, was dominated by A.N. Richards [27, 49, 50] (fig. 5). These studies started with the puncture of single amphibian glomeruli and demonstrated that the composition of the fluid collected and the hydrostatic pressures in glomerular capillaries satisfied the ultrafiltration theory of Ludwig [49]. The mapping of the main sites of solute transport along amphibian tubules followed [49]. Micropuncture studies in Richards laboratory culminated in 1941 with the first exploration of the transport properties of mammalian tubules [51, 52]. World War II interrupted further investigations.

The second period in micropuncture studies began after World War II with Gottschalk [53, 54] (fig. 6) and subsequently by similar efforts in a number of laboratories. As a consequence there has been a significant broadening of our understanding of fluid and electrolyte transport and of the factors that regulate renal blood flow. Solute transport along the nephron could now be explored in great detail, the mechanism of urine concentration and dilution studied at critical sites along the nephron, and the nature of many transport processes clarified [28].

The development of techniques of microperfusion of tubules and their peritubular capillaries [55] and especially the perfusion of isolated tubules in vitro [56] have provided important additions to the study of the function of single nephrons. The latter method makes possible the investigation of tubule segments not accessible to puncture on the surface of the cortex or the exposed papilla and complete control of the composition of the fluids in the lumen and peritubular (bath) environment. Such studies have been further complemented by refinement of enzymatic analyses and electrophysiological approaches that make possible precise measurement of the forces driving ion transport across individual cell membranes [57].

Conclusion

Our knowledge of the function of the kidney has come a long way during the last century and at an accelerating pace since World War II, and it is safe to say that American laboratories have made a major contribution to this progress. The international attendance at the annual meetings of the American Society of Nephrology suggests that this is widely recognized.

References

1 Flexner A: Medical Education in the United States and Canada. New York, Carnegie Foundation for the Advancement of Teaching, 1910.

2 Addis T, Watanabe CK: The rate of urea excretion – First paper. A criticism of Ambard and Weill's laws of urea excretion. J Biol Chem 1916;24:203–220.

3 McLean FC: The numerical laws governing the rate of excretion of urea and chlorides in man. I. An index of urea excretion and the normal excretion of urea and chlorides. J Exp Med 1915;22:212–236.

4 Folin O, Denis W: New methods for the determination of total non-protein nitrogen, urea and ammonium in blood. J Biol Chem 1912; 11:527–536.

5 Van Slyke DD, Rhoads CP, Hiller A, Alving AS: Relationships between urea excretion, renal blood flow, renal oxygen consumption, and diuresis. The mechanism of urea excretion. Am J Physiol 1934;109:336–374.

6 Ambard L, Weill A: Les lois numériques de la sécrétion de l'urée. J Physiol Pathol Gen 1910; 12:209–219.

7 Marshall EK Jr: A rapid clinical method for the estimation of urea in urine. J Biol Chem 1913; 14:283–296.

8 Hastings AB: Donald Dexter Van Slyke, 1883–1971. Managing Editor 1914–1925. J Biol Chem 1972;247:1635–1640.

9 Rowntree LG, Geraghty JT: An experimental and clinical study of the functional activity of the kidneys by means of phenolsulphonephthalein. J Pharmacol Exp Ther 1909–1910; 1:579–661.

10 Marshall EK Jr, Vickers JL: The mechanism of the elimination of phenolsulphonephthalein by the kidney – A proof of secretion by the convoluted tubules. Bull Johns Hopkins Hosp 1923; 34:1–6.

11 Marshall EK Jr, Crane MM: The secretory function of the renal tubules. Am J Physiol 1924;70:465–488.

12 Marshall EK Jr: The secretion of phenol red by the mammalian kidney. Am J Physiol 1924;70: 465–488.

13 Peters JP, Van Slyke DD: Quantitative Clinical Chemistry. Baltimore, Williams & Wilkins, vol 1: Interpretations, 1931, rev 1946; vol 2: Methods, 1932, rev 1943.

14 Paul JR, Long CN: John Punnett Peters. Biogr Mem Natl Acad Sci 1958;31:347–375.

15 Lavietes PH: John Punnett Peters: An appreciation. Yale J Biol Med 1956;29:175–182.

16 Epstein FH: The contributions of John P. Peters to nephrology. Yale J Biol Med, in press.

17 Peters JP: Renal excretion of water and inorganic salts; in Thomas CC (ed): Body Water. Springfield, Thomas Books, pp 274–341.

18 Hald PM: The flame photometer for the measurement of sodium and potassium in biological materials. J Biol Chem 1947;167:499–510.

19 Loeb RF: James Lawder Gamble. Biogr Mem Natl Acad Sci 1962;36:146–160.

20 Gamble JL: Companionship of water and electrolytes in the organization of body fluids; in Lane Medical Lectures. Stanford, Stanford University Press, 1951, vol 5, pp 1–90.

21 Gamble JL: Chemical Anatomy, Physiology and Pathology of Extracellular Fluid, ed 6 (lecture syllabus). Cambridge, Harvard University Press, 1954.

22 Chasis H: History of collaboration by Department of Physiology at New York University School of Medicine. Physiologist 1983;26:64–70.

23 Rector F: Presentation of the George M. Kober Medal to Donald W. Seldin. Trans Assoc Am Physicians 1985;98:132–147.

24 Epstein F: Presentation of the first John P. Peters Award to Donald W. Seldin. Semin Nephrol 1983;4:107–112.

25 Epstein FH: A Laboratory by the Sea: The Mount Desert Island Biological Laboratory, 1989–1998. River Press, Rhinebeck, 1998.

26 Maren T: An historical account of the Mount Desert Island Biological Laboratory: 1898–1993. Bull Mt Desert Isl Biol Lab 1994;33:3–20.

27 Gottschalk CW: A history of renal physiology to 1950; in Seldin DW, Giebisch G (eds): The Kidney: Physiology and Pathophysiology, ed 2. New York, Raven Press, 1992, pp 1–29.

28 Gottschalk CW, Berliner RW, Giebisch GH: Renal Physiology: People and Ideas. Bethesda, American Physiological Society, 1987.

29 Marshall EK Jr: The aglomerular kidney of the toadfish *(Ospanus tau)*. Bull Johns Hopkins Hosp 1929;45:95–101.

30 Smith HW: The excretion of the non-metabolized sugars in the dogfish, the dog, and man; in Berglund H, Meds G (eds): The Kidney in Health and Disease. Philadelphia, Lea & Febiger, 1935, pp 92–110.

31 Burger JW, Hess WW: Function of the rectal gland in the spiny dogfish. Science 1960;131: 670–671.

32 Schmidt-Nielsen K: The salt-secreting gland of marine birds. Circulation 1960;21:955–967.

33 Forster RP, Hong SK: In vitro transport of dyes by isolated renal tubules of the flounder as disclosed by direct visualization. Intracellular accumulation and transcellular movement. J Cell Comp Physiol 1956;51:259–272.

34 Chambers R, Kempton RT: Indications of function of the chick mesonephros in tissue culture with phenol red. J Cell Comp Physiol 1933;3:131–167.

35 Forster RP: Use of thin kidney slices and isolated renal tubules for direct study of cellular transport kinetics. Science 1948;108:65–67.

36 Forster RP, Taggart JV: Use of isolated renal tubules for the examination of metabolic processes associated with active cellular transport. J Cell Comp Physiol 1950;36:251–270.

37 Rehberg RB: Studies on kidney function. I. The rate of filtration and reabsorption in the human kidney.Biochem J 1926;20:447–460.

38 Mayrs EB, Watt JM: Renal blood-flow and glomerular filtration. J Physiol 1922;56:120–124.

39 Bradley SE: Clearance concept in renal physiology; in Gottschalk CW, Berliner RW, Giebisch GH (eds): Renal Physiology: People and Ideas. Bethesda, American Physiological Society, 1987, pp 63–100.

40 Smith HW: Newer methods of study of renal function in man; in Lectures on the Kidney. Lawerence, University of Kansas, Extension Div, 1943, p 39.

41 Richards AN, Westfall BB, Bott PA: Renal excretion of inulin, creatinine and xylose in normal dogs. Proc Soc Exp Biol Med 1934;32: 73.

42 Smith HW: Highlights in the history of renal physiology. Georgetown Med Bull 1959;13:4–48.

43 Smith HW: The Physiology of the Kidney. New York, Oxford University Press, 1937, p 25.

44 Smith HW: Renal physiology between two wars; in Lectures on the Kidney. Lawernce, University of Kansas, Extension Div, 1943, pp 63–82.

45 Smith HW: The Kidney: Structure and Function in Health and Disease. New York, Oxford University Press, 1951.

46 Smith HW, Goldring W, Chasis H: The measurement of the tubular excretory mass, effective blood flow and filtration rate in the normal human kidney. J Clin Invest 1938;17:263–278.
47 Smith HW, Goldring W, Chasis H, Ranges HA, Bradley SE: The application of saturation methods to the study of glomerular and tubular function in the human kidney. J Mt Sinai Hosp 1943;10:59–108.
48 Berliner RW: Homer Smith: His contribution to physiology. J Am Soc Nephrol 1995;5:1988–1992.
49 Richards AN: Urine formation in the amphibian kidney. Harvey Lect Ser 1934–1935;30:93–118.
50 Gottschalk CW: Dr. A.N. Richards and kidney micropuncture. Ann Intern Med 1969;21:28–37.
51 Walker AM, Oliver J: Methods for the collection of fluid from single glomeruli and tubules of the mammalian kidney. Am J Physiol 1941; 134:562–579.
52 Walker AM, Bott PA, Oliver J, MacDowell MC: The collection and analysis of fluid from single nephrons of the mammalian kidney. Am J Physiol 1941;134:580–595.
53 Blythe WB: In memoriam: Carl William Gottschalk (1922–1997). Kidney Int 1998;53:1–2.
54 Gottschalk CW: Renal tubular function: Lessons from micropuncture. Harvey Lect 1962–1963;58:99–124.
55 Burg MB: Introduction: Background and development of microperfusion technique. Kidney Int 1982;22:417–424.
56 Windhager EE: Micropuncture and microperfusion; in Gottschalk CW, Berliner RW, Giebisch GH (eds): Renal Physiology: People and Ideas. Bethesda, American Physiological Society, 1987, pp 101–129.
57 Giebisch G: Transport of electrolytes across renal tubules; In Gottschalk CW, Berliner RW, Giebisch GH (eds): Renal Physiology: People and Ideas. Bethesda, American Physiological Society, 1987, pp 165–216.

American Journal of Nephrology

Am J Nephrol 1999;19:274–281

The Contribution of French-Speaking Scientists to the Origins of Renal Physiology and Pathophysiology (1790–1910)

Gabriel Richet

Académie Nationale de Médecine, Paris, France

Key Words

Potassium · Uremia · Edema · Urea · Lesion

Abstract

Some contributions: (1) urinary urea, its chemical composition and physiological meaning, Fourcroy and Vauquelin (1790–1808); (2) in binephrectomized animals blood urea is high and chemically identical to that of urine, Prevost and Dumas (1821); (3) urea level in renal vein blood is 50% of that in the arteries, Picard (1856); (4) retained potassium is the uremic poison, Feltz and Ritter (1881); (5) polyuria induced by intravenous injections of sugars or urea, Richet and Moutard Martin (1880); is the kidney in command of the concentration of the blood? Using cryoscopy, Hédon got the clue, the osmotic load (1900); (6) methylene dye excretion measures the global renal function and thus the degree of renal failure, Achard and Castaigne (1897); (7) the disentanglement of chronic uremia and edema, Widal and Achard (1900–1910); (8) evaluation of the global renal function by the ratio plasma urea/urine urea output, Ambard's Constant (1905), initial step of the concept of clearance; (9) a circulating nephropoietic factor in one-kidney animals, Carnot (1910). In bled animals he also disclosed a hemopoietic factor which later became the renal erythropoietin.

L'expérience anime les scientifiques de tous les pays, les éclaire et forme entre eux un nouveau lien social à jamais indissoluble.[1]

F. Magendie (Précis élémentaire de physiologie, ed 2. Paris, 1825, Preface, p VI)

The contributions to renal physiology presented here are interwoven with those of English, German and Italian laboratories. New facts emerged from animal and clinical investigations, the latter particularly in France.

This account focuses on three points: (1) urea chemistry and physiology; (2) individualization of the excretory functions of the kidney, and (3) renal physiology in relation to urological surgery.

Urea Chemistry and Physiology

Fourcroy and Vauquelin

Around 1790, at the same time as W.H. Wollaston (1766–1826) in London, two chemists, the physician Antoine François Fourcroy (1755–1809), a faithful disciple of Lavoisier (1743–1794), and the pharmacist Nicolas Vauquelin (1763–1829), were studying renal calculi [1]. They were convinced that the calculi originated from urinary solutes [2]. Fourcroy and Vauquelin made a chemical inventory of the constituents of urine and in addition to the mineral solutes, they studied the 'soapy substance' first observed by H. Boerhaave (1668–1738) [3] and later by H. Rouelle (1718–1779) [4]. They isolated and cristallized it, as did W. Cruickshank in 1798, named it urea, gave its composition, and published their results between

1 Experiments are the foundation of the scientific community of all countries, they enlighten them and bind them in an indissoluble link.

KARGER

Fax + 41 61 306 12 34
E-Mail karger@karger.ch
www.karger.com

© 1999 S. Karger AG, Basel

0250–8095/99/0192–0274$17.50/0

Accessible online at:
http://BioMedNet.com/karger

Dr. Gabriel Richet
76, rue d'Assas
F–75006 Paris (France)

1797 and 1808 [6–9]. They considered that urea gave rise to ammonia which C. Berthollet (1760–1822) had just shown to be rich in nitrogen, and that urea was the main cause of the difference in density between urine and distilled water. The principal findings was its high nitrogen content (35.3%). Historically these researches were a critical step for the development of modern clinical chemistry [5].

The Physiological Significance of Urea. For Fourcroy and Vauquelin urea was an essential substance in the metabolism of an animal. Without any knowledge of the nitrogen cycle they assumed its existence and called its fixation into tissues 'animalization of nitrogen' [10]. They considered that urea was nitrogen's final metabolic stage, which needed to be disposed off each day in a controlled manner [11], and the kidney to be its natural exit as the lungs are for carbon [12], and they insisted that its elimination was obligatory. They suggested that urea is separated from the blood flowing into the renal artery, a process which assures that the concentration of urea in the blood remains in equilibrium. They advised clinicians to note the kidney's ability to denitrogenate the blood and probably to dispose of excess solids [13].

Where does urea come from? To find it out, Fourcroy and Vauquelin suggested that the conent of urea in the renal arterial blood should be compared to that in the renal vein [14]. *Can urea have a pathological role?* They proposed that, though there was no direct evidence, an impaired ability to eliminate a nitrogenous substance as urea might cause a rise in its concentration in body fluids that might cause disease [15].

Other discoveries made by Fourcroy and Vauquelin. They determined the composition of many urinary, biliary and intestinal stones, the chemistry of the urine of all the animals of the zoo of the Jardin du Roi and of many plant extracts. Fourcroy found that the salts in edema fluid were the same as in plasma and that it contained a variable amount of albumin which increased with the duration of the edema [16].

Fourcroy, a Public Man

Fourcroy was the son of a modest pharmacist in Paris, established in the 'Quartier Latin'. During his medical studies he was interested in chemistry and joined Lavoisier's group. His lucid exposition of the new chemical theories and his books *(Philosophie Chimique* and *Système des connaissances Chimiques)* singled him out. As a scientist in the tradition of the Age of Enlightment, it was not his nature to compartmentalize advances in scientific knowledge from current thoughts and activities. He launched a journal, *La médecine éclairée par les sciences physiques* [17], which lasted only a year and vainly proposed that either a department of chemistry or a hospital should be devoted to the study of chemistry in disease. But at that time there was an ingrained vogue to confine medical research to a search for the origins of clinical signs in life by examining the organs after death. Fourcroy was also a politician and a manager. From 1794 to 1808 he organized a new national teaching network from primary school to higher education. In medicine he created three 'Ecoles de Santé' in which a basic knowledge of the sciences, anatomical dissection and an active participation in hospital care were imposed on both physicians and surgeons, at last blended. His memory is clouded by a shadow: did he do all he could to save Lavoisier's life?

Vauquelin, a Chemist at the Laboratory Bench

Vauquelin was born in Normandy to a poor family. Before coming to Paris he assisted in a country pharmacy. He joined Fourcroy's laboratory and thereafter was never deflected from his experiments. Beside his studies of urine and stones, he isolated chromium and beryllium and explored animal and vegetable substances. Under his deanship, the laboratories of the 'Faculté de Pharmacie' played an important role in the chemical elucidation of the alkaloids and plant drugs [18].

Removing the Kidneys to Establish whether the Kidney Synthetises Urea

Whether a substance was only excreted by an organ or also synthesized by that organ was a hotly debated question [19]. A possible approach was to measure the concentration of urea in the blood before and for 2 or 3 days after a bilateral nephrectomy. In practice this was also difficult because, even if the blood urea rose, the rise had to be sufficient to be detected by the methods then available.

In 1803, J.N. Comhaire (1778–1837) performed this experiment. He hoped thereby to insert the 'scientific simplicity of chemistry' into the ongoing medical debate. The kidneys were removed one at a time on separate occasions [20]. Of 65 dogs only 2 survived the first nephrectomy and no rise in blood urea was detected when the second kidney was removed, although they smelled of urine. A severe blow. Nevertheless, Comhaire made important observations. He established that it was possible to survive with only one kidney and was probably the first to note the phenomenon of compensatory hypertrophy. The survival of 2 dogs for a few days after bilateral nephrectomy also made him think of certain therapeutic possibilities and, almost 'en passant' he noted that the urine of dogs does not contain uric acid. Subsequently his work was only quoted by Rayer [21]. Comhaire, a Belgian, came to Paris to study medicine where he was impressed by the work of Xavier Bichat (1771–1802) and Fourcroy. At the beginning of his thesis, he hoped to be able to add a fourth organ, the functional failure of which would immediately lead to death, in addition to the heart, lungs and brain [22]. Back in Liège he organized a course of medicine which later led to the birth of the faculty. All in all as an expert in public health and an organizer, he played a decisive role in his home town [23].

J.L. Prevost and J.B. Dumas repeated the work in 1821 following the same protocol as Comhaire, but with improved surgical techniques and a more sensitive method to measure urea [24]. The experiments were carried out on dogs, cats and rabbits. Following the second nephrectomy the postoperative immediate mortality was low and the animals survived for 5–6 days. Nothing of note was detected at autopsy. Blood sampled just before death was dried, washed, treated with alcohol and the urea cristallized by means of nitric acid. Its concentration was raised and its composition was almost identical to that in urine. Blood urea contained: nitrogen 42.2%; carbon 18.2%; hydrogen 9.9%, and oxygen 29.6%; and urine urea contained: nitrogen 43.4%; carbon 19.4%; hydrogen 10.8%, and oxygen 26.4%. They stated, 'We believe it permissible to conclude that urea in blood is identical to that in urine. This urea is synthesized outside the kidney which acts as an eliminating surface'. In addition they suggested that the concentration of uric acid in the blood was probably raised in gout and that of glucose in diabetes, and they thought that it was very likely that other diseases were also 'associated with humoral disturbances'. It is noticeable that in the title of their paper bilateral nephrectomies and blood measurements are not mentioned. This was possibly because they wished humoral changes in disease to be considered as a major biological discovery, even greater than the techniques used for its revelation. In effect it was a directional change in experimental pathology, a new way of thinking of biology in diseases [25, 26].

Jean Louis Prevost (1780–1850) was born in Geneva, to which he returned in 1820 after studying in Paris and Edinburgh. There he met Jean Baptiste Dumas (1800–1884) a penniless young man who in 1816 had walked from Alès near Montpellier to Geneva in order to continue his studies while an apprentice to a pharmacist named Tingry. In the evenings naturalists, chemists and doctors from Geneva, such as N.T. de Saussure (1767– 1845), G. de la Rive (1770–1834), P. de Candolle (1778–1841), and J.F. Coindet (1774–1834), met in the pharmacy. There were also other eminent birds of passage [27].

Prevost and Dumas had a wide range of research interests. Using J.B. Amici's (1784–1863) achromatic microscope they described the morphology of blood constituents, the formation of spermatozoa and the site of impregnation. Prevost became an influential figure in the medical school and political life in Geneva. Dumas left Geneva shortly after the nephrectomy study. He was enticed to Paris by A. Humbolt (1769–1859) who had travelled to Geneva expressly to lure him away. Humbolt was a naturalist of Darwinian stature who lived and worked in Paris from 1789 to 1825, where he was known as 'the most Parisian of the German scientists'. Dumas became a leading organic chemist and a powerful politician. He persuaded Pasteur to study an epidemic among silkworms, and thus Pasteur identified two diseases, the first due to definite microbial infections. L. Gmelin, F. Tiedemann and R. Marchand confirmed that urea was synthesized in nonrenal sites, but this was only accepted after the experiments of F.T. Frerichs (1824–1885) [28]. Urea is not a toxic. Vauquelin and Ségalas (1792–1875) soon followed upon Prevost and Dumas's findings. They made a futile attempt to show that the intravenous administration of urea was toxic. In their disappointment they paid little attention to the diuresis which they recorded as missing and thereby the first observation of an osmotic diuresis [29].

Renal Arteriovenous Gradient in Animals and the Concentration of Blood Urea in Human Diseases

The normal blood urea. As a young intern in Strasbourg in 1856 J. Picard (1834–1895) modified Liebig's method for the measurement of urea and increased its sensivity [30], and was thus able to measure its concentration in only 50–100 ml of blood. Though it was criticized by Recklinghausen [31], the advantages of this modification to physiology and clinical medicine were substantial.

Picard established four biological norms: (1) human normal venous blood contains 0.016–0.035 g urea/100 ml, he was one of the first to make this measurement; (2) horse arterial and venous blood contain 0.02 and 0.04 g urea/100 ml, except for renal venous blood similar results were obtained in dogs; (3) in 2 dogs renal arterial and venous blood urea was 0.036 and 0.040 and 0.018 and 0.020 g/100 ml, respectively, and (4) the urea in blood and in nonrenal secretions is the same.

Blood urea in disease. Picard also observed that in severe acute dehydration conditions such as cholera the blood urea rose and then returned to normal after recovery. Thus a high blood urea does not necessarly imply irreversible uremia. He noted that in chronic renal diseases, as revealed by a long-standing albuminuria, the concentration of urea in the blood might bear little relation with the clinical state. It might be normal or raised up to 0.200 g/100 ml (latent renal insufficiency). In terminal uremia the blood urea was very high, less in cases of associated cerebrovascular accident when at autopsy there was only moderate atrophy of the kidneys. Perhaps Picard, before it was possible to measure blood pressure, was noting a distinction between the clinical uremia of terminal renal failure and that sometimes associated with essential severe hypertension. Though often quoted by Claude Bernard [32], Picard's work was ignored by clinicians.

J. Picard was born in Wissembourg, Alsace. His interpretation of the chemical data he had made at the age of 22 and their relation to the autopsy findings was remarkable for its lucidity. His interests were not in line with those of his superior E. Kuss (1815–1871) who nevertheless presided over the jury who assessed his thesis. He was helped by E. Hepp (1819–1871) who had created a laboratory of clinical chemistry at the hospital in 1845. Picard, having failed in his attempt to work in an academic department, went into practice in Guebviller where he became an authority on public health. He retired near Nancy in 1895 where he died the next year.

Claude Bernard

Claude Bernard (1811–1878) was interested in what happened to urea in the gut of the anephric dog. This was a minor contribution in contrast to his concept of the 'milieu intérieur' which increasingly occupied him from 1854 until his death. But the principle of the constancy of 'milieu intérieur' came to dominate thinking about both normal and pathological renal function.

Potassium Is Uremic Poison

This discovery was made in Nancy in the 1870s by V. Feltz (1835–1895) and E. Ritter (1837–1884). Though their protocol was simple, it involved a multitude of laborious experiments. Dogs on a constant diet were injected intravenously with urine or with each of its various constituents. This technique had been used by Frerichs to demonstrate the absence of toxicity of urea in nephrectomized dogs [28].

There were 2 groups of dogs, with normal renal function and made anuric by a bilateral ligature of the renal pedicles in which death occurred in about 3 days. The intravenous administration of 1 day's urine output from a normal dog to anuric dogs shortened their survival from 72 to 36 h or less, whereas when administered to normal dogs, it had no detectable effects. In other words normal urine is toxic when given intravenously to anuric dogs but not to dogs with normal renal function. Then instead of normal urine, the anuric dogs were given either plain water or water in which were dissolved various organic solutes such as urea, uric acid, hippuric acid, creatine, creatinine, leucine, tyrosine, guanosine, xanthine, hypoxanthine and taurine in amounts equivalent to a normal output in 24 h. Each of these did not affect survival but, when an extract of the urinary minerals was given, the anuric dogs died within a few hours. The minerals responsible were potassium salts either extracted from the urine or chemically pure. It is true that the toxicity of potassium salts had been suspected, but it was Feltz and Ritter who first provided the evidence that they were [33].

V.T. Feltz (1835–1893), born in Colmar (Alsace), was Professor of Pathological Anatomy in 1863. He was as obsessed by physiology as he was by bacteriology. In 1866, E. Ritter (1837–1884), born in Strasbourg, became Professor of Medicine. He was also interested in chemistry. After the Franco-Prussian War of 1870–1871 they left Strasbourg for Nancy. There they continued their studies on experimental uremia until the early 1880s.

Individualization of the Excretory Functions of the Kidney

The Osmotic Load, a Nonhemodynamic Factor in Water Excretion

In 1880 Charles Richet (1850–1935) and R. Moutard Martin (1850–1926) were studying the effect of intravenous injections of milk in animals submitted to a large blood loss. A paradoxal polyuria occurred inspite of the hypotension produced by the loss of blood. This turned out to be due to the lactose of the milk. Other sugars such as saccharose, levulose and dextrose also induced a rise in urine flow which began as the sugar appeared in the urine. The urine flow depended on the total amount of sugar that was administered and not on the concentration in the fluid that was injected. Urea had the same effect. They concluded that '... the kidney controls the concentration of the blood; thus an increase in the concentration of a dialyzable substance in the blood causes a polyuria regardless of the blood pressure or renal innervation' [34]. The previous observations of Wöhler (1800–1882) and the work of C. Ustimowitsch were acknowledged [35]. Wöhler noted that polyuria is occasioned by nonmetabolized foreign substances, and Ustimowitsch, a pupil of Ludwig, found, to his and Ludwig's surprise, that an intravenous injection of urea to hypotensive anuric dogs induced a rise of urine flow [36].

Twenty years later E. Hédon (1863–1933) in Montpellier put forward a unifying explanation. He observed that polyuria of sugars and urea was related to the osmotic load administered, as measured by freezing point depression [37].

R. Moutard Martin was a clinician who thereafter was no longer interested in research. Charles Richet, acknowledged as a 'Renaissance humanist', had an independent mind and wide interests. The range of his inquiries engendered a certain amount of humor among his colleagues. Nevertheless in 1902 with P. Portier (1866–1962) he discovered anaphylaxis for which he was awarded the Nobel Price in 1913. Both the poluria study and the discovery of anaphylaxis began by an unexpected result, a rational explanation emerging from further experiments. Richet enjoyed studying paradoxal results, especially if it was in a blank page of science [38].

Disentanglement of Chronic Uremia and Edema by the Teams of F. Widal and C. Achard: A Piece of a Paneuropean Effort

Attempts to deduce the origin of clinical abnormalities in uremia and edema simply from an examination of the kidney at autopsy finally came to an end around 1890. Within the next 20 years the Hungarian A. Korànyi (1866–1944), the German H. Strauss (1866–1944), the Austrian R. Jaksch (1855–1935) and in France F. Widal (1862–1929), A. Lemierre (1875–1956), Ch. Achard (1860–1944), J. Castaigne (1871–1951) and J. Winter [39] advanced the subject by applying physiological principles to distinguish the two main renal syndromes in chronic kidney diseases [40].

The techniques used were: Strauss's needle for sampling blood from a vein (1898), a tool that opened up clinical blood chemistry; the use of the freezing point depression for measuring the molecular concentration of a solution, established by F.M. Raoult (1830–1901) in Grenoble (1880); dye excretion tests (1897); improved techniques for measuring blood urea, and the concept of metabolic balance at last accepted.

In 1896 Winter confirmed H. Dreser's (1860–1925) results in Tübingen. When measuring the ability of the kidneys to concentrate the urine by dehydration, Dreser had shown that the freezing point depression of urine could fall as much as –2.40°C in contrast to that of the blood which remained constant. Koranyi in 1897 applied this technique to investigate the maximal capacity of the kidney to concentrate the urine in health and renal failure where isosthenuria is usual. He called his method 'funktionell Nierendiagnostik'.

In the years that followed the particular pathophysiological features of each of the two main syndromes of 'chronic nephritis' were distinguished.

One was terminal renal failure without edema but with hypertension and small kidneys. Widal and his team pointed out that the characteristic biological disturbance in this syndrome was a progressive and relentless retention of nitrogen as witnessed by the rise in blood urea. Having delineated this syndrome they wanted to understand the underlying mechanism. They performed balance studies on patients with moderate renal failure in a relatively stable state. They found that a low protein diet changed the blood urea to a lower steady-state level, whereas increasing it gradually raised the blood to a higher plateau. When, with either of the diets, the blood urea had leveled out it was found that the intake of nitrogen was equal to its urinary output. They concluded that on a constant input of nitrogen: (1) the concentration of urea in the blood is directly related to the kidney's capacity to excrete it in the urine, and (2) the concentration of urea in the blood controls the amount of urea that is excreted. Moreover they noticed that the content of sodium chloride in the diet did not appear to affect the excretion of urea and that varying the intake of protein did not affect the excretion of sodium chloride.

In 1897, Achard and Castaigne, for their part, were studing the 'renal permeability' of a dye, methylene blue. After injection it was not metabolized and, whatever the renal function, it was all excreted by the kidneys into the urine even in patients with chronic renal failure, though it took longer. The delay was related to the severity of the renal failure.

The studies of the two Parisian teams blended with that of Koranyi and his urine concentration test and that of Strauss who also put forward the measurement of blood urea. Between them they defined the principal biological features of terminal renal failure which at that time was labelled 'interstitial nephritis'.

The other nephropathological entity was chronic edema with heavy proteinuria, usually without a rise of blood pressure, which at autopsy was associated with large white kidneys and was known as 'parenchymatous nephritis'. In these cases there was no retention of urea and the excretion of methylene blue was normal or nearly so [41]. Further evidence showed that retention of urea and edema were independent. It was clinically evident that the edema fluid occupied subcutaneous spaces and the body cavities, and it was known that sodium and chloride were situated mainly outside the cells. The Parisian teams established that in such patients plasma chloride was normal but chloride balances were abnormal. The methods used were relatively coarse but adequate. Body weight, the output of urine and its content of chloride were measured whereas the chloride content of the food was assessed with the use of tables. Widal's group demonstrated that a diet low in chloride diminished edema, whereas the chloride content in a normal diet was not totally excreted in the urine and edema became worse. Edema was due to salt retention and the accompanying retention of water was to maintain the osmolality of the blood within normal physiological limits.

It was not long before it became obvious that the intake of salt was the common denominator of all forms of edema and, more importantly perhaps, that it was also related to hypertension. Subsequently these two seminal observations were forgotten for more than 20 years, mainly because physicians would not measure the weight, the daily urinary output of salt and control its dietary intake accordingly. Achard was particularly interested in the space in which salt and water accumulated which he named the 'lacunar system' [42], a step towards the concept of extracellular space.

In Berlin H. Strauss was also studying the physiological basis for interstitial and parenchymatous nephritis and came to identical conclusions as Widal. Nevertheless, as is so often the case, the clinicians' attitude was identical to that of their predecessors, one century before, postmortem morbid anatomy for ever!

Besides his work on kidney function in renal disease, Widal made important contributions to the serological diagnosis of typhoid fever (Eberth bacillus), the interpretation of the cells of serosal effusion and the anaphylactic manifestations in man, shock, asthma and urticaria. He died in 1929 at the hight of his ability and renown. Achard's interest in medicine was part and parcel of his interest in biology. The *Nouveaux Procédés d'Exploration* published in 1902 emphasized the necessary change in medical thinking that was taking place: 'there is a need to study function of organs in order to supplement anatomical data with physiological investigation' [43].

Widal and Achard had a pronounced influence on French medicine.

Around 1900 Ambard Measures the Global Renal Function by the Ratio Plasma Urea/Urine Urea Output, a Better Idea than Its Formulation

Leo Ambard (1876–1962) was a physician fascinated by renal physiology. Early in the 20th century he was in charge of a laboratory attached to a Department of Urology. His surgical colleagues were anxious to know the risks of operating on their patients. Ambard thus studied renal function in dogs and humans to evolve a test which would measure the kidney's capacity to excrete urea. For 10 years he covered a great deal of ground beginning with the capacity to concentrate urea. This led him to measure the amount of urea excreted by the kidney in a unit of time and to consider the ratio between the plasma concentration of urea and its output as a measure of overall renal function. From an extensive accumulation of experimental and clinical data, and his passion for mathematics, Ambard empirically deduced a rather complicated equation which in a simplified form has a familiar look:

$$K = P/\text{sqr } UV,$$

where K was Ambard's constant, P plasma urea, U the concentration of urea in the urine and V the 24-hour urine volume. A K value of 0.08 was normal, when it was >0.20 uremia could appear during the postoperative period. Ambard's studies were performed and published before the First World War [44].

Was the 'Ambard constant' the initial step in the emergence of the concept of clearance [45]? In the 1920s at the Rockfeller Institute, D.D. Van Slyke (1883–1971) who was also studying urea excretion, came up with the equation UV/P which was more suitable for clinicians and had its well-known physiological meaning. On December 7, 1926, in a memorable rebuttal in support of Ambard, Van Slyke wrote a letter to the editor of a French journal which ended: 'Credit is to be given to Ambard for having been the first to show that a more precise idea of the renal function could be obtained in studying the ratio between the blood urea level and urea excretion than in considering only the blood urea concentration. Honor has to be paid to him for having also been the first to set up a method for studying this ratio by a quantitative formula' [46]. In a personal letter to Ambard, Van Slyke added: 'I hope that this note will assure you the honor and priority in the work of urea secretion which assuredly belongs to you' [47].

Once again a major advance in physiology, the concept of clearance, stemmed from a clinical need.

Ambard was an acute observer, gifted with a penetratingly original mind. He was the first to discard (with ridicule) the then fashionable myth that hypertension was due to the retention of mysterious unidentifiable byproducts of protein metabolism. He is perhaps best known for his suggestion, based on the results of chloride balances in hypertensive individuals, that hypertension is a renal disease related to the ingestion of sodium chloride [48]. After nearly a century of diminished opposition this brillant deduction is now generally accepted.

Ambard was head of the laboratory of the Urology Department at the Hôpital Necker. In 1919 he was appointed to the Chair at Strasbourg and focused his activity on enzymatic disturbances in diabetes. He retired soon after the end of the Second World War.

Renal Physiological Queries Raised by Urological Surgery

At the end of the 19th century before they decided to operate, urologists wanted to know the answer to two questions: (1) will renal compensatory hypertrophy aid survival after a total or partial nephrectomy, and (2) individual renal functions and unilateral lesions.

Compensatory Hypertrophy and a Circulating Nephropoietic Factor

Théodore Tuffier (1857–1929) in the introduction to his book on experimental surgery of the kidney [49], summarized his results in a concise surgical manner: 'The extend of a nephrectomy must be based on how much renal tissue is necessary for life. It is the first idea I tried to establish. By means of repeated partial nephrectomies I have been able to remove an amount of kidney tissue by weight equal to that of the two normal original kidneys, without killing the animal. I have demonstrated that this paradoxical result is due to the kidney's almost inexhaustible ability to regenerate and hypertrophy. Having thus shown how little normal kidney is necessary for life, I promoted and perfected operations which were aimed at conserving this tissue' [50].

In dogs on a constant diet, Tuffier first performed a right nephrectomy followed some weeks later by successive partial nephrectomies of the left kidney. The weight of the right kidney was compared to the sum of the resected fragments of the left kidney added to its postmortem remnants. After each operation there was a fall in urine urea output followed by a return to the preoperative level. This was the only biological measurement made. Tuffier was an eminent surgeon who, during World War I, was one of the first to operate on the lungs and heart.

A circulating nephropoietic factor. Paul Carnot (1869–1956) in the early 1900s was looking for the humoral control of the capacity of organs to regenerate [51]. He noted that when the blood of an animal that had recently undergone a unilateral nephrectomy was injected into a control animal, renal hypertrophy occurred with cellular proliferation. Carnot named this unidentified circulating substance 'néphropoïétine'. Carnot's experiments on organ regeneration indirectly led fifty years later to the discovery of an important physiological renal function. He and Deflandre [52] reported that the blood of animals that had been bled stimulated the production of erythrocytes. They named the circulating substance 'hématopoëtine'. It became 'renal erythropoietin'.

Individual Renal Functions and Lesions

This was one of Joachim Albarran's (1860–1912) areas of research. He was a Cuban who qualified in Madrid at the age of 18 and came to Paris for a few months of relaxation. But after several adventures, he decided to stay and joined the Faculté de Médecine. An exceptionally skilled surgeon, fond of experimental pathology he carried out experiments which made him famous. In rabbits with an experimental injury of the urinary tract, he induced an infection on the kidney(s) upstream of the lesion with an intravenous injection of *Escherichia coli*. He thus demonstrated the role of an existing urological lesion in the development of pyelonephritis [53]. Albarran was anxious he might induce uremia in performing a nephrectomy for renal tuberculosis, the treatment of choice for what was at that time a common complaint. Two questions needed to be answered. Were the lesions unilateral or bilateral, and what was the probable functional capacity of the remaining kidney? He pointed out that to answer these questions it was necessary to collect and compare the urine from each ureter. He improved the intravesical illumination provided by the existing cystoscopes and added a better guiding device to enable uretheric catheterization. In this way he could study both the chemistry and the bacteriology of the urine from each kidney. Renal function was assessed from the concentration of urea and the response to a dilution test. He thus knew if the tuberculosis infection was uni- or bilateral and if uremia was likely to follow a nephrectomy [54]. In this way the uncertainties of surgery were diminished.

If one wants to demonstrate how, before 1914, medical research in France on the kidney was based predominantly in hospitals, one only has to recite the French contributions to renal physiology, both normal and pathological. After 1945 basic laboratories expanded in line with the needs of research. And this expansion was often instigated by clinicians. The period from 1895 to 1910 was critical for renal physiology. It was then that the ancestors of the syndrome era of clinical nephrology set up a series of investigations identifying in an almost scientific manner renal functions, comparing them in health and disease, before the specialized laboratories gave birth to modern renal physiology.

Acknowledgements

The author is deeply indepted to the librarians of the Académie de Médecine and the Bibliothèque Interuniversitaire de Médecine, Mrs. F. de Sainte Marie, J. and M. Chapuis and B. Molitor who dug out the documents from their archives.

References and Notes

1 Scheele KW (1742–1786) identified uric acid and calcium phosphate in urinary stones.
2 Richet G: The chemistry of urinary stones around 1800: Kidney Int 1995;48:876–886.
3 Boerhaave H: Elementa Chimiae, Paris, 1733, p 37. Eléments de chimie, Amsterdam, 1752, pp 77–78.
4 Rouelle H: Observations sur l'urine humaine, etc. J Méd Chir 1773;IX:451–468.
5 Carillo (de Sevilla) JL: Hacia una medicina de laboratorio. Del Programa de A.F. Fourcroy (1784) a la obra de R. Bright (1827). Medicina e Historia, Barcelone, 1988, no 21, p I–XVI. Richet G. See also Fourcroy et son décret. Création de l'enseignement de la médecine moderne, clinique et chimique, in Bernard J, et al, L'acte de naissance de la médecine moderne. vol 1, 1995, pp 41–47.
6 Fourcroy AF, Vauquelin N: Premier mémoire pour servir à l'histoire naturelle, chimique et médicale, de l'urine humaine contenant quelques faits nouveaux sur son analyse et son altération spontanée. Ann Chim 1799;31:48–71 (first appearance of the word *urea* on p 69).
7 Fourcroy AF, Vauquelin N: Mémoire pour servir à l'histoire naturelle chimique et médicale de l'urine humaine. Mém Inst 1797;2:431.
8 Fourcroy AF, Vauquelin N: Second mémoire pour servir à l'histoire naturelle chimique et médicale de l'urine humaine, dans lequel on s'occupe spécialement des propriétés de la matière particulière qui la caractérise. Ann Chim 1799;32:80–161.
9 Fourcroy AF, Vauquelin N: Nouvelles expériences sur l'urée. Ann Mus Hist Nat 1808;11: 226.
10 Animalization: the incorporation of nitrogen to animal matter.
11 Ref 8, p 152.
12 ibid, p 153.
13 ibid, pp 153–154.
14 ibid, p 158.
15 ibid, pp 153–154.
16 Fourcroy AF: Expériences sur l'eau des hydropiques. J Soc Pharm Paris, 1797, pp 103–105.
17 Medicine enlightened by basic sciences.
18 For more information and references on Fourcroy and Vauquelin see Ref 2.
19 Bostock J: An Elementary System of Physiology, 3 vol. London, 1824, vol 2 pp 370–380.
20 Comhaire JN: Dissertation inaugurale sur l'extirpation des reins, mêlée à quelques recherches physiologiques sur ces organes et les fluides qu'ils sécrètent. Thèse Paris, 1803.
21 Rayer P: Traité des Maladies des Reins. Paris, Baillière, 1839, vol I, p 52.
22 Bichat X: Recherches physiologiques sur la vie et la mort, 1 vol, 384 pp, Paris, 1800.
23 Richet G: Le début de la néphrologie expérimentale: Les néphrectomies bilatérales de J.N. Comhaire en 1803. Néphrologie 1990;11:1–3.
24 Prevost JL, Dumas JB: Examen du sang et de son action dans les différents phénomènes de la vie. Ann Chim Phys Paris 1823;XXIII:90–104.
25 Mani N: La découverte de l'urémie expérimentale par J.L. Prevost et J.B. Dumas. Méd Hyg 1963;21:408–409.
26 Richet G: Early history of uremia. Kidney Int 1988;33:10–13.
27 Details in Richet G: Osmotic diuresis before H.W. Smith. Kidney Int 1994;45:1242–1243.
28 Frerichs FT: Die Bright'sche Nierenkrankheit und ihre Behandlung. Braunschweig, 1851, 286 pp.
29 Ségalas d'Etchepare: Sur de nouvelles expériences relatives aux propriétés médicamenteuses de l'urée; Lettre à Magendie. J Physiol Exp Pathol 1822;II:354–363.
30 Picard J: De la présence de l'urée dans le sang et de sa diffusion dans l'organisme. Thèse Médecine Strasbourg, 1856.
31 Recklinghausen F.v: Über Picard's Bestimmungsmethode des Harnstoffes im Blute. Virchovs Arch 1858;XIV:476–478.
32 Bernard C: Les liquides de l'organisme. 1859, vol II, p 31.
33 Feltz V, Ritter E: De l'urémie expérimentale. Paris, Berger Levrault, 1881, 1 vol, 347 pp.
34 Moutard-Martin R, Richet Ch: Recherches expérimentales sur la polyurie. Arch Phys Norm Pathol 1881;8:1–48.
35 A comprehensive litterature in Richet G: Osmotic diuresis before Homer W. Smith. Kidney Int 1994;45:1241–1252; An unrecognized renal physiologist: Friedrich Wöhler. Am J Nephrol 1995;15:528–532.
36 Brunton L: Ludwig's and other theories of the secretion of urine and the action of diuretics. Proc R Soc Med Ther Pharmacol Sect 1912;5: 133–151, see pp 139–141.
37 Hédon E, Arrous J: Des relations existant entre les actions diurétiques et les propriétés osmotiques des sucres. C R Acad Sci Paris 1900; CXXIX;778–781.
38 Wolf S: Brain, Mind, and Medicine. Charles Richet and the Origins of Physiological Psychology. N. Brunswick, Transaction, 1963, 1 vol, 214 pp.
39 Winter J: Head of Prof. Hayem's laboratory. Birth and death dates and places are unknown.
40 For detailed references see: Richet G: Edema and uremia from 1827 to 1905. The first faltering steps of renal pathophysiology. Kidney Int 1993;43:1385–1396.
41 Bard L, Bonnet L: Recherches et considérations cliniques sur les différences de perméabilité rénale dans les diverses espèces de néphrites. Arch Gén Méd Chir 1898;VIII:129–163.
42 Achard Ch: Système Lacunaire. Paris Masson, 1924, 124 pp.
43 Achard, et al: Nouveaux procédés d'exploration. 1903, 2nd ed, 1 vol, 436 pp.
44 Ambard L: Physiologie normale et pathologique des reins. Paris, 3 ed, 1914–1920–1931, Masson.
45 Gottschalk CW, Berliner RW, Giebisch GH: Renal physiology. Am Physio Soc, 1987;Bradley SE: Clearance concept in renal physiology, p 63.
46 Van Slyke's statement was written in French: C'est à Ambard que revient l'honneur d'avoir été le premier à montrer qu'on pouvait obtenir une idée plus précise de l'état de la fonction rénale en étudiant le rapport entre la teneur du sang en urée et l'excrétion d'urée dans l'urine qu'en considérant l'urée du sang isolément. C'est à lui également que revient l'honneur d'avoir été le premier à proposer une méthode permettant d'étudier ce rapport au moyen d'une formule quantitative.
47 The copy of these documents were conveyed to me by the late Dr D. Ambard, Léo Ambard's son.
48 Ambard, Beaujard: Causes de l'hypertension artérielle. Arch Gén Méd 1904;81(1):520–533, and Ambard L: Origine rénale de l'hypertension artérielle permanente. Semin Méd 1906; 26:361–366.
49 Tuffier Th: Etudes expérimentales sur la chirurgie du rein. 1 vol, Paris, 1889.
50 Tuffier, ibid, p 8.
51 Carnot P, Lelièvre A: Sur l'activité néphropoïétique du sang au cours des régénérations rénales. C R Acad Sci Paris 1907;144:718–720.
52 Carnot P, Deflandre C: Sur l'activité hémopoïétique du serum au cours de la régénération du sang. C R Acad Sci Paris 1906;143:432–435.
53 Albarran J: Etude sur le rein des urinaires. Thèse Paris, 1889.
54 Albarran J: Exploration des fonctions rénales. Paris, Masson, 1905.

Origins of Renal Physiology
(Dedicated to Carl Gottschalk)

American Journal of Nephrology

Am J Nephrol 1999;19:282–289

The Low Countries – 16th/17th Century

Marc E. De Broe[a] Dirk L. De Weerdt[a] Dirk K. Ysebaert[b]
Sven R. Vercauteren[b] Kathleen E. De Greef[b] Luc C. De Broe[c]

Departments of [a]Nephrology and [b]Experimental Surgery, University of Antwerp, and [c]Zeneca Pharma, Ghent, Belgium

Key Words
Vesalius · Van Helmont · Urine analysis · Edema

Abstract
Andreas Vesalius and Jan Baptist Van Helmont are the two major personalities who contributed substantially and in a different way to the early development of renal anatomy/physiology of the 16th/17th century in the Southern Low Countries. The importance of A. Vesalius' publication *'de humani corporis fabrica libri septem'* cannot be overestimated. The kidney was an intriguing organ to Vesalius, the function of which he could not fully grasp. J.B. Van Helmont was the first to demonstrate the importance of the measurement of the specific gravity of the urine and relating it to physiological and pathophysiological conditions. He made accurate clinical observations supported by autopsy examinations concerning the role of the kidney in the generation of dropsy.

When analyzing the contribution of scientists to the renal anatomy-physiology of the 16th/17th century in the Southern Low Countries, two figures step forward: Andreas Vesalius and Jan Baptist Van Helmont (fig. 1).

According to Gottschalk [1] 'the great advance in our knowledge of human anatomy was provided in 1543 by Andreas Vesalius (1514–1564), with the publication of his "de humani corporis fabrica libri septem" (1543). Based on actual dissection of the human body its importance cannot be overestimated'. In contrast it is remarkable that a scientist such as J.B. Van Helmont is almost unknown to the general and scientific community. This text will focus on the view of Andreas Vesalius concerning the anatomy and physiology of the kidney, and the important contribution of J.B. Van Helmont in the understanding of renal physiopathology will be demonstrated.

Vesalius' View on Anatomy and Physiology of the Kidney

Vesalius' views are clearly exposed in the main section dealing with the kidney in his major book 'de Humani corporis fabrica Libri septem' (1543). In book 5, entitled 'Organis nutritioni', chapter 10 'de renibus' is entirely devoted to the kidney and consists of three and a half pages [2]. The chapter starts by describing the localization of both kidneys in the abdominal cavity. In the second part, Vesalius formulates his own ideas concerning kidney architecture and function. Furthermore, he dwells extensively and with passion on the misconceptions and misin-

KARGER
Fax + 41 61 306 12 34
E-Mail karger@karger.ch
www.karger.com

© 1999 S. Karger AG, Basel
0250–8095/99/0192–0282$17.50/0

Accessible online at:
http://BioMedNet.com/karger

Marc E. De Broe, MD, PhD
Department of Nephrology-Hypertension
University Hospital of Antwerp, Wilrijkstraat 10
B–2650 Edegem/Antwerpen (Belgium)
Tel. +32 3 821 3421, Fax +32 3 829 0100

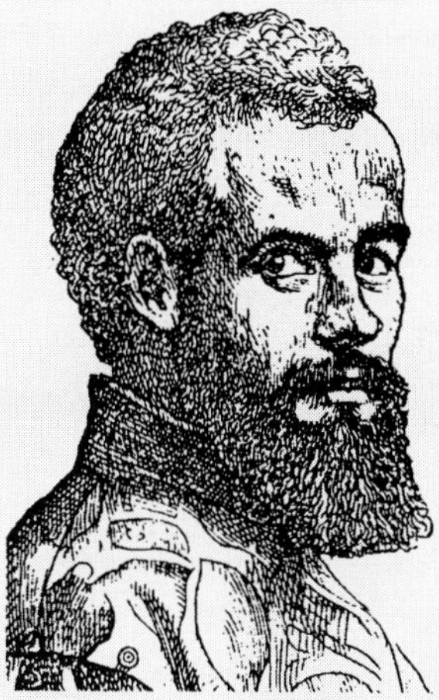

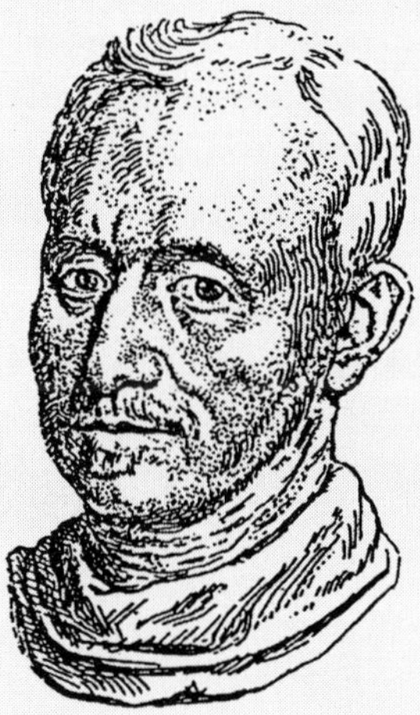

Andreas Vesalius	Europe - The World
	1438 Gutenberg makes first printing press
	1477 dead of the last Burgundian duke
	1492 Columbus-America / fall of Granada
	1498 V. da Gama in Calicut
1514 born in Brussels	1517 M. Luther - Wittenberg
1526 T. Moore "Utopia"	
1533-36 studied in Paris	1536 war between Charles V and François I
1537 graduated in medicine Padua	
1538 "Tabulae sex, Tabulae anatomicae"	
1540 public anatomy Bologna	1540 foundation of the "Societas Jesu" sj
1543 "De humani Corporis Fabrica" "Epitome" (Basel)	
1546 married to Anna Van Hamme	
1556 nominated earl	1556 abdication of Charles V → Philips II
1564 died in Zante, Greece	
J.B. van Helmont	
1579 born in Brussels	1579 separation of the Netherlands
	1582 Gregorian calendar
1599 graduated in medicine in Leuven	1598 abdication of Philips II
1609 married to Margareta van Ranst	1615 G. Galilei in conflict with inquisition
	1619 J. Kepler "Harmonices Mundi"
	1620 F. Bacon "Novum Organum Scientiarum"
	1628 W. Harvey "De Motu Cordis et Sanguinis"
1634 conflict with inquisition / house arrest	
1644 "Opuscula Medica Inaudita" (Köln) Died in Brussels	1643 F. Torricelli invents mercury barometer
1648 "Ortus Medicinae" (Amsterdam)	1648 peace treaty of Munster
1659 "Dageraad ofte opkomst der Geneeskonst" (Amsterdam)	

Fig. 1. Time table of Andreas Vesalius' and Jan Baptist Van Helmonst's lives besides important events in their age.

terpretations of his contemporaries, concerning the kidneys (fig. 2A–C).

Vesalius makes short work, in more than clean wording, of the 'perforated membrane theory', the contemporary notion of his colleagues concerning the formation of the urine in the kidney (fig. 3A, B). For the demonstration of his own view on the anatomy and physiology of the kidneys, he used a dog kidney, which he considered very close to the human kidneys and moreover, having less fat, hence more useful to demonstrate that the 'sieve' theory of the urine formation was absurd (fig. 4, 5).

Vesalius also described 'two cavities which have been constructed by nature however in a totally different way from what the doctors think'. By repeating step by step the dissection of a dog kidney we tried to better understand Vesalius' views (fig. 6A–G).

The kidney was an intriguing organ to Vesalius '(quod incredible artificium ut videas') the function of which, particularly regading to the production of urine, he did not fully grasp [3]. 'It is the renal mass itself, which according to an inborn capacity and within appropriate and correct proportions ("ac propria ad iustitia temperie") will filter the serous drag out of the arterial and venous blood distributed over the renal mass and bringing the filtrate into the cavity, it will leave the kidney through the urinary conduct' [Fabrica, p. 516, lines 7–9].

A

maximè quum tot fabulæ de renum oſtijs, ſinibus, membranis, & quæ in renibus diſtribuuntur uaſis, antehac cæteris diſſectionis profeſſoribus efficta ſint. Galenus inquit ſimpliciter, uenas ac arterias per renis corpus diſtribui, & per ſpiſſam duramque renum ſubſtantiam, retento ſanguine, urinam cum bilis quæ ſanguini adeſt portione tranſmitti, inque urinarium meatum effluere.

there are so many concoctions invented by professors of anatomy concerning the functions, structures, membranes and vessels splitting up in the kidneys. Galen claims that the vessels (vein and arteries) split up in the kidney mass where the blood is retained within the renal mass during which the urine together with part of the bile present in the blood is passed through and discharged in the urine.

B

Noſtrorum medicorum, & qui Galenum ſequuti ſunt omnium, hæc exprimere ſtudentium, alij perperam oſcitanterque renis fabricam aggredientes, & quæ hæc uaſorum ſit diſtributio & ſitus non obſeruantes, neſcio quas colatorias membranas ementiuntur. Alij ſectionem auerſati, & in altis cathedris ſedentes, ſibique ipſis mirificè placentes Promethei, abundè ſuo munere ſe perfunctos eſſe arbitrantur, ſi diſcipulis imaginatione hominem cõfingant.

Our doctors, who follow Galen's ideas, describe however the structure of the kidney in an uncritical and false way. Where they do not take into account the distribution and localization of the vessels they invent many things, among them sieving membranes. Others, having an aversion to the practice of dissection sit on their high chairs, self-sufficient as Prometheuses and consider their assignment as fulfilled after having created a human body by means of their imagination.

C

Atque hinc illud eſt, quod præcipuos noſtræ ætatis medicos & docuiſſe & ſcripſiſſe ſcio, nobis triplicem, quo urina à ſanguine in renibus diſcernitur modum excogitari poſſe: non addentes interim, quid in ipſa hominis ſectione appareat, ſed ſibi ſinus & ductus ſuo arbitratu effingunt.

As an example, today's important doctors have taught and written that there is a threefold process in the separation of the urine from the blood. They do not argue based on what they observe by themselves dissecting a human body, but they invent, according to their own pleasure, cavities and tracks.

Fig. 2A–C. Extracts from Fabrica, pp. 515–516 (1543), with translation into English.

A

DVABVS præſentibus figuris medicorum de urinæ excolatione commentum exprimere conatus ſum, ac ſuperiori figura renem ab ipſius gibbo uerſus ſinum cauum uedissectum finxi, inferiori autem renis duntaxat media ſpectatur portio. Cæterùm quid ſingulis indicetur, ipſe characterum Index in hunc modum edocebit.

A *Vena & arteria ſeroſum ſanguinem reni offerentes.*

B, B *Sinus, in quem medici uenam & arteriam nuper dictas ſeroſum ſanguinem profundere docent.*

C, C *Sinus, in quem urina ex iam dicto ſinu colaretur.*

D *Renis ſubſtantia orbiculatim ſinus hos amplectens.*

E *Beatum & nugaciſsimum renis colatorium, ſeu membrana cribri modo peruia, & urinam ex ſinu B indicato in ſinum C inſignitum unà cum bile promanare ſinens.*

F *Vrinam è rene ad ueſicam deferens meatus.*

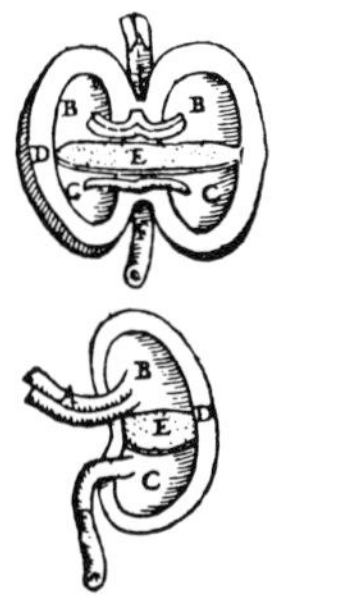

In those two figures, I have attempted to represent the false teaching ('commentum exprimere') of doctors on the straining ('excolatione') of the urine. In the upper figure, I have sketched the kidney dissected from its hump towards the sinus or hollow, but in the lower, only the central portion is seen. The other concepts will be indicated one by one.

A The vein and artery which brings the serous blood to the kidneys.

B The sinus in which the just-mentioned vein and artery let the serous blood flow, as taught by the doctors.

C Sinus, in which the urine from the aformentioned sinus is filtered.

D Circular renal mass which embraces both sinuses.

E A naive and ridiculous presentation of the kidney function as if the urine together with the bile is allowed to flow from the sinus indicated by B into the sinus indicated by C through a membrane behaving as a sieve.

F The excretory way towards the bladder of the urine leaving the kidneys.

B

Profectò ſagaciſſimus ille rerum Opifex tãtum munus uni membranulæ cribri modo perforatæ non tribuerit, neque in renibus eandem extruxerit.

It is obvious that the eminent Creator of the things has not assigned such an important function to that single thin membrane perforated like a sieve and that, furthermore, he never even constructed such a membrane in the kidney.

Fig. 3A, B. Extracts from Fabrica, pp 515–516 (1543), with translation.

Jan Baptist Van Helmont (1579–1644) – 'Doctrina, labor, disciplina'

Short Biography

J.B. Van Helmont (fig. 7, left) was born in Brussels (1579) and died in the same city on 3rd December 1644. At a very young age he went to the University of Leuven and followed the courses in the seven arts (magister septem artium). In 1599 he obtained his doctoral degree in medicine and was appointed as professor to teach the surgeons. He resigned very soon after, considering that he had only theoretical knowledge and dramatically missed practical experience.

From 1600 to 1602 he travelled through Germany, Switzerland and Italy and had his first contact with the scientific approach of Paracelsus (1493–1541), the founder of the iatrochemistry. Iatrochemistry or medical chemistry was the name given to the fusion of alchemy, medicine and chemistry, as it was practised by the followers of Paracelsus in the 16th and 17th centuries. This was an alternative to the new mechanistic philosophy, which eventually dominated modern science. According to this theory all expression of life and disease are based on chemical processes and diseases have to be treated by chemical way.

In 1609, J.B. Van Helmont married Margaretha Van Ranst. They settled in Vilvoorde, where Van Helmont

Quod incredibile artificium ut uideas, caninum renem utpote macilentum, & nulla, quemadmodum humanus eſt, pinguedine oppletum, ad manum tibi eſſe uelim, illumque uti renis adminiſtrationem ad præſentis libri calcem ſubiungam, te primum aggredi. Poſt aliquot enim obitas ſectiones (dummodo prima non ſuffecerit) duos in renibus ſinus adinuenies, ſecus multo ac noſtri arbitrantur medici, à Natura formatos.

I suggest that, in order to understand this unbelievable masterpiece of nature, you take the kidney of a dog since it is lean and in contrast to the human kidney not covered with fat. Since after performing a couple of sections, in the case a first attempt would not be succesful; you will also find two cavities which have been constructed by nature however in a totally different way from what the doctors think.

Fig. 4. Extracts from Fabrica, p. 516 (1543), with translation.

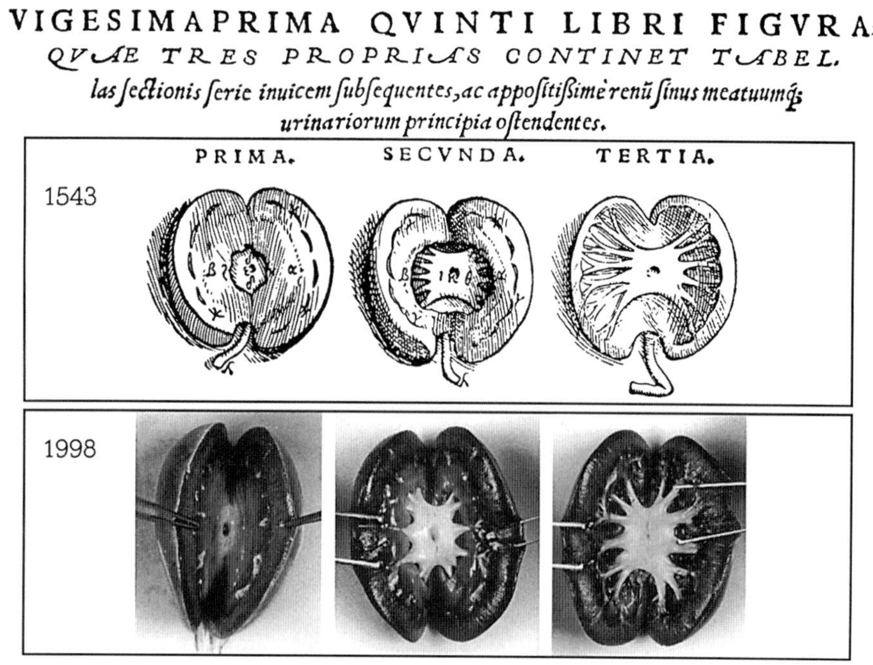

Fig. 5. Top panel consists in the original figures of Vesalius' dissection of the dog kidney (Fabrica, p. 371, 1543). The bottom panel is a careful dissection of a dog kidney performed according to the text in the Fabrica (p. 372), translated below (from *Prima*). The twenty-first figure of the fifth book consists of three small special plates which follow one another in the sequence of dissection and show very clearly the sinus of the kidneys and the origin of the urinary passage. *Prima:* The first figure demonstrates a section in the sense of the length of the kidney passing through its hump and deep enough so that the second cavity is attained in the absence however of ablation any part of the renal mass. The α indicates the anterior side of the right kidney, the β posterior side. The γ and γ are openings of the branches of the first renal cavity or the membranous body itself, where the different branches come together. Obviously, due to dissection, the branches are separated where they come together. The δ and δ mark the membranous body of the first cavity wherein the renal artery and vein end. ε Indicating the small hole is the origin of the urinary tract, λ is a piece of the urinary tract. On top of this membranous membrane, indicated by δ and δ, is situated the second renal cavity. In this particular dissection only the internal part close to the membranous body appears. The parts of this cavity formed at both sides from the partition out of renal substance and which cut the cavity in two parts, cannot be seen, except if a small instrument is introduced under the places indicated by ζ and χ. In this dissection this partition appears as separated in two parts, and anterior one and a posterior one indicated respectively by χ, and ζ. *Secunda:* Everything which has been mentioned in the first figure also holds for the second one, except that the renal mass, which constitutes this partition, has been cut circularly using a small scalpel. Here the complete second cavity of the kidney can be seen. However, not separated in two parts, since I have removed the partition which separates this cavity of her external side. The α, and the β, the γ and the δ, indicate the same as in the first figure, since the circle drawn between α and β indicates the second cavity of the kidney. The θ indicates indeed the anterior side of the first cavity or of the membranous body, where this part separates in different branches. The ι indicates the posterior part of this membranous body, consequently the θ and the ι together indicate the membranous body or the first cavity of the kidney. The χ indicates however the starting point of the urinary tract. *Tertia:* The third figure shows all branches of the first cavity or of the membranous body. Indeed, the renal mass, which merges with the terminal parts of the branches of this cavity, has been extensively removed. The figure speaks for itself without the help of letter symbols.

started building up a small laboratory. Van Helmont became increasingly dissatisfied with the bookish galenic medicine practised in the schools and eventually took up a career of private researcher. He performed numerous experiments in chemistry and studied thoroughly the texts of among others Paracelsus. His opposition to the established doctrines of medicine and to the medical teachings of churchmen (the Jesuit Jean Roberty) brought him in conflict with the Spanish inquisition, which badgered him throughout much of his life.

His most important writings were edited in 1642, in Antwerp: 'Febrium doctrina inaudita'. In 1644 in Köln appeared four combined texts: 'Opuscula medica inaudita de lithiasi, de febribus, de humoribus galeni et de peste'

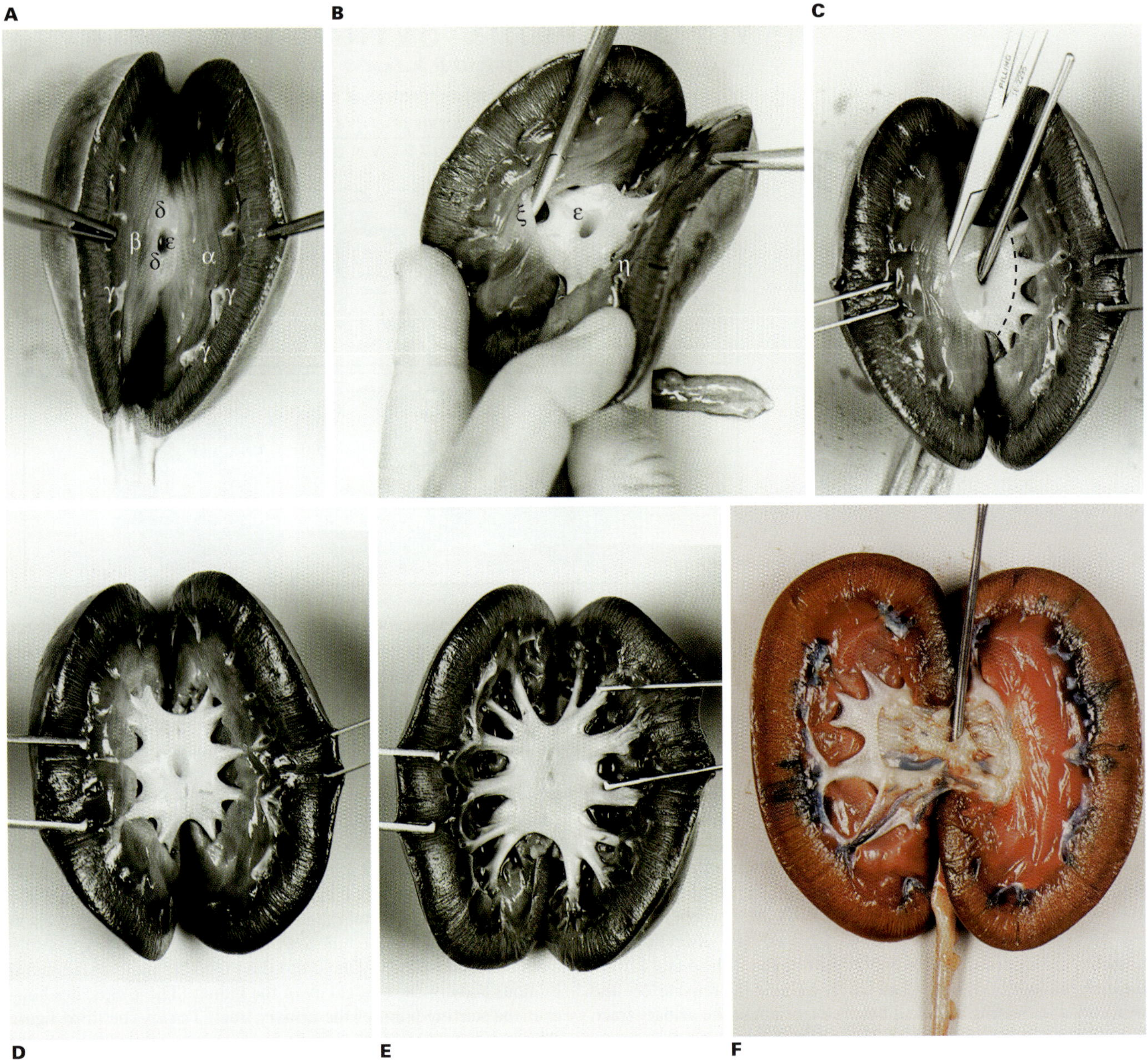

G

Sinus hic inter diſſecandum ſubhumidus exanguisq; omnino occurrit, corpus autem illud membraneum cum ſuis ramis omnibus, aut primus ſinus (ſi ita corpus id appellare uiſum ſit) ſanguine plenus ſemper inuenitur.

This (second) cavity seems somewhat wet and not containing blood, the membranous body with all his ramifications, so called the first cavity, is always full of blood.

Fig. 6. Dissection of a dog kidney according to Vesalius. **A** The dog kidney is incised longitudinally, through cortex and medulla, until a white membranous pouch is reached. In the middle of the white membrane, one can see the opening of the ureter (ε). The α marks the ventral side of the kidney, β the dorsal side. The first cavity described by Vesalius, consists of the white membranous 'body', together with its branches. γ and γ are the openings of the branches of the membranous body. These branches are obviously cut in two at the place where they come together during the dissection. δ and δ mark the membranous body of the first cavity. The second cavity described by Vesalius is formed by the medullary tissue on the one side, and the membranous body on the other side. This is illustrated on the next picture. **B** The instrument is placed in the second cavity. By lifting the instrument, the branches of the membranous body become clearly visible. The membranous body and its branches form the bottom of the second cavity. Above the tip of the instrument, one can see the medullary tissue with the papilla communis, constituting the partition of the second cavity. This partition is cut in two due to the dissection, with η indicating the ventral side and ξ the dorsal side. The urine comes out of the papilla communis, falls down on the branches of the membranous body, and is guided to the ureter (ε). **C** The gauging rod is inserted in the ureter. On the ventral side of the kidney, the papilla communis is excised (marked by the dotted line). **D** This figure corresponds with the second picture of Vesalius. The

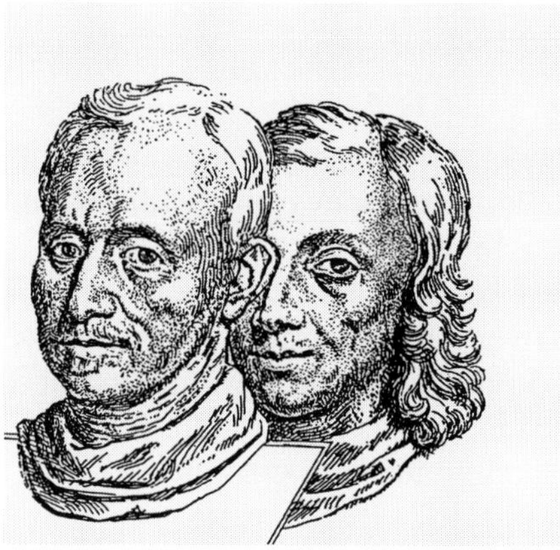

Fig. 7. J.B. Van Helmont and his son.

Ick ſchrijve dit in mijn vaderlandtſche tael, op dat mijnen naeſten in 't gemeyn daer af geniete, verſtaende dat de waerheyt nergens naeckter en verſchijnt, dan daer ſy van alle cieraet ontbloot is. Anderſins ſchrijvende alleen voor de Geleerden, ſtaet te beduchten, dat naedemael de letter opblaeſt, mijnen arbeydt mocht gedyen als in menige andere, alwaer de ſtrijdt-reden alles verſtroyt.

Soo heeft het my goet gedacht te ſchrijven in een ſpraecke, waer in de gemeynte my ten beſten verſtonde.

I write in my national language in order that my compatriots can use and understand easily and clearly the truth, which is exposed without any ornament. If I should have written only for the scholars, one can expect that my texts will be interpreted in a wrong way and will be diluted by many discussions. (-) Accordingly, it seems obvious for me to write in a language in which the common people can understand me.

Fig. 9. Extract from 'Degeraad ofte Nieuwe Opkomst der Geneeskonst', Amsterdam 1659, with translation.

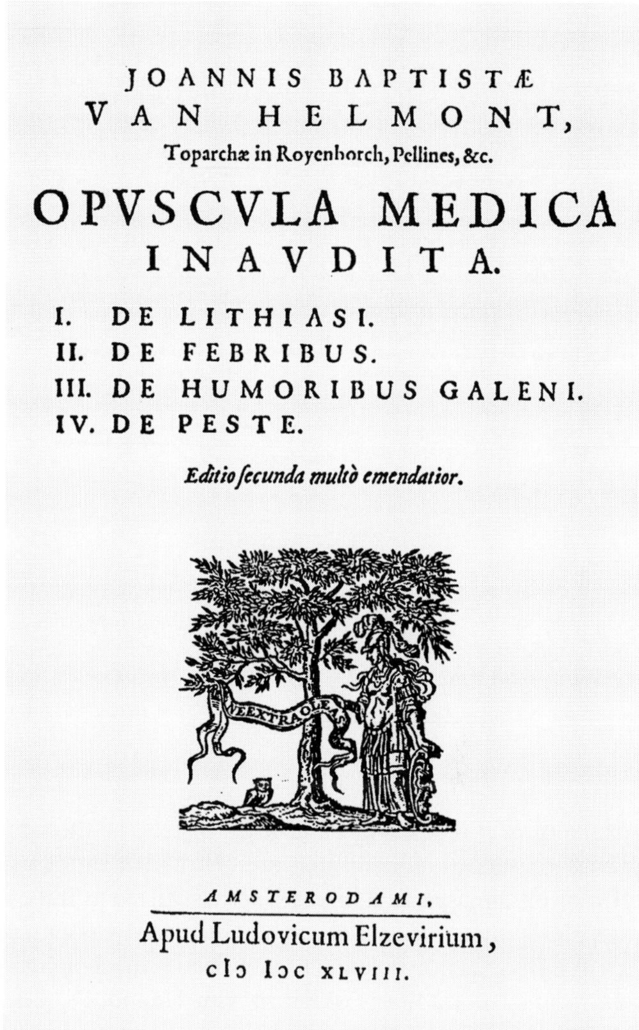

JOANNIS BAPTISTÆ
VAN HELMONT,
Toparchæ in Royenborch, Pellines, &c.
OPVSCVLA MEDICA
INAVDITA.
I. DE LITHIASI.
II. DE FEBRIBUS.
III. DE HUMORIBUS GALENI.
IV. DE PESTE.
Editio ſecunda multò emendatior.

AMSTERODAMI,
Apud Ludovicum Elzevirium,
cIɔ Iɔc XLVIII.

Fig. 8. Front page of 'Opuscula medica ...', Amsterdam 1648.

partition of the second cavity is cut away circularly. The membranous body with its ramifications is clearly visible. Within this first cavity the renal artery and vein branch and follow the ramifications of the membranous body. **E** This figure corresponds with the third picture of Vesalius. The medulla, connected to the offshoots of the first cavity, is entirely excised. As such, the three-dimensional aspect of the membranous cavity becomes visible. **F** The gauging rod is inserted in the ureter. The membranous body is opened, so that its two layers become visible. Methylene blue is injected in the arteria renalis, visualizing the ramifications within the branches of the membranous body. The blue pigment flows out of the opening of the branches (γ and γ) of the first cavity at the transition cortex-medulla. Hence, the membranous body is not a real cavity, but a bilayered membrane, in which the ramifications of the vessels run, and forms the bottom of the second cavity, thus forming an estuary guiding the urine to the ureter. **G** *De humani corporis fabrica* (p. 516, line 41, *Liber V* 1542), with translation.

(fig. 8). After his death in 1644 his son edited several of his texts written in Latin and Flemish. Among them is 'Dageraad ofte Nieuwe Opkomst der Geneeskonst' (Amsterdam 1659). In the introduction of this text, Van Helmont explicitly mentioned why he wrote in his mother language (fig. 9). At several places throughout the text he discusses the issue why he has chosen the Flemish language to explain his scientific findings. It is remarkable that at the same time several outstanding scientists in other disciplines than medicine in Flanders wrote their texts in their mother language (Simon Stevin, Mercator, Dodoens).

Van Helmont believed that the basic substances of the world were not the four elements of Aristotle and Galen,

Tuta eſt interim methodus, examinandi urinas per pondus. Uncia nimirum, pendeat 600 grana. Vas autem vitreum habui, anguſti colli, pendens grana 1354. Repletum autem aqua pluvia; pendente inſuper grana 4670. Inventa eſt urina ſenis, pendere eodem vaſe, 4720 grana. Sive ſuperare pondus aquæ pluviæ, 50 granis. Urina autem mulieris ſanæ, ætatis annorum 55, pependit 4745 grana. Urina juvenis ſani, annorum 19, pependit grana 4766. Alterius autem juvenis paris, abſtemii à potu, pependit 4800 grana. Juvenis 36 annorum, tertianam tolerantis cum tuſſi, pependit 4763 grana. Præfatus autem juvenis 19 annorum, cum tertiana duplici, nocte præcedente, parum biberat: pependit autem urina ejus, 4848 grana. Quod fuit 82 granis amplius, quàm dum ſanus eſſet. Virgo, cordis palpitationem paſſa, minxit inſtar aquæ pluviæ, quæque ideo æquiponderabat aquæ pluviæ. Urina tepens, ſemper ſe ipſa frigida, paucis granis levior, ut & extenſior. Sitque idcirco vas colli brevis, & acuminati, ut fere in puncto urinam dimetiatur.

The method examining the weight of the urine is a safe one: one ounce of urine weigheth 600 grains*, but it had a glassen vessel of a narrow neck weighing 1,354 grains, but it was filled with rain-water weighing besides 4,670 grains. The urine of an old man was found to weigh in the same vessel 4,729 grains, or to exceed the weight of the rain-water 50 grains. But the urine of a healthy woman 55 years old weighed 4,745 grains. The urine of a healthy man of 19 years old weighed 4,766 grains. But that of another young man of a like age being abstemious from drink weighed 4,800 grains. The urine of a young man 36 years old, undergoing a tertian ague with a cough weighed 4,763 grains. But the aforesaid youth of 19 years old with a double tertian had drunk little in the night aforegoing, but this urine weighed 4,848 grains, which was 82 grains more than while he was healthy. A maid having suffered the beating or passion of the heart made a water like unto rain-water, and the which therefore was of equal weight with rain-water. A luke-warm urine is always a few grains lighter and also more extended than itself, being cold. And therefore let the vessel be of a short neck and sharp pointed that it may measure the urine almost to a point.

*20 grains weigh about 1 gram

Fig. 10. Extract from: Ortus Medicinae, Opuscula Medica Inaudita, II De Febribus, p. 108, 1648, Apud Ludovicum Elzevirium Amsterdami. Translation from: The evolution of urine analysis, Lecture Memoranda BMA meeting, p. 49, Birmingham, 1911.

nor the three principles of Paracelsus. Instead he thought that all matter was reducible to water. He had an ontological view on diseases. In it diseases are visualized as if they were real beings, objects that can be considered and classified like any other object. Such a view is in radical opposition to ancient tradition which in Van Helmont's time ruled absolutely in medicine [4].

J.B. Van Helmont and the Kidney

The contribution to nephrology of this gifted original scientist of the end of the 16th, early 17th century, is that he was the first to demonstrate the importance of the measurement of the specific gravity of the urine, and relating it to physiological and pathophysiological conditions (fig. 10).

Van Helmont introduced the concept of concentrated/diluted urine depending on particular clinical condition, based on simple experimental data he collected in patients and normal subjects. Van Helmont was aware of the fact that the temperature of the specimen (the urine) makes a slight difference in weight and insisted very strongly to use rain water as a standard weight for comparison with urinary samples.

The second contribution of Van Helmont to the renal physiopathology consists in his views on dropsy. The nature of dropsy by the galenic medicine of that time was unknown. One distinguished three types of dropsy: (1) anasarca or aqua intercus; (2) ascites, and (3) tympanitis or gaseous dropsy.

The galenic medicine was not making a clear-cut distinction between anasarca and ascites and attributed the primary cause of these clinical settings to the liver.

Van Helmont disagreed with this view.

It is true that the liver may, in certain conditions, be the starting point of dropsy, however, it will not occur if the kidneys are functioning sufficiently well. 'Adeoque non pecat hepar, generando urinam, quantum renes pecant, non emulgendo eam' [5].

Even the main cause for dropsy resides in the kidney instead of in the liver. 'Quapropter vitium potius in rene mihi subsistere visum, quam in hepate' [5].

He performed several autopsies of patients who died from ascites, without finding macroscopic lesions of the liver. An officer died of dropsy following dysentery and the liver appeared to be perfectly normal. The same was true for a young woman who died from dropsy associated with a gynecological pathology. He found, however, that the kidneys were decreased in volume, had a size of a hazel nut, in this dropsy patient. A banker died from dropsy. His kidneys were inflammatory and hardened. He claimed that this clinical condition does not go along with renal obstruction, but that the extravascular blood is the cause for this occasional hydrops. 'Obstructio renis non est causa occasionalis hydrops, set cruror extra venatus' [6]. He concluded that the kidney was the architect of dropsy: 'ren artifex hydropsys'. He observed that during dropsy urinary secretion is dramatically decreased and on the other hand if one is successful in increasing the urinary output one can see that there is a decrease in the dropsy.

How does Van Helmont interpret his observations of the role of the kidney in particular form of dropsy? Dropsy is a disease which starts by a depravation of the blood following an 'idea indignationis' induced by the renal archeus. Indeed, according to Van Helmont in the body the principal of life is the 'archeus'. Every organ has its own archeus. Disease acts by the 'idea indignationis' which makes the 'archeus' acting in the wrong direction.

Under influence of this wrong-acting archeus there is an obstruction of the renal circulation in the kidney. The blood undergoes some alterations in the kidney, which permits its fluid part to be discharged in the peritoneal cavity.

His view on this clinical setting was completely in contradiction to that of his colleagues. It is remarkable that this clinical scientist already at the beginning of the 17th century made clinical observations which were supported by autopsy examinations concerning the role of the kidney in the generation of dropsy. The kidneys in fact conceive, make and maintain dropsy 'renes actualiter hydropem concipiunt, fabricant et continent' [7].

The idea that at the beginning of the 19th century it had not yet been realized that there could be a causal relationship between kidney disease and dropsy, may be reconsidered [8].

References

1 Gottschalk CW: A history of renal physiology to 1950. The Kidney: Physiology and Pathophysiology (2nd edition); in Seldin DW, Giebisch G (eds). New York, Raven Press, 1992, pp 1–29.

2 Andreas Vesalii Bruxellensis, scholae medicorum Patavinae professoris, de Humani corporis fabrica Libri septem. Basilea, ex officina Joannis Oporoni. Anno salutis reparatae 1543. Mense Junio.

3 Roth M: Andreas Vesalius Bruxellensis. Berlin, Reimer, 1892.

4 Pagel W: Jan Baptista Van Helmont. Reformer of Science and Medicine. Cambridge, Cambridge University Press, 1982.

5 Van Helmont JB: Ortus Medicinae, Ignotus Hydrops, p 509, Amsterdam, 1648.

6 Van Helmont JB: Ortus Medicinae, Ignotus Hydrops, p 513, Amsterdam, 1648.

7 Van Helmont JB: Ortus Medicinae, Ignotus Hydrops, p 514, Amsterdam, 1648.

8 Fine LG, English JA: John Blackall (1771–1860). Failure to see the obvious in dropical patients with coaguable urine? Am J Nephrol 1994;14:371–376.

Origins of Renal Physiology
(Dedicated to Carl Gottschalk)

American Journal of Nephrology

Am J Nephrol 1999;19:290–294

Vitalism and Synthesis of Urea

From Friedrich Wöhler to Hans A. Krebs

E. Kinne-Saffran R.K.H. Kinne

Max-Planck-Institut für molekulare Physiologie, Dortmund, Germany

Key Words
Vitalism · Wöhler · Urea · Krebs · Henseleit

Abstract
In 1828, Friedrich Wöhler, a German physician and chemist by training, published a paper that describes the formation of urea, known since 1773 to be a major component of mammalian urine, by combining cyanic acid and ammonium in vitro. In these experiments the synthesis of an *organic* compound from two *inorganic* molecules was achieved for the first time. These results weakened significantly the vitalistic hypothesis on the functioning of living cells, although Wöhler, at that time, was more interested in the chemical consequences of isomerism than in the philosophical implications of his finding. However, the chemical synthesis observed by Wöhler does not represent the reaction which is employed in the mammalian liver for urea synthesis. The mechanism of this process was elucidated by the German physician Hans A. Krebs and his medical student Kurt Henseleit in 1932 and was shown to include the ornithine cycle. This 'urea cycle' is only observed in living cells; this apparently vitalistic phenomenon is caused by the compartmentalization of the various enzymatic reactions in mitochondria and cytosol, respectively.

Vitalism

The doctrine of vitalism implies that the functions of living organisms are fueled by a vital principle, 'vis vitalis', 'spiritus vitalis', or 'soul', distinct from the physicochemical forces governing the nonanimated world. Aristotle used the term 'entelechy' for the distinction between matter and form. Thus, in the case of a living organism one might distinguish the mere matter of the organism from a certain essence or inner activity without which it would not be a living organism at all. This ancient school of thought was revitalized during the renaissance, the transitional movement between medieval and modern times, marked by the revival of classical influence and by the beginning of modern science. Its most prominent proponent was Paracelsus (1490–1541), who attributed the cause of sickness in man to the 'failure of Archeus', an occult vital force, 'to perform its function of separating the useful compounds of the body from the poisonous compounds'. Even during the nineteenth century, the concept of the nature of life as resulting from a vital force prevailed.

Gradually though, vitalism lost its prestige and influence as the chemical and physical nature of more and more biological phenomena could be demonstrated by a new generation of physiologists, physicists and chemists who founded and developed an experimentally oriented

KARGER

Fax + 41 61 306 12 34
E-Mail karger@karger.ch
www.karger.com

© 1999 S. Karger AG, Basel
0250–8095/99/0192–0290$17.50/0

Accessible online at:
http://BioMedNet.com/karger

Dr. E. Kinne-Saffran
Max-Planck-Institut für molekulare Physiologie
Rheinlanddamm 201
D–44139 Dortmund (Germany)
Tel. +49 231 12 06 482, Fax +49 231 12 06 494

science. This group of highly motivated men which dared to implement the laws of physics and chemistry as the only forces in physiological processes includes Theodor Schwann (1810–1882), Emil du Bois Reymond (1818–1896), Hermann Helmholtz (1821–1894) and, above all, Carl Ludwig (1816–1895). A contemporary of these scientists was Friedrich Wöhler.

Friedrich Wöhler

Wöhler (the portrait given in figure 1 shows him at the age of about 40) was born in 1800 in Eschersheim, near Frankfurt/Main, and went to school in Frankfurt. He was not a particularly outstanding student because he was more fascinated by chemistry than by any other topic. Following the suggestion of his father, he started to study medicine in Marburg in 1820. The next year, he moved to Heidelberg and came under the influence of the most prominent German chemist of that time, Leopold Gmelin (1748–1804). Gmelin recognized Wöhler's abilities and advised him to make chemistry his career. And, indeed, after receiving a medical degree in 1823, he decided to take up studies in chemistry. He moved to Stockholm and joined the laboratory of Berzelius (1779–1848), the leading chemist of Europe at that time. He worked with Berzelius for nearly a year acquiring techniques of chemical analysis and became interested in the chemistry of new elements, an area for which Berzelius was famous. The two became close friends. Wöhler later translated the major reviews and textbooks of Berzelius from Swedish into German.

Upon his return to Germany, he accepted a position as a teacher of chemistry at a municipal technical school in Berlin which offered the possibility of extended periods of experimentation in the laboratory. During this time, he made his observations on the artificial formation of urea. At about the same time, he also made another major discovery in developing a method for the production of metallic aluminum; later, he was instrumental at expanding it to an industrial process.

As time went on, the teaching load became heavier and heavier, encroaching on his desire to perform experiments. When cholera struck Berlin in 1831, he moved his family to Kassel, the town his wife's family originated from. There, his wife died in 1832 after giving birth to their second child. In this adverse situation, Justus von Liebig invited him to come to Giessen and to work together with him in his laboratory. There, another lifelong friendship developed. The two took up the study of the chemistry of benzaldehydes found in the oil of bitter almonds. From these investigations came the theory of radicals, one of the first attempts to understand the reactivity of organic molecules.

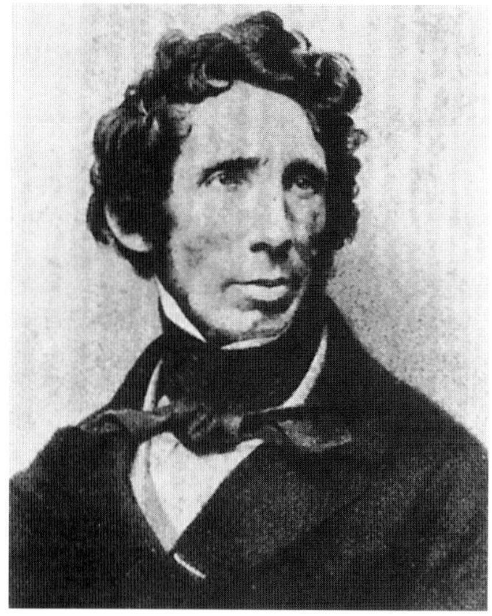

Fig. 1. Friedrich Wöhler (taken from [12] with kind permission).

In 1836, Wöhler was appointed Professor of Chemistry at the University of Göttingen, where he remained for the rest of his life. He continued his studies in both inorganic and organic chemistry, including investigations of compounds of physiological importance such as uric acid, which is the equivalent to urea in the excrements of birds and land-dwelling reptiles.

During this period in Wöhler's life, the revolution of 1848 against the established order and royalty, and the creation of the German Empire in 1871, took place. Wöhler, however, was never involved in any political affairs and never leaned towards 'liberal circles'; activities because of which many of his contemporaries in science, such as Jacob Henle and Carl Ludwig, had to seek refuge in Switzerland or Austria in order to escape the mounting interest and persecution by the authorities. Wöhler was happy at work in the laboratory. In his later years, teaching and training his numerous students became his major interest. His modesty and generosity are documented in an extensive correspondence with his former students.

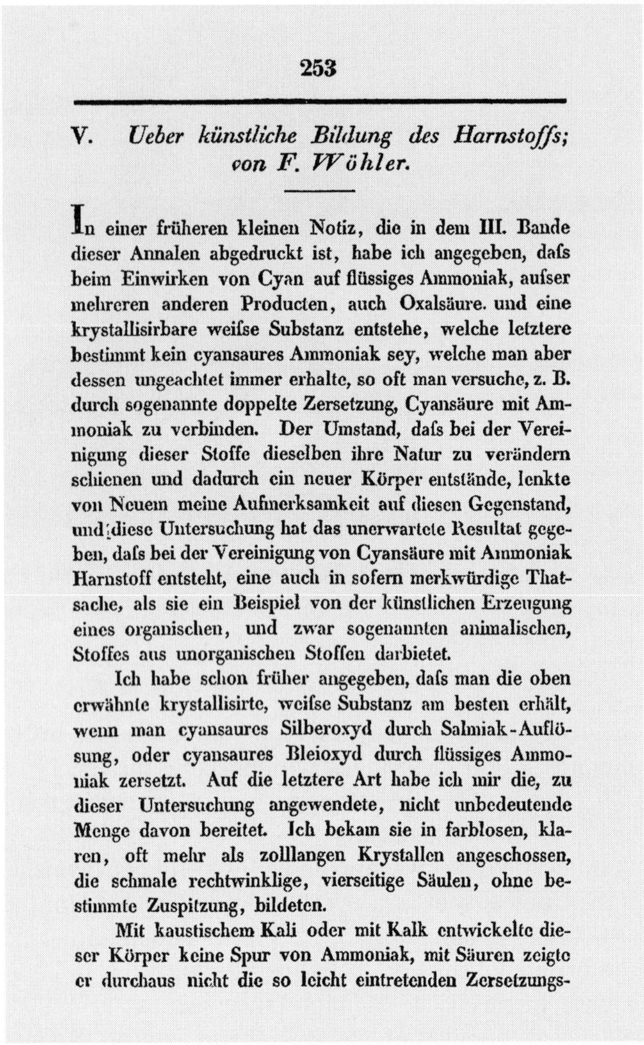

253

V. *Ueber künstliche Bildung des Harnstoffs; von F. Wöhler.*

In einer früheren kleinen Notiz, die in dem III. Bande dieser Annalen abgedruckt ist, habe ich angegeben, dafs beim Einwirken von Cyan auf flüssiges Ammoniak, aufser mehreren anderen Producten, auch Oxalsäure. und eine krystallisirbare weifse Substanz entstehe, welche letztere bestimmt kein cyansaures Ammoniak sey, welche man aber dessen ungeachtet immer erhalte, so oft man versuche, z. B. durch sogenannte doppelte Zersetzung, Cyansäure mit Ammoniak zu verbinden. Der Umstand, dafs bei der Vereinigung dieser Stoffe dieselben ihre Natur zu verändern schienen und dadurch ein neuer Körper entstände, lenkte von Neuem meine Aufmerksamkeit auf diesen Gegenstand, und diese Untersuchung hat das unerwartete Resultat gegeben, dafs bei der Vereinigung von Cyansäure mit Ammoniak Harnstoff entsteht, eine auch in sofern merkwürdige Thatsache, als sie ein Beispiel von der künstlichen Erzeugung eines organischen, und zwar sogenannten animalischen, Stoffes aus unorganischen Stoffen darbietet.

Ich habe schon früher angegeben, dafs man die oben erwähnte krystallisirte, weifse Substanz am besten erhält, wenn man cyansaures Silberoxyd durch Salmiak-Auflösung, oder cyansaures Bleioxyd durch flüssiges Ammoniak zersetzt. Auf die letztere Art habe ich mir die, zu dieser Untersuchung angewendete, nicht unbedeutende Menge davon bereitet. Ich bekam sie in farblosen, klaren, oft mehr als zolllangen Krystallen angeschossen, die schmale rechtwinklige, vierseitige Säulen, ohne bestimmte Zuspitzung, bildeten.

Mit kaustischem Kali oder mit Kalk entwickelte dieser Körper keine Spur von Ammoniak, mit Säuren zeigte er durchaus nicht die so leicht eintretenden Zersetzungs-

Fig. 2. First page of the publication by F. Wöhler in 1828 entitled: 'On the artificial formation of urea (reprinted from [1]).

The Discovery of Urea

Urea, the major organic compound excreted by the kidneys had first been isolated from urine in 1773 by the French chemist Hilaire-Marin Rouelle as an alkaline nitrogenous compound which yielded carbonic acid and ammonia on bacterial fermentation (urease). He coined the name 'urée' for the substance. Subsequently, Antoine Fourcroy (1755–1809) and Louis Vauquelin (1763–1829) prepared urea nitrate from urine in 1798, and the isolation of pure urea from the same source was first accomplished by Joseph Louis Proust (1754–1826) in 1821 under the guidance of his teacher Rouelle.

The Artificial Formation of Urea

In 1828, Wöhler published a paper in volume 12 of Poggendorf's *Annalen der Physik und Chemie* called 'Über künstliche Bildung des Harnstoffs' or 'On the artificial formation of urea', artificial meaning here that urea was formed by 'man's effort and not by nature' [1].

In the introduction to his paper, shown in figure 2, Wöhler notes that '... This investigation gave the unexpected result that by combining cyanic acid and ammonia urea is generated, quite a peculiar fact in that it represents the artificial (in vitro) formation of an organic compound, so-called 'animalischem Stoff' out of inorganic compounds.'

He then describes some properties of the unknown product and observes: 'This similarity (of the product obtained) with urea prompted me to perform comparative experiments with pure urea isolated from urine which demonstrated unambiguously that urea of urine and the former crystallized matter or the ammonium cyanate, if it could be called that way, are completely identical compounds.'

In discussing his findings Wöhler remarks: 'If, however, by combining cyanic acid and ammonia really only urea is generated, urea must have the same composition (of elements) as that obtained when calculating it from the formula of cyanic acid salts; which, indeed, is the case ...'

And he concludes: 'Thus, without demonstrating the generation of urea from cyanic acid and ammonia experimentally, one could have also calculated in advance that ammonium cyanate together with one atom of water has the same composition as urea.'

Urea Synthesis in vivo

Thus, Wöhler had delineated a chemical reaction by which urea could be formed in vitro; however, the question how urea was synthesized in vivo remained undeciphered for about another 100 years. By the middle of the nineteenth century, physiological chemists had already assumed that the urea excreted in the urine was the nitrogenous endproduct of the breakdown of tissue proteins. In 1877, Ernst Salkowski [2] speculated that two cyanic acid molecules could, in the presence of water, form urea. Since this reaction was not known to occur outside the organism, he turned to a formation à la Wöhler, where two cyanic acid molecules and two ammonia molecules were postulated to form two urea molecules. These conclusions were based on the observation by Woldemar von

Knierim [3] that ammonium salts added to the diet of animals increased the formation of urea. Already in 1872, Otto Schultzen and Marceli Nencki [4] had shown that when glycine or leucine were added to the diet of an animal, the amount of urea excreted increased. Because these amino acids contain only a single nitrogen atom, whereas urea contains two, they inferred that 'the formation of urea is in part ... a synthetic process'. Without mentioning Wöhler, they speculated that the amino acids upon degradation gave rise to cyanate groups which might combine with ammonia produced simultaneously from protein to generate urea. Even in 1930, Robert A. McCane [5] wrote in *Physiological Reviews*: 'All are agreed upon that mammals excrete 80 to 90 percent of the protein they metabolize as urea ... The details of this process, however, form some of the most baffling problems in biochemistry'.

Little did he know that this particular problem would be solved 2 years later. One hundred and sixty years after the first discovery of urea in 1773, Hans Krebs (1900–1981) and his medical student associate Kurt Henseleit (born 1907) [6] reported in 1932 in a paper published in Hoppe Seyler's *Zeitschrift für physiologische Chemie*, volume 210, 'that formation of urea is brought about by what is now called urea cycle' (Harnstoff-Kreislauf) and which Hans Krebs himself called 'the ornithine cycle of urea synthesis'.

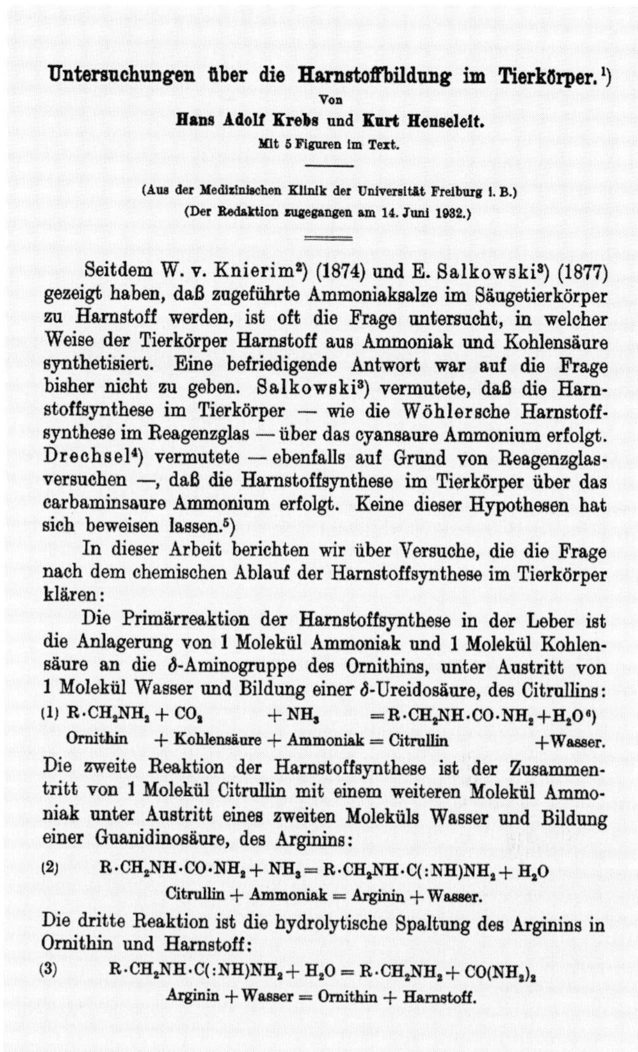

Untersuchungen über die Harnstoffbildung im Tierkörper.[1])

Von

Hans Adolf Krebs und **Kurt Henseleit.**

Mit 5 Figuren im Text.

(Aus der Medizinischen Klinik der Universität Freiburg i. B.)

(Der Redaktion zugegangen am 14. Juni 1932.)

Seitdem W. v. Knierim[2]) (1874) und E. Salkowski[3]) (1877) gezeigt haben, daß zugeführte Ammoniaksalze im Säugetierkörper zu Harnstoff werden, ist oft die Frage untersucht, in welcher Weise der Tierkörper Harnstoff aus Ammoniak und Kohlensäure synthetisiert. Eine befriedigende Antwort war auf die Frage bisher nicht zu geben. Salkowski[3]) vermutete, daß die Harnstoffsynthese im Tierkörper — wie die Wöhlersche Harnstoffsynthese im Reagenzglas — über das cyansaure Ammonium erfolgt. Drechsel[4]) vermutete — ebenfalls auf Grund von Reagenzglasversuchen —, daß die Harnstoffsynthese im Tierkörper über das carbaminsaure Ammonium erfolgt. Keine dieser Hypothesen hat sich beweisen lassen.[5])

In dieser Arbeit berichten wir über Versuche, die die Frage nach dem chemischen Ablauf der Harnstoffsynthese im Tierkörper klären:

Die Primärreaktion der Harnstoffsynthese in der Leber ist die Anlagerung von 1 Molekül Ammoniak und 1 Molekül Kohlensäure an die δ-Aminogruppe des Ornithins, unter Austritt von 1 Molekül Wasser und Bildung einer δ-Ureidosäure, des Citrullins:

$$(1)\quad \mathrm{R{\cdot}CH_2NH_2 + CO_2 + NH_3 = R{\cdot}CH_2NH{\cdot}CO{\cdot}NH_2 + H_2O}$$ [6])

Ornithin + Kohlensäure + Ammoniak = Citrullin + Wasser.

Die zweite Reaktion der Harnstoffsynthese ist der Zusammentritt von 1 Molekül Citrullin mit einem weiteren Molekül Ammoniak unter Austritt eines zweiten Moleküls Wasser und Bildung einer Guanidinosäure, des Arginins:

$$(2)\quad \mathrm{R{\cdot}CH_2NH{\cdot}CO{\cdot}NH_2 + NH_3 = R{\cdot}CH_2NH{\cdot}C(:NH)NH_2 + H_2O}$$

Citrullin + Ammoniak = Arginin + Wasser.

Die dritte Reaktion ist die hydrolytische Spaltung des Arginins in Ornithin und Harnstoff:

$$(3)\quad \mathrm{R{\cdot}CH_2NH{\cdot}C(:NH)NH_2 + H_2O = R{\cdot}CH_2NH_2 + CO(NH_2)_2}$$

Arginin + Wasser = Ornithin + Harnstoff.

Fig. 3. First page of the publication by H.A. Krebs and K. Henseleit entitled: 'Investigations on the formation of urea in animals' (reprinted from [6]).

Investigations on the Formation of Urea in Animals by Krebs and Henseleit

Figure 3 shows the first page of the article called 'Investigations on the formation of urea in animals' in which the state of knowledge as detailed above is summarized – citing the work of Knierim, Salkowski and Wöhler. Krebs, who had worked in the laboratory of Otto Warburg during 1926–1930, preferred for his studies on cellular metabolism the method of thin tissue slices over the organ perfusion method established by Carl Ludwig in the late nineteenth century. For him, the main advantages of tissue slices were adequate supply of the tissue with nutrients, especially with oxygen, and sufficient removal of metabolic endproducts. This page also depicts the three critical reactions that had been observed by Krebs and Henseleit in their studies on the formation of urea in thin liver slices. Two amino acids not commonly found in proteins are involved in these reactions: ornithine and citrulline.

The most significant observation made by the authors, which according to Krebs provided the key for the elucidation of the urea synthesis, was the so-called ornithine effect.

As stated by the authors: 'In experiments on the formation of urea from amino acids we discovered a surprising, unexpected fact. If the medium (used for the incubation of the liver slices) contains simultaneously ammonia and d-ornithine we find an extraordinary high formation of urea'.

It might be interesting in this context to ask the question why Krebs used ornithine in his experiments. According to Krebs himself, 'I think it was really a blind or unprejudiced collection of facts' [7].

Now the question arose how ornithine stimulated urea synthesis. Studies on the concentration dependence of the effect and measurements of the rate of disappearance of ornithine showed that it acted like a catalyst – being active at low concentrations and not changing significantly in concentration during the experiments.

They thus deduced that a cyclic process occurs in which one molecule of ornithine combines with one molecule of ammonia and one molecule of CO_2 to form citrulline. A second amino group is added to citrulline to form arginine which is then hydrolyzed to yield urea, with regeneration of ornithine. Ornithine is then ready for the next turn of the urea cycle. In this context, it is noteworthy that citrulline had just been characterized in 1931 and was provided to Krebs by Dankwart Ackermann [8] who had recently described the transformation of ornithine into citrulline.

Vitalism and Urea Synthesis

Wöhler's achievement has long been hailed as an important step in the overthrow of the doctrine of vitalism. But at the time when Wöhler reported on the artificial formation of urea, he was more concerned with the chemistry of urea than with the philosophical significance of its synthesis from inorganic substances. He was mainly interested in isomerism, i.e. in the fact that substances with the same element composition showed strikingly different properties, suggesting different structural arrangements of the elements. Yet, in a letter to his teacher and friend, Berzelius in Sweden, dated from February 22, 1828, he is less inarticulate. He writes 'that he kind of cannot hold his chemical water if he wouldn't inform him about the fact that he (Wöhler) is capable of producing urea requiring neither kidneys nor any animal, may it be man or dog. Ammonium cyanate is urea ... and it is by no chemical means different from urea of the urine, which I have produced all by myself' [9].

Berzelius, himself a stern believer in the doctrine of the 'vis vitalis' without which no organic compounds could be generated, nevertheless acknowledged the accomplishment and congratulated Wöhler with 'Indeed, the Doctor has mastered the art to make his name immortal' [10]. Other contemporaries, such as Jean Baptiste Dumas (1800–1884), realized the implications of Wöhler's experiment for the doctrine of vitalism and wrote: 'All chemists have applauded Wöhler for his magnificent discovery of the artificial formation of urea and I do ... sincerely hope that the same principle will also be used for other causes' [11].

At the end of his publication, Krebs refers to Wöhler and describes one experiment where he tested whether ammonium and cyanate are transformed into urea in liver slices, as observed by Wöhler in vitro. The result was that no urea was formed. Krebs also observed that urea synthesis did not occur in tissue homogenates, but only in vital cells; thus a certain factor unique to the living cell appeared to be essential for the cycle to operate. Can we consider this as a rebirth of vitalism? In his publication, Krebs does not discuss this fact in further detail, but we know now that the need for an intact and vital cell is due to the compartmentalization of the various steps of the complete urea cycle which requires the proper arrangement of mitochondrial and cytoplasmic reactions.

Acknowledgments

The competent help in securing the original publications by the staff of our library, the library of the University of Dortmund and the Department of History of Medicine at the Ruhr University of Bochum is gratefully acknowledged. This paper is dedicated to Professor Richard P. Kreher, companion and combattant in joining chemistry and biology. We also thank the unit for scientific documentation at our institute for their skillful electronic art and D. Mägdefessel and P. Jurczynski for their expert secretarial help.

References

1 Wöhler F: Über künstliche Bildung des Harnstoffs. Ann Phys Chem 1828;12:253–256.
2 Salkowski E: Ueber den Vorgang der Harnstoffbildung im Thierkörper und den Einfluss der Ammoniaksalze auf denselben. Z Physiol Chem 1877;1:1–5.
3 Knierim W: Beiträge zur Kenntnis der Bildung des Harnstoffs im thierischen Organismus. Z Biol 1874;10:263–294.
4 Schultzen O, Nencki M: Die Vorstufen des Harnstoffs im thierischen Organismus. Z Biol 1872;8:124–138.
5 McCane RA: Degradation of protein nitrogen. Physiol Rev 1930;11:2–52.
6 Krebs HA, Henseleit K: Untersuchungen über die Harnstoffbildung im Tierkörper. Z Physiol Chem 1932; 210:33–66.
7 Holmes FL: Hans Krebs. Oxford, Oxford University Press, 1991.
8 Ackermann D: Über den biologischen Abbau des Arginins zu Citrullin. Z Physiol Chem 1931;203:66–69.
9 Wallach O: Briefwechsel zwischen J. Berzelius und F. Wöhler im Auftrage der Königlichen Gesellschaft der Wissenschaften zu Göttingen. Leipzig, 1901, vol 1, p 206.
10 Wallach O: Briefwechsel zwischen J. Berzelius und F. Wöhler im Auftrage der Königlichen Gesellschaft der Wissenschaften zu Göttingen. Leipzig, 1901, vol 1, p 208.
11 Dumas JB: Über die Zusammensetzung des Harnstoffs. Ann Physik Chemie 1830;19:487–493.
12 Bugge G: Friedrich Wöhler; in Das Buch der grossen Chemiker. Weinheim, Verlag Chemie, 1965, vol 1, p 31–52.

Origins of Nephrology – The Modern Era

American Journal of Nephrology

Am J Nephrol 1999;19:295–303

Evolution of Nephrology

The Caldron of Its Organizations

George E. Schreiner

Great Falls, Va., USA

Key Words

International Society of Nephrology · American Society of Nephrology · National Kidney Foundation · Macy Foundation · American Society for Artificial Internal Organs

Abstract

Nephrology in America was the first and largest of the new internal medical specialties to emerge after World War II. It was a novel fusion of traditional basic sciences and new clinical tools such as renal biopsy, new imaging, molecular target drugs, dialysis, hemoperfusion and transplantation. The immediate roots were provided by great scientists/clinicians like John Peters, Homer Smith and Tom Addis. The caldron was formed by the tensions arising from newly formed organizations such as the AHA (including NYHA and WHA), NIH, ISN, ASN, ASAIO and NKF. Without these tensions, nephrology might have become a much smaller and narrower specialty of clinical physiology, salt and water and acid-base metabolism. The evolution was rapid from attendance 100+ at the first ISN in Evian, France in 1960 to the 1998 ASN meeting in Philadelphia which drew more than 10,000 nephrologists. This is a personalized history of those tensions and their interactions written by the only nephrologist who has been President of the WHA, ASN, ISN, ASAIO and the NKF.

Nephrology was the first of new medical specialties to emerge in the reconstruction after World War II. It was a novel fusion of disparate elements of basic science, particularly physiology, the development of clinical tools to understand and treat renal disorders, dedicated physicians applying science to clinical syndromes, and the desire of philanthropic people to associate for needs not met by the medical organizations then dealing with renal disease. It was formed in a caldron of revolutionary changes in medicine, biology, and the social order. Its evolution broke down old barriers that had prevented a unified, complex, multidisciplinary approach needed for the delineation of renal pathophysiology, the rational design of therapy and the bold step of renal replacement. The organizations that helped nephrology evolve were them-

Abbreviations for Organizations

AEC = Atomic Energy Commissions; AFIP = Armed Forces Institute of Pathology; Heart Associations: AHA = American; NYHA = New York; WHA = Washington; APS = American Physiology Society; ASPT = American Society for Pharmacology and Therapeutics; ASAIO = American Society for Artificial Internal Organs; ASCI = American Society for Clinical Investigation; ASN = American Society of Nephrology; EDTA = European Dialysis and Transplant Association; ISN = International Society of Nephrology; JAMA = Journal of the American Medical Association; MDIBL = Mt. Desert Island Biological Laboratory, Maine; NIH = National Institutes of Health; NKF = National Kidney Foundation; NKDF = National Kidney Disease Foundation; NNF = National Nephrosis Foundation; NYU = New York University; RA = Renal Association (UK); SSCI = Southern Society for Clinical Investigation.

KARGER

Fax + 41 61 306 12 34
E-Mail karger@karger.ch
www.karger.com

© 1999 S. Karger AG, Basel
0250–8095/99/0192–0295$17.50/0

Accessible online at:
http://BioMedNet.com/karger

George E. Schreiner, MD
PO Box 199
Great Falls, VA 22066 (USA)
Tel. +1 703 759 2447, Fax +1 703 759 2465
E-Mail boppadoc@aol.com

selves built in fits and starts. There were blind alleys, and not all participants knew the eventual outcome. But, they were all committed to solving the mysteries of renal physiology and the sorrows of renal pathology, each in its own way and with its own perspective. This is the story of some of the pioneers in the birth of nephrology with emphasis on their organizations.

In the post-WWII scientific ferment, there were a handful of gifted clinicians who were able to interface with the mushrooming advances of basic science. There was an outpouring of medical research support from all sources: foundations, industry, universities and federal governmental agencies, the military, the Manhattan project, etc. New York City even had a Research Institute. Homer Smith and Jim Shannon and others had worked on an anti-malarial project involving the Goldwater and NYU[1] Laboratories. They were able to learn from and work with the chemical and physical scientists, as surgeons had done with the anatomists and pathologists. Engineering and math came in swiftly.

Early clinical nephrologists were largely drawn from cardiology. Many were involved with circulatory physiology and were fascinated by the intricate mechanisms of the kidney. They sought to learn more about the complex syndromes produced by legions of separate kidney diseases. The research oriented, turned largely to physiology, chemistry, and pharmacology for the tools of their quest. Immunology was a waif at the window waiting to be invited. Genetics was but a curious dream. Dana Atchley, Thomas Addis, and William Goldring all came out of cardiology. When NYU Dean Wyckoff ushered in the golden era of NYU, he chose leaders for divisions. He simply told Goldring: 'You take care of the kidney!' Goldring quickly set up what was to be a lifelong collaboration with Homer Smith who had been Chairman of Physiology at Virginia, and in 1928 was brought to NYU as Chair of Physiology. A young internist, Herbert Chasis took a PhD with them at NYU. Their seminal paper [1] ushered in an era of widespread objective measurement of renal functions in scores of healthy states from sleep to stress and starvation and in many renal and systemic diseases.

A few master clinicians could then tie at last these objective measurements of function with the earlier morphologic gains beginning with the likes of Vesalius (1514–1564) and Malpighi (1628–1694), up to Bright [2] and Volhard [3] who had refined in a globally recognized way some of the causal connections between Pathology and clinical kidney disease. When I started kidney rounds with Goldring, Chasis and Baldwin, we would marshall history, physical and lab with imaging data and discuss every facet of the putative lesion. If the patient died, the diagnosis was reviewed with the insights from pathology. If the patient lived, the final diagnosis was picked by Dr Goldring whose skills had been honed by clinical research at Bellevue. Percutaneous needle biopsy [4, p 339] changed the nephro-world. Specific diagnoses could be made in hours or days. Some diagnoses like IGA nephropathy, and a host of immune diseases would be recognized later when immunostaining and electron microscopy became available. Added to the tide in structure and function were new imaging techniques, growth of immunology and genetics and the insights provided by specific drugs and knock-out enzymes on precise renal mechanisms that were to come much later.

The interfaces of metabolism with the kidney were fleshed in by giants such as Fuller Albright and John P. Peters and the host of Fellows trained who latterly entered nephrology such as Donald W. Seldin and Louis G. Welt. Insights were added by epidemiological and demographic research. Proof of insights was provided by the success of therapies such as drugs, dialysis and transplants. The ingredients in the caldron were strong and the impeccable fruits of science. The bubbling was provided by a huge class of patients with hypertension, diabetes and an index of kidney diseases which numbered more than 200 specific diagnoses when I tried to classify Uremia in 1961 [4]. We grouped them into diseases of: infection, circulation, hypersensitivity, metabolism, development, neoplasms, tubular necrosis, tubular syndromes and miscellaneous. Only a decade later after thousands of renal biopsies, could we specify, in 1971 [5], over 60 causes of just the nephrotic syndrome. The post-War medical specialty out of the caldron was tentatively named renal medicine, renology, kidney and electrolyte medicine, and ultimately nephrology (néphrologie in France, nephrologia in Spain) [26, p xi] with its own fellowships, boards and journals.

Some subspecialists formed in the caldron around a specific technology, e.g., dialysis, transplant, apheresis, biopsy, renal imaging, etc. But every application of a new technique to an individual patient had ultimately to be done by a clinician needing a broad base of training and experience. 'The responsibility and the opportunity for maintaining normal physiology is in the hands of the physician' [6].

It is impossible to overestimate the influence of Homer Smith (fig. 1) when he espoused marrying science and the bedside. He vowed to eliminate the false barrier between

[1] All medical organizations in text are abbreviated. Alphabetical list is given before the references.

the two halves of Medical School. Sir George Pickering said: 'Smith saw that the scientific method had been developed by the laboratory sciences.... clinical science had not yet accepted it. He had a clear and practical idea of how clinicians could be trained as scientists.... he was one of the most attractive writers of my generation. He combined a clear mind, imagination and precision of thought; and these were all evident in his writings. I would say he was one of the great men of our generation.' There is no complete record of how many scientists Smith personally influences, besides the thousands who devoured his classic publications [7, 14].

I have reviewd a partial list of co-workers compiled at his retirement in July, 1961. He had sent 28 Scientists to the NYU faculty, 6 to the NIH, including Jim Shannon, its legendary Director, more than 50 renal scientists to 33 different US schools of whom 13 in 1962 had already become Chairmen of Physiology or Medicine and had sent Professors to 11 different countries. Smith went to the mountain in 26 major lectureships and visiting professor tours between 1936 and 1960. The breadth of his biology was sculpted in 24 years as trustee of the Bermuda Biological Station and 11 years as president and guru of the MDIBL where he built a house and laboratory and spent most summers. He was also associated with the Museum of Natural History and the NY Zoological, and as a Guggenheim Fellow went on scientific expeditions to Central Africa (1928) and Siam and Malaysia (1930). Smith's laboratory door was always open, his support unfailing, financially meager but boundless in inspiration, enthusiasm and opportunity. Exciting visitors came to NYU in a steady stream. In the 3 years I served on his faculty, I have vivid memories of conversations with Thomas Addis who took his vacations from California in New York, spent his days with the fellows, attended conferences and luncheons, and his nights on Broadway in what he called a 'cultural shower'. There was Trueta of the kidney a–v shunt fame; André Cournand who brought his catheters to NY, and went on to win the Nobel prize; Julian Huxley whose father fed Smith's agnosticism and Domingo Gomez who was exiled from Cuba after heading its Cardiac Research Institute. I inherited Robert Pitts' Lab who had just gone to Cornell. While doing a dog experiment, I answered a knock on the lab door to be startled by the unmistakeable face of Albert Einstein who asked to be taken to Gomez because 'I need help with an equation!' I must have looked startled for he went on; 'don't you know he is one of the 5 or 10 best mathematicians in the world?' Weeks later I heard Gomez figure out in about 3 minutes in the hall, the formula and method for

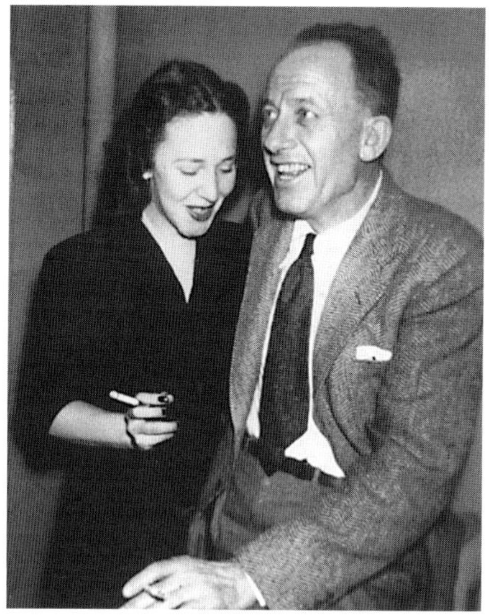

Fig. 1. Homer Smith and his second wife Margaret at a lab party in Physiology lab at NYU. (photo in 1949 by G. Schreiner). Note smoking. Smith suffered from its pulmonary and cardiac toxicity.

doing the inulin space as a measure of extracellular fluid. There were at least 4 Nobel Prize winners working within 300 feet of Smith's office during those days. His authentic genius worked in a heady aura.

Smith was an unmistakeable leader among cardiac scientists. He became a towering figure in the NYHA, and through it to the AHA. Smith's collegiality together with 15 years on the Fellowship Board of the NRC and later (1956), the NIH led to the allocation of research and fellowship support toward kidney research. In have no hard figures but perhaps as much as a third of AHA research was kidney directed – particularly in the overlap areas of hypertension and diabetes. The AHA developed a renal section and John P. Merrill became one of its chairmen. He had returned to Harvard and the Brigham from the Air Force and Thorn appointed him as Chief of Hypertension and Renal.

I had interiewed George Thorn for the Canisian paper when he was in Pediatrics in Buffalo and first used ACTH. In 1944, I made rounds with him. We saw a Patient with acute uremia. Thorn said he had lost similar patients, just as urine output was rising. He predicted that we would be saving patients by transplanting kidneys or using some form of dialysis to gain time. In 1946 he asked C. Hufnagel and intern D. Hume to attach a fresh cadaver kidney to such a patient's brachial artery and vein. It was bathed in Ringers and warmed with a gooseneck lamp and made urine. I was an intern at the Boston City and went over to see it. Meanwhile, G. Murray at Toronto had built his artificial kidney at home using over USD 8,000 of his own funds and use it on postoperative acute uremia. I saw the Murray Kidney in Baltimore in 1946.

When Kolff came to NY Mount Sinai to demonstrate his wooden-slatted rotating drum, I visited his exhibition from NYU where I was already working with Smith after coming from MDIBL. Thorn either attended or heard about it and invited Kolff to the Brigham. He introduced Kolff to Carl Walter who had a bioengineering friend, Edward Olsen who took Kolff's blueprints and rebuilt Kolff's drum in stainless steel, lucite and plastic-lined rotating couplings. The first one went to the Brigham. The second came to Georgetown, the third to J. Kiley at Albany. H. Jeghers and L. Kyle acquired Georgetown's on an NIH grant to study barbiturate intoxication. In 1938, Reginald Cutting and Theodore Koppanyi [15] (my teachers in physiology and pharmacology, respectively) showed that rapid isotonic expansion of extracellular fluid lowered tissue levels of barbiturate and lightened sedation in animals. This suggested blood level was governing. Rapid lowering might be therapeutic. Koppanyi and Linegar [16] joined the circulations of severely poisoned dogs with normal partners. They recovered in 27 min. Control dogs without cross-circulation took 29 h. With prescience, they wrote, 'Probably an apparatus could...provide a slow continuous bleeding of the poisoned individual and replacement...with plasma or compatible blood'. Hemodialysis met that principle and in 1955 we published the first successful dialysis of aspirin intoxication in a controlled human experiment [17]. And in 1956 [18], we reported 2 years of experience treating 7 patients with severe barbiturate poisoning. We worked out clearances and distribution spaces.

Thorn appointed Merrill to set up dialysis and the rest is modern renal history. Merrill and Murray also started a transplant program. John took a sabbatical in London to augment his immunology and worked with Medawar. While there, he spent time in Paris with Jean Hamburger. Hamburger had worked with Homer Smith at NYU, had set up Hopital Necker as a premier kidney Center, and had done human transplants using total body radiation. They became close friends.

The clinical kidney medicine had developed in a more organized fashion in Europe thanks to the British Renal Society, the traditions of Claude Bernard and such giants as Alwall. Perhaps because the War was so much more destructive in Europe, there was need to build new unifying institutions in place of divisive ones. Europe moved faster to build the new specialty of nephrology. Indeed, the first functional dialyzer was developed by Kolff in Holland in the midst of the inferno. Alwall rapidly followed. In many American universities, there was a kind of mental Chinese wall between 'basic' and clinical scientists.

The International Society of Nephrology

While in Europe, John Merrill met with European nephrologists including Jean Hamburger and Gabriel Richet. They decided to start a society as a forum for the kidney and its diseases. They wrote a constitution and commissioned a large boat model which was restored in Washington after the Prague Congress. The ship was damaged again in transport and restored and exhibited in glory by Robert Adkins at the Sydney Congress in 1997. They decided on a First Congress for Evian on September 1–4, 1960, Congress President was Hamburger; Richet and Cottet were Secretaries. Organizing Societies were listed as: La Société de Néphrologie, The Scandinavian Society for Kidney Research, The ASCI, the Societa Italiana di Nefrologia (Italy) and the RA (UK). The ASN did not exist, The NYHA and AHA were visibly absent. At least 4 of the key individuals had close ties to Homer Smith.

The meeting was attended by a few hundred including myself and was sponsored by Evian water. There were 14 presentations on tubular ion exchange, 11 on the kidney in shock, 3 round tables on morphology of ultrafiltration, stop-flow and diuretics; 3 lectures – one by Wirz on his controversial counter-current multiplier hypothesis; 14 papers on recent advances, and 37 brief communications. A 728-page book was edited by Richet and published by Karger. There were 217 'nephrologists' listed in the author index. They elected Jean Hamburger as ISN President (1960–1963), Jan Brod to organize the 2nd congress in Prague. This was an interesting venture behind the Iron Curtain. Europeans could drive through the border but it required 2½ days, and over 16 permits for me to rent a Skoda so my wife, 2 children and I could tour to Bratislava. There were lines many blocks long in front of every gas station in Prague. Driving in rural areas was dicey and sometimes required barter for fuel. It was a tribute to Jan Brod's standing in the party that when we limped into Prague on empty the day before the congress, all stations were stocked and lines gone.

Claus Brun (Den) was elected president with John Merrill to follow. They chose Washington DC for the 3rd

Fig. 2. Herodotus Atticus Theatre near Parthenon, at Athens Congress of the ISN. L to R – Gabriel Richet, Past-President Jean Hamburger, President George E. Schreiner and Madame K. Hamburger. Photo by Peter Schreiner.

Fig. 3. Founding and first meeting of the Australasian Society of Nephrology on steps of the Kanamatsu at Sydney Hospital. Priscilla Kincaid-Smith is in foreground, face turned away from camera. Photo by G. Schreiner.

2

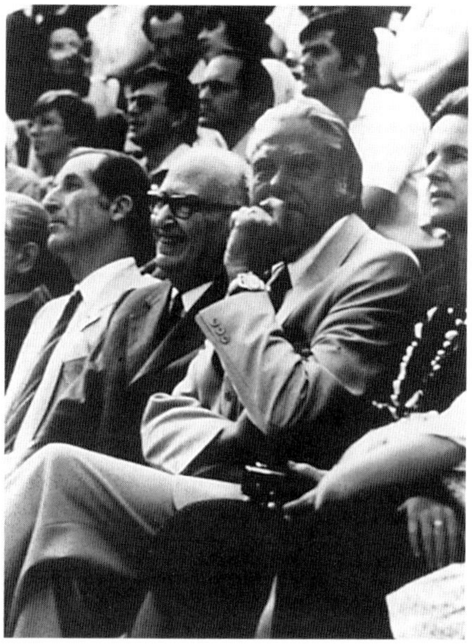

3

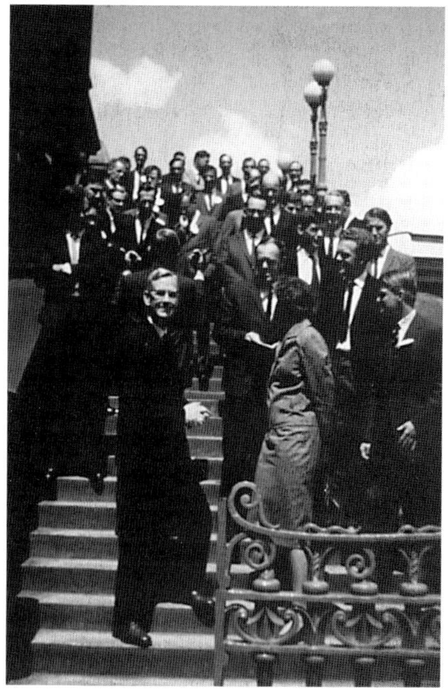

Congress, and considered revising the constitution. The Greek nephros had clearly won out over its Latin renal root, and national Societies of Nephrology were forming all over the globe. The notable exception was the USA. The reason lay in the rivalries in the NNF, the NKDF, the AHA and the lack of resources in the ISN. The Prague Congress with its communist support had not really provided any forward continuity for the ISN as a world organization.

There was much overlap in the leadership of the Renal Section of the AHA and the SAB of the NKF as well as the boards of its most successful affiliates. For example, I had worked with Goldring, Kossman, Bradley and others on the still famous book on the NYHA classification of cardiac disability. I jointed the AHA at NYU, the WHA in 1957, became a director in 1958, chairman of the Renal Section and Scientific Council in 1959, President-elect in 1968 and president in 1969. I joined the NKF in 1963, attended most of the conferences at Princeton and was recruited as president in 1969 by Bricker and Welt. Many of the research oriented members of the Renal Section, AHA...had loyalty to the AHA, or NYHA and some feared that a new organization would drive a wedge into the AHA, reduce its grant support and be competitive in fund raising. Some foresaw formation of a National Kidney Institute which would disrupt the structure placing the kidney in the Heart Institute under Bob Berliner. Offstage, the caldron bubbled. John Merrill became Chairman of the Renal Section, AHA, and the ISN-EC extended to the AHA the invitation to organize the 3rd Congress in Washington with Bob Berliner as president and George E. Schreiner as secretary-general. The task was made difficulty by controversy in the background but at the same time, the caldron was energizing.

The Third International Congress of Nephrology

The 1966 congress deadline loomed despite the stalemate on an ASN. We hired Helena Lemp from the Federated Societies as manager. A new Washington Hilton was planned. As the hole was being dug, we signed a contract for all 1,000 rooms at an unprecedented USD 10/day including suites. This enabled us to offer a low 'mean' room rate. The architect assured me that the planned egg-shaped ballroom would have impeccable acoustics. That enabled us to sign the Washington Symphony for its first-ever formal concert outside its home Consititution Hall. The concert was hailed by orchestra, critics and the audience as a smash success. Prize Napa and Sonoma Valley vintages dazzled even the Italian and French delegates.

I will never forget the planning moment when Bob Berliner and the Committee directed me to send out 'to the nephrologists of the world', a preliminary announcement of the 3rd Congress. What was a nephrologist? Who were such people? Where did they work or live? How would we find them? I was given estimates from 200 to 2,000. I worried about our commitment for 1,000 rooms. No lists were available from the two previous congresses which were heavily European and quite small. I had lists of the APS and ASPT, to both of which I belonged. But they were huge. We could not afford indiscriminate mailing and subjective culling would miss the younger workers on the kidney who were not yet members. I went to the AFIP for lists of pathologists who had worked on kidney projects. I went to the AHA, the NKF and all the nephrology societies around the world. Many were unedited for address changes and antiquated. Then came one of my better inspirations:

I took a short leave of absence from Georgetown and went through every stack in our and some in the National Library of Medicine. I looked at every article for the past 3 years that had anything to do with kidney. I copied addresses of every author including the most junior and scanned the bibliography for leads to more obscure journals. All were added to our lists and purged for duplicates and variants. Fired up, I later wrote Hugh Hussey, who had been my teacher, Chairman and Dean and had become Editor of JAMA. The abbreviations for a periodic survey of US specialists had no mention of nephrology, or place to register. Either through a droll sense of humor or inability to read my handwriting, Hugh wrote back: 'George, I didn't realize you had become a Neurologist'. We were in the next survey!

The final list was more than 10,000. The response of over 50% to a first mailing was beyond anything that Helena Lemp or any of the convention professionals had ever seen or calculated. The tangible results were 2,134 scientists registered for the full week, 624 abstracts submitted, 75 invited papers and 224 brief communications presented. Including exhibitors, guests, press, visitors and single day trippers, attendance at some functions exceed 3,500. Intangibles were even greater: new ideas appreciated, constructive criticisms received, new directions indicated, new friendships created and old ones confirmed. The results were published in three volumes: I Physiology, II Morphology, Immunology, Urology, and III Clinical Nephrology. J. Handler, R. Heptinstall and E.L. Becker were subeditors for the individual volumes [20]. This very division emphasized the roots of the new nephrology. Separate categorial volumes were unique at the time. The 3rd Congress of the ISN was widely judged successful on all counts: scientifically, socially and financially. Its six-figure profit was used to fund the up-front costs for the 1984 ISN Congress in Los Angeles and then given to the ASN to administer. The 3rd Congress 'presented the only currently available inventory of the range of Nephrology in 1966' [20, p. X]. I don't believe that anything I have done in nephrology has had such a lasting effect with the possible exception of training almost 200 nephrologists. The 3rd Congress almost instantly established nephrology as a broad-based medical and research specialty throughout the world. It was the kind of base Homer Smith envisioned.

Bob Berliner and I actually invented a new format for the meeting. Each day would begin with state-of-the art plenary sessions on a major theme to develop the general knowledge of the entire audience. There would then be a limited breakup to simultaneous symposia with little overlap. From there the audience would break to a larger number of free oral communications and thence to poster sessions, thus preserving a logic tree from the general to the specific. This 'unfolding' concept has been used for more than 25 years for the ASN annual meeting [5, p. 7]. The format was used at the first ASN meeting because Bricker and I ran the meeting and lifted it from the ISN. Berliner and I originated the format for the 3rd Washington Congress of the ISN. It has since been adopted by many Societies for large meetings.

The American Society of Nephrology

Embarrassed at last by the missing silhouette of ANY American Society and forced by the timeline of the 3rd Congress, 18 nephrologists gathered under the aegis of the NYHA. They came largely from both the Council on Circulation of the AHA and the SAB of the NKF. Over one third had worked closely with Homer Smith. At least 3, that I know of worked with John Peters. They were : Barnett, Berliner, Bradley, Bricker, Earle, Glenn, Good, Kleeman, Malvin, Merrill, Papper, Petersdorf, Schreiner, Scribner, Seldin, Tosteson, Vernier and Welt.

Fire raged beneath the Caldron between basic and clinical; optimist and pessimist; gregarious and loner; provincial and expansionist, liberal and less liberal. Discussion became so heated that at one point Stan Bradley resigned and walked out. He later recanted and asked me to propose him for membership in ASN. Obviously, he was unanimously approved.

They got the job done. The ASN was founded in 1966 with a Constitution: 'to advance the knowledge of nephrology and to foster the dissemination of this knowledge through national scientific meetings...cooperation with other national societies...and by other means approved.' Membership was to be open and inclusive and not elitist. The first annual meeting was held in the Ambassador Hotel in Los Angeles, October 18–19, 1967.

The executive committee asked Bricker and me to prepare for 200–300. Neal whispered to me, 'go for 500+.' I went for 900. The attendance was above 1,250. Meetings have been held yearly since then except for 1972 when the ISN Congress was in Mexico City. By 1991, there were 4,000 members and attendance; the Baltimore meeting surpassed 6,000, and Philadelphia in 1998 had 10,000+. From the Founding Group, Bricker, Welt, Seldin, Berliner, Schreiner, Scribner, and Vernier would later become Presidents of the ASN. The NYHA had established a Homer Smith Award in 1964 for achievement in renal physiology and in 1971 offered to share sponsorship with the ASN. Since then, the award has been presented yearly at the ASN. In 1983, the ASN established a John P. Peters Award for excellence in clinical research. Of the ASN founding group, Seldin, Merrill, Scribner, Barnett, Schreiner and Bricker have received Peters Medals, as have Hamburger and Habib from the ISN pioneers.

The National Kidney Foundation

The NKF had a bifid root. In 1948, Jack Metcoff and Henry Barnett started in Boston a conference on Research on the Nephrotic Syndrome. It was dominated by pediatricians and early immunologists. In 1961, it changed to the Annual Kidney conference and its function was subsumed by the NFK. Some of the 3 dozen or so early members, mostly pediatricians, were organized into a Medical Advisory Board (MAB) and fused with clinicians who cared for Robert Lee DeBold, an infant stricken with nephrosis. In November, 1950, the child's parents, Mr. and Mrs. Harry DeBold of Tuckahoe, N.Y. convened a 'Commitee for Nephrosis Research' which 2 weeks later became a charitable foundation in NY named 'National Nephrosis Foundation' (NNF). This patient/parent orientation is important because in 1952, the NNF took steps to become national. Its first booklet entitled *Nephrosis, Nature of the Disease* was prepared by Janeway and in 1953 some 5,000 copies were distributed. In 1954, a plan was made to go national and form state and regional chapters. The first national fund raising was 1956. It was supported by 35 state Governors as a Governor's Council and many notables such as Dr. Spock, Steve Allen, Art Linkletter, Perry Como, David Garroway, Helen Hayes, James Thurber, Rosemary Clooney, etc. They raised USD 400,000. Mrs Mamie Eisenhower became National Chairperson in 1957 and USD 600,000 was raised. Many heated conflicts arose which kept the caldron bubbling. They were principally between state and regional, weak and strong, wealthy and poor chapters, between chapters and national, between local and national legislators, between laymen and physicians, the merger with the AHA; and ego conflicts between talented professional trying to forge nephrology [21]. The local energy, once a source of conflict, became a boon (Tip O'Neill said 'all politics is local'). Ira Griefer and E. Lovell Becker were particularly effective in NY. When Becker became President 'he appointed me chair of a newly formed National Legislative Committee, supported by Charles Plante whom I had previously hired as a Washington representative.' The complex events leading up in the passage of ESRD Legislation [25] were extensively reviewed in 'How ESRD Developed' in the May *Seminars in Nephrology* [25]. Most of the nephrology community except for the government was supportive. Certainly, the NKF played the central role in the passage of this unique and historic legislation. The cooperative spirit had started earlier in the resolution of conflicts which had helped delay the start of an ASN. A compromise resulted in a promerger group, joined by Michigan, agreeing to reorganization for 1 year with reevaluation, and support for the 3rd Congress. I breathed a sigh of relief, the remnant MAB of the NKDF was expanded to an NSAB to which I was invited. From them would come most of the founding group which would later vote to form an ASN by constitutional means and then dissolve itself.

Macy Foundation Conference on Renal Failure

The Macy Foundation held conferences for integration of science over 2 days for 5 years. You can feel their breadth by looking at their 13 fields: aging, adrenal cortex, biological oxidants, blood clotting, connective tissues, cybernetics, blood pressure, infancy and childhood, metabolic interrelations, nerve impulse, problems of consciousness, liver injury and renal function. For each, 15 scientists were selected as members. Invited speakers and discussors expanded to a strict limit of 25. The Renal panel was packed with talent: Pitts, Bradley, Berliner, Binkley, Bott, Darrow, Dock, Fishberg, Forster, Grafflin, Luetscher, Oliver, Selkurt, Shannon, Shock, Taggert and Thorn. Topics included ion and water transport, effect of corticoids and hormones in the kidney, etc. The flavor of give and take discussions was preserved by Stan Bradley, their Editor. Reading them helps to understand the trepidation with which Bradley and many of his colleagues faced the prospect of larger kidney organizations.

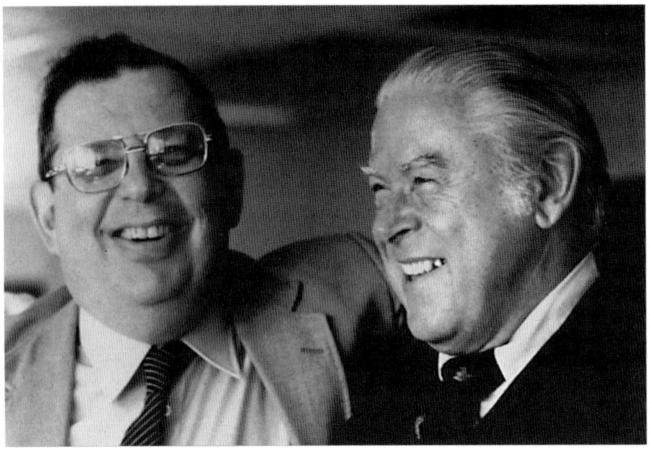

Fig. 4. Drs. Eli Friedman and George E. Schreiner at the turning over of the editorship of the transactions of the ASAIO after 29 years. Photo by Dr. Friedman's camera.

The American Society for Artificial Internal Organs (ASAIO)

The ASAIO had its first national meeting in the Hotel Chelsea in Atlantic City, N.J. on June 5th, 1955. The idea for an organization devoted to bioengineering and clinical research in artificial organs, especially hearts, kidneys and related hardware came out of boardwalk conversations during Federated Societies and AFCR meetings. Peter Salisbury, an inventor, a friend of Kolff and a sort of free-lance clinical dialyzer suggested that a society with a name like ASAIO should be formed for rapid exchange of ideas between engineers, basic scientists and clinical 'organists' and to solve publication problem that arose from the long delays (often 1 year) between submission of a paper and its publication. Pioneers in the field were making advances every few months. Also bioengineering was alien to the more traditional medical journals, resulting in uninformed reviewing and editing decisions, delays and even refusals to publish what would later emerge as pivotal advances. Salisbury defined 'socitey' in the words of Daniel [22] 'many shall run to and fro and kowledge shall be increased.' I made a personal attempt to secure a rapid, dedicated section on artificial organs in some ongoing journals like the *Journal of Applied Physiology* but was rebuffed. To a clinical investigator and a teacher, the prospect of such a disparate and innovative group was exciting and I hastened to join. It would be the first medical society I could join where a non-physician could be a member, on a committee or even an officer. Pim Kolff invited people to submit abstracts; a steering committee was selected of Clarence Dennis, Pim Kolff and Peter Salisbury. On 12/4/54 a '3rd circular letter' issued a formal call for papers. By early April, 1955, there were 47 'nominee members' intending to be present. The constitution called for approval at the annual meeting. I have no official attendance record. I do have a list, dated 1/1/56 listing 67 members approved at the first meeting. Peter's wife, June who is still alive and reads the transactions annually, collected manuscripts in the back of the hall. I helped her and would estimate over 125 people in the Chelsea for that first meeting.

With a cast so stellar, it is dangerous to name names, but the original speaker's list contained such as Gibbon who built the first successful pump oxygenator, Dennis who used one early on, Bailey who invented finger valve fracture for mitral stenosis, Hufnagel the first to install an artificial aortic valve for repair of aortic stenosis and/or regurgitation, G. Murray from Toronto, who built the first dialyzer in North America, and Kolff of artificial kidney and heart fame. Kolff brought a large number of fellows (perhaps 8 or 10) and had them sleep two to a bed in a motel in the Atlantic City boondocks. He also brought a dozen of his new coil dialyzers for human use and gave them away – including one to me. I used it, cleaned it, saved it and was able to give it to the Artificial Organs Museum in Cleveland as the only surviving sample of Kolff's first batch with gray screening.

The first 5 presidents of the ASAIO were Kolff, Dennis, Salisbury, Clowes and Schreiner. All were present at that first meeting. June Salisbury transcribed the first transactions with typewriter and Peter published the first transactions with ditto machine. About 100 were printed and mailed. George Clowes was the second editor with me as assistant. I was named editor for volume III which was accepted by *Index Medicus* after adapting to offset printing with half-tones. I remained as editor for 29 years until Dr. Eli Friedman took over on volume XXXII, kindly naming me for life: 'Editor Emeritus' (fig. 4). Lippincott is now publisher. Volume XXXI included a supplement with memorable selections and a 30-year index.

The transactions cut a whole new swath in scientific communication that directly contributed to the explosive advances in artificial organs. It aimed for a 90-day after-the-meeting mailing. One volume made it in 59 days. The citation index rating was meteoric. Such data was unavailable from existing journals and greatly facilitated timely cross-fertilization. A good example was the classic 1960 publication of Scribner's first report on chronic dialysis [24]. This work was not finished in time to submit an abstract. It was printed within a few weeks by editorial privilege. We estimated it reached the indexed, published world fully 14–16 months before it would have by conventional methods. The ASAIO was an icon for the splintering of academic societies into ever more specialized and more technical groups. The events detailed in [25] have now kept more than 200,000 persons artificially alive in programs exceeding USD 10 billion and an industrial-research complex exceeding USD 100 billion. The ASAIO developed a vastly larger interest in bioengineering and research in medical devices such as artificial hearts, ventricular assist, pancreas, gut, eyes, ears, liver, nerve stimulators, pacemakers, etc. With them came a huge array of organizations such as the ISAO and societies for peritoneal dialysis, blood pumps, apheresis, membrane research, hemoperfusion, etc. The specific societies of one generation have become the general societies of the next.

I shall be criticized for giving this history an American slant. Certainly, the EDTA, the ISAO, The Australasian, The Latin-American and the many national Societies of Nephrology have made innovations and I hope that someone with personal experience will research and report on them. I have chosen to stick with organizations in which I have had extensive work and experience.

While researching my memories, I came upon this couplet written on a flyleaf in my own handwriting. I remember not whether I composed or copied it. Anyone who knows the author, please contact me:

Old men who can't remember last week
On strident tongues destroy the meek,
With memories flung by crossing winds,
Recounting all their meanest sins.

However, after a delightful rereading of Homer Smith's essays, I prefer to end with a paraphrase of his immortal words: 'We are what we are because we have the kind of kidneys we have.' Nephrology, today, is what it is because we have the kind of organizations we have. And we have the kind of organizations we have because we had the kind of early nephrologists we have as our everlasting endowment!

Acknowledgements

The author thanks Charles Plante and Drs. George F. Schreiner and Garabed Eknoyan for reading drafts of this manuscript, and making suggestions. Willian P. Schreiner gave valuable technical support.

References

1 Smith HW, Goldring W, Chasis H: The measurement of the tubular excretory mass, effective blood flow and filtration rate in the normal human kidney. J Clin Invest 1938;17:263–278.
2 Bright R: Reports of Medical Cases, Selected with a View of Illustrating the Symptoms and Cure of Diseases by a Reference to Morbid Anatomy. London, Longman, Rees, Orne, Brown & Green, 1827–31, vol 1, pp 1–231.
3 Volhard F: Uremia, chap 39; in Berglund H, Medes G (eds): The Kidney in Health and Disease. Philadelphia; Lea & Febiger, 1935, pp 1–754.
4 Schreiner GE, Maher JF: Uremia: Biochemistry, Pathogenesis and Treatment. Springfield, Thomas, 1961, pp 24–28.
5 Schreiner GE: The nephrotic syndrome; in Strauss MB, Welt LG (eds): Diseases of the Kidney, ed 2. Boston, Little, Brown, 1971, pp 503–636 + index.
6 Bradley SE: The Pathologic Physiology of Uremia in Chronic Bright's Disease. Springfield, Thomas, 1948, pp 1–69.
7 Smith HW: The Kidney Structure and Function in Health and Disease. New York, University Press, 1951, pp 1–1049.
8 Smith HW: Lectures on the Kidney. Porter Lectures Ser 9, 1943.
9 Smith HW, Chasis H, Goldring W, Ranges HA: Glomerular Dynamics in the Normal Human Kidney. J Clin Invest 1940;19:751.
10 Smith HWE: Kamongo. New York, The Viking Press, 1932, revised ed 1949.
11 Smith HW: Plato and Clementine. Bull NY Acad Med 1947;23:352.
12 Smith HW: From Fish To Philosopher. Boston, Little, Brown, 1953.
13 Smith HW: Highlights in the history of renal physiology. Bull Georgetown Univ Med Center 1959;13:4.
14 Smith HW: Complete Bibliography, pp 259–268; in Homer William Smith, ScD, New York.
15 Cutting RA, Koppanyi T: Effect of massive intravenous infusions of the course of barbiturate narcosis. Arch Int Pharmacodyn Ther 1938;60:395–409.
16 Koppanyi T, Linegar CR: Cross-circulation as a method of studying drug fixation and poisoning. Science 1942;96:562–563.
17 Schreiner GE, Berman LB, Griffin J, Feys J: Specific therapy for salicyclism. N Eng J Med 1955;253:213–217.
18 Berman LB, Jeghers HJ, Schreiner GE, Pallotta AJ: Hemodialysis: An effective therapy for acute barbiturate poisoning. JAMA 1956;161: 820–827.
19 Tannen RL: A quarter century of nephrology. ASN 1992:1–360.
20 Schreiner GE: Proceedings of the Third International Congress of Nephrology. Basel, Karger, 1967 vol 1, p 288, vol 2, p 363, vol 3, p 382.
21 Massry SG (ed): The National Kidney Foundation: The First 40 Years. Philadelphia, Saunders, 1990, pp 1–179.
22 Holy Bible, book of Daniel 12: 4 year of original publication unknown.
23 Schreiner GE: Trans Am Soc Artif Int Organs 1986;XXXI:1–185.
24 Scribner BH, Buri R: Caner JEZ, Hegstrom R, Burnell JM: The treatment of chronic uremia by means of chronic intermittent hemodialysis. Trans Am Soc Artif Intern Organs 1960;VI: 114–122.
25 Schreiner GE: How end-stage renal disease (ESRD) developed. Semin Nephrol 1997;17: 152–159.
26 Hamburger J, Crosnier J, Grunfeld JP: Nephrology. New York, Wiley-Flammarion, 1979, pp 1–1393.

Origins of Nephrology – The Modern Era

American Journal of Nephrology

Am J Nephrol 1999;19:304–307

Contributions of Camillo Golgi to Renal Histology and Embryology

Ilaria Dal Canton Alessandro L. Calligaro Francesca Dal Canton
Moris Frosio-Roncalli Alberto Calligaro

Nephrology Unit and Institute of Histology and General Embryology, IRCCS Policlinico San Matteo and University of Pavia, Italy

Key Words
Golgi · Renal hypertrophy · Tubular cell · Nephron dissection

Abstract
Camillo Golgi was awarded the Nobel prize in 1906 for his studies on the fine anatomy of the central nervous system. His wide present popularity depends on his discovery of the cell apparatus, the tendon mechanoreceptor and the tactile corpuscles of the fingertips that are named after him. However, Golgi also made important contributions to nephrology. In 1882, he published novel observations on the mechanism of renal hypertrophy, which he understood to be due to renal cell proliferation. Two years later, he described tubular cell mitoses in the kidney of a patient with tubulointerstitial nephritis, which he interpreted as an essential part of the repair process. His most important findings, published in 1889, were obtained by studying the microscopic anatomy of the kidney with an original technique that allowed the isolation of whole intact nephrons. He discovered that the ascending limb of Henle's loop always returned to the glomerulus from which the tubule originated, and he realized that the early distal tubule passed between the glomerular arterioles. In addition, applying the same method to dissect nephrons in progressive phases of development, he identified exactly what tubular segments originated from the various parts of the metanephric early S-shaped structure.

Notes on Camillo Golgi

The name of Camillo Golgi is one of the most frequently evoked in biological science. In fact, entering his name in a Medline search, one can find more than 22,000 citations, 700 of which appeared in the last year. The man destined to such a popularity was born in 1843 in Corteno, a small mountain village in the north of Lombardy, where his father served as municipal doctor. However, Golgi was only 7 years old when he left his native village to attend school in Pavia, a town that was the site of an ancient university with an outstanding tradition of biomedical research. Here, Golgi was enrolled in the Faculty of Medicine in 1859, just in the year in which Pavia was liberated from Austria. The political revolution that fol-

KARGER

Fax +41 61 306 12 34
E-Mail karger@karger.ch
www.karger.com

© 1999 S. Karger AG, Basel
0250–8095/99/0192–0304$17.50/0

Accessible online at:
http://BioMedNet.com/karger

Ilaria Dal Canton, PhD
Nephrology Unit and Institute of Histology and General Embryology, IRCCS
Policlinico San Matteo and University of Pavia
P. le Golgi, 2, I–27100 Pavia (Italy)
Tel. +39 382 422037, Fax +39 382 526341

lowed the incorporation of Pavia into the state of Italy was accompanied by changes in the organization of the Medical Faculty (Casati's act, 1859), the institution of new chairs (including General Pathology, Physiology, Clinical Neurology), and a thrust toward the experimental methods in medical research [1]. Actually, in Pavia this process of renovation met an old naturalistic tradition, previously sustained by Marcantonio Della Torre (1478–1511), Girolamo Cardano (1501–1576), Lazzaro Spallanzani (1729–1799) and Antonio Scarpa (1752–1832), and created great chances for young students interested in research. In fact, other students contemporary with Golgi were to become famous investigators: Enrico Sertoli (1842–1910), who gave his name to the cells in the testicles and Giulio Bizzozero (1846–1901) who discovered the platelets.

Golgi graduated in medicine in 1865, and after a short internship in neurology, he started working in the laboratory of General Pathology, where he soon devoted himself to studying the histology of the nervous system. In 1872, financial difficulties forced Golgi to accept a position in a modest province hospital in Abbiategrasso, not far from Pavia. However, he did not renounce research, and he transformed the kitchen of his modest apartment into a rudimentary laboratory. It was here, in this period of solitary work, distant from the Academy, that Golgi made his first important discovery. In fact, he prepared sections of nervous tissue colored with a completely original method, based on the use of a solution of silver nitrate, by which he could obtain black images of nerve cells and their prolongations never seen before. The 'black reaction' was the right instrument in the right hands, and Golgi, in the next few years, began to publish papers on the microscopic anatomy of the nervous system that rapidly introduced him to the scientific community as a respected investigator. In 1876, his reputation was so great that he gained a position of ordinary professor of Histology at the University of Pavia. Here he worked (later as professor of General Pathology) until he retired.

In 1906, Golgi was awarded the Nobel Prize for his studies on the nervous system. The prize acknowledged his contributions to understanding the fine anatomy of the brain, the cerebellum, the cord and to describing the nervous cell types that are still named for their discoverer. However, Golgi's outstanding contributions to the progress of biomedical science include the discovery of the cell apparatus that is named from him, of the tendon mechanoreceptor and of the tactile corpuscles of the fingertips. In addition, Golgi made important studies on malaria that led to the demonstration of the relation between the fever curves and the life cycle of the parasite (the *Plasmodium malariae* was first classified by Golgi).

Contributions of Golgi to Nephrology

In 1882, Golgi published his first paper on the kidney, which dealt with the mechanism of compensatory hypertrophy of the organ [2]. At that time, the increase in weight and volume occurring in the remnant kidney after unilateral nephrectomy was well known, but the opinions on its mechanism were contradictory. In fact, a few months before the publication of Golgi's paper, Ribbert concluded his studies on renal hypertrophy admitting that 'the anatomical conditions of a kidney enlarged after destruction or excision of the contralateral one are not yet clarified'. The prevalent opinion was still based on the old statement of Valentin (1839) that the increase in kidney weight is exclusively due to an increase in its content of blood and urinary fluid. An alternative theory was formulated by Rosenstein (1877). This author compared the dimensions of the tubules and of Malpighi's corpuscles in normal and hypertrophic kidney and, since he could find no difference, he concluded that there was no dilatation due to blood and urine accumulation. Therefore, he hypothesized that kidney enlargement was due to an increase in the number of tubules and glomeruli, that is, to the formation of new renal elements. The same idea was supported by Tizzoni and Pisenti (1882), who supposed that the new tubules originated from cells of the interstitium, in agreement with the current opinion that the tubules were 'passive', i.e. that tubular cells could not proliferate. The approach of Golgi to the problem was modern and elegant and was based on his exceptional ability at the microscope. Golgi was aware of the recent discovery that specific nuclear changes accompany and characterize cell proliferation, the changes described by Schleicher as 'Karyokinesis' and by Flemming as 'Indirecte Kernvermehrung'. Thus, he conceived that if he could find these nuclear changes in the kidney undergoing hypertrophy, he could understand both the mechanism and the cells responsible for the phenomenon. The results of his studies on the remnant kidney of uninephrectomized rabbits are depicted in figure 1 that is taken from Golgi's original paper. In the figure, Golgi reproduced the various phases of cell division occurring in the tubules, thus demonstrating that tubular cell proliferation can take place (the kidney is not 'passive') and actually accounts for renal hypertrophy.

1

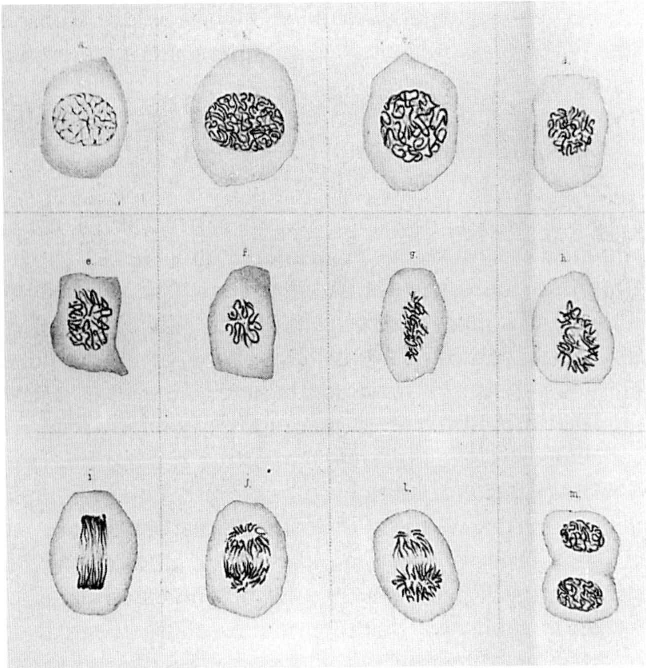

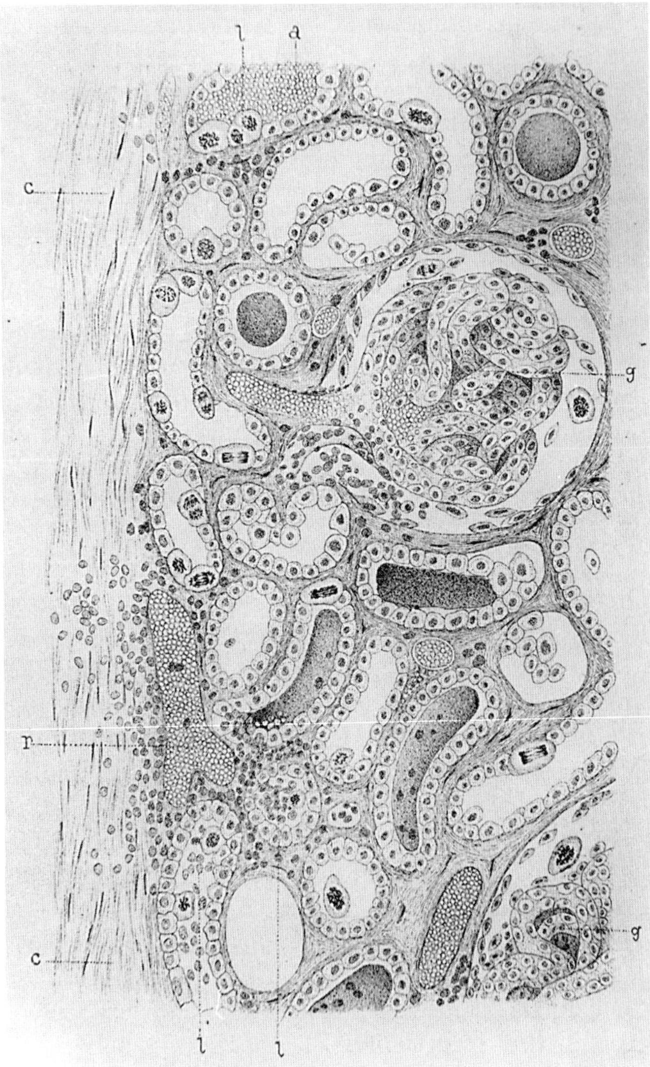

2

Fig. 1. Drawing taken from Golgi [2], showing mitotic figures observed in tubular cells of the remnant kidney after experimental unilateral nephrectomy.

Fig. 2. Drawing taken from Golgi [3], showing the histopathological picture of the kidney of a patient with Bright's disease. Letters are part of the original drawing; a, r = tubular casts; c = subcapsular space with inflammatory cell infiltrate; g = glomerulus; l = mitoses.

Two years later, Golgi applied the same methods to studying Bright's disease [3]. At that time, the diagnosis of Bright's disease was extended to any patient with edema, oliguria, hematuria and urinary casts and probably included both patients with glomerulonephritis and patients with tubulointerstitial disorders. Golgi had the chance to follow the clinical course of a patient with symptoms of Bright's disease and urinary casts made of tubular cells. The patient died of pneumonia 40 days after the appearance of renal symptoms, i.e. when the renal disease was in its recovery phase. Golgi made a histopathological study on the kidney and demonstrated that several tubular cells were undergoing mitosis (fig. 2), thus proving that the necrotic, detached cells forming the casts were replaced by new cells. Golgi studied another patient who died in the acute phase of Bright's disease and could not find mitotic figures in his kidney. Thus, he concluded that tubular cell proliferation was part of the repair process and not a consequence of tubular cell stimulation due to renal inflammation.

In 1889, Golgi published his most important contribution to histology and embryology of the kidney [4]. As the 'black reaction' was the tool that disclosed the structure of the nervous system, a new technique allowed Golgi's original observations on the fine anatomy and the development of the nephron. Traditionally, the shape of the nephron and the spatial relations of its various segments were reconstructed from sequences of microscopic sections of

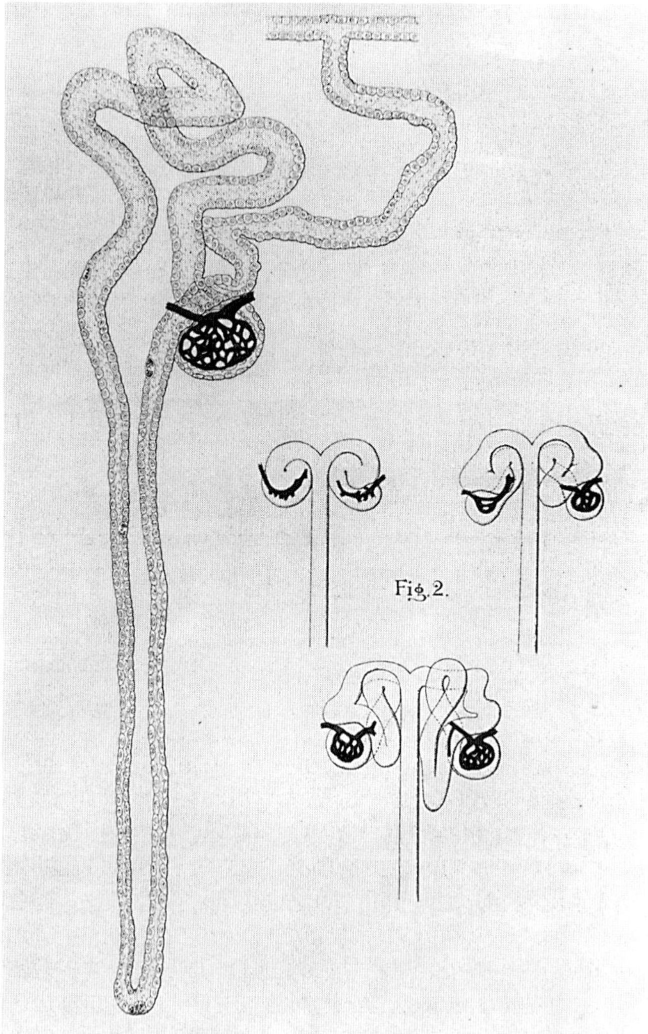

Fig. 3. Drawing taken from Golgi [4]. Figure 2 within the drawing refers to the number of the figure in the original paper. The drawing on the left shows the anatomical relation of the ascending limb of Henle's loop with the vascular pole of the glomerulus, and the drawings on the right show progressive stages of the developing nephron, starting from the early S-shaped metanephric formation.

the kidney. Golgi used a new approach consisting of studying whole intact nephrons obtained through an original process of maceration-hardening in an alcoholic solution of arsenic acid. Dissecting intact nephrons, he made the important discovery that the ascending limb of Henle's loop always returns to the glomerulus from which the tubule originates (he wrote 'con legge invariabile', with invariable law), and he precisely realized that the early distal tubule passes between the glomerular arterioles (fig. 3). These observations were absolutely new and contrasted with the current opinion based on Ludwig's authority that the ascending branch of Henle's loop 'avoids the labyrinth' (labyrinth means the cortex) and is always external to the glomerulus with respect to the descending one.

Applying the same method to dissect nephrons in progressive phases of development, Golgi could describe exactly from what parts of the S-shaped metanephric early structure the various definitive tubular segments originate (fig. 3). In addition, he associated tubule dissection with vascular dye injection, and he stated that glomerular capillaries form within Bowman's capsule, i.e. they do not push the capsule from outside as a 'fist pushes a deflated ball of caoutchouc'.

References

1 Mazzarello P: La Struttura Nascosta. La vita di Camillo Golgi, Capitolo Terzo. Bologna, Istituto Editoriale Universitario, 1996, pp 17–42.
2 Golgi C: Sulla ipertrofia compensatoria dei reni. Arch Sci Med 1882;6:346–356.
3 Golgi C: Neoformazione dell'epitelio dei canalicoli oriniferi nella malattia di Bright. Arch Sci Med 1884;8:961–971.
4 Golgi C: Annotazioni intorno all'istologia dei reni dell'uomo e di altri mammiferi e sull'istogenesi dei canalicoli oriniferi. Rendiconti R Accad Lincei 1889;5:545–557.

Origins of Nephrology – The Modern Era

American Journal of Nephrology

Am J Nephrol 1999;19:308–312

Renal Growth Factors: Past, Present and Future

F.P. Schena G.F.M. Strippoli P. Wankelmuth

Department of Intensive Care and Transplantation, Division of Nephrology, University of Bari, Polyclinic, Bari, Italy

Key Words
Growth factors · Renal hypertrophy · Chronic renal failure · Gene therapy

Abstract
It is known that a series of mediators, so-called growth factors, are able to induce hypertrophy of the kidney in a patient after uninephrectomy. The first investigator who demonstrated this phenomenon was C. Sacerdotti, an Italian pathologist of Bizzozero's School in Turin, who published an important report in 1896. He attempted to explain how compensatory renal hypertrophy occurred and how this hypertrophy might be induced in a normal dog. Interestingly, he demonstrated that when the kidneys of a normal dog received a blood transfusion from uni- or binephrectomized dogs several mitoses appeared in the renal epithelium. These mitoses, expression of renal hypertrophy, were more evident in dogs receiving several blood transfusions for 6–7 days. He concluded that hypertrophy was induced by specific substances circulating in the blood of uni- or binephrectomized dogs. This hypothesis was in the next 100 years confirmed by the discovery of renal growth factors such as epidermal growth factor, insulin-like growth factor-1, hepatocyte growth factor, platelet-derived growth factor and others. The pathogenic role of these mediators is evident in the recovery of tubules after acute tubular necrosis and in the remnant glomeruli after glomerular damage. Today, attempts to use these growth factors for improving renal function in patients with acute tubular necrosis and to block their action in the progression of renal damage in chronic glomerulonephritides are under investigation. Future trends in these growth factors will be set by drug companies designing specific therapies such as gene therapy. In conclusion, the outstanding observation by Sacerdotti, over a century ago, remains an important step in nephrologic history for prognosis and therapy of renal diseases.

Renal growth factors are soluble mediators synthesized by cells and released to influence the function of the cells that produce them (autocrine action) or the cells in the immediate vicinity (paracrine action). These intercellular messengers, by binding specific cell surface receptors on the target cell, trigger a cascade of events that influence cellular function. Thus, they modulate their own synthesis and secretion as well as the synthesis and secretion of other mediators such as cytokines.

A number of growth factors are synthesized within the kidney. They are normally involved in the renal development in many physiological regenerative processes such

KARGER

Fax + 41 61 306 12 34
E-Mail karger@karger.ch
www.karger.com

© 1999 S. Karger AG, Basel
0250–8095/99/0192–0308$17.50/0

Accessible online at:
http://BioMedNet.com/karger

F. Paolo Schena, MD
Division of Nephrology, Polyclinic
Piazza Giulio Cesare, 11
I-70124 Bari (Italy)
Tel. +39 80 5592237, Fax +39 80 5575188

as renal hypertrophy and tissue repair after tubular necrosis, and in pathological conditions, e.g glomerulonephritis, puromycin- and Adriamycin-induced nephrosis, diabetes and obstructive nephropathy [1].

This brief review summarizes the evolution of the meaning of renal growth factor in this century.

Past: Renal Hypertrophy

The search for renal growth factors has been pursued for over a century. In 1896, Sacerdotti, an assistant of the pathologist Bizzozero who was chief of the Institute of Pathology at the University of Turin, first demonstrated that the infusion of blood from uni- or binephrectomized dogs induced renal growth in normal dogs [1].

In the late 19th century, scientific investigators proposed several theories on renal hypertrophy. Cohnheim [2] suggested that renal hypertrophy was caused by the increased renal blood flow after uninephrectomy. Nothnagel [3] hypothesized that after uninephrectomy, many substances such as nutrients and catabolic products arrived in the remnant kidney and caused the proliferation of renal cells. The theory of Ziegler [4], however, was more acceptable than others. In his paper *Über die Ursachen der pathologischen Gewebsneubildungen,* he wrote that compensatory renal hypertrophy was characterized by the proliferation of resident cells induced by the catabolic substances arriving in the remnant kidney. On the other hand, Ribbert [5] suggested that hyperemia and the altered relationship between cells and the extracellular compartment were more important factors responsible for renal hypertrophy.

Sacerdotti moved from these theories to organizing his own experiments in dogs. Under the guidance of Bizzozero, he focused on comprehending how compensatory hypertrophy developed when urine excretion was reduced, and whether it was possible to induce renal hypertrophy in animals without uninephrectomy or other renal trauma.

He performed his experiments prevalently in dogs because they were more resistant than others to postnephrectomy infections. In a pilot study, he achieved uninephrectomy in several dogs and did not find the cessation of urine excretion other contemporary investigators had reported [6, 7]. He concluded that after uninephrectomy the remnant kidney compensated for lost function, since no accumulation of catabolic substances occurred. In addition, after a few days the remnant kidney exhibited compensatory renal hypertrophy. In a second study, Sacerdotti performed uninephrectomy in dogs with acute inanition and demonstrated that even in the presence of reduced urine excretion and a concomitant reduction of catabolic urinary substances, renal cell mitoses were present. Finally, Sacerdotti demonstrated that the continuous infusion of blood from bilaterally nephrectomized dogs for 5–6 days into normal dogs induced renal cell mitoses and hyperplasia of tubular cells in Henle's loop. These phenomena were not evident in normal dogs receiving blood transfusions from other normal dogs. This conclusive data demonstrated clearly that unknown substances occurring in uni- or total nephrectomized dogs were able to induce renal cell hyperplasia and hypertrophy in normal dog kidneys.

Subsequently, several investigators, in various time frames, demonstrated the occurrence of renal hypertrophy in uninephrectomized animals. Differences in results were due to the variable techniques, strain and age of animals and environmental conditions. The amount and rate of compensatory hypertrophy varied greatly with the age of the animal; in fact, in young animals the amount of hypertrophy was greater than in older animals.

The possibility that endocrine factors may influence the kidney was suggested by Selye and Friedman [8], who found that after ligation of one ureter, the kidney did not show atrophy if testosterone was administered. Zecker [9] first investigated the effect of various hormones on the amount of compensatory hypertrophy and discovered that thyroidectomy did not affect the amount of hypertrophy. Further, Astarabadi and Essex [10] found that the pituitary gland exerted some control over the amount of compensatory hypertrophy following uninephrectomy, since in hypophysectomized rats the kidney's weight only increased its value of about 15% while in control animals the increase was 83%.

There is no doubt that local factors or humoral agents with possible pituitary connections may influence compensatory renal hypertrophy after uninephrectomy. In 1964, in his thesis for a Bachelor of Science, Davison [11] discussed the early effects of uninephrectomy in the rat and demonstrated that in rat serum, after uninephrectomy, two proteins may be related to compensatory renal hypertrophy. Lowenstein and Stein [12] found that serum, taken after 48 h uninephrectomy and injected into normal animals, induced an increase in the uptake of tritiated thymidine by renal cells; thus, some humoral agents may be responsible for compensatory hyperplasia. Ogawa and Nowinski [13] found that if at day 2 postuninephrectomy serum was added to kidney explants in tissue culture, mitotic activity was stimulated. They found that the

Table 1. Main renal growth factors and their preferential action on renal cells

Growth factors	Synthesis sites	Target sites
IGFs	G, PCT	G, PCT
FGFs	G, I	G, I
PDGFs	G, DCT, CD	G, I
TGF-β	G, PCT, CD	G, I
VEGF	G, CD	G
ETs	G, PCT, DCT, CD	G, PCT, TAL
EGF	TAL, DCT	G, PCT, DCT, CD
TGF-α	TAL, DCT	G, PCT, DCT, CD
NGF	CD	G, CD
A II	PCT	PCT, I
Ost.	PCT, TAL, DCT	I
HGF	I	PCT

IGFs = Insulin-like growth factors; FGFs = fibroblast growth factors; VEGF = vascular endothelial growth factor; ETs = endothelins; EGF = epidermal growth factor; TGF-α = transforming growth factor-α; NGF = nerve growth factor; A II = angiotensin II; Ost. = osteopontin; HGF = hepatic growth factor; G = glomerular; PCT = proximal convoluted tubule; TAL = thick ascending limb of Henle loop; DCT = distal convoluted tubule; CD = collecting duct; I = interstitium.

Table 2. Renal pathological conditions with increased production of local growth factors

Glomerulonephritis
Acute tubular necrosis
Acute tubulointerstitial nephritis
Obstructive nephropathy
Acute renal rejection

constituent of the serum responsible for this was heat-stable at 56°C for 30 min but heat-labile at 100°C for 20 min and nondialyzable.

Present: Progression of Chronic Renal Failure

A number of growth factors synthesized within the kidney have been discovered during the past 100 years. Table 1 lists the main renal polypeptide growth factors and their preferential action on glomerular and tubular cells, the interstitium and the renal parenchymal vessels. Table 2 shows the renal pathological conditions in which there is an increased production of local growth factors.

In the remnant kidney this increase is mandatory to trigger compensatory growth of the remaining nephrons. The permanent and progressive loss of functioning nephrons, after the glomerular filtration rate decreases halfway from the normal level, leads to functional adaptations in the remaining nephrons. This phenomenon is very common in experimental and human glomerulopathies, and is characterized by nephron hypertrophy and an increase in the glomerular filtration rate in single nephron-meeting excretory demands [14].

Recent studies have shown that the expression and local synthesis of growth factors are increased after nephron reduction [15]. Progression of renal damage is characterized by glomerular and tubular cell injury which leads to local production and release of mitogenic growth factors, platelet-derived growth factor (PDGF) for resident cells, transforming growth factor-β (TGF-β) and fibroblast growth factor for fibroblasts and smooth muscle cells. These renal mediators are meant to play a role in the pathogenesis of glomerular sclerotic injury and tubulointerstitial fibrosis. In addition, other growth factors have recently been reviewed for the progression of renal damage and include angiotensin II, osteopontin and endothelin [16]. Angiotensin II promotes systemic and glomerular hypertension, increases macromolecular flow into the mesangium, increases proteinuria and stimulates tubular cells to produce and release growth factors into the interstitium, thus promoting interstitial fibrosis.

The beneficial effect of inhibiting angiotensin II on renal deterioration has been well established in experimental renal disease and in patients with chronic glomerulonephritis [17–19]. Recently, maneuvers for attenuating the effects of angiotensin II have been done by administering angiotensin-converting enzyme (ACE) inhibitors and angiotensin II receptor antagonists. Clinical trials in primary and secondary glomerulonephritides have been carried out and the results obtained show a decrease in the progression of renal damage [20–22]. In experimental models, the administration of ACE inhibitors demonstrated that these drugs had a renoprotective effect when the treatment started early in the course of the disease [23].

Future: Therapeutic Strategies

Measures to reduce the overproduction of growth factors in the partial ablation of the renal parenchyma and in the progressive loss of nephrons in chronic renal failure have been considered by several investigators [24].

Beneficial effects may be obtained by using several strategies (table 3).

The process by which these short-living factors are produced and exert their actions is divided into three stages: (1) interaction of these factors with their specific cell surface receptors, (2) transmission of the external signal in the cell by the signal transduction process, and (3) synthesis and secretion of growth factors. Therefore, it is necessary to develop new therapeutic strategies able to interfere with these three biological events.

A variety of natural and synthetic molecules can competitively inhibit the binding of growth factors to their specific cell surface receptors, thus blocking their interaction. Trapidil, an antiplatelet drug, can compete with the interaction between PDGF and its receptor and therefore, inhibit PDGF's mitogenic effect [25]. Its administration in the anti-Thy-1 experimental glomerulonephritis significantly improved the clinical and histopathological changes noted [26].

In rats with mesangioproliferative glomerulonephritis, administration of an antibody against TGF-β has been shown to improve the course of the disease, since a reduction of extracellular matrix production and an accumulation in the injured glomeruli resulted after use of the antibody [27]. In the same model of glomerulonephritis, however, a natural inhibitor of this growth factor, decorin, may also antagonize TGF-β actions, thus obtaining the same results [28].

The blockade of the intracellular signalling may be another valuable tool for inhibiting the effect of growth factors excessively produced in pathological conditions. Hydroxy-methylglutaryl CoA reductase inhibitors can inhibit PDGF-induced mesangial cell proliferation or LPS-stimulated NF-kB activation in mesangial cells through the inhibition of p21 ras [29, 30] which is a small intracellular protein playing a central role in the signal transduction pathways of most growth factors. Instead, Cyclosporin A and FK506 bind to calcineurin which is a critical factor of the T cell activation pathway regulating the T-cell-specific transcription factor, NF-AT [31]. A specific inhibitor of PKC-β can significantly reduce glomerular hyperfiltration and microalbuminuria in rats with diabetes [32].

Current strategies involve the use of either modified or attenuated retro- or adenoviruses or DNA-liposome mixtures as vectors for carrying genetic material into the cell. The best way to achieve local production of a specific factor is by ex vivo gene therapy. This approach consists of removing target cells from the body, introducing the new genetic material in vitro, and replacing the 'modified' cells in the body, where they can produce the desired protein. In rats affected with anti-Thy-1 nephritis, Kitamura et al. [33] infused mesangial cells transfected with TGF-β1 into the kidney via renal artery injection and achieved recovery of acute glomerular injury by reducing mitogenesis of resident cells.

Expression of specific growth factor genes may be blocked using antisense oligonucleotides which inhibit the synthesis of a given factor by hybridizing to target sequences within the mRNA coding for that factor, destabilizing the target mRNA and consequently decreasing its translation into protein. Akagi et al. [34] treated rats with anti-Thy-1 nephritis by administrating TGF-β antisense oligonucleotides and demonstrated a reduced expression of this growth factor with a concomitant reduction of extracellular matrix synthesis and deposition.

Considering the results of growth factor studies, published within the last 100 years, encouraging progress has been made in understanding the role of these mediators in promoting physiological processes such as renal hypertrophy and the progression of damage in renal diseases. Now investigators must concentrate on applying more qualitative approaches for improving the response to therapy which consists in the blockade of renal damage.

Table 3. Therapeutic strategies for controlling the renal overproduction of growth factors

Experimental models	Neutralizing antibodies Antisense oligonucleotides Natural inhibitors
Experimental models and human diseases	Low protein diet ACE inhibitors Receptor antagonists

References

1 Sacerdotti C: Über die compensatorische Hypertrophie der Nieren. Virchows Arch Pathol Anat 1896;146:267–297.

2 Cohnheim: Vorlesungen über allgemeine Pathologie, 1882, vol 1.

3 Nothnagel H: Über Anpassungen und Ausgleichungen bei pathologischen Zuständen. Z Klin Med 1886;11.

4 Ziegler: Über die Ursachen der pathologischen Gewebsneubildungen. Virchow's Festschrift 1891;2.

5 Ribbert: Das pathologische Wachsthum der Gewebe bei der Hypertrophie, Regeneration, Entzündung und Geschwulstbildung. Bonn, 1896.

6 De Paoli: Della resezione del rene. Studio sperimentale. Perugia, 1891.

7 Tuffier: Etudes expérimentales sur la chirurgie du rein. Paris, 1889.

8 Selye H, Friedman SN: Beneficial action of testosterone in experimental renal atrophy caused by ligation of ureter. Endrocrinology 1941;29: 80.

9 Zecker IT: Compensatory growth of the kidney after unilateral nephrectomy in thyroidectomized rats. Am J Physiol 1945;145:681.

10 Astarabadi T, Essex H: Effect of hypophysectomy on compensatory renal hypertrophy after unilateral nephrectomy. Am J Physiol 1953; 173:526.

11 Davison AM: Early Effects of Uninephrectomy in the Rat. Bachelor of Science, Edinburgh University, 1964.

12 Lowenstein LH, Stern A: Serum factor in renal compensatory hyperplasia. Science 1963;142: 1479.

13 Ogawa K, Nowinski WN: Mitosis stimulating factor in serum of unilaterally nephrectomized rats. Proc Soc Exp Biol 1958;99:350.

14 Hostetter TH, Troy JL, Brenner BM: Glomerular hemodynamics in experimental diabetes mellitus. Kidney Int 1981;19:410–415.

15 Fine LG, Hammerman MR, Abboud HE: Evolving role of growth factors in the renal response to acute and chronic disease. J Am Soc Nephrol 1992;2:1163–1170.

16 Johnson RJ: Cytokines, growth factors and renal injury: Where do we go now? Kidney Int 1997;52(suppl 63):2–6.

17 Ruiz-Ortega M, Gonzales S, Jeron D, Condom E, Bustos C, Largo R, Gonzales E, Oritz A, Egido J: ACE-inhibition reduces proteinuria, glomerular lesions and extracellular matrix production in a normotensive rat model of immune-complex nephritis. Kidney Int 1995;48: 1778–1791.

18 Ruilope LM, Miranda B, Morales JM, Rodicio JL, Romero JC, Raij L: Converting enzyme inhibition in chronic renal failure. Am J Kidney Dis 1989;13:120–126.

19 Gansevoort RT, Sluiter WJ, Hemmelder MH, De Zeeuw D, De Jong DE: Antiproteinuric effect of blood-pressure lowering: A meta-analysis of comparative trials. Nephrol Dial Transplant 1995;10:1963–1974.

20 Lewis EJ, Hunsicker LG, Bain RP, Rohde RD: The effect of angiotensin-converting enzyme inhibition on diabetic nephropathy. N Engl J Med 1993;329:1456–1462.

21 Maschio G, Alberti D, Janin G, Locatelli F, Mann JFE, Motolese M, Ponticelli C, Ritz E, and the Angiotensin-Converting-Enzyme Inhibition in Progressive Renal Insufficiency Study Group: Effect of the angiotensin-converting enzyme inhibitor benazepril on the progression of chronic renal insufficiency. N Engl J Med 1996;334:939–945.

22 The Gisen Group (Gruppo Italiano Studi Epidemiologici in Nefrologia): Randomized placebo-controlled trial of effect of ramipril on decline in glomerular filtration rate and progression to terminal renal failure in proteinuric non-diabetic nephropathy. Lancet 1997;349: 1857–1863.

23 Perico N, Amuchastegui SC, Colosio V, Sonzoni G, Bertani T, Remuzzi G: Evidence that an angiotensin-converting enzyme inhibitor has a different effect on glomerular injury according to the different phase of the disease at which the treatment is started. J Am Soc Nephrol 1994;5:1139–1146.

24 Schena FP, Gesualdo L, Grandaliano G, Montinaro V: Progression of renal damage in human glomerulonephritides: Is there sleight of hand in winning the game? Kidney Int 1997; 52:1439–1457.

25 Gesualdo L, Di Paolo S, Ranieri E, Schena FP: Trapidil inhibits human mesangial cell proliferation: Effect on PDGF β receptor binding and expression. Kidney Int 1994;46:1002–1009.

26 Futamura A, Iida H, Izumino K, Entani C, Takata M: Effect of platelet-derived growth factor antagonist trapidil on rat mesangial cell proliferation (abstract). J Am Soc Nephrol 1992;3:588.

27 Border WA, Okuda S, Languino LR, Sporn MB, Ruoslahti E: Suppression of experimental glomerulonephritis by antiserum against transforming growth factor-β. Nature 1990;346: 371–374.

28 Border WA, Noble NA, Yamamoto T, Harper JR, Yamaguchi Y, Pierschbacher MD, Ruoslahti E: Natural inhibitor of transforming growth factor-β protects against scarring in experimental kidney disease. Nature 1992;360: 361–364.

29 Grandaliano G, Biswas P, Choudhury GG, Abboud HE: Simvastatin inhibits PDGF-induced DNA synthesis in human glomerular mesangial cells. Kidney Int 1993;44:503–508.

30 Guijarro C, Kim Y, Schoonover CM, Massy ZA, O'Donnell MP, Kasiske BL, Keane WF, Kashtan CE: Lovastatin inhibits lipopolysaccharide-induced NF-kB activation in human mesangial cells. Nephrol Dial Transplant 1996; 11:990–996.

31 Bennett WM, Demattos A, Meyer MM, Andoh T, Barry JM: Chronic cyclosporin nephropathy: The Achilles' heel of immunosuppressive therapy. Kidney Int 1996;50:1089–1100.

32 Ishii H, Jirousek MR, Koya D, Takagi C, Xia P, Clermont A, Bursel SE, Kern TS, Ballas LM, Heath WF, Stramm LE, Feener EP, King GL: Amelioration of vascular dysfunction in diabetic rats by an oral PKC β inhibitor. Science 1996;272:728–731.

33 Kitamura M, Burton S, English J, Kawachi H, Fine LG: Transfer of a mutated gene encoding active transforming growth factor-β1 suppresses mitogenesis and IL-1 response in the glomerulus. Kidney Int 1995;48:1747–1757.

34 Akagi Y, Isaka Y, Arai M, Kaneko T, Moriyama T, Kaneda Y, Ando A, Orita Y, Kamada T, Ueda N, Imai E: Inhibition of TGF-β1 expression by antisense oligonucleotides suppressed extracellular matrix accumulation in experimental glomerulonephritis. Kidney Int 1996; 50:148–155.

Origins of Nephrology – The Modern Era

American Journal of Nephrology

Am J Nephrol 1999;19:313–319

A History of Eclampsia, Toxemia and the Kidney in Pregnancy

Mabel L. Purkerson Lilla Vekerdy

Renal Division, Department of Medicine, and The Bernard Becker Medical Library, Washington University School of Medicine, St. Louis, Mo., USA

Key Words
Pregnancy · Eclampsia · Toxemia · Proteinuria

Abstract
Eclampsia, accompanied by convulsions, is one of the most dangerous complications of pregnant women. This condition was known to the ancient Greeks, who named it eclampsia. Prior to the 18th century, the term eclampsia was used only to refer to the visual phenomena which accompanied the neurologic aspects of the malady. Rayer's landmark contribution (1839–1841) provided evidence for renal involvement with the observation of protein in the urine of pregnant, edematous women. Lever (1843) reported finding proteinuria in eclampsia and concluded that disappearance of proteinuria after delivery of the child was evidence that eclampsia was different from Bright's disease.

Toxemia is a symptom complex that consists of hypertension, proteinuria, edema, and central nervous system irritability. Typically toxemia occurs in late pregnancy. It has been classified into eclampsia (if the above symptoms are present and convulsions occur) and pre-eclampsia (if the symptom complex is present and convulsions are absent) [1]. For this article, we will refer to the symptom complex as toxemia. In theory, resolution of all symptoms will occur following delivery, unless renal disease or hypertension were pre-existing conditions before the pregnancy. More is known today about toxemia of pregnancy, and the kidney in pregnancy than ever before, but even so, knowledge remains incomplete concerning the exact etiology and factors which determine severity of clinical manifestations of this entity peculiar to pregnancy. Current research focuses on the possible etiological role of prostaglandin deficiency, uteroplacental ischemia, intravascular coagulation, and immunological factors [2]. Depending upon which possible theory has been advocated to best explain mechanisms of the disease process, it has appeared under various headings: puerperal convulsions, puerperal nephritis and albuminuria, puerperal albuminuria and convulsions, eclampsia, pre-eclampsia, and more recently as pregnancy-induced hypertension. In the present study, we will present information concerning what was known of the early history of toxemia of pregnancy up to and including 19th century evidence for involvement of the kidney.

Ancient Beginnings

Eclampsia was familiar to the ancients. The danger of convulsions in pregnancy was noted in the literature of the ancient Egyptians and Chinese. Eclampsia is alluded to in the pre-Hippocratic *Coan Prognosis*: 'In pregnancy, drowsiness and headache accompanied by heaviness and convulsions, is generally bad' (XXXI, 507). Pre-eclampsia

KARGER
Fax + 41 61 306 12 34
E-Mail karger@karger.ch
www.karger.com

© 1999 S. Karger AG, Basel
0250–8095/99/0192–0313$17.50/0

Accessible online at:
http://BioMedNet.com/karger

Mabel L. Purkerson, MD
Box 8132, Washington University School of Medicine
660 South Euclid Avenue, St. Louis, MO 63110-1093 (USA)
Tel. +1 314 362 4234, Fax +1 314 362 6839
E-Mail purkerm@msnotes.wustl.edu

1

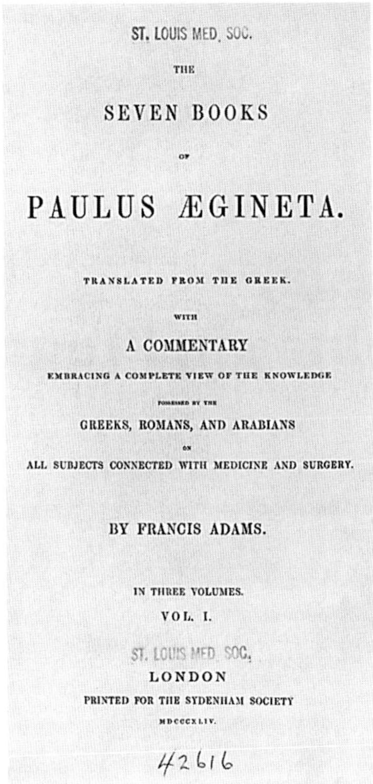
ST. LOUIS MED. SOC.

THE

SEVEN BOOKS

OF

PAULUS ÆGINETA.

TRANSLATED FROM THE GREEK.

WITH

A COMMENTARY

EMBRACING A COMPLETE VIEW OF THE KNOWLEDGE

POSSESSED BY THE

GREEKS, ROMANS, AND ARABIANS

ON

ALL SUBJECTS CONNECTED WITH MEDICINE AND SURGERY.

BY FRANCIS ADAMS.

IN THREE VOLUMES.

VOL. I.

ST. LOUIS MED. SOC.

LONDON

PRINTED FOR THE SYDENHAM SOCIETY

MDCCCXLIV.

42616

2

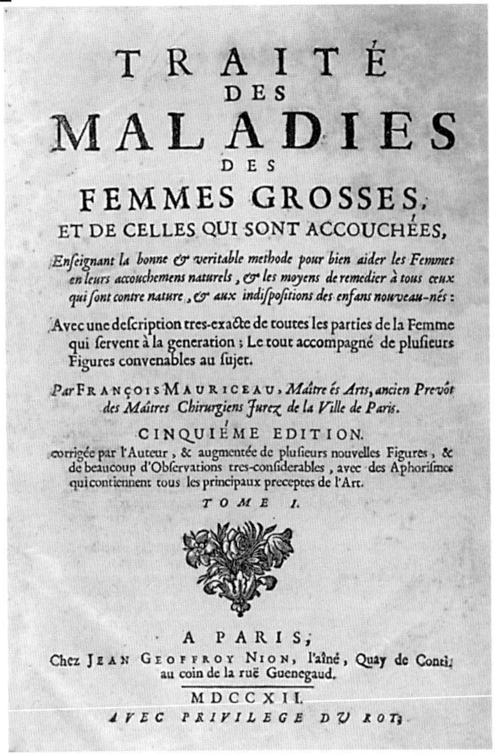
TRAITÉ

DES

MALADIES

DES

FEMMES GROSSES,

ET DE CELLES QUI SONT ACCOUCHÉES,

Enſeignant la bonne & veritable methode pour bien aider les Femmes en leurs accouchemens naturels, & les moyens de remedier à tous ceux qui ſont contre nature, & aux indiſpoſitions des enfans nouveau-nés :

Avec une deſcription tres-exacte de toutes les parties de la Femme qui ſervent à la generation ; Le tout accompagné de pluſieurs Figures convenables au ſujet.

Par FRANÇOIS MAURICEAU, *Maître és Arts, ancien Prevôt des Maîtres Chirurgiens Jurez de la Ville de Paris.*

CINQUIÉME EDITION.

Corrigée par l'Auteur, & augmentée de pluſieurs nouvelles Figures, & de beaucoup d'Obſervations tres-conſiderables, avec des Aphoriſmes qui contiennent tous les principaux preceptes de l'Art.

TOME I.

A PARIS,

Chez JEAN GEOFFROY NION, l'aîné, Quay de Conti, au coin de la ruë Guenegaud.

MDCCXII.

AVEC PRIVILEGE DU ROY.

Fig. 1. Title page of Paulus Aegineta's *De re medica* in the translation of Francis Adams, published in three volumes in 1844–47 [reproduced from 6] (courtesy of the Bernard Becker Medical Library, Washington University, St. Louis).

Fig. 2. Title page of François Mauriceau's *Traité des maladies des femmes* ... This fifth edition was published in 1712 [reproduced from 12] (courtesy of the Bernard Becker Medical Library, Washington University, St. Louis).

possibly was described in another line from the same work: 'In pregnancy, the onset of drowsy headaches with heaviness is bad; such cases are perhaps liable to some sort of fits at the same time' (XXXI, 523) [3]. Chesley [4] in discussing the origin of the word 'eclampsia' notes that most textbooks of obstetrics credit its derivation from a Greek word, 'eklampsis' which means 'shining forth', so called because it referred to the sudden appearance of convulsions. We are uncertain when this term was introduced, or to whom it should be attributed. Though some have written that Hippocrates wrote on this subject, the Adams translation of *The Genuine Works of Hippocrates* [5] does not mention eclampsia anywhere, nor does Hippocrates in his book, 'On the Sacred Disease', about epilepsy, describe pregnancy associated with convulsions. The well-respected 7th-century Greek physician, Paulus Aegineta (625–690) wrote a medical epitome in seven books (fig. 1), compiling the complete view of medical and surgical knowledge possessed by the Greeks, Romans and Arabians up to his time. Paul mentioned this condition in writing about 'epilepsy' (the term used by many ancients to refer to convulsions). He notes (Book iii, Chapter xiii): 'It has also been seen to proceed from the uterus in females at the time they were pregnant, for after delivery it ceased' [6].

It was recognized that in some cases children might be delivered live, despite the death of the mother during convulsions in childbirth, if the uterus were opened immediately after the death of the woman. However, during this period, all such Cesarian sections were only permitted postmortem. Mettler notes a 'lex regia' (instituted ca. 600 BC). This law provided 'that no pregnant woman dying in childbirth might be buried without abdominal section to remove the product of conception'. Mettler credits 'this law to Numa Pompilius, second legendary king of Rome (715–672 BC). This law represented one of those customs existing before Rome, which was sanctified by time'. The operation was never performed on the living mother. It is not until the 16th century that we have evidence of the performance of an abdominal extraction in a living woman [7].

Medieval Medicine

A dearth of activity appears to have surrounded the field of obstetrics and gynecology during the period of the Middle Ages. Chesley [8] notes that it is not surprising there are so few references to eclampsia in the older writings because obstetrics still was largely in the hands of

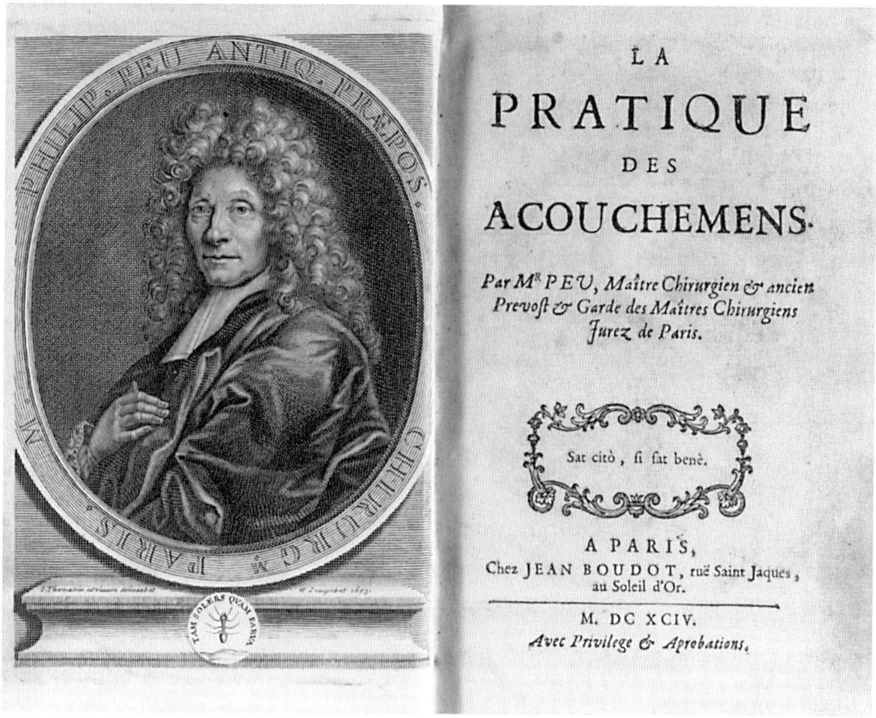

Fig. 3. Frontispiece portrait and title page of Philippe Peu's *La pratique des accouchements* [reproduced from 16] (courtesy of the Bernard Becker Medical Library, Washington University, St. Louis).

midwives and eclampsia still had not been differentiated from epilepsy.

Midwives of this time were said to have written procedures (now lost) which were followed. They may have compiled these works or the writings may have been physicians' communications to the midwives. Midwives consulted physicians regarding their patients when complications developed. 'In 1452 the city of Regensburg instituted a midwifery code, and, gradually, the examination of midwives by the members of the medical profession became an established Continental practice' [9].

Sixteenth and Seventeenth Centuries

It is during the 16th century that Cesarian operations to deliver difficult labors were begun in the living mother [10]. There still was no differentiation between convulsions associated with epilepsy and those observed with eclampsia in late pregnancy. The literature of eclampsia really begins in the 17th century, when male French physicians entered the field and exerted a positive influence on obstetrics [11].

François Mauriceau's (1637–1709) book, *Traité des maladies des femmes grosses et accouchées* [12], was first published in 1668 (fig. 2). The celebrated French obstetrician and leading representative of obstetric knowledge of the time, wrote on the diseases of pregnant and puerperal women. The book was considered to be the state-of-the-art in its time, giving a good account of normal labor, employment of version and management of placenta previa. In this book, he mentions only convulsions associated with severe obstetric hemorrhage and writes that this was the cause of his sister's death. His aphorisms in subsequent editions show definite familiarity with the problem of eclampsia [13]:

> The mortal danger to mother and fetus is greater when the mother does not recover consciousness between convulsions (number 228); Primigravidas are at far greater risk of convulsions than are multiparas (number 229); Convulsions during pregnancy are more dangerous than those beginning after delivery (number 230); Convulsions are more dangerous when the fetus is dead than when it is alive (number 231).

Even though Mauriceau was unable to clearly differentiate eclampsia from epilepsy, he probably recognized its existence, when he credited the convulsions 'to an excess of hot blood flowing from the uterus to stimulate the nervous system, with aggravation by cervical irritation'. In addition, he assumed that 'when the fetus dies, malignant vapors arising from the dead and decomposing fetus might cause convulsions' [14]. Mauriceau's book was translated into English by Hugh Chamberlen, Sr. He retitled it *The Accomplisht Midwife* and in 1673 published it under his name [15].

A pupil of Mauriceau, Philippe Peu (d. 1707), a Paris obstetrician and chief surgeon in the Hôtel Dieu published his *Pratique des accouchements,* in 1694 [16] (fig. 3). In this book he wrote about clonic spasms in pregnancy. Even though *Pratique des accouchements* received scathing criticism from Mauriceau, Peu maintained an excellent professional reputation, due to his experience with four to five thousand deliveries [17].

It is apparent that convulsions associated with pregnancy had been recognized for a long time. Mauriceau's discussions and descriptions of them were excellent. However, it would be the 19th century before real advances and a further understanding of the condition would be made.

Eighteenth Century

During the period of the 18th century, the battle to understand the cause and to conquer puerperal fever occupied much attention. Throughout the century, obstetricians continued to write concerning benefits of induction of premature labor to speed delivery in cases of convulsions associated with pregnancy. Early in the 18th century (1721), Guillaume Manquest de la Motte (1665–1737) recognized the beneficial effect of delivery for patients with convulsions for he noted, 'I delivered the mother, and the convulsions immediately ceased'. De la Motte was almost 70 years old when he published his *Traité complet des accouchements* [18] (fig. 4). He was a country practitioner and his book was a compilation of observations and reflections based upon his more than 30-year-long practice. Thomas Denman (1733–1815) writing first in his book, *Essays on Puerperal Fever and on Puerperal Convulsions* (1768) [19], and later in *An Introduction to the Practice of Midwifery* (1788) [20], discussed medical management versus termination of pregnancy. Difficult deliveries were assisted through development and understanding of measurements of the pelvis. Forceps extractions [not actually a late invention for early use of forceps was traced to Avicenna (980–1037)] and podalic version of the fetus to facilitate delivery were definite advances to assist in treating the mechanical process of labor [21]. Forceps were useful for delivery of cases where convulsions threatened mother and child; where there was cessation of labor; and in cases of threatened hemorrhage. The first distinction between epilepsy and

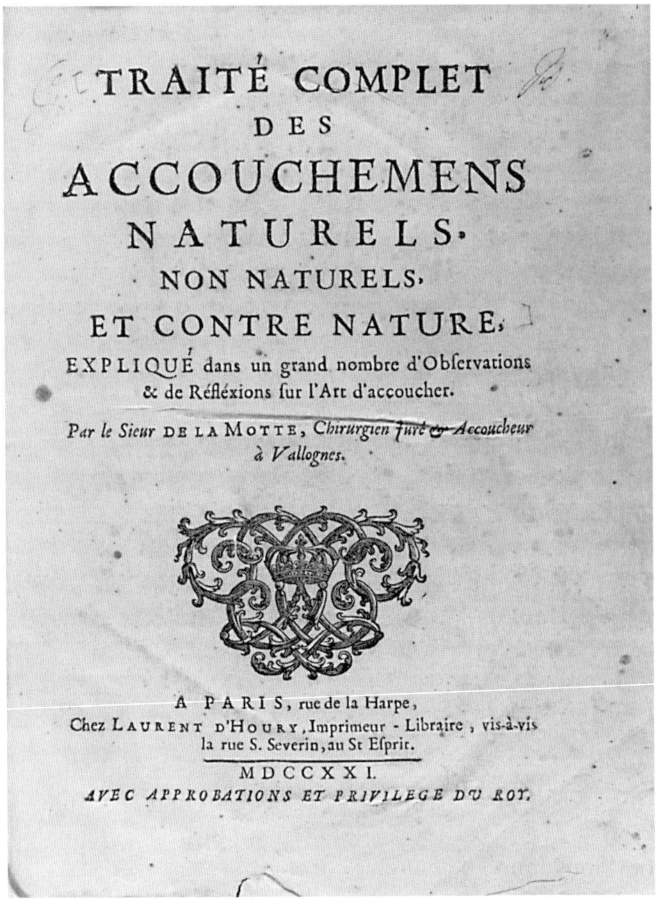

TRAITÉ COMPLET
DES
ACCOUCHEMENS
NATURELS,
NON NATURELS,
ET CONTRE NATURE,
EXPLIQUÉ dans un grand nombre d'Obſervations & de Réflexions ſur l'Art d'accoucher.

Par le Sieur DE LA MOTTE, *Chirurgien Juré & Accoucheur à Vallognes.*

A PARIS, rue de la Harpe,
Chez LAURENT D'HOURY, Imprimeur - Libraire, vis-à-vis la rue S. Severin, au St Eſprit.
MDCCXXI.
AVEC APPROBATIONS ET PRIVILEGE DU ROY.

Fig. 4. Title page of Guillaume Mauquest de la Motte's *Traité complet des accouchements naturels, non naturels et contre nature* ... [reproduced from 18] (courtesy of the Bernard Becker Medical Library, Washington University, St. Louis).

eclamptic convulsions was made by François Boissier de Sauvages (1706–1767) when in 1739 he published *Pathologia methodica* [22]. De Sauvages [23] considered epilepsy a chronic disorder and eclampsia an acute disorder, describing the two entities as two separate problems. Later, de Sauvages (1763) used the term 'eclampsia parturiemtium' for convulsions in pregnancy and 'eclampsia ab ischuria' for uremic convulsions [24]. Garrison [25] described the 18th century medicine as an age of theorists and system-makers. Some of these system-makers, following Sydenham's suggestion that the natural history of disease should be studied in the same spirit that natural objects were studied, felt obliged to classify diseases just as plants and animals were classified, i.e., classes, orders, and genre. De Sauvages was one of the 'system-makers' and he initiated the movement with his publications. It appears that others of his time were reluctant to change

5

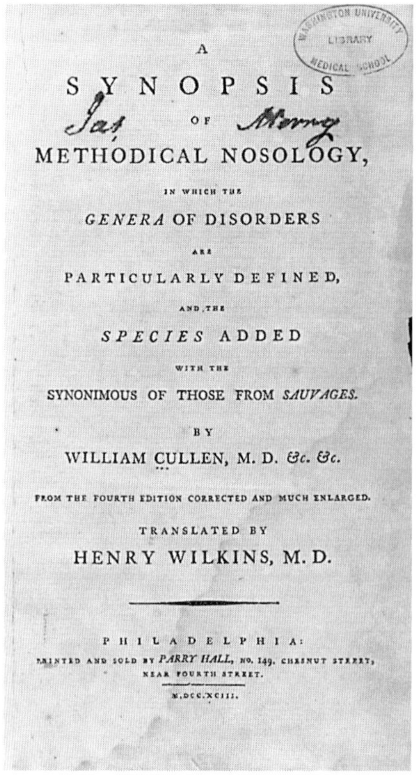

A
SYNOPSIS
OF
METHODICAL NOSOLOGY,
IN WHICH THE
GENERA OF DISORDERS
ARE
PARTICULARLY DEFINED,
AND THE
SPECIES ADDED
WITH THE
SYNONIMOUS OF THOSE FROM *SAUVAGES*.
BY
WILLIAM CULLEN, M. D. &c. &c.
FROM THE FOURTH EDITION CORRECTED AND MUCH ENLARGED.
TRANSLATED BY
HENRY WILKINS, M. D.
PHILADELPHIA:
PRINTED AND SOLD BY *PARRY HALL*, NO. 149, CHESNUT STREET, NEAR FOURTH STREET.
M.DCC.XCIII.

6

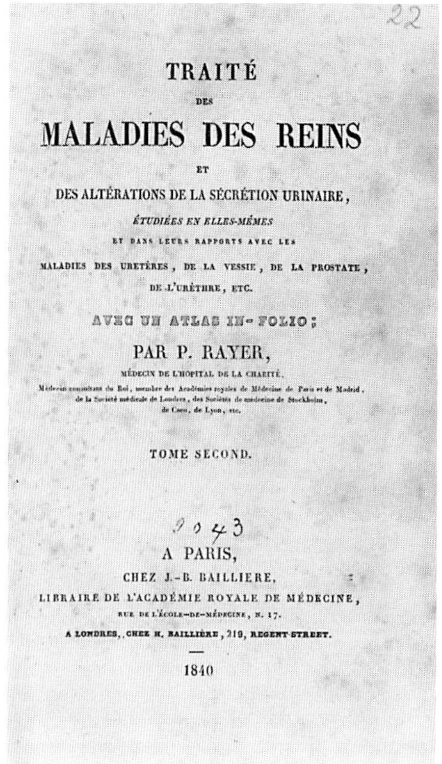

TRAITÉ
DES
MALADIES DES REINS
ET
DES ALTÉRATIONS DE LA SÉCRÉTION URINAIRE,
ÉTUDIÉES EN ELLES-MÊMES
ET DANS LEURS RAPPORTS AVEC LES
MALADIES DES URETÈRES, DE LA VESSIE, DE LA PROSTATE, DE L'URÈTHRE, ETC.
AVEC UN ATLAS IN-FOLIO;
PAR P. RAYER,
MÉDECIN DE L'HOPITAL DE LA CHARITÉ.
TOME SECOND.
A PARIS,
CHEZ J.-B. BAILLIERE,
LIBRAIRE DE L'ACADÉMIE ROYALE DE MÉDECINE,
RUE DE L'ÉCOLE-DE-MÉDECINE, N. 17.
A LONDRES, CHEZ H. BAILLIÈRE, 219, REGENT-STREET.
1840

Fig. 5. William Cullen, *A synopsis of methodical nosology* ... published in 1793; title page [reproduced from 23] (courtesy of the Bernard Becker Medical Library, Washington University, St. Louis).

Fig. 6. Pierre François Olive Rayer, *Traité des maladies des reins et des altérations de la sécrétion urinaire*; title page [reproduced from 30] (courtesy of the Bernard Becker Medical Library, Washington University, St. Louis).

opinions and acceptance of his distinction between eclampsia and epilepsy does not seem to have been gained quickly. As late as 1793, in William Cullen's (1710–1790) classification [26] (fig. 5) we find eclampsia and epilepsy still discussed together. Cullen [27], an eminent clinician, who led Edinburgh University Medical School to greatness, wrote:

> But as it is always difficult to fix the limits between acute and chronic disorders, and as the eclampsia of Sauvages for the most part exactly agrees with epilepsy, in cause as well as symptoms, I could by no means receive it for a different genus.

'In 1797, Demanet wrote that all six of his eclamptic patients had anasarca and suggested that edema be added to the three recognized causes of convulsions: depletion, repletion, and the pains of labor' [28].

Nineteenth Century

While little or no progress was made during the 19th century in management of the toxemias of pregnancy, the recognition that these conditions were definitely associated with the pregnant state and not just incidental illnesses was an advance for that time. Improvement of the microscope now allowed microscopic examination of the patient's urinary sediment.

In 1840, the well-known French pathologist Pierre François Rayer (1793–1867) demonstrated proteinuria in 3 edematous pregnant women. Prof. Richet has reviewed [29] the *Preface* and the *Prolegomenas* of Rayer's *Treatise (Traité des Maladies des Reins et des Altérations de la Sécrétion Urinaire* [30] (fig. 6) and has provided us excellent insight into the methods Rayer developed for scientific study and his comprehensive approach to clinical problems of nephrology. Giant steps were made in understanding toxemia with recognition that proteinuria was associated with eclampsia and pre-eclampsia.

John Charles Lever (1811–1858), of London, was struck by the resemblance of his eclamptic patients and those who had nephritis on the service of his colleague Richard Bright. This prompted him to examine the urine of the eclamptic patients for proteinuria. He made the important observation that convulsing pregnant women with edema, blurred vision and headaches had albuminuria in their urine. He reported his findings for 14 cases (these were collected between 1834 and 1843) of puerperal convulsions in a 1843 publication from Guy's Hospital (fig. 7). His suspicion was confirmed that the above symptoms were part of the same disorder and signs of impend-

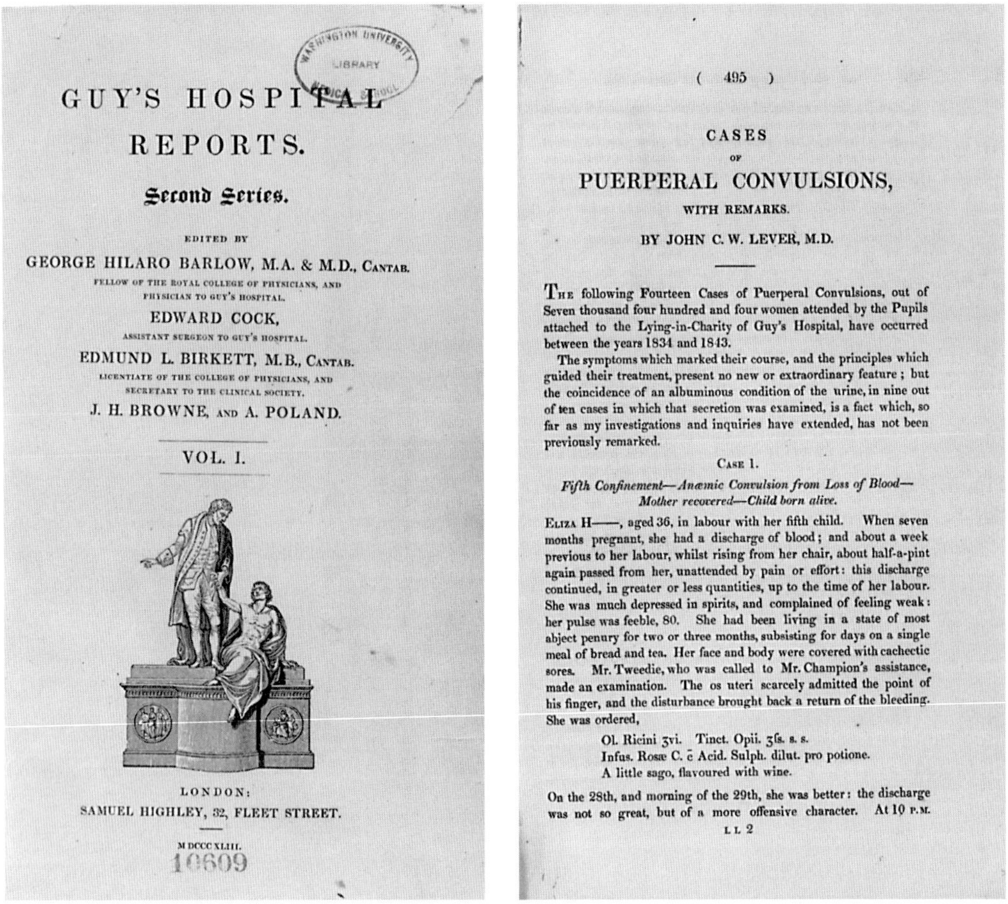
GUY'S HOSPITAL
REPORTS.

Second Series.

EDITED BY
GEORGE HILARO BARLOW, M.A. & M.D., CANTAB.
FELLOW OF THE ROYAL COLLEGE OF PHYSICIANS, AND PHYSICIAN TO GUY'S HOSPITAL.
EDWARD COCK,
ASSISTANT SURGEON TO GUY'S HOSPITAL.
EDMUND L. BIRKETT, M.B., CANTAB.
LICENTIATE OF THE COLLEGE OF PHYSICIANS, AND SECRETARY TO THE CLINICAL SOCIETY.
J. H. BROWNE, AND A. POLAND.

VOL. I.

LONDON:
SAMUEL HIGHLEY, 32, FLEET STREET.

MDCCCXLIII.

(495)

CASES
OF
PUERPERAL CONVULSIONS,
WITH REMARKS.

BY JOHN C. W. LEVER, M.D.

THE following Fourteen Cases of Puerperal Convulsions, out of Seven thousand four hundred and four women attended by the Pupils attached to the Lying-in-Charity of Guy's Hospital, have occurred between the years 1834 and 1843.

The symptoms which marked their course, and the principles which guided their treatment, present no new or extraordinary feature; but the coincidence of an albuminous condition of the urine, in nine out of ten cases in which that secretion was examined, is a fact which, so far as my investigations and inquiries have extended, has not been previously remarked.

CASE 1.

Fifth Confinement—Anæmic Convulsion from Loss of Blood—Mother recovered—Child born alive.

ELIZA H——, aged 36, in labour with her fifth child. When seven months pregnant, she had a discharge of blood; and about a week previous to her labour, whilst rising from her chair, about half-a-pint again passed from her, unattended by pain or effort: this discharge continued, in greater or less quantities, up to the time of her labour. She was much depressed in spirits, and complained of feeling weak: her pulse was feeble, 80. She had been living in a state of most abject penury for two or three months, subsisting for days on a single meal of bread and tea. Her face and body were covered with cachectic sores. Mr. Tweedie, who was called to Mr. Champion's assistance, made an examination. The os uteri scarcely admitted the point of his finger, and the disturbance brought back a return of the bleeding. She was ordered,

Ol. Ricini ʒvi. Tinct. Opii. ʒſs. s. s.
Infus. Rosæ C. c̄ Acid. Sulph. dilut. pro potione.
A little sago, flavoured with wine.

On the 28th, and morning of the 29th, she was better: the discharge was not so great, but of a more offensive character. At 10 P.M.

L L 2

Fig. 7. Main title page of the 1843 *Guy's Hospital Reports* together with the first page of Lever's article [reproduced from 31] (courtesy of the Bernard Becker Medical Library, Washington University, St. Louis).

ing eclampsia. He found albuminuria in 9 out of 10 of the convulsing pregnant women but 'in upwards of 50 women during labor, in no case have I detected albumen, except in those in which there have been convulsions, or in which symptoms have presented themselves, and which are readily recognised as the precursors of puerperal fits' [31]. Lever observed that the proteinuria of eclampsia and preeclampsia disappeared following delivery and therefore concluded that eclampsia was not nephritis.

Sir James Young Simpson (1811–1870), a Scotsman, was professor of obstetrics at Edinburgh University. He made numerous contributions to his area of specialization [32]. He was the first to use chloroform in obstetrics. The contribution we wish to emphasize is the distinction that Simpson shares with John Lever. Both men, working independently, observed albumin in the urine of patients with eclampsia. Simpson wrote in the *Monthly Journal* for 1843: '(I) had publicly taught for the last two sessions, viz., that patients attacked with puerperal convulsions had almost invariably albuminous urine, and some accompanying, or rather preceding dropsical complication, and hence probably granular renal disease' [33]. Both authors reported this finding the same month, November, 1843, and both realized that the presence of albumin preceded the convulsions in eclamptic women, and both observed that the albuminuria cleared after completion of the delivery.

Urinalysis would become a routine office procedure as would routine monitoring of blood pressure in pregnant women but that would not occur until the 20th century. The measurement of blood pressure as a regular clinical procedure did not begin until around 1906–1910.

The debt of gratitude owed these investigators from the 19th century by subsequent generations is an enormous one. The observation of albuminuria in pregnant women was a milestone and provided a tool that could be used to predict toxemia. This tremendous advance allowed earlier diagnosis and successful treatment of toxemia, and the most dreaded complication of pregnancy, convulsions, could be prevented.

References

1 Ferris TF: Toxemia and hypertension; in Burrow GN, Ferris TF (eds): Medical Complications during Pregnancy, ed. 2. Philadelphia, Saunders, 1982, pp 1–35.
2 Lindheimer MD, Katz AI: The kidney in pregnancy; in Brenner BM, Rector FC (eds): The Kidney, ed 3. Philadelphia, Saunders, 1986, pp 1253–1288.
3 Chesley LC: A short history of eclampsia. Obstet Gynecol 1974;43:599–602.
4 Chesley LC: The origin of the word 'eclampsia'. Obstet Gynecol 1972;39:802–804.
5 Adams F (tr): The Genuine Works of Hippocrates. London, Sydenham Society, 1849, 2 vol.
6 Adams F (tr): The Seven Books of Paulus Aegineta. London, Sydenham Society 1944–47, 3 vol, 1:376.
7 Mettler CC: Obstetrics and gynecology; in History of Medicine. Philadelphia, Blakiston, 1947, p 938.
8 Chesley LC: Historical developments; in Friedman EA (ed): Blood Pressure, Edema and Proteinuria in Pregnancy. New York, Liss, 1976, p 22.
9 Mettler CC: Obstetrics and gynecology; in History of Medicine. Philadelphia, Blakiston, 1947, p 949.
10 Ibid, pp 952–953.
11 Chesley LC: History and epidemiology of preeclampsia-eclampsia. Clin Obstet Gynecol 1984;27:802.
12 Mauriceau F: Traité des maladies des femmes. Paris, Nion, 1712.
13 Chesley LC: History and epidemiology ..., p 802.
14 Ibid, p 802.
15 Mauriceau F, Chamberlen H (tr): The Accomplisht Midwife. London, J Darby, 1673.
16 Peu P: La pratique des accouchements. Paris, Boudot, 1694.
17 Dexter L, Weiss S: Preeclamptic and Eclamptic Toxemia of Pregnancy. Boston, Little, Brown, 1941, pp 10–11.
18 Mauquest de la Motte G: Traité complet des accouchements naturels, non naturels et contre nature ... Paris, d'Houry, 1721, pp 377–378.
19 Denman T: Essays on the Puerperal Fever, and on Puerperal Convulsions. London, Walter, 1768.
20 Denman T: An Introduction to the Practice of Midwifery. London, s.n., 1788.
21 Mettler, pp 952, 960.
22 Sauvages F de: Pathologia methodica. Montpellier, Martel, 1739.
23 Cullen W: A Synopsis of Methodical Nosology ... Philadelphia, Hall, 1793, p 103.
24 Dexter L, Weiss S: p 11.
25 Garrison F: An Introduction History of Medicine. Philadelphia, Saunders, 1960, p 310.
26 Cullen, pp 103–105.
27 Ibid, p 103.
28 Chesley LC: History and epidemiology ... Clin Obstet Gynecol 1984;27:802.
29 Richet G: From Bright's disease to modern nephrology. Kidney Int 1991;39:787–792.
30 Rayer PFO: Traité des maladies des reins et des altérations de la sécrétion urinaire. Paris, Baillière, 1839–1841.
31 Guy's Hospital Reports: Second series, vol 1, pp 495–517.
32 Garrison, p 606.
33 Simpson JY: London and Edinburgh Monthly Journal of Medical Science, Nov. 1843, p 1015.

Origins of Nephrology – The Modern Era

American Journal of Nephrology

Am J Nephrol 1999;19:320–322

Hyposthenuria: Sándor Korányi's Concept of Renal Insufficiency

S. Sonkodi

First Department of Medicine, Albert Szent-Györgyi Medical University, Szeged, Hungary

Key Words

Korányi · Urine · Freezing point depression · Renal insufficiency

Abstract

Around the turn of the 19th century, the Hungarian physiologist and clinician, Sándor Korányi, started to use physicochemical methods to estimate renal function. In parallel with the deterioration of renal function, he found characteristic changes in the freezing point depression of urine, which he termed hyposthenuria. On the basis of these findings, he was the first to introduce the functional concept of renal insufficiency.

Before the 19th century, the main approach to the study of diseases was the morphological concept. Virchow, in one of his major presentations [1], promulgated the anatomical concept 'seek the answer to the question: ubi est morbis?'

One of the most famous proponents of the structural concept was Morgagni, who was working and teaching in Padua. In the second half of the 18th century, a revolutionary change occurred with the identification of functional changes in relation to the morphological changes observed in diseases. The pioneer and most famous representative of this concept was Claude Bernard [2].

Sándor Korányi, the Hungarian physiologist and clinician, was greatly impressed by the functional concept and fundamental works of Claude Bernard. Korányi's most important research activity was in renal physiology and pathophysiology.

The method of cryoscopy had been used to measure the freezing point depression (FPD) of fluids for the estimation of osmotic pressure. In 1892 Dreser [3] and in 1896 Winter [4] published their findings that the FPD in the blood of normal subjects was rather constant (0.56 °C), but varied in the urine over a fairly wide range (from 0.45 to 2.40 °C). Korányi confirmed these observations [5], but he made further steps by using cryoscopy in patients with kidney disease and in experimental animals. He found that the FPD changes characteristically in certain circumstances and pathophysiological conditions and observed that in rabbits fluid loads produced an increased urine flow. The urine became lighter, the volume increased and the FPD values came closer to the lower limit (0.08), but if the animal was restricted in its fluid uptake, the FPD values moved close to the higher limit observed [5].

He made his probably most important observations in connection with studies of the changes in renal function. He observed that when there was a deterioration in renal

KARGER

Fax + 41 61 306 12 34
E-Mail karger@karger.ch
www.karger.com

© 1999 S. Karger AG, Basel

0250–8095/99/0192–0320$17.50/0

Accessible online at:
http://BioMedNet.com/karger

Prof. S. Sonkodi
First Department of Medicine, Albert Szent-Györgyi Medical University
Korányi fasor 10
H–6720 Szeged (Hungary)
Tel. +36 62 454 000, Fax +36 62 455 185

function, the spontaneous changes in the FPD shrank, and with changes in the hydration there was an inability to modify the urine osmolality appropriately. Eventually the FPD and the values approached the plasma values. To this pathophysiological condition he gave the name 'hyposthenuria'. This is described in his text in the following way: 'Bei Krankheiten kann die Kraft, mit welcher die Nieren eine Veränderung in der osmotischen Spannung der sie passierenden Flüssigkeit hervorbringen, abnehmen. Dann nähert sich die Gefrierpunktserniedrigung des Harnes derjenigen des Blutes, und befindet sich zwischen 0,56–1,3°: es entsteht Hyposthenurie' [6].

Table 1 illustrates the results of his investigations of a patient with hyposthenuric polyuria caused by nephrosclerosis.

At the time when Korányi was practising as a clinican, it was not rare for surgeons to connect the ureter of the diseased kidney to the abdominal wall. In these cases, Korányi made separate renal function studies [7]. These were very good opportunities to compare the functions of the normal and the diseased kidney. The impaired renal function was indicated by the hardly changeable FPD and correlated with the decreased excretion of sodium, chloride, phosphate and urea with the urine.

These observations led Korányi to the view that the kidney function is responsible for keeping the osmolality and FPD of the blood stable. If the renal function is deteriorating, the kidneys cannot function appropriately and excrete materials properly, which leads to an impairment of renal function (i.e. hyposthenuria develops and the osmolality and the FPD in the blood should be elevated. To quote one of the findings of Korányi referring to this: '... die Erkrankung der Niere so hochgradig ist, dass die gesamte Nierenfunktion darunter leidet. Es handelt sich in diesen Fällen um eine Niereninsufficienz', i.e. 'the renal disease had progressed so much that the total renal function had nearly stopped. In such cases, renal insufficiency developed'.

Franz Volhard, the famous German nephrologist, in a lecture given in 1938 under the title 'Über Niereninsufficienz' states [8]: 'The idea of renal insufficiency is fairly new. ... The concept was first formulated by v. Korányi at the beginning of this century.'

Gabriel Richet, dealing with the history of renal pathophysiology, recently wrote as follows [9]: 'In 1897, Korányi measured the FPD of the urine during water restriction. He found that in advanced renal disease it was lower than the normal, approaching that of the plasma, a phenomenon which he named isosthenuria. He introduced the concept of renal insufficiency when, whatever the lesions, the urinary excretory function does not adapt to the needs of the body'.

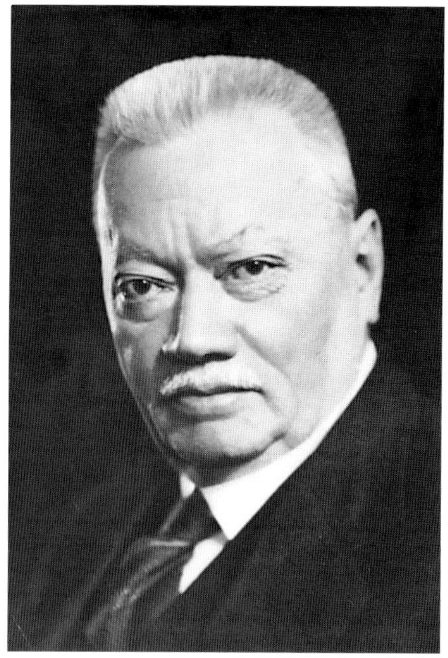

Fig. 1. Sándor Korányi.

Table 1. Results of functional studies on a patient with hyposthenuric polyuria (Dg.: Essential hypertension, 'benign nephrosclerosis')

Stunde	Harnmenge cm^3	Spez. Gewicht	Kochsalzgehalt, %	Gefrierpunkt, °
6	90	1012	0,22	0,84
7	36	1012	0,20	0,78
8	52	1012	0,19	0.78
9	32	1012	0,36	0,78
10	80	1012	0,36	0,74
1	160	1012	0,35	0,76
4	194	1012	0,32	0,77
7	212	1012	0,29	0,78
nachts	960	1012	–	–
–	1816	–	–	–

Vorlesungen über funktionelle Pathologie und Therapie der Nierenkrankheiten A. v. Korányi, Springer Verlag, Berlin, 1929.

Sándor Korányi (fig. 1) was born in Budapest (Hungary) on 18 June 1866. His father was professor of medicine in Budapest. He studied medicine and received his medical diploma in Budapest in 1888. He made several study trips to France and Germany. In Strasbourg, while spending several months under the tutelage of Hoppe Seiler, he conducted studies on physicochemical methods in physiological conditions. In 1909, he was appointed a full professor of internal medicine and chairman at the Department of Medicine at Budapest University. He died in 1944.

To summarize, Korányi's most important contribution to nephrology was the introduction of functional diagnostics into nephrology through the use of physicochemical methods for estimation of the renal function. In doing so, he became the first to introduce the functional concept of renal insufficiency.

References

1 Virchow R: Morgagni der anatomische Gedanke. C.r. XI Internat Med Kongr Roma, 1894.

2 Bernard Cl: Introduction á l'étude de medicine experimentale. Paris, 1865.

3 Dreser H: Über Diurese und Beeinflussung durch pharmakologische Mittel. Arch Exp Pathol Pharmakol 1892;29:303–319.

4 Winter J: De l'equilibre moléculaire des humeurs. Etude de la concentration des urines, ses limites. Arch Physiol Normale Pathol 1896, pp 114, 287, 296, 529.

5 Korányi A: Physiologische und klinische Untersuchungen über den osmotischen Druck thierischer Flüssigkeiten. Z Klin Med 1897;33: 1–54.

6 Korányi A: Physiologische und klinische Untersuchungen über den osmotischen Druck thierischer Flüssigkeiten. Z Klin Med 1898;34: 1–57.

7 Korányi A: Vorlesungen über funktionelle Pathologie und Therapie der Nierenkrankheiten. Berlin, Springer, 1929.

8 Volhard F: Nierenerkrankungen und Hochdruck. Eine Sammlung klinischer Vorträge. Leipzig, Barth, 1942 (newer edition 1956).

9 Richet G: Edema and uremia from 1827 to 1905: The first faltering steps of renal pathophysiology. Kidney Int 1993;43:1385–1396.

Origins of Nephrology – The Modern Era

American Journal of Nephrology

Am J Nephrol 1999;19:323–332

Inference of the Existence of High Blood Pressure as a Cause of Renal Disease in the Mid-19th Century: Observations on Vascular Structures in the Kidney

Nina M. Newton Leon G. Fine

Department of Medicine, Royal Free and University College Medical School, University College, London, UK

Key Words
Bright's disease · Hypertrophy · Blood pressure · Nephrology · Toynbee · Johnson · Gull · Traube · Ewald · Renal disease, 19th century

Abstract
Histological examination of the kidney was well under way by the mid-19th century. Pathological changes noted to be present in Bright's disease gave rise to considerable debate in the literature of the time. Toynbee was perhaps the first to note medial hypertrophy and intimal narrowing of blood vessels in the kidney, while Johnson, around the same time, thought that kidney disease was the cause of compressed vessels. Although he later proposed a causal relationship between contraction of vessels and hypertrophy, Johnson never went beyond the insights articulated by Bright himself and failed to make the link between hypertrophy of vessels and persistently raised blood pressure. Traube considered the possibility that cardiac and renal disease could be the consequences of the same unknown disease, but rejected hypertrophy per se as a causal factor. Gull and Sutton disagreed strongly with Johnson and proposed the presence of a general disease which leads to both cardiac hypertrophy and renal disease. But it was Ewald, writing in Germany, who was able to ascribe both cardiac and vascular hypertrophy to increasing tension in the arterial system and he was the first to articulate the effect of hypertension on the kidney.

Introduction

Towards the end of his career, Richard Bright [1] wrote a letter to the *London Medical Gazette*, pointing out that during the previous 2 years his colleague, Mr. John Toynbee, had made microscopic observations on over 1,000 specimens from the minutely injected kidneys of nearly 100 individuals which enabled him 'to trace out the gradual change which the structure of the kidney undergoes during the successive stages of the complaint [i.e., kidney disease], and by the aid of engravings, the proof impressions of which are now before me, we shall be able to show that one of the most interesting features in the morbid anatomy of this disease is to be found in the condition of the corpora Malpighiana' [glomeruli].

This statement is the very first indication that histological examination of the kidney was being pursued in the

KARGER

Fax +41 61 306 12 34
E-Mail karger@karger.ch
www.karger.com

© 1999 S. Karger AG, Basel
0250–8095/99/0192–0323$17.50/0

Accessible online at:
http://BioMedNet.com/karger

Prof. Leon G. Fine
5th Floor, Jules Thorn Institute
Middlesex Hospital, Mortimer Street
London W1N 8AA (UK)
Tel. +44 171 504 9441, Fax +44 171 380 9117

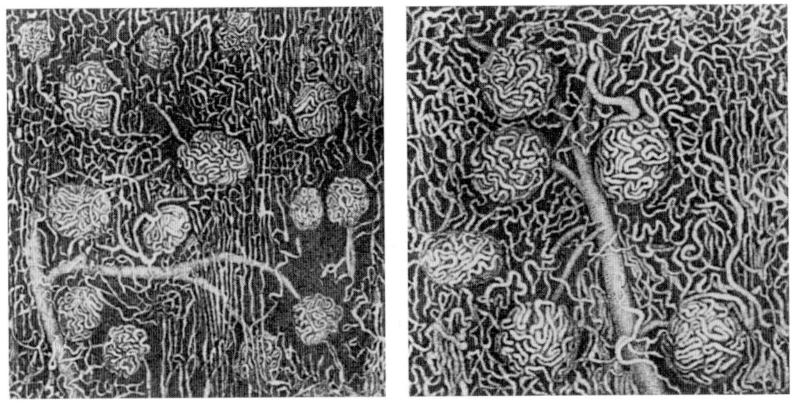

Fig. 1. Toynbee's illustrations of the glomeruli and vasculature of the diseased kidney. Figure 1: Vascular plexus of the Malpighian body in a healthy state. Figure 2: Vascular plexus enlarged and its component vessels dilated. [From ref. 2.]

mid-19th century, and it is interesting to speculate what led to the writing of the letter by Bright. He indicates that it is 'incumbent upon [him] to beg [the Editor] to insert in [his] columns the following brief statement of what Mr J Toynbee has been doing during the last two years, in co-operation with myself, on this interesting subject ...' [1, pp. 707–708]. One wonders if a certain Mr. George Robinson, who prompted this plea by dedicating his investigation on the pathology of the kidney and its secretion of albuminous urine to Bright, was also engaged in such work, and that Bright generously wished to obtain precedence for Toynbee.

John Toynbee (1815–1866)

Whatever the case, Toynbee [2] published his observations in 1846 and makes it clear that he agrees with Bright and Robinson that the congested state of the kidney blood vessels gives rise to albuminous urine. He attributes the presence of albumin in the urine to 'an obstructed condition of the blood vessels of the organ' [2] and then goes on to describe three stages of the disease, since referred to as 'Bright's disease'. He states:

> 'The condition of the arteries is visibly changed, even at this early period: the artery entering the corpus being actually twice or thrice its natural size which is the case also with the Malpighian tuft.' He also points out that 'an injection [of dye], in this stage, cannot very easily be made to pass through the tuft and fill the capsule of the corpus, – a circumstance which almost always attends injection in the later stages of the disease' [2, p. 320].

In the second stage of the disease, he observes that 'the artery of the corpus Malpighianum becomes so greatly enlarged, that frequently it equals the dimensions of the tube itself, and is eight or ten times its natural size. It is tortuous and dilated, and sometimes, previous to entering the capsule of the corpus, presents analogous swellings to those of varicose veins' [2, p. 321]. In the third stage of the disease, he says that the arteries are in a more contracted state than in the second and that the greater part of the vessels is incapable of being injected (fig. 1). '... The difficulty has its origin in the great pressure, which is exerted on the whole of the arterial system, by the contraction and hardening of the organ' [2, p. 323]. He attributes the difficulty to inject to the external compression on the vasculature – possibly the first allusion to medial hypertrophy and intimal narrowing, known to occur in the condition.

George Johnson (1818–1896)

Around this time George Johnson entered the medical debate. Born in Kent on 29 November 1818, he graduated in medicine at King's College London in 1843, where he became its first resident medical tutor. In 1887 he was appointed Vice-President of the Royal College of Physicians and, in 1889, Physician-Extrordinary to the Queen. He was knighted in 1892. An authority on kidney disease, he was nicknamed both 'Kidney Johnson' and 'Castor Oil Johnson', the latter for his treatment of cholera. He was a man of outspoken, if not intolerant, viewpoint which led in part to his quarrel with Gull in 1876 (on a matter of medical etiquette) in which the Royal College of Physicians adjudicated (in his favour). He died in 11, Saville Row, London, Bright's old house, on 3 June 1896 [3, 4].

Johnson's observations on the pathology of the kidney had, in fact, preceded those of Toynbee. In 1845 he published a paper entitled 'On the minute anatomy and pathology of Bright's Disease of the kidney, and on the

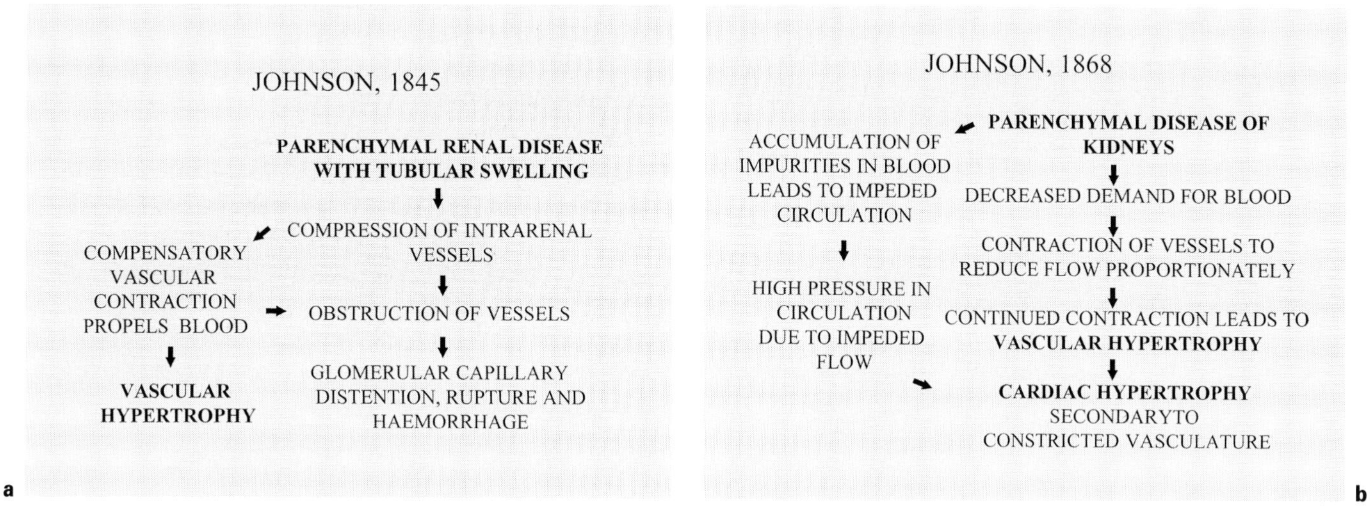

Fig. 2. a Johnson's view of the pathogenesis of vascular wall hypertrophy from his early writings, ca. 1850. **b** His later formulation, ca. 1870.

relation of the renal disease to those diseases of the liver, heart, and arteries, with which it is commonly associated' [5]. In this paper Johnson, too, describes the vasculature of the diseased kidney. Talking of Bright's disease he maintains that [5, pp. 5–6]

> 'Any one having a clear conception of the anatomy of the kidney cannot fail to perceive the effect upon the circulation through the glands which must result from the changes which I have described as primarily and essentially constituting Bright's Disease of the kidney. The fat accumulates in the epithelial cells to such an extent as to produce engorgement and dilatation of the cells, and of the tubes which are lined by them; the consequence is, compression of the capillary plexus surrounding the tubes, giving rise to congestion of the Malphighian plexus. This passive congestion of the Malphighian plexus leads to transudation of the serum of the blood, and sometimes to rupture of the delicate vessels of the plexus, and the consequent escape of the colouring matter and fibrin of the blood. These constituents of the blood pass into the tubes, and so become mixed with urine. Their escape from the blood-vessels is the result of a mechanical impediment to the return of the blood consequent on compression of the veins by an accumulation of fat in the tubes.'

His thesis in 1845 is, therefore, that disease is causing compression of the vessels. He additionally refers to the presence of a 'fibro-cellular' matrix (by which he means the interstitial fibrosis) in these kidneys and notes that the vessels constituting the 'portal plexus' of the kidney are contained in the substance of this tissue. '... It is evident that a dilatation of the tubes will lead to compression of the fibro-cellular net-work which surrounds the tubes, and of the vessels contained within the tissue' [5, p. 8]. Johnson also noticed that the arteries of these kidneys are, 'very commonly affected by those changes to which the terms *atheroma* and *steatoma* have been applied ... This fatty degeneration of the arteries is by no means confined to subjects who are affected with Bright's disease; on the contrary, it is in various degrees an extremely common morbid appearance in persons above the age of 30 who die in London hospitals' [5, p. 12]. Having observed the generality of this condition, Johnson refers to another frequent concomitant of Bright's disease, hypertrophy of the heart. In raising the question as to why the heart becomes hypertrophied, however, he was unable to give a plausible answer other than that the fatty matter is 'an indication of general perverted nutrition of the artery, by which, probably, its elasticity is impaired ... And perhaps in this way may be explained some of those cases of hypertrophy and dilatation of the heart which are not accounted for by the existence of any visible obstacle to the circulation either at the orifices of the heart or in the course of the arteries' [5, pp. 13–14]. He certainly does not, in 1845, take the link further (fig. 2a).

Johnson held sway in the field of renal pathology in Britain, but even as late as 1859 he had not made further comment in terms of developing his hypotheses further [6]. More than 20 years later however, Johnson wrote two further papers entitled: I. 'On Certain Points in the Anatomy and Pathology of Bright's Disease of the Kidney' and II. 'On the influence of the Minute Blood-Vessels upon the Circulation' [7]. In the first, he refers to his earlier, 1845, paper quoting his comment that 'the remarkable hypertrophy of the muscular coats of [the arteries] seems

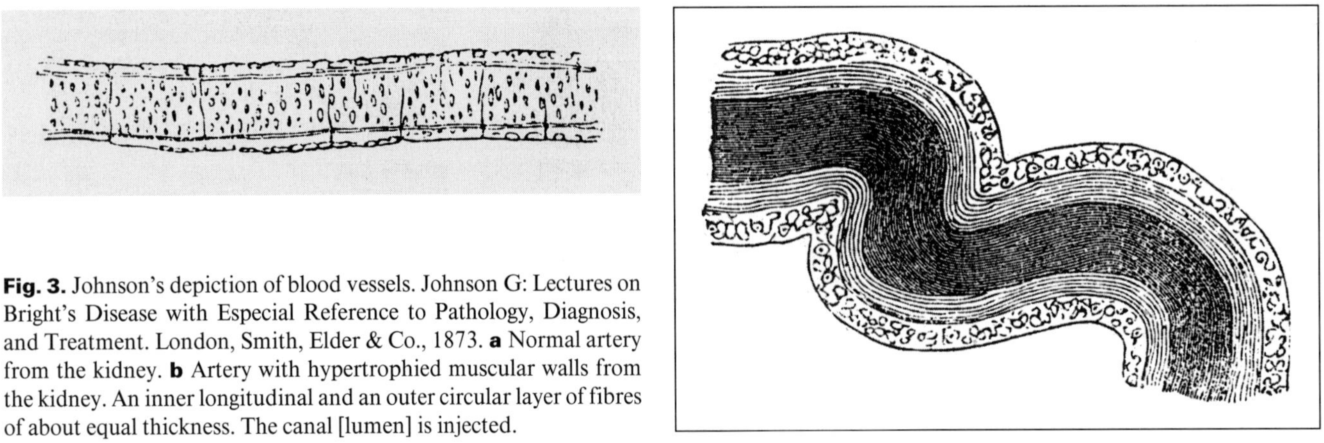

a

b

Fig. 3. Johnson's depiction of blood vessels. Johnson G: Lectures on Bright's Disease with Especial Reference to Pathology, Diagnosis, and Treatment. London, Smith, Elder & Co., 1873. **a** Normal artery from the kidney. **b** Artery with hypertrophied muscular walls from the kidney. An inner longitudinal and an outer circular layer of fibres of about equal thickness. The canal [lumen] is injected.

to have for its object to assist in driving the blood onwards through the intertubular vessels in which the impediment exists' (fig. 3a, b) but continues: 'I have long been aware that this explanation of the phenomena is physiologically untenable ... Having recently been engaged in making a careful revision of the morbid anatomy and pathology of Bright's disease in its various forms and stages, I believe that I am now in a position to give the true physiological explanation of the hypertrophy of the muscular walls of the small renal arteries, which is so constant a phenomenon in the advanced stages of all forms of chronic Bright's kidneys'. Johnson's explanation was as follows [7, p. 61]:

> '... In proportion to the destruction of the renal gland-cells, and the consequent diminution of the secretory power of the kidney, there is less demand for blood to be acted upon by the gland; the small arteries consequently contract upon their contents, so as to maintain the balance between the blood supply and the diminished secretory action of the kidney. *This continued over-action of the small arteries in antagonism to the heart results in hypertrophy of their muscular walls.* I believe that all the facts will be found to harmonise with this theory.'

Johnson' revised view is depicted in figure 2b. Although a cause-and-effect relation is drawn, no mention is made of tension within the vessels. Johnson thus fails to provide any insight beyond that articulated by Bright himself who felt that the minute capillary circulation was affected by the quality of the blood in kidney disease and that this led to the need for a greater force to maintain the local circulation. Bright had also pointed out that hypertrophy of muscular tissue occurs at two opposite extremities of the arterial system, i.e., the heart and the resistance arteries. Neither Bright nor Johnson went beyond attributing this to some qualitative change in the circulating blood and certainly never alluded to blood pressure as a cause of the hypertrophy. Johnson, however, does say that there is 'evidence of impeded transit through the minute arteries in the full, hard, throbbing pulse, which is a very common phenomenon in the advanced stage of chronic Bright's disease' [7, p. 64]. He goes on to mention Sanderson's recently published *Handbook of the Sphygmograph* which, he points out, states that, in cases of chronic Bright's disease with hypertrophy of the left ventricle, the sphygmograph affords decided evidence of increased arterial pressure.

We are thus in a position to see that Johnson has missed his opportunity to forge the necessary link between high blood pressure and arterial and cardiac hypertrophy. He maintained that nephritis (Bright's disease) leads to less demand for blood by the kidney with consequent contraction of the vessels. Cardiac hypertrophy is secondary to the constricted vasculature in the kidney. Nowhere does he attribute the cardiac hypertrophy to high blood pressure, and nowhere does he make the link that hypertrophy of the vessels is due to persistently increased blood pressure.

Ludwig Traube (1818–1876)

It is now appropriate to turn briefly to Ludwig Traube writing in Germany in 1856. Born to Jewish parents he had studied under both Purkinje and Schönlein. Although remembered for his routine introduction of the thermometer in patient examination, his description of *pulsus bigeminus*, and his monograph on experimental pathology, he had also studied the effects of vagus nerve section on pulmonary function and the relationship between cardiac and renal disease [8]. Here, we find a similar train of thought to that of Johnson, i.e., that kidney disease causes vascular hypertrophy and does so by impeding flow of blood through its parenchyma and by diminishing the removal of fluid from the circulation. However, Traube specifically points to the fact that consequent upon diminished urine output, an increase in arterial pressure occurs and maintains that this leads to an increase both in vascular resistance and cardiac hypertrophy. He rejects the fact that cardiac hypertrophy could be the cause of the renal disease and considers the possibility that cardiac and renal diseases could be the consequences of the same unknown cause. Traube rejects hypertrophy, per se, as a causal factor, arguing the implausibility of something causing hypertrophy in the heart being able to cause atrophy simultaneously in the kidney [9, 10].

Elaborating on his hypothesis, he argues that, as a result of increasing tension in the arterial system, more urea is freely excreted through the existing remnant of the intact parenchyma than would be excreted for an equivalent portion of renal parenchyma under normal circumstances. This is perhaps the first statement of renal adaptation in chronic renal disease (fig. 4).

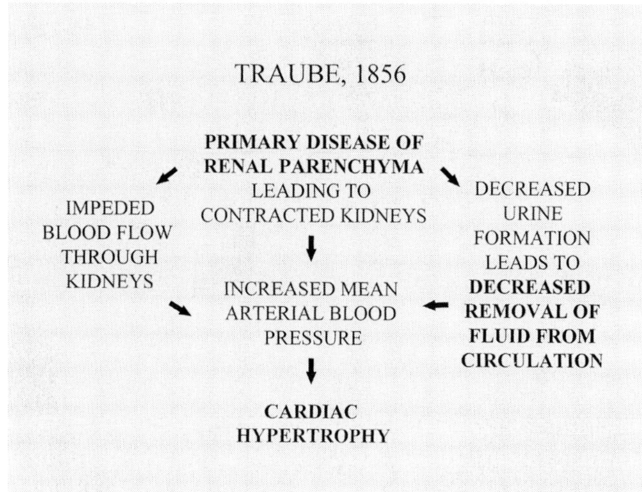

Fig. 4. Traube's postulate [9] for the pathogenesis of vascular and cardiac muscle hypertrophy in renal disease.

William Gull (1816–1890)

In 1872 William Gull published a landmark paper co-authored with his colleague, Henry Sutton of the London Hospital, entitled 'On the Pathology of the Morbid State Commonly Called Chronic Bright's 'Disease with Contracted Kidney' [11]. Born on 31 December 1816, he graduated from Guy's Hospital in 1841. He held several posts in the hospital at the same time as achieving outstanding success in private practice, becoming consulting physician at Guy's in 1871. He was elected F.R.S. in 1869. Invited by Jenner to attend the Prince of Wales, gravely ill with typhoid fever, he was rewarded with a baronetcy by the Queen and, like Johnson after him, appointed Physician-Extrordinary in 1872. He became Physician-in-Ordinary in 1887 and was several times a crown member of the G.M.C. He was known for his unhurried thoroughness, flair for diagnosis, and tenacity. It is interesting to note that his interest in patients extended beyond physical symptoms to hereditary and environmental factors and that he was the first to differentiate anorexia nervosa in medical terms. Among other things, he was a pioneer in diseases of the spinal cord, the first to describe myxoedema, and was openly sceptical of all but a very few drugs. Notwithstanding his masterful teaching and flamboyant assertiveness of manner, many colleagues were riled by his airs of superiority and carelessness in ignoring their part in consultations [12]. He is thought to have been the richest physician in London of his day and, by some at least to have been involved with Jack the Ripper [13].

In the paper of 1872 [11], Gull and Sutton appended a subtitle in parentheses (Arterio-Capillary Fibrosis), indicating their fundamental disagreement with Johnson who, they claimed, was describing a post-mortem artifact or 'congestion', seen '... in by far the majority of post-mortem examinations ... It appears to us, therefore, that Dr Johnson had attached undue importance to these slight changes in the epithelial tissue' [p. 329]. Their thesis, in contrast, was that fibroid or hyaline fibroid deposition in the intertubular compartment leads to hyaline-fibroid involvement of blood vessels. It is contraction of this hyaline-fibroid substance which compresses the tubules and leads to renal atrophy. They additionally maintain, albeit cautiously, that the observed changes are entirely secondary phenomena. '... Our observation ... seems to show that the visible morbid changes in granular contracted kidneys are due to the primary formation of 'fibroid' or 'hyaline-fibroid' substance in the intertubular parts, including the vessels, and to atrophy of the tubular and intra-tubular structures of the kidney' (fig. 5).

Gull and Sutton [11] further showed that the same fibroid and hyaline-fibroid formation is seen in meningeal arteries. 'Our examinations have shown us that this hyaline-fibroid formation commences, as regards the pia

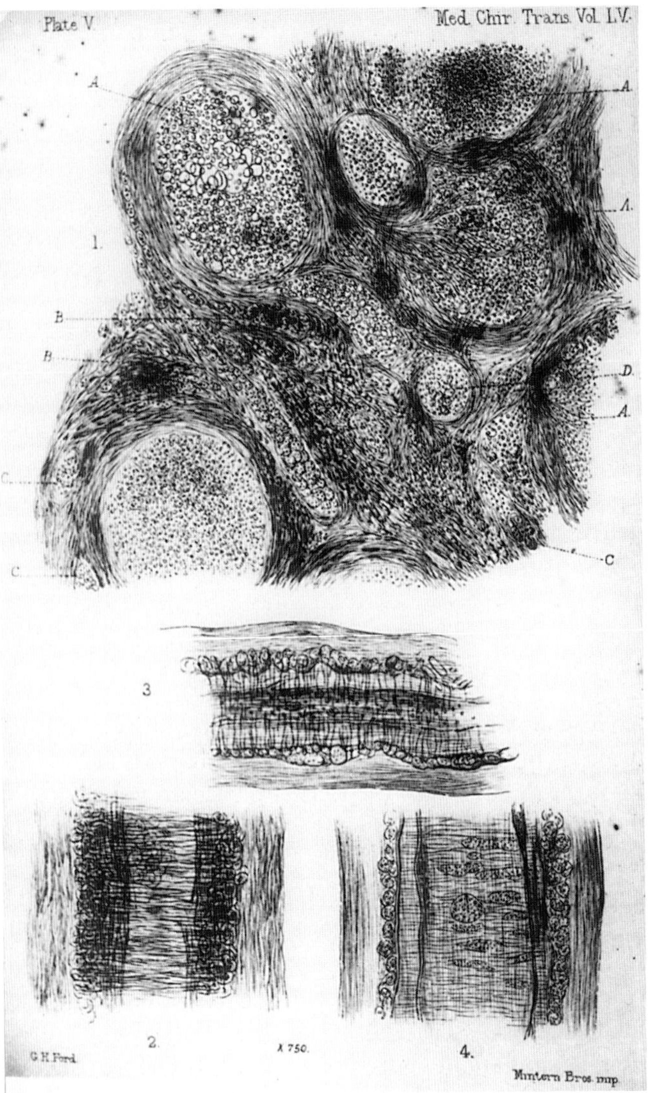

Fig. 5. Gull and Sutton's illustration [11] of the microscopic appearance of the granular contracted kidney. Figure 1: The microscopic appearances seen in very granular contracted kidneys. From a girl aged 9 years. The letter A points to six Malphighian bodies which are lying clustered together and surrounded by a quantity of fibroid material. These bodies contain numbers of fat and other granules. A convoluted tubule indicated by D is seen coming down from one of the Malpighian bodies with its epithelial cells destroyed. The letters B mark tubules which are lined with epithelial cells for the most part healthy. C points to isolated wasted tubules, containing shrivelled, ill-defined epithelial cells, and in some, in place of epithelium, nothing but fat-granules remain. Figure 2: Arteriole much thickened by coarse fibroid changes outside muscular layer; tunica intima thickened also. Figure 3: Tunica adventitia and intima thickened by fibroid changes. Figure 4: Arterioles of the pia mater. Fibroid changes outside the muscular nuclei.

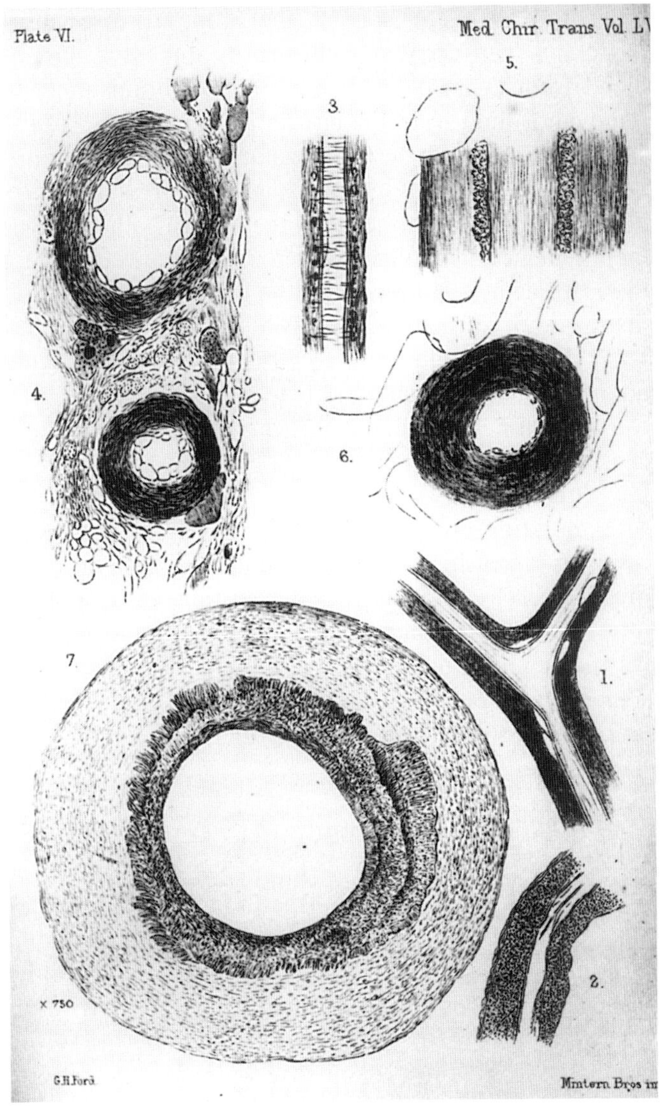

Fig. 6. Gull and Sutton's illustration [11] of capillaries of the pia mater, thickened by a homogeneous hyaline substance. Figure 1: A capillary of the pia mater much thickened by a homogeneous hyaline substance. Figure 2: Capillary very much thickened by a granular substance. Figure 3: Hyaline-fibroid thickening outside the wasted muscular layer. Figure 4: The arterioles in the choroid greatly thickened by the formation of fibroid material outside the so-called muscular nuclei. The dark parts represent choroid pigment. Figure 5: Arterioles of the skin thickened by fibroid formation outside muscular layer. Figure 6: Arteriole lying amongst muscular tissue of heart greatly thickened by the fibroid material. Figure 7: Minute artery of the kidney greatly thickened by hyaline-fibroid changes in the outer layer of the vessels.

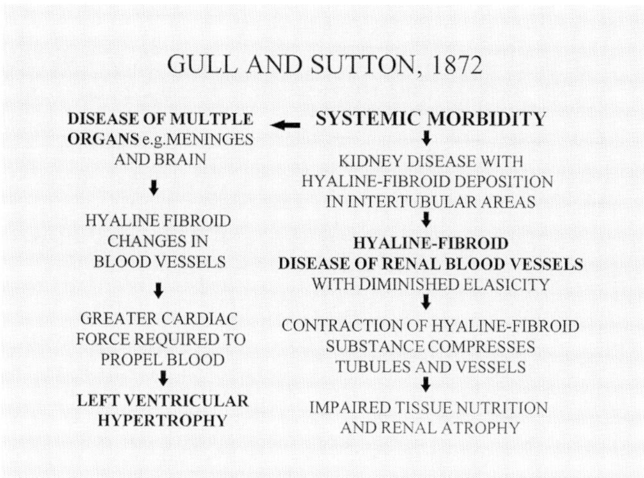

Fig. 7. The sequence of events leading to structural changes in small vessels as formulated by Gull and Sutton [11] in 1872.

mater (fig. 6), in the outer coats of the arterioles and in the walls of the capillaries themselves; and in observing that the same kind of formation occurs in the arterioles and capillaries of the kidney, we are led to infer that this change begins in the kidney as in the pia mater in the walls of the arterioles and capillaries, and subsequently extends to the surrounding structures' [p. 331]. They summarize their microscopic findings (fig. 7) thus:

'1. That the arterioles throughout the body in that condition usually called chronic Bright's disease with contracted kidney are more or less altered.

2. That this alteration is due to a "hyaline-fibroid" formation in the walls of the minute arteries, and a "hyaline-granular" change in the corresponding capillaries.

3. That this change occurs chiefly outside the muscular layer, but also in the tunica intima of some arterioles.

4. That the degree in which the affected vessels are altered, and the extent to which the morbid change is diffused over the vascular system of the different organs, vary much in different cases.

5. That the muscular layer of the affected vessels is often atrophied in a variable degree' [p. 336].

This is a very clear allusion to the arterial pathology being of a primary nature and extending outwards beyond the arterial wall. Whereas Johnson had restricted himself to hypertrophy of the muscular coating of vessels, Gull and Sutton are now saying that this is due to hyaline-fibroid formation. They state:

'We are led to conclude that the kidney disease does not give rise to the vascular change. Our investigations show the disease under the following forms:

1. Kidneys often much contracted, heart much hypertrophied, minute arteries and capillaries proportinately thickened by "hyaline-fibroid" formation.

2. Kidneys little contracted, but heart much hypertrophied, and minute arteries and capillaries much thickened by "hyaline-fibroid" substance.

3. Kidneys healthy, whilst heart much hypertrophied, and minute arteries and capillaries much thickened by "hyaline-fibroid" substance ... the absence of such lesions [i.e., kidney changes] of the kidneys proves that they do not constitute an essential and indispensible part of the general process' [p. 338].

Here, for the first time, Gull and Sutton [11] raise the observation that there is a morbid state which affects blood vessels and causes cardiac hypertrophy *in the absence of any kidney disease.*

Moving to the issue of cardiac hypertrophy, that Bright attributed to impurity in blood, and Johnson, as we have seen, attributed to impeded circulation, Gull and Sutton [11] suggest an alternative hypothesis, namely that *there is a more general disease which leads both to cardiac hypertrophy and to renal disease.* The data they present appear to show that, in granular contracted kidneys, the cardiac hypertrophy is not caused by renal disease per se, but by morbid changes in minute arteries and capillaries. It was their view that in a number of cases in their sample, 'the hypertrophy [of the left ventricle] would appear to have been the older and preceding condition' [p. 341]. Importantly and crucially, they have stated that when there is an impediment to the elasticity of the vessel wall, it may be shown experimentally that a greater force of contraction is required to propel fluid along the vessel.

'The "hyaline-fibroid" material in the walls of the arterioles must be an impediment to elasticity, and it can be experimentally shown that greater force is required to propel a fluid continuously through a non-elastic than through an elastic tube. The left ventricle therefore, owing to this diminished elasticity of the arterial walls, has of necessity to contract with greater force to carry on the circulation' [p. 342].

They produced an interesting table showing how the number of granular-to-healthy kidneys increases with increasing age (fig. 8). Gull and Sutton do not, however, begin to address what this disease, mysteriously beginning in other parts of the body, could possibly be.

Carl Anton Ewald (1845–1915)

Carl Anton Ewald [14] published an important paper on the vasculature of the kidney in 1877. Born on 30 October 1845 in Berlin, Ewald studied in Vienna, Heidelberg, and Bonn. He worked for his PhD in Berlin in 1870,

From the age of	The total number of deaths from all causes.	The number of those cases in which the kidneys had undergone granular degeneration.	The proportion of granular to healthy kidneys in each decennial period of life.
10—20 years........	44	1	1 granular kidney in 44 healthy ones.
20—30 "	69	2	1 ditto in 34 ditto.
30—40 "	84	10	1 ditto in 8·4 ditto.
40—50 "	82	31	1 ditto in 2·6 ditto.
50—60 "	39	28	1 ditto in 2·3 ditto.
60—70 "	13	12	1 ditto in 1·08 ditto.
70—80 "	5	4	1 ditto in 1·2 ditto.

Fig. 8. Table depicting the increasing prevalence of granular kidneys in each decade of life [from ref. 11].

qualifying as physician in medicine in 1874. He became director of the Medical Faculty of the Kaiserin Augusta Hospital and was made professor in 1883. He was named Honorary Professor in 1909. Apart from numerous additions to the understanding of the physiology and pathology of the digestive system, he enriched the field in terms of diagnosis and therapy. In particular, he was the first to widen the use of soft gastro-intestinal tubing as a diagnostic tool (*Probefrühstück* – literally meaning 'trial breakfast') and made important representations of thyroid disease. He died in Berlin on 20 September 1915 [15].

Ewald studied isolated vessels which were fixed in such a way that lumen and wall thickness could be measured. He studied these with a drawing prism and used a micrometric method to express the data. His most important observations were performed on preparations of pia mater vessels.

Ewald [14] first addressed a central question: 'How is it to be decided whether the lumen of a vessel is normal, increased, or decreased in character?' His answer was that the only measurement possible is the relation of thickness of the wall to that of the lumen. Importantly he recognized that a thickened wall could be due to contraction of the muscular layers or to simple hypertrophy of these layers. However, since contraction cannot continue after death, the thickening in post-mortem specimens must represent true hypertrophy. Ewald could not support views which he attributed to Johnson and to others which put vessel hypertrophy later in time than hypertrophy of the heart (although Johnson did not, in fact, say this) or regard it as the consequence of active contractions of smaller vessels, 'designed to aid the heart's activities' (i.e., to propel blood flow). He believed that hypertrophy could only occur, if there were rhythmical contractions synchronous with the pulse. In fact, he argued, such contractions could only make it more difficult to propel blood forward because of increased resistance at the site of contraction. In contrast, widening of the vessels with consequent lowering of resistance 'would ease the activity of the heart'. Therefore, the theory of the 'backing up' contraction of arterioles he believed to be without foundation.

The only remaining possibility was that the 'heightened side pressure' (i.e., stretch) is responsible for the mechanical movement. Ewald further recognized that clinicians agreed that the condition most likely to cause heightened tension of the arteries was chronic nephritis with contracted kidneys. 'Nowhere else, are such strong loads exerted on the sensing lever of the sphygmograph or the sensory finger on the rope-like remittance of the pulse' [14]. This remark makes it quite clear that Ewald was aware of the concept of blood pressure, although its clinical relevance at the time was obscure.

Ewald goes on to argue that the small arteries are thus subjected 'to an abnormally high or abnormally sustained side pressure which would widen the lumen excessively if they [the vessels] did not confront this through tension of the muscular apparatus to maintain a normal lumen' [14] during the course of the nephritis. He points out that this is the fundamental difference between blood vessels and elastic pipes, i.e., their contractility which occurs indepen-

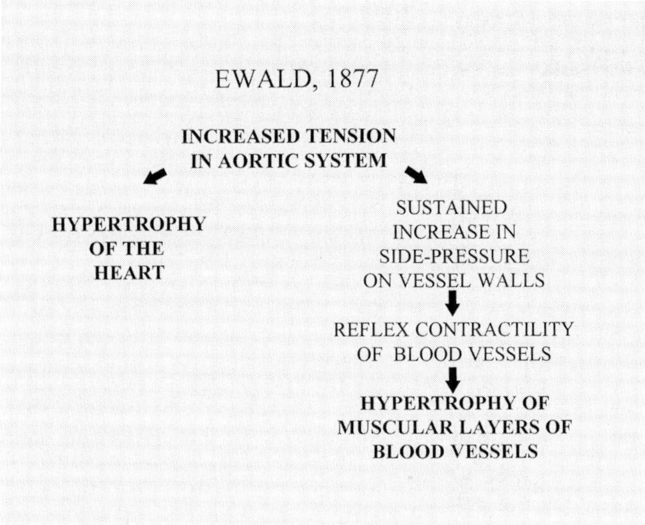

Fig. 9. Ewald's overview [14] of cardiac and vascular wall hypertrophy consequent upon increased tension in the arterial system.

dently of the central nervous system and as a 'mechanical consequence of heightened pressure'. He notes that experiments have shown that the mechanism 'tires' but that this is an experimental situation which may not apply in vivo.

Having ascribed both cardiac hypertrophy and vascular hypertrophy to increasing pressure (tension) in the arterial system, he finally addresses the question of the cause of the heightened arterial pressure. He concluded that it must be due to increasing resistance at the level of the capillaries. What the reason for this could be, he does not yet know [14].

By stating that a primary increase in tension in the aortic system later leads to hypertrophy of the muscular vessels, Ewald can lay claim to being the first to articulate the effect of hypertension on the kidney. Moreover, he not only asks why this is manifest, but why the hypertrophy is more pronounced in some locations. In addressing the question of why there is heterogeneous, rather than homogeneous, involvement of vessels, he points out that, 'since, in a networked system of pipes, sudden changes of character or other sharp bends cause sudden changes in speed with consequetial losses of pressure, it is here that one must seek for the reason for the hypertrophy which is likely to follow the changes in pressure' [14]. An overview of Ewald's theory is shown in figure 9.

Conclusions

It is clear that although Gull and Sutton have commonly been credited with the 'discovery' of high blood pressure as a cause rather than the consequence of renal disease, they did not, in fact, allude to high blood pressure in their writings. What they did do was to postulate the existence of a common disease affecting the heart and the kidneys. Traube, on the other hand, does recognize that an increase in pressure must occur within the vascular system and attributed this both to a resistance to flow through the kidneys and an increase in vascular volume secondary to decreased urine formation. It was Ewald, however, who had the first insight that this common disease could be an increase in systemic arterial pressure.

Was Ewald more insightful than his predecessors, or was it possible that this deduction related to the fact that clinical medicine had come to include thoughts about blood pressure more routinely? To answer these questions a review of the history of blood pressure measurement is finally necessary. It is clear that routine measurement of the blood pressure as a clinical tool was not in place in Ewald's time. Karl Vierordt was measuring blood pressure as early as 1855 in Germany, and Frederick Mohamed was using a sphygmomanometer from 1870. But it was only in 1876 that Marey introduced blood pressure measurement into clinical medicine, and by 1881 von Basch had introduced the first accurate and practical measurement by obliterating the arterial pulse [16].

It seems highly unlikely, therefore, that Ewald's unique insight, published in 1877 and based upon observations during the preceding decade, was conditioned by a specific clinical environment. We conclude that his deductions were based on his ability to make systematic measurements, on his powers of observation, on his understanding of physiology, and upon his flair for lateral thinking.

References

1 Bright R: Pathology of the kidney. London Med Gaz 1842;29:707–708.
2 Toynbee J: On the intimate structure of the human kidney and on the changes which its several component parts undergo in 'Bright's Disease'. Med Chir Trans 1846;29:304–326.
3 Brown GH: Munk's Roll: Lives of the Fellows of the Royal College of Physicians of London 1826–1925. London, Royal College of Physicians of London, 1955, pp 60–61B.
4 Cameron JS: The nephrotic syndrome: A historical review; in Cameron JS, Glassock RJ (eds): The Nephrotic Syndrome. New York, Dekker, 1988, pp 3–56.
5 Johnson G: On the minute anatomy and pathology of Bright's disease of the kidney, and on the relation of the renal disease to those of the liver, heart, and arteries, with which it is commonly associated. Med Chir Trans 1845; 29:1–24.
6 Johnson G: On the forms and stages of Bright's disease of the kidneys, with especial reference to diagnosis and prognosis (fourth communication). Med Chir Trans Second Series 1859;24: 153–167.
7 Johnson G: I. On certain points in the anatomy and pathology of Bright's disease of the kidney. II. On the influence of the minute blood-vessels upon the circulation. Med Chir Trans 1868;51: 59–76.
8 Firkin BG, Whitworth JA: Dictionary of Medical Eponyms. Carnforth, Parthenon Publishing, 1987, p 531.
9 Traube L: Concerning the interrelation between cardiac and renal diseases. Delivered before the Society for Scientific Medicine in Dec. 1855 and Jan. 1856. Published in Gesammelte Beiträge zur Pathologie und Physiologie. Clinical Investigations. Berlin, Hirschwald, 1871, vol II, pp 290–353. Reproduced in Nowinski WW (ed): A Monograph in American Lectures in Classics, Science and Medicine: Classics in Arterial Hypertension. Springfield, Thomas, 156, pp 188–196.
10 Traube L: Supplementary observations concerning the interconnection of cardiac and renal diseases. From a report delivered to the Society of Scientific Medicine, May 2, reprinted from Goeschen's Deutsche Klinik, 1859, Nos. 31 and 32. Published in Gesammelte Beträge zur Pathologie und Physiologie, I. Clinical Investigations. Berlin, Hirschwald, 1871, vol II, pp 421–437. Reproduced in Nowinski WW (ed): A Monograph in American Lectures in Classics, Science and Medicine: Classics in Arterial Hypertension. Springfield, Thomas, 1956, pp 197–198.
11 Gull W, Sutton H: On the pathology of the morbid state commonly called chronic Bright's disease with contracted kidney ('arterio-capillary fibrosis'). Med Chir Trans 1872;55:325–371.
12 Brown GH: Munk's Roll: Lives of the Fellows of the Royal College of Physicians of London 1826–1925. London, Royal College of Physicians of London, 1955, pp 50–51.
13 Cameron JS, Hicks J: Frederick Akbar Mohamed and his role in the description of hypertension at Guy's Hospital. Kidney Int 1996;49: 1488–1506.
14 Ewald CA: On the changes of small vessels in Bright's disease and the theories dealing with them. Arch Pathol Anal Physiol Klin Med 1877;80:453–491.
15 Fischer I: Biographisches Lexikon der hervorragenden Ärzte der letzten fünfzig Jahre. Berlin, Urban & Schwarzenberg, 1932, pp 380–381.
16 Major RH: The history of taking the blood pressure. Ann Med Hist 1930;II:47–55.

American Journal of Nephrology

Am J Nephrol 1999;19:333–335

Experimental Nephritis: One of the Earliest Publications on the Subject by a Pioneer of Neohippocratism

Spyros G. Marketos Demetrios A. Koutras

Athens University Medical School, Athens, and the International Hippocratic Foundation of Kos, Greece

Key Words
Alexander Cawadias · Antikidney antibodies · Autoimmune reactions · Kidney damage · Masugi-type nephritis · Renal antigens

Abstract
From the beginning of the 20th century, cumulative experimental work has provided considerable evidence for the possible immune mechanisms by which certain diffuse glomerular diseases develop. The first classic well-documented studies are attributed to Masugi and his research team (1933), whose experimental model involved the induction of glomerulonephritis by the administration of antikidney sera. However, 23 years earlier, in 1910, Alexander Cawadias had published a monograph on the same subject, for which he was honored with the Medal of the Paris University School of Medicine. In his study, Cawadias concluded that the mechanism of experimental nephritis was multifactorial and that the progression and the aggravation of uremic disease was caused by the production of nephrotoxins and/or antibodies against renal tissue. Cawadias referred to 'a new colloid substance', a kind of autoantibody in the context of anaphylaxis; he can be credited with foreseeing the modern era of the autosensitivity and immunology of renal diseases. Although Cawadias is well-known as a pioneer of Neohippocratism, his contribution to experimental nephritis has not been amply appreciated; he merits better recognition as one of the pathfinders in the field of renal immunopathogenesis.

Cawadias and the Neohippocratic Movement

The Greek physician Alexander P. Cawadias (1884–1971) was a leading exponent of the doctrine of Neohippocratism in Britain [1–3]. He was educated in Athens and at the Universities of Paris, Montpellier, Bonn, Heidelberg and London and graduated as an M.D. in 1910. He held hospital posts in Paris and in 1914 became senior physician and lecturer on internal diseases at Evangelismos Hospital, Athens. In 1926 he went to England and entered practice on Harley Street; he was also endocrinologist to the St. John Clinic and the Institute of Physical Medicine in London. He was president of the Section of History of the Royal Society of Medicine during 1937–1939 and of the International Congress of Neohippocratic Medicine in 1938. He was Thomas Vicary lecturer of the Royal College of Surgeons in 1941. He became F.R.C.P. in 1935. He later returned to Athens and was appointed Honorary Professor of Medicine at the Athens University Medical School in 1946. He was well known for his work

KARGER
Fax + 41 61 306 12 34
E-Mail karger@karger.ch
www.karger.com

© 1999 S. Karger AG, Basel
0250–8095/99/0192–0333$17.50/0

Accessible online at:
http://BioMedNet.com/karger

Spyros G. Marketos, MD, PhD
20 Patr. Ioakeim
GR–106 75 Athens (Greece)
Tel. +30 1 7219534, Fax +30 1 7246162

1 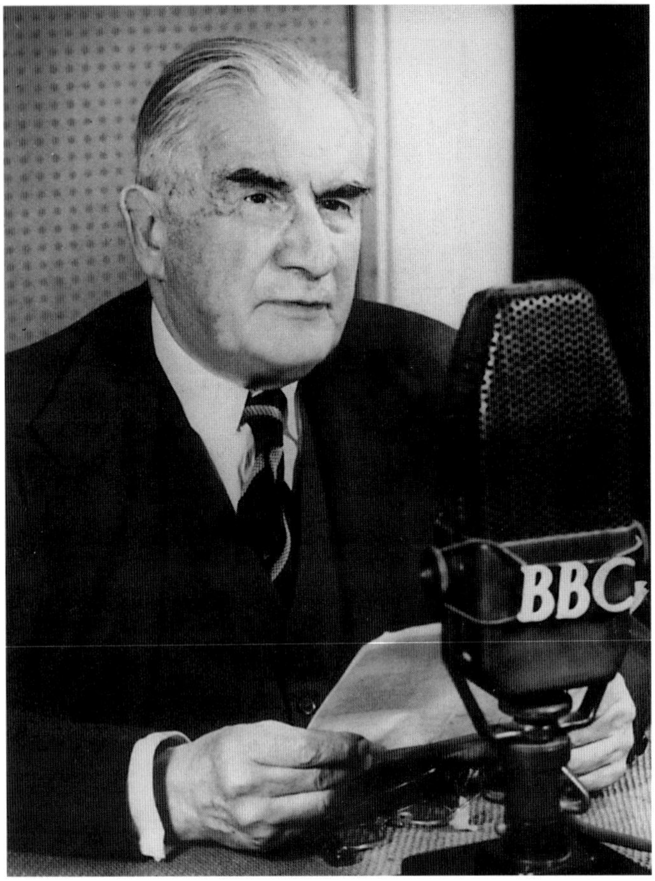

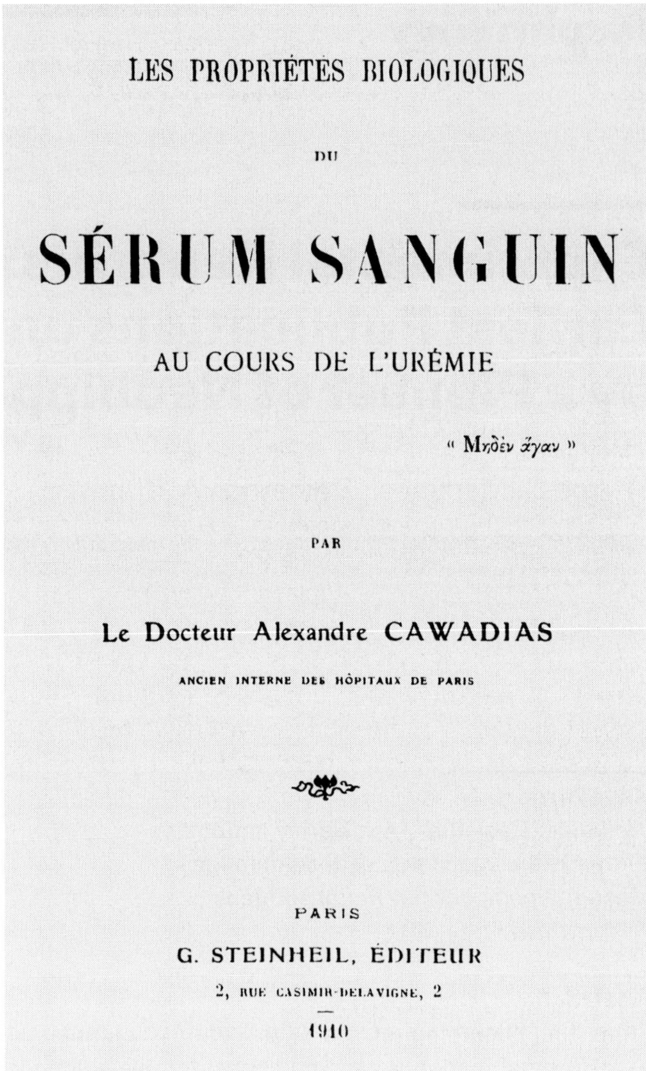

LES PROPRIÉTÉS BIOLOGIQUES

DU

SÉRUM SANGUIN

AU COURS DE L'URÉMIE

« Μηδὲν ἄγαν »

PAR

Le Docteur Alexandre CAWADIAS

ANCIEN INTERNE DES HÔPITAUX DE PARIS

PARIS

G. STEINHEIL, ÉDITEUR

2, RUE CASIMIR-DELAVIGNE, 2

1910

2

Fig. 1. Alexander Cawadias at the BBC in London (1943).
Fig. 2. The front cover of Cawadias' monograph [13].

on behalf of the Greek Red Cross of which he was president. His fascinating historical publications include a broad range of topics, ranging from ancient Greece [4] to modern medicine [5–9], as well as interesting papers on medicine and the humanities [10] and on medical thought and education [11] – and his monumental 1937 Presidential address on Neohippocratism to the Section of the History of Medicine of the Royal Society of Medicine in London [12].

In the aforementioned address [12], Cawadias (fig. 1) emphasized that:

> 'The contemporary conception, which is not pure speculation but has been demonstrated by precise experimental and clinical work, is that preceding all local manifestations there are disturbances of psycho-neuro-endocrine equilibrium, which ultimately result in modification of the body chemistry, a disturbance of the humors if we wish to preserve the Hippocratic terminology. This could easily be deduced from what we know of biology. Through the psycho-neuro-endocrine system the organism adapts itself to its environment. Disease is a struggle of adaptation to a changed environment, and thus the first manifestation must be psycho-neuro-endocrine, that is, general constitutional, metabolic, or "humoral".'

Cawadias and Experimental Nephritis

Cawadias' study on experimental nephritis entitled 'Biological Properties of Blood Serum during the Course of Uremia' [13] was published in Paris in 1910 (fig. 2). The 110-page text is divided into eight chapters and is followed by the author's critique on clinical and laboratory experiments performed in four medical centers: the Sorbonne, Hôtel-Dieu, Beaujon, and Lariboisière. His original publication was honored with the Medal of the Paris University School of Medicine.

The simplest definition of uremia is that of a 'syndrome due to a dynamic imbalance between the organism's current metabolism and its appropriate renal function' [14]. During the first two decades of the 20th century, even though numerous investigators conceded that the pathogenesis of experimental uremia might be related to the retention of metabolites, there were some who doubted that kidney damage and all metabolic disorders could be so explained. In some of the laboratory models using animals, glomerulonephritis was developed by repeated injections of foreign serum proteins [14, 15]; at about this time, Cawadias, using the Bordet and Gengou method, was attempting to explain the mechanism of uremia experimentally by the production of cytotoxins (nephrotoxins) and/or specific antibodies against renal tissue (hypersensitivity nephritis). The results of Cawadias' study strongly supported the view that the underlying mechanism by which certain glomerular diseases develop is multifactorial and poorly understood. Furthermore, Cawadias stressed the role of a 'colloid substance', a kind of autoantibody in the context of anaphylaxis, which is involved in mediating the renal tissue injury.

The earliest experimental demonstration that immunologic reactions may participate in the damage to kidney tissue is attributed to the classic studies of Masugi et al. [16] which were published in 1933. Masugi's experimental model showed the presence of specific circulating anti-kidney autoantibodies or pathogenic antigen-antibody complexes which are responsible for the pathogenetic mechanism of the glomerular damage. The model of Masugi-type nephritis was later amplified and more thoroughly investigated by numerous other authors [17–20].

Conclusions

Alexander Cawadias was a brilliant clinical physician who had tremendous interest in medical history and in the Neohippocratic Movement and who achieved recognition in these areas. However, his early contribution to experimental nephritis (1910) has not been amply appreciated; he merits better recognition as one of the pathfinders in the field of renal immunopathogenesis.

References

1 Aschner B: Neohippocratism in everyday practice. Bull Hist Med 1941;10:260–271.
2 Marketos SG, Pournaropoulos CG: Professor Alexander P. Cawadias (1884–1971) a pioneer of Neohippocratism. Mater Med Greca 1984; 12:503–508.
3 Marketos SG, Androutsos GJ: Professeur Alexandre P. Cawadias (1884–1971). Un pionnier du Néohippocratisme. In: Actes XI Congrès International de Médecine Humaniste Néo-Hippocratique. Rome, Eurostampa, 1996.
4 Cawadias AP: From Epidauros to Galen: The principle currents of Greek medical thought. Ann Med Hist 1931;3:501–514.
5 Cawadias AP: Thomas Linacre and the early scholar physicians of Oxford. Br Med J 1936;ii: 550–552.
6 Cawadias AP: Harvey in Padua. In: Proceedings of the Harvey Tercentenary Congress. Oxford, Blackwell, 1958.
7 Cawadias AP: The history of endocrinology. Proc R Soc Med 1940;34:25–30.
8 Cawadias AP: The early nineteenth century school of Paris and the development of clinical science. St Marys Hosp Gaz 1960;66:149–153.
9 Cawadias AP: The Royal College of Physicians of London on the occasion of its recent bombing. Proc R Soc Med 1941;34:811–822.
10 Cawadias AP: Medicine and the humanities. Med Illustr 1952;6:468–472.
11 Cawadias AP: Medical thought and education. Med Illustr 1953;7:422–426.
12 Cawadias AP: Neohippocratism. Proc R Soc Med 1937;31:29–38.
13 Cawadias AP: Les propriétés biologiques du sérum sanguin au cours de l'urémie. Paris, Steinheil, 1910.
14 Schreiner GE, Maher JF: Uremia: Biochemistry, Pathogenesis and Treatment. Springfield, Thomas, 1961.
15 Longcope WT: Production of experimental nephritis by repeated protein injections. J Exp Med 1913;18:678–682.
16 Masugi M, Sato Y, Tomizuk Y: Über die experimentelle Glomerulonephritis durch das spezifische Antinierenserum: Ein Beitrag zur Pathogenese der diffusen Glomerulonephritis. Beitr Pathol Anat 1933;92:429 –436.
17 Lange K, Gold MMA, Weiner D, Simon V: Autoantibodies in human glomerulonephritis. J Clin Invest 1949;28:50–58.
18 Stoloff IL, Stout R, Myerson RM, Haven WP Jr: Production of antibody in patients with uremia. N Engl J Med 1958;259:320–323.
19 Gajdusek DC: An autoimmune reaction against human tissue antigens in certain acute and chronic diseases. 1. Serological investigations. Arch Intern Med 1958;101:9–16.
20 Dixon FJ, Feldman JD, Vazquez JJ: Experimental glomerulonephritis. The pathogenesis of a laboratory model resembling the spectrum of human glomerulonephritis. J Exp Med 1961; 113:899–903.

Origins of Nephrology – The Modern Era

American Journal of Nephrology

Am J Nephrol 1999;19:336–339

Diagnosis of Renal Disease at the Beginning of the 20th Century

M. Cioffi L. Esposito D. De Santo P. Giannattasio F. Cappabianca S. Mangiacapra T. Materiale G. Conte

Chair of Nephrology, Second University of Naples, Italy

Key Words

Renal diseases · Diagnosis · Urine · Urea · Animal models · Autopsy

Abstract

At the beginning of this century, the diagnosis of various renal diseases was made with relative accuracy although neither plasma markers of glomerular filtration nor renal biopsy nor imaging were available. Renal edema was identified by high albuminuria, hyalin cylinders, high urine density and oliguria. Renal hematuria was detected by cylinders of erythrocytes. Hallmarks of chronic renal insufficiency, recognized at autopsy by atrophic kidneys, were hyposthenuria, polyuria and slight albuminuria without edema associated with arterial hypertension, anemia, retinopathy and left ventricular hypertrophy. The detection of increased plasma volume in experimental toxic nephritis by St. Moscati proposed the underlying mechanism of arterial hypertension. Experimental and clinical research in the preinsulin era indicated the central role of the kidney in the functional alterations induced by diabetes. Indeed, glucosuria was known to appear only when glycemia was relatively high. The kidney appeared enlarged and hyperemic, i.e. the so-called glomerular hyperfiltration. Glucosuria was directly correlated with diuresis but it markedly decreased in renal insufficiency. In diabetes complicated by nephropathy, tolerance to carbohydrates improved. Correction of glucosuria by dietary treatment was followed by a prompt rise in body weight, due to retention that counterbalanced the previous losses. Diabetic ketoacidosis, determined by the measurement of urinary ketonic body excretion, was treated with sodium bicarbonate (30–50 g/day in severe acidosis) up to achieving an alkaline urine pH. It was known that high doses of sodium bicarbonate might induce edema which gradually disappeared with a reduction in the alkaline administration. Clinical significance of sodium balance was, in fact, recognized: the external NaCl balance between alimentary ingestion and urinary excretion was neutral in normal conditions and became positive at high body temperature or negative during reabsorption of exudates.

Introduction

At the beginning of this century, diagnosis of various renal diseases was possible with relative accuracy, although neither markers of glomerular filtration nor renal biopsy or imaging were available in clinical practice. The main media to know the renal pathology were represented by anamnestic and clinical evaluation, laboratory measurements, and experimental and autopsy findings.

KARGER

Fax + 41 61 306 12 34
E-Mail karger@karger.ch
www.karger.com

© 1999 S. Karger AG, Basel

0250–8095/99/0192–0336$17.50/0

Accessible online at:
http://BioMedNet.com/karger

Dr. Mario Cioffi
Cattedra di Nefrologia, Seconda Università di Napoli
Via M. Longo 50
I–80130 Napoli (Italy)
Fax +39 081 254 9409

Anamnestic and Clinical Evaluation

The clinical history of the patient was examined in relation to lifestyle (excessive nutrition, alcoholism), to professional activity (lead intoxication), to administration of nephrotoxic substances (lithium, salicylic acid, antipyrine, quinine, etc.), to infective diseases (tuberculosis, syphilis, scarlet fever, diphtheria, etc.), and to metabolic diseases (diabetes, gout, amyloidosis, etc.) [1]. The observation of renal and urinary symptomatology implied the evaluation of type, localization, radiation, and intensity of pain (renal colic, serious pain) and was almost similar to that observed today in clinical practice. The clinical significance of nocturia and the changed circadian rhythm of diuresis from day to night in renal diseases was well recognized [2]. Specifically, it was observed that a healthy man produced more urine during the day than during the night and that the ratio ranged from 3.2 to 8.2. The reduction of this ratio below 3.2 was associated with a pathological condition [2]. Therefore, it was considered useful to separate the urine of the day from that of the night.

The physical characteristics of urine (appearance and color) were carefully identified. Symptoms such as pyuria, pain, and fever were investigated to prove renal infections (pyelonephritis, abscess of the kidney). Extrarenal symptoms of arterial hypertension (left ventricular hypertrophy, dyspnea, visual damage, headache, etc.) and uremia (anorexia, dyspepsia, tonic-clonic seizures, itching, paleness, etc.) were evaluated in renal patients [1, 2]. Renal dropsy was initially searched on the face, particularly on the eyelids, and then on malleoli, legs, and scrotum before development of anasarca [1]. Renal sclerosis (chronic renal failure) slowly develops: polyuria of low specific density, modest urinary abnormalities, no edema, arterial hypertension with left ventricular hypertrophy, anemia, and retinopathy were often associated [1].

In preinsulin era, the different clinical outcomes of diabetes were well identified; in youth, the syndrome is severe and quickly progressive, whereas in advanced age (above 30–40 years), it is mild and generally stable for decades [3]. Moreover, it was observed that muscular exercise improved the clinical picture [3].

Laboratory Measurements

The chemical and microscopic analysis of urine was well advanced [4]. The presence of protein in the urine was determined by several reactions: heat reaction (clouding after heating up to boiling plus addition of acetic acid), reaction of Heller (clouding after nitric acid administration), heat reaction with acetic acid and potassium iron cyanide, and biuret reaction. A high level of coagulable protein in the urine indicated glomerular disease: during nephrosis 20–30 g/l [5, 6]. In patients with renal sclerosis, moderate alterations of albuminuria were generally evidenced [1]. In advanced diabetes mellitus, the presence of albuminuria (more than 0.5 g/l) was well documented [1]. The detection of albuminuric retinopathy indicated the association between glomerulopathy and retinopathy in diabetics [1].

Microscopic hematuria in association with cylinders of blood cells was diagnostic of glomerulonephritis [5]. The urinary cylinders were in fact considered products of renal tubules [1]. Microscopic hematuria in combination with pyuria suggested the diagnosis of renal tuberculosis ascertained by the detection of Koch bacilli in the urine [1, 5].

The urine density ranges between 1,015 and 1,025 under normal conditions, but decreases down to 1,002 in renal diseases and diabetes insipidus and increases up to 1,060 in diabetes mellitus. In diabetic patients, it was possible to deduce from the value of urine density the entity of glycosuria [1]. If the urinary excretion of glucose was equal to 10–20 g, the output of urine was in the normal range of 1,500–2,000 ml/day, whereas if the glycosuria was greater, the daily diuresis generally increased [1]. After high body temperature, the urine density is high [1]. In renal sclerosis there is an increase of urine that appears pale and has a low density [1]. It was demonstrated that in advanced renal failure, the freezing point depression is lower than normal, approaching that of plasma, identifying the so-called isosthenuria [7, 8]. It was suggested that in renal insufficiency the urinary excretory function does not adapt to the needs of the body: the maximal urine concentration was not modified by water restriction. The measurement of the urine density during water restriction allowed the detection of a latent stage of renal insufficiency before its full symptomatic development [8].

Urea in blood, under normal conditions 20–50 mg%, increases in the renal lesions, when the permeability of the kidney is decreased [1]. Urea increases also in several acute pathologies, associated with exaggerated disintegration of the tissues (the so-called endogenous hypercatabolism); however, its increase is typical of renal lesions and specifically of chronic uremic nephritis [1]. In normal subjects, the daily urine production of urea ranges from 20 to 40 g. This value increases by an animal protein based diet or by a large endogenous consumption, such as in diabetes mellitus (up to 100 g/day) or hyperpyrexia (up to 50 g/day) etc., but decreases by a low-nitrogen diet, in uremia, and acute atrophy of the liver etc. [1]. Nitrogen, present in the urine, is excreted not only as urea, but also as other nitrogen substances: it was useful to measure the total amount of nitrogen and not that of urea to calculate the organic composition of albuminoid substances [1]. It was also noted that the degree of the urea plasma concentration was not always proportional to the seriousness of uremic symptoms: the lack of a relationship between urinary nitrogen retention and plasma nitrogen accumulation may be due to an endogenous nitrogen hyperproduction with or without an altered renal function [5].

The role of salt, initially measured in terms of its anion chloride, began to be appreciated by the middle to late 19th century [9]. The daily urinary amount of NaCl ranges from 11 to 15 g and mainly depends on NaCl contained in the food [1]. The clinical significance of NaCl was, in fact, recognized: the NaCl balance between alimentary ingestion and urinary excretion is neutral in healthy subjects and becomes positive at high body temperature or negative during rapid reabsorption of exudates [1]. This last clinical condition could increase the urinary excretion of NaCl to up to 55 g/day [1]. In diabetic patients, high doses of sodium bicarbonate administered to counterbalance acidosis could induce edema, that gradually disappeared by reduction in alkaline administration: to determine the dose of sodium bicarbonate better tolerated by these patients, the body weight and the degree of the edema must be controlled [1]. In patients with severe diabetes, a prompt rise of the body weight followed the prescription of a dietary regimen with reduction of glycosuria: this rise was due to the retention of water that counterbalanced the previous losses [1].

The main parameters of acid-base assessment and their measurements were known. The urine reaction was normally acidic but became neutral or slightly alkaline when HCl was lost by repeated vomiting. In uremic or diabetic acidosis, the breath was very deep and/or more frequent, and the content of CO_2 in the blood was very decreased: alkali treatment was used both in uremia and in diabetes. In diabetic acidosis, glycosuria implied loss of carbohydrates and, therefore, markedly changed the process of fat acid oxidation: consistent amounts of β-hydroxybutyrate and diacetate acid appeared in the urine as products of this altered oxidation [1]. Acetone was mainly formed from the diacetate contained in the urine [1]. In the healthy subject, the urinary excretion of acetone was determined to be equal to 1–3 cg/day, and the air expiration of acetone is normal at up to 50 mg/day [1]. During diabetic coma, the production of high levels of acids was persistent, and the increased excretion of acetone was evidenced by typical halitosis. Therefore, it was necessary to administer alkali substances (sodium bicarbonate 30–50 g/day) until the achievement of an alkaline urine pH [1]. In severe diabetic acidosis, a loss of sodium and potassium was also observed [1].

Table 1. The main diagnoses of renal diseases and their hallmarks

Renal sclerosis (chronic renal failure)	Low-density polyuria Moderate urinary abnormalities Almost never edema Hypertension with left ventricular hypertrophy and retinopathy Anemia
Nephrosis (nephrotic syndrome)	High urinary protein levels
Acute uremic nephritis (acute renal failure)	Transitory oliguria and hyperazotemia, generally postoperative
Glomerulonephritis	Microscopic hematuria and cylinders of blood cells, generally postinfective
Pyelonephritis	Pyuria, pain, and fever
Interstitial nephritis	Administration of nephrotoxic drugs Autoptic findings
Diabetic nephropathy	Reduction of glycosuria Albuminuria (more than 0.5 g/l) Sodium retention Improved carbohydrate tolerance Hyperemic and enlarged kidneys
Renal tuberculosis	Microscopic hematuria, pyuria, and Koch bacilli in the urine
Unilateral renal hypertrophy	Experimental studies on animals Study of separated functions of kidneys by ureteral catheterisation

Experimental and Autopsy Findings

The experimental studies of animals and the autopsy findings provided evidence of renal hypertrophy when the contralateral kidney was absent or severely damaged [5]. Furthermore, it was known that the time necessary to develop a compensatory hypertrophy of one kidney after interruption of renal function in the contralateral kidney was not short: in a patient with a recent unilateral renal infection, the surgeon had to wait until the healthy kidney became hypertrophic before of unilateral nephrectomy

[5]. In such clinical conditions, it was suggested to study separate function of the kidneys by ureteral catheterization: the acute consumption of water induced a greater excretion of water, urea and Cl from the undamaged kidney [5, 6].

Several experimental models were designed to better determine the physiopathology of renal insufficiency and diabetes. In 1922, Moscati and Napolitano proposed an optical method to determine the amount of blood in experimental nephrotoxicity induced by subcutaneous injections of uranium acetate in dogs [10]. The aim of the paper, as suggested in the Introduction, was to assess whether the pathogenesis of altered blood pressure was due to the altered state of the vascular wall or to the altered rate of hypervolemia. In an experimental model of nephritis, the effective rise of plasma volume was considered completely different from the plethoric states associated with edema and transudates [10]. To our knowledge, the detection of hypervolemia in nephritis as an underlying mechanism of arterial hypertension, proposed by Moscati and Napolitano [10] in 1922, is the first reported observation of this very important issue.

Experimental research in the preinsulin era indicated the central role of the kidney in the functional alterations induced by diabetes. Indeed, glucosuria was known to appear only when glycemia was relatively high, i.e., greater than 0.17 g% [1]. At autopsy, the kidney appeared enlarged and hyperemic, i.e., the so-called glomerular hyperfiltration [1]. Glycosuria was directly correlated with diuresis, but it markedly decreased in renal insufficiency. In diabetes complicated by nephropathy, the tolerance to carbohydrates improved [1]. Moreover, the experimental model of diabetes mellitus induced by pancreatectomy and its prevention by subcutaneous implantation of pancreatic fragments established that the pancreas played a central role in this disease and probably performed its action by a substance secreted by itself [3]. Finally, the administration of phlorizin to animals induced glycosuria without hyperglycemia, i.e., an experimental model of renal diabetes [3].

Diagnosis of Renal Diseases

Table 1 lists the main diagnoses of renal diseases described at the beginning of the 20th century with their more relevant clinical hallmarks. In conclusion, it is extraordinary to observe that the main renal diseases were identified despite the absence of relevant laboratory and technical methods, such as renal clearance, renal biopsy or imaging, and the faltering of renal pathophysiology [7]. Few clinical pioneers were working in isolation from the main body of their colleagues: the medical science had not yet developed an international language [7]. Indeed, renal knowledge was poorly integrated into clinical medicine which was essentially based on the empirism rather than on scientific methods [11]. However, it is important to understand how the careful observation of the anamnestic and clinical findings allowed to define the body of renal diagnosis.

References

1 De Carolis A: Prontuario per il medico pratico, ed 2. Bologna, Garagnani, 1910, p 668.
2 Rassegna della stampa Italiana ed estera; in Rummo A (ed): La riforma medica anno XXXVIII. Napoli, Muca, 1922, p 472.
3 Mohr L, Staehlin R: Diabete mellito; in: Trattato di medicina interna. Milano, Società Libraria, 1913–1914, vol 8, pp 664–723.
4 Ritz E, Kuster S, Zeier M: Clinical nephrology in 19th century Germany. Am J Nephrol 1994; 14:443–447.
5 Lanzillotta R: I metodi di indagine nella funzinalità renale. Napoli, Trinchera, 1921, p 200.
6 Zina A: Ricerche sul ricambio intermedio ed esterno nei nefritici ed uremici; in Rummo A (ed): La riforma medica anno XXXVIII. Napoli, Muca, 1922, pp 243–246.
7 Richet G: Edema and uremia from 1827 to 1905: The first faltering steps of renal pathophysiology. Kidney Int 1993;43:1385–1396.
8 Koranyi A: Physikalisch-chemische Methoden und Gesichtspunkte in ihrer Anwendung auf die pathologische Physiologie der Nieren; in Koranyi A, Richter PF (eds): Physikalische Chemie und Medizin. Leipzig, Thieme, 1907, pp 133–190.
9 Eknoyan G: A history of edema and its management. Kidney Int 1997;51(suppl 59):118–126.
10 Moscati G, Napolitano G: La determinazione della quantità del sangue con il metodo ottico. Studio sulla quantità del sangue in alcune nefriti; in Rummo A (ed): La riforma medica anno XXXVIII. Napoli, Muca, 1922, pp 435–438.
11 Conte G: Empiricism versus science in the teaching of nephrology. Am J Nephrol 1994;14: 257–258.

Origins of Nephrology – The Modern Era

American Journal of Nephrology

Am J Nephrol 1999;19:340–342

The History of Science: Defending Epistemology with New Technologies

G. Aliotta[a] G. De Angelis[a] N.G. De Santo[b] J. Sepe[c] V. Stingo[a]

[a]Dipartimento di Scienze della Vita, [b]Cattedra di Nefrologia, Dipartimento di Pediatria e [c]Centro di Ricerca Interdipartimentale di Scienze Computazionali e Biotecnologiche, Seconda Università di Napoli, Italia

Key Words

CD-ROM · Epistemology · Life sciences history

Abstract

The leap in scientific discoveries made with new computer technologies can be compared to the invention of the printing press and expanding scientific thought in the 16th century. Nowadays, new communication technologies offering a multimedia contribution illustrate the fascinating reality of scientific exploration even for individuals who can otherwise not be reached. Since rare books are usually kept in libraries with limited access, the strict safekeeping, however, often overrides the need for academic consultation. Moreover, rare manuscripts are often illustrated with figures that are just as important as the written texts, but which are also unavailable. We combined our expertise in biology, medicine and multimedia to produce a CD-ROM with a hyperlinked text on the scientific revolution of the 16th century, focusing on the early conceptualization of life sciences in Europe. In this paper we show the first page of Malpighi's *Epistle II* (De pulmonibus – on the Lungs) as it appeared in *Opera Omnia* published in London (1686) by the Royal Society.

Introduction

What is science? When did it begin? What are its methods and objectives? These questions may seem banal, but they are often neglected. Given that progress implies having a history, science also grew out of mythology and classical philosophy and continues to change. It is therefore a valid subject for historians. Since science involves a continuous effort to understand the world and ourselves, the history of science is first a record of scientific problems and attempts to solve them, and second a collection of principles. Not all historians of science provide answers to 'six basic questions of science' needed to critically describe scientific progress: who?, when?, where?, what?, how?. why? Depending on which question is chosen to be answered, we can have a chronological chain of events, a biographical account, or a cultural and social history [1].

When attempts are made to describe the history of principles, attention is focused on the scientists and their conceptual background. What were the scientific problems of their period? What were the theoretical tools and methods they had to solve problems? What were the ideas of the period that influenced their choices? A novel way to cope with these questions has been opened up by multimedia. Indeed, the leap in scientific discoveries made with new computer technologies can be compared to the invention of the printing press and expanding scientific thought in the 16th century. The printed page rapidly changed the way in which information was processed in almost every field of study. Multiple copies of printed scientific illustrations produced by xylography and chal-

KARGER

Fax + 41 61 306 12 34
E-Mail karger@karger.ch
www.karger.com

© 1999 S. Karger AG, Basel

0250–8095/99/0192–0340$17.50/0

Accessible online at:
http://BioMedNet.com/karger

Dr. Giovanni Aliotta
Dipartimento di Scienze della Vita
Seconda Università di Napoli, Via Arena
I–81100 Caserta (Italy)
Tel. +39 0823 275 225, Fax +39 0823 275 219, E-Mail aliotta@cds.unina.it

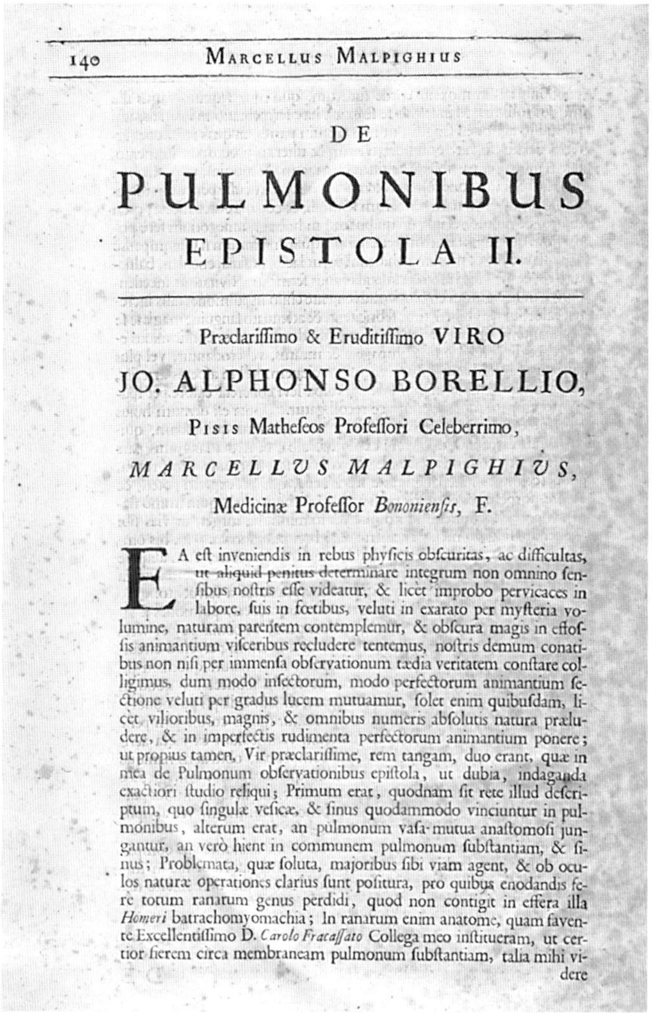
140 MARCELLUS MALPIGHIUS

DE
PULMONIBUS
EPISTOLA II.

Præclariſſimo & Eruditiſſimo VIRO
JO. ALPHONSO BORELLIO,
Pisis Matheſeos Profeſſori Celeberrimo,
MARCELLUS MALPIGHIUS,
Medicinæ Profeſſor *Bononienſis*, F.

EA eſt inveniendis in rebus phyſicis obſcuritas, ac difficultas, ut aliquid penitus determinare integrum non omnino ſenſibus noſtris eſſe videatur, & licet improbo pervicaces in labore, ſuis in fœtibus, veluti in exarato per myſteria volumine, naturam parientem contemplemur, & obſcura magis in effoſſis animantium viſceribus recludere tentemus, noſtris demum conatibus non niſi per immenſa obſervationum tædia veritatem conſtare colligimus, dum modo infectorum, modo perfectorum animantium ſectione veluti per gradus lucem mutuamur, ſolet enim quibuſdam, licet vilioribus, magnis, & omnibus numeris abſolutis natura præludere, & in imperfectis rudimenta perfectorum animantium ponere; ut propius tamen, Vir præclariſſime, rem tangam, duo erant, quæ in mea de Pulmonum obſervationibus epiſtola, ut dubia, indaganda exactiori ſtudio reliqui; Primum erat, quodnam ſit rete illud deſcriptum, quo ſingulæ veſicæ, & ſinus quodammodo vinciuntur in pulmonibus, alterum erat, an pulmonum vaſa mutua anaſtomoſi junguntur, an verò hient in communem pulmonum ſubſtantiam, & ſinus; Problemata, quæ ſoluta, majoribus ſibi viam agent, & ob oculos naturæ operationes clarius ſunt poſitura, pro quibus enodandis ferè totum ranarum genus perdidi, quod non contigit in effera illa *Homeri* batrachomyomachia; In ranarum enim anatome, quam faventе Excellentiſſimo D. *Carolo Fracaſſato* Collega meo inſtitueram, ut certior fierem circa membraneam pulmonum ſubſtantiam, talia mihi videre

Fig. 1. First page of Malpighi's *Epistle II* (De pulmonibus – On the Lungs) sent to his mentor Giovanni Alfonso Borelli.

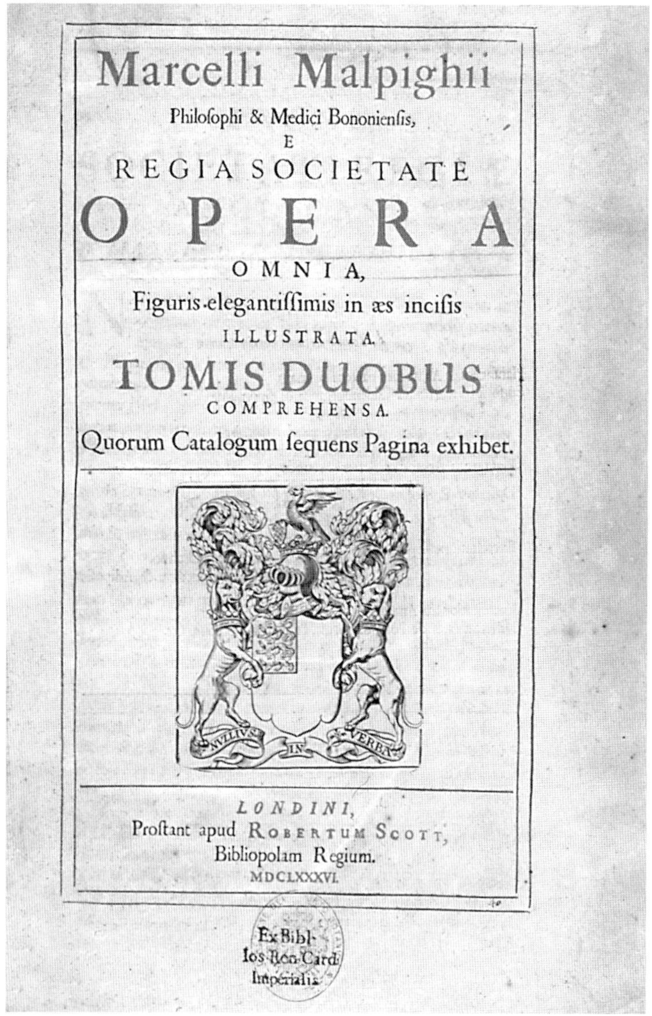
Marcelli Malpighii
Philoſophi & Medici Bononienſis,
E
REGIA SOCIETATE
OPERA
OMNIA,
Figuris elegantiſſimis in æs inciſis
ILLUSTRATA.
TOMIS DUOBUS
COMPREHENSA.
Quorum Catalogum ſequens Pagina exhibet.

NULLIUS IN VERBA

LONDINI,
Proſtant apud ROBERTUM SCOTT,
Bibliopolam Regium.
MDCLXXXVI.

Ex Bibl. Ios. Ren. Card. Imperialis

Fig. 2. Title page of Malpighi's *Opera Omnia* published in London (1686) by the Royal Society.

cography could finally be examined and studied by scholars at different times and locations.

It this context, communication technologies can better illustrate the reality of scientific exploration even for individuals who can otherwise not be reached and make a new socially oriented science available to everyone [2]. Since rare books are usually kept in libraries with limited access, the strict safekeeping, however, often overrides the need for academic consultation. Moreover, rare manuscripts are often illustrated with figures that are just as important as the written texts, but which are also unavailable.

We have combined our expertise in biology, medicine and multimedia to produce a CD-ROM with a hyperlinked text on the scientific revolution of 16th century, focusing on the early conceptualization of life sciences in Europe.

The Origin of Science: Places and Dates

The hyperlinked text presented is neatly woven with the thread of places and dates of major events in the scientific revolution occurring when alchemy was the last flower of a dying plant and mathematics the first flower of a perennial plant. The science historian Rossi claimed that there was no specific birth place of modern science in Europe. It began everywhere at roughly the same time. Copernicus was Polish, Vesalius Flemish, Bacon, Harvey and Newton English, Cartesio, Fermat and Pascal French, Tycho Brahe Danish, Paracelsus, Kepler and Leibniz German, Huygens Dutch, and Galilei, Borelli and Malpighi Italian. These scientists were linked in a world without frontiers, in a republic of science built with great difficulty at a time of social and political upheaval [3].

The following are just a few important dates for life sciences.

1530. The botanist Otto Brunfels published the *Herbarum Vivae Icones* containing the first scientific illustrations made by Hans Weidtz, a pupil of the celebrated painter Albrecht Dürer [4, 5].

1543. Two books appeared that challenged long-held convictions about the nature of the heavens and the human body: *De Revolutionibus Orbium Coelestium* by Nicolaus Copernicus and *De Humani Corporis Fabrica* by Andreas Vesalius. This double publication supported the view that 1543 was the beginning of the scientific revolution [6].

1545. The Padua Botanical Garden was founded designed to grow medicinal plants. This was the first of its kind worldwide. Its location and layout have been maintained over the years. The garden has had an educational tradition with a strong commitment to university instruction and research [7].

1558. Giambattista Della Porta published the *Magia Naturalis.* Della Porta started the oldest Scientific Society in the world, Academia Secrotorum Naturae, whose members met at his house in Naples. This group took the important step of asking potential members to present a new fact in natural sciences as a condition for admission [3].

1628. William Harvey described the cardiovascular system in his *De Motu Cordis* [6].

1661. Marcello Malpighi discovered the capillaries in the lung of a frog. He described his experiment in two letters addressed to his mentor Giovanni Alfonso Borelli [8, 9] (fig. 1).

1667. The Royal Society of London invited Malpighi to undertake its scientific correspondence and offered to have all his work set in type. We found in Naples an original published copy of *Opera Omnia* by Malpighi [10] (fig. 2) that belonged to the famous physician Domenico Cotugno (1736–1822), who was the first to reveal albumin in urine. As reported by Schena [11] Cotugno had a large collection of books and antiquities. Much of his library was lost after his death or burned by his wife for unknown reasons. Fortunately, Malpighi's *Opera Omnia* was purchased by the founder of Naples Botanical Garden, Michele Tenore, who left his library to the University of Naples.

1680. The famous text *De Motu Animalium* by Giovanni Alfonso Borelli was published after his death. Borelli applied mathematical interpretations to animal physiology [12, 13].

These events are presented in a hyperlinked text with period music which allows movement within the application from one place in time to another without loss of orientation.

Conclusions

Although science and technology are of fundamental importance in the complex modern world, there is a serious imbalance in our approach to a general education. Our culture allows and excuses widespread scientific illiteracy, exacerbates differences between the sciences and humanities, and encourages overspecialization within all disciplines. Studies of the history of science might do much to bridge the gap between scientists and nonscientists and encourage the scientific literacy that will be needed to deal with the increasing powerful tools of molecular biology. In the past, the term 'scientific revolution' was generally limited to the physical sciences, but today we are living in the midst of a biological revolution which requires scientific awareness.

Acknowledgement

We are grateful to Professors V. Mezzogiorno, F. Mazzocca and Dr A.M. Ciarallo who provided manuscript reprints and encouragement.

References

1 Mayr E: The Growth of Biological Thought. Cambridge, Harvard University Press, 1982.
2 Negroponte N: Being Digitals. New York, Sperling & Kupfer, 1995.
3 Rossi P: The Origin of Science in Europe. Oxford, Blackwell, 1996.
4 Morton AG: History of Botanical Science. London, Academic Press, 1981.
5 Toresella S: Le xilografie botaniche e la nascita della scienza. Erboristeria Domani 1997;1:48–58.
6 Magner LN: A History of the Life Sciences. New York, Dekker, 1994.
7 Levorato M: The context of the Botanical Garden of Padua, from its foundation to the beginning of this century (in Italian). Museol Sci 1998;14/1:179–187.
8 Mezzogiorno A, Mezzogiorno V: Marcello Malpighi (1628–1694). Am J Nephrol 1997;17: 269–273.
9 Andreae L, Fine LG: Unravelling dropsy: From Marcello Malpighi's discovery of the capillaries (1661) to Stephen Hales' production of oedema in an experimental model (1733). Am J Nephrol 1997;17:359–368.
10 Malpighi M: Opera Omnia. Londini, apud Robert Scott, 1686.
11 Schena FP: Domenico Cotugno and his interest in proteinuria. Am J Nephrol 1994;14:325–329.
12 Borelli GA: On the Movement of Animals (translation P Macquet). Berlin, Springer, 1989.
13 Mezzogiorno V: Giovanni Alfonso Borelli. Naples, Arte Tipografica, 1991.

American Journal of Nephrology

Am J Nephrol 1999;19:343–345

Josep Trueta (1897–1977): Military Surgeon and Pioneer Investigator of Acute Renal Failure

Ori S. Better

Dr. Rebecca Chutick Crush Syndrome Center and Faculty of Medicine, Technion – Israel Institute of Technology, Haifa, Israel

Key Words
J. Trueta · Posttraumatic acute renal failure · Military medicine

Abstract
The great Spanish military and orthopedic surgeon J. Trueta gained his field and clinical experience in the Spanish civil war (1936–1939) and in Britain during World War II. As part of his major contribution to traumatology, he searched for the causes of the characteristic oliguria of combat casualties. For this purpose he studied the effect of induced ischemic myopathy on renal perfusion in the rabbit. He and his coworkers demonstrated conclusively that in this model there was an extreme renal cortical vasoconstriction with preservation of the medullary circulation. This early first demonstration of posttraumatic vasomotor nephropathy was independently confirmed 20 years later in the USA when 'preferential renal cortical ischemia' was demonstrated in acute renal failure in man. Thus, Trueta discovered in the early 40s the circulatory component of acute renal failure as part of his monumental contribution to military medicine.

The first pioneers of the study and management of patients and casualties with acute renal failure (ARF) were Trueta [1, 2], Bywaters [3; cited in ref. 4], and Kolff [5]. Their remarkable studies were conducted under the extreme stress and personal hardship during early Second World War when the course of the war and its final outcome were in doubt. Their combined contribution is the foundation of our current knowledge on ARF.

Josep Trueta, MD and Hon. DSc (Oxon), was born 1897 in Barcelona and graduated as an MD from the Faculty of Medicine, University of Barcelona in 1921. He was an orthopedic and military surgeon on the loyalist side in the Spanish civil war (1936–1939). Following the defeat of the republicans he was exiled from Spain in 1939 when he was invited to Britain to give advice and help in civil defense to the British home front in anticipation of the imminent Second World War. He then moved as a senior orthopedic surgeon to the Radcliffe Hospital in Oxford (1940) which was later incorporated into the Nuffield Orthopedic Center, Oxford, which with the help of Trueta became the leading orthopedic hospital in the UK at that time. In 1967 he returned to Barcelona and became president of the Catalan Society of Biology (1971–1973). Trueta died in Barcelona in 1977.

The bibliography of Trueta includes 11 books and 149 articles, many of them in prestigious journals such as *The Lancet, British Medical Journal, British Journal of Hae-*

KARGER
Fax + 41 61 306 12 34
E-Mail karger@karger.ch
www.karger.com

© 1999 S. Karger AG, Basel
0250–8095/99/0192–0343$17.50/0

Accessible online at:
http://BioMedNet.com/karger

Ori S. Better, MD
POB 9649 Bat Galim
Haifa 31096 (Israel)
Tel. +972 4 8295263, Fax +972 4 8520751

matology, Journal of Bone and Joint Surgery [British Volume], Surgery, Gynecology and Obstetrics, etc. One of his books summarizes the Catalan historic-cultural heritage. Based on his personal experience in the Spanish civil war his publications covered a wide spectrum of subjects, including: surgery of combat casualties [1], organization and activation of rescue and salvage operations during air raids on cities, osteomyelitis, coagulation of blood, and the circulation of the bones and of the kidneys [1, 2].

His papers and book on war surgery [1] had a worldwide impact at the time and were considered the classic definitive treatises on the subject in the early 40s. As a result, Trueta was widely considered the father of modern traumatic orthopedic surgery.

Trueta was one of the first (1936–1939) to search for the reasons of the posttraumatic oliguria seen early in combat casualties [1, 2]. This search led him and his associates to conduct extensive angiographic studies mainly in the rabbit of posttraumatic ARF, induced by a tourniquet placed for 4.5 h on one hind limb to cause postischemic muscle damage. This ischemic myopathy in turn resulted in an intense swelling of the affected limb musculature followed by renal cortical ischemia as proved by renal angiography. In this postmyopathy experimental model, the renal artery was markedly constricted, whereas the renal vein was dilated and the intrarenal transit time of the blood circulation shortened (from the normal of 2.7 s to 1.65 s) [2]. Moreover, the renal venous blood appeared arterialized. In contrast to the conspicuous renal cortical ischemia, the juxtamedullary circulation and the medullary circulation remained intact and even showed a tendency of engorgement. Taken together, these results showed for the first time the local and systemic deleterious effects of extensive muscle injury. Trueta proposed that ischemic muscular injury, at least in the rabbit, probably via exaggerated adrenergic tone caused extreme renal cortical vascular constriction. Such cortical constriction and increased vascular resistance diverted the renal blood flow to the low-resistance beds of the medulla and juxtamedullary glomeruli, thus by-passing the cortical circulation. Trueta felt that similar posttraumatic renal cortical vascular spasm in man was responsible for the typical oliguria seen after combat casualties.

It is interesting to note from today's perspective some of the peculiarities of the rabbit model. The muscles of the rabbit do not contain myoglobin, so that this specific species is free from the nephrotoxicity of myoglobin [6] aggravated by arterial hypotension, oliguria, and aciduria. Also, the early appearance of contrast medium as observed in the rabbit with posttraumatic ARF [2] was not seen in man with ARF [7], suggesting species differences between man and rabbit in intrarenal circulatory anatomy and physiology and their response to circulatory stress.

It appears that the phenomenon of posttraumatic renal cortical ischemia with preservation of the medullary circulation, first suggested by Trueta 1943 and proven angiographically by him in 1947 in the rabbit, was reproduced some 20 years later in man by Hollenberg et al. [7] in 1968 who demonstrated 'preferential cortical ischemia' (their terminology) in 20 patients with oliguric renal failure secondary to shock, acute glomerulonephritis, renal allograft ischemia, or allograft rejection. Renal perfusion in these patients with ARF [7] was monitored by selective angiography, radioactive xenon tracer studies, and in some open renal biopsy specimens (which showed a reduced renal bleeding tendency). Similar extreme renal cortical ischemia was seen in a patient with the hepato-renal syndrome [8] (reversible on postmortem renal perfusion).

Hollenberg et al. [7] postulated in 1968 that increased adrenergic tone and activation of the renin-angiotensin II system caused preglomerular cortical vasoconstriction and oliguria in their patients with ARF. Today one would add to the list posttraumatic hemodynamic, toxic, or immune activation of additional renal vasoconstrictor systems (in parallel with increased α-adrenergic tone), such as with arginine vasopressin, thromboxane, and endothelin. Hemodynamic or ischemic activation of endothelin is a particularly appealing possibility, since this most potent of the vasoconstrictors acts preferentially in the renal cortex, while sparing the medullary circulation, partially through activation of the medullary nitric oxide synthase system and nitric oxide production as well as prostaglandin generation, both medullary vasorelaxants [9, 10].

It appears that the statement of Trueta made in 1943 [1, p. 122] that posttraumatic ARF in casualties is 'probably due to the spasm of the renal arteries' and to preferential cortical ischemia with sparing of the medulla withstood the test of time and was reproducible in man with ARF 20 years later [7]. Starting from such fundamental simple field and bedside observations, Trueta thus postulated the concept of acute vasomotor nephropathy. Trueta aptly dedicated his 1947 book on the renal circulation [2] to William Bowman, Claude Bernard and Richard Bright, thus affiliating himself with and ushering in the nascent field of Nephrology. This drive led him to visit in the early 50s the laboratories of Homer Smith in New York where he presented his views on the circulation of the kidney [Schreiner, personal commun].

References

1 Trueta J: The Principles and Practice of War Surgery. London, Hamilton Medical Books and Heinemann Medical Books, 1943.
2 Trueta J, Barclay AE, Daniel PM, Franklin KJ, Prichord MML: Studies of the Renal Circulation. Oxford, Blackwell, 1947.
3 Bywaters EGL: 50 years of the crush syndrome. BMJ 1990;301:1412–1415.
4 Better OS: History of the crush syndrome: From the earthquakes of Messina, Sicily 1909 to Spitak, Armenia 1988. Am J Nephrol 1997; 17:392–394.
5 Kolff WJ: First clinical experience with the artificial kidney. Ann Intern Med 1965;62: 608–619.
6 Bywaters EGL, Stead JK: The production of renal failure following injection of myohemoglobin. Q J Exp Physiol 1944;33:53–70.
7 Hollenberg NK, Epstein M, Rosen SM, Basch RI, Oren DE, Merril J: Acute oliguric renal failure in man: Evidence for preferential cortical ischemia. Medicine (Baltimore) 1968;47:455–474.
8 Epstein M, Bork DP, Hollenberg NK, et al: Renal failure in the patient with cirrhosis: The role of active vasoconstriction. Am J Med 1970;49:175–185.
9 Brezis M, Rosen S: Hypoxia of the renal medulla. Its implications for disease. N Engl J Med 1995;332:647–655.
10 Abassi Z, Gurbanov K, Rubinstein I, Better OS, Hoffman A, Winaver J: Regulation of intrarenal blood flow in experimental heart failure: Role of endothelin and nitric oxide. Am J Physiol 1998;274:F766–F774.

History of Dialysis and Transplantation

American Journal of Nephrology

Am J Nephrol 1999;19:346–349

A Note on the Early History of Renal Transplantation: Emerich (Imre) Ullmann

Judit Nagy

Nephrological Center and Second Department of Medicine, University Medical School of Pécs, Hungary

Key Words
Transplantation · Kidney · Ullmann

Abstract
In January 1902 at the Vienna Medical Society Meeting, the surgeon Emerich Ullmann reported the first case of renal autotransplantation performed in the neck of a dog. In the same year, he presented the first xenotransplantation of the kidney (a goat with a dog's kidney). These publications immediately had a great impact on the medical word. After his failed attempt to transplant a pig's kidney into a young uraemic woman he stopped his research in this field in order to devote himself to other lines of surgical research. However, his idea survived him, because, nowadays, nearly 100 years later, pigs appear to be the most suitable donors for human renal xenotransplantation. Ullmann was born in Pécs, Hungary, on February 23, 1861. After a distinguished undergraduate career in 1878 his father (being also a medical doctor) sent him to study medicine at the world-famous Vienna Medical School. He graduated in 1884 and was immediately invited to the Surgical Department where Billroth worked. Next year, because of his interest in bacteriology he visited Pasteur in Paris and successfully volunteered to serve as a healthy subject to prove the effectiveness of Pasteur's antisera against rabies. Although Ullmann did not succeed in doing a human transplantation he gave birth to the era of the organ transplantation, stimulated vascular surgery and the development of transplantation immunology.

Replacing a diseased, non-functioning organ with a healthy one from another individual – dead or alive – is an attractive solution to the problem of organ failure. Replacing a non-functioning kidney was a forerunner in the field, although there was a long time between the dream and the reality of giving a new life to the patients with end-stage renal failure.

The beginnings go back to the mythology of ancient Egypt and Greece where there are countless examples of metamorphoses, symbolic incarnations, demons, sirens, tritons or centaurs which can be considered as prefigurations of transplantations or grafting. In reality, however, these creatures were the products of limitless imagination that enjoyed the mixing or transformation of different species.

The works of Ovid and Homer contain several examples of these mythological hybrids. For example, Ovid in the fifth book of his *Metamorphosis* mentions a hunter, Actaeon, who surprised Artemis while she was bathing. For this offense, he was transformed into a stag by the goddess and was torn to pieces by his own dogs who could no longer recognize him (fig. 1). With some imagination,

KARGER

Fax + 41 61 306 12 34
E-Mail karger@karger.ch
www.karger.com

© 1999 S. Karger AG, Basel
0250–8095/99/0192–0346$17.50/0

Accessible online at:
http://BioMedNet.com/karger

Judit Nagy
Nephrological Center and Second Department of Medicine
University of Medical School of Pécs, Pacsirta u. 1
H–7624 Pécs (Hungary)
Tel. +36 72 324 122/2265, Fax +36 72 333 533, E-Mail nagyju@bel2.pote.hu

1

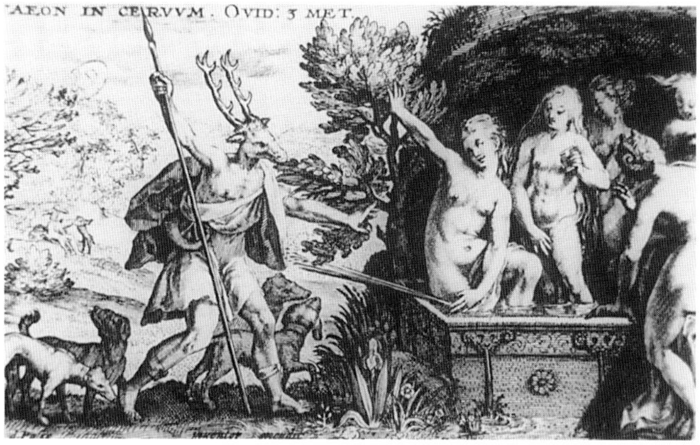

2

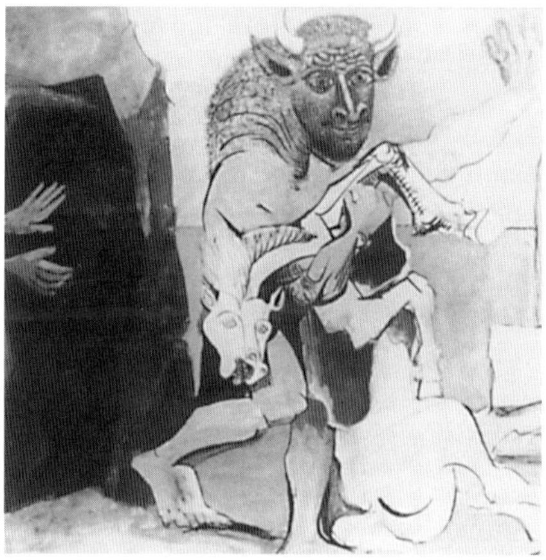

Fig. 1. Actaeon from the fifth book of Ovid's *Metamorphosis* (17th century engraving). Bibliothèque des Arts Décoratifs.
Fig. 2. Picasso: *Guernica* (detail with the Minotaur). Musée Picasso, Paris.

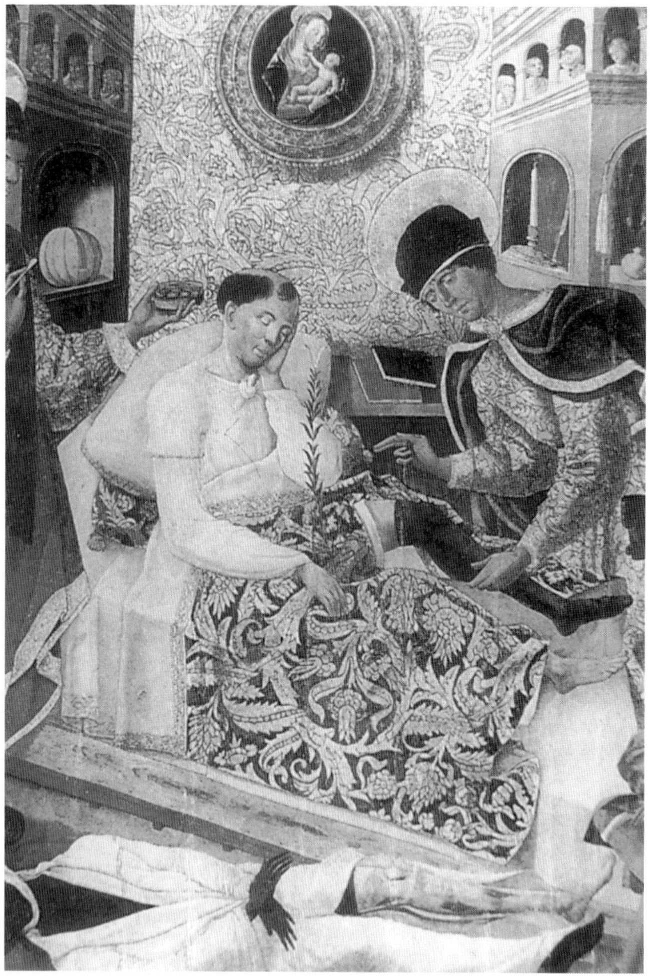

Fig. 3. Fra Angelico: Saint Cosmas and Saint Damian grafting a leg taken from a cadaver on a sexton.

this can be considered as the first literary evidence of transplantation and rejection immunology! This archival but miraculous mythological world has been a favourite theme of different painters. For example, in Picasso's *Guernica* we can see the Minotaur with a bull's head, a rendering of whole body segment transplantation (fig. 2).

Later, in the Christian era myths and legends gave way to miracles based on acts of faith. In connection with transplantation the most famous miracle was recorded in the 13th century, in the golden legend of the 'Lives of Saints'. It was performed by Saint Cosmas and Saint Damian during the reign of Diocletian in 280. On the basis of the legend they grafted a leg taken from the cadaver of a Moor on a sexton (fig. 3).

However, all these metamorphoses, symbolic incarnations and miraculous transplantations were the product of boundless imagination. During the long period that followed, animal experiments were performed to solve the problem of acute transplantation. Experiments were done with almost every type of organ, but soon, the kidney was adopted as the best experimental model. And in 1902 at a meeting of the Vienna Medical Society Emerich Ullmann reported the first successful renal transplantation [1–5].

Imre (the Hungarian name for Emerich) Ullmann (fig. 4) was born in 1861 and grew up in Pécs [6–8]. His name is recorded in the parish birth registry of Pécs (fig. 5, 6). At that time, German was the official administrative language in Hungary, which is the reason why the registry

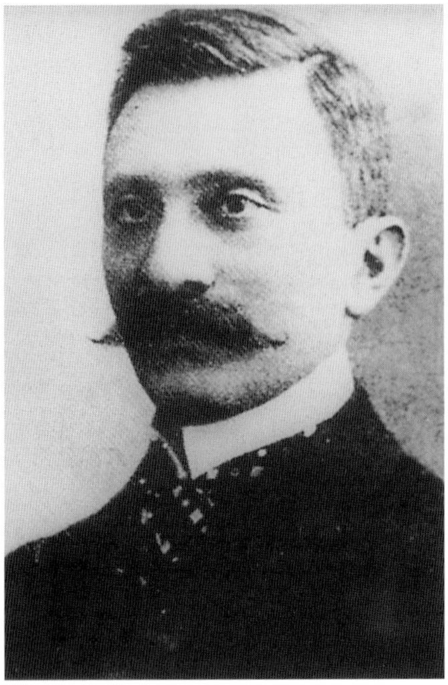

4

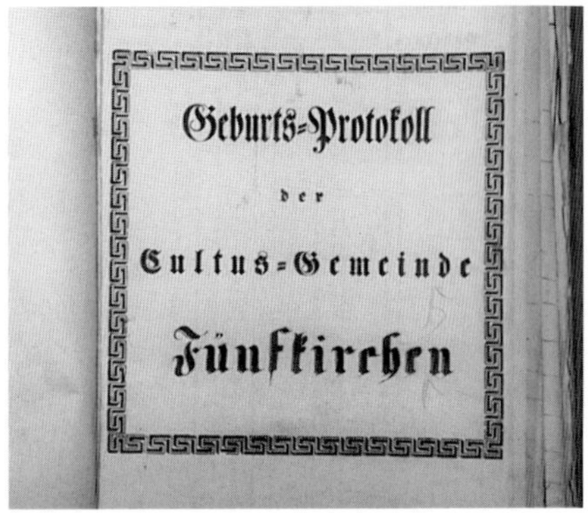

5

Fig. 4. Emerich (Imre) Ullmann. Institute for the History of Medicine, Vienna University.

Fig. 5. The cover page of the parish birth registry of Pécs in 1861.

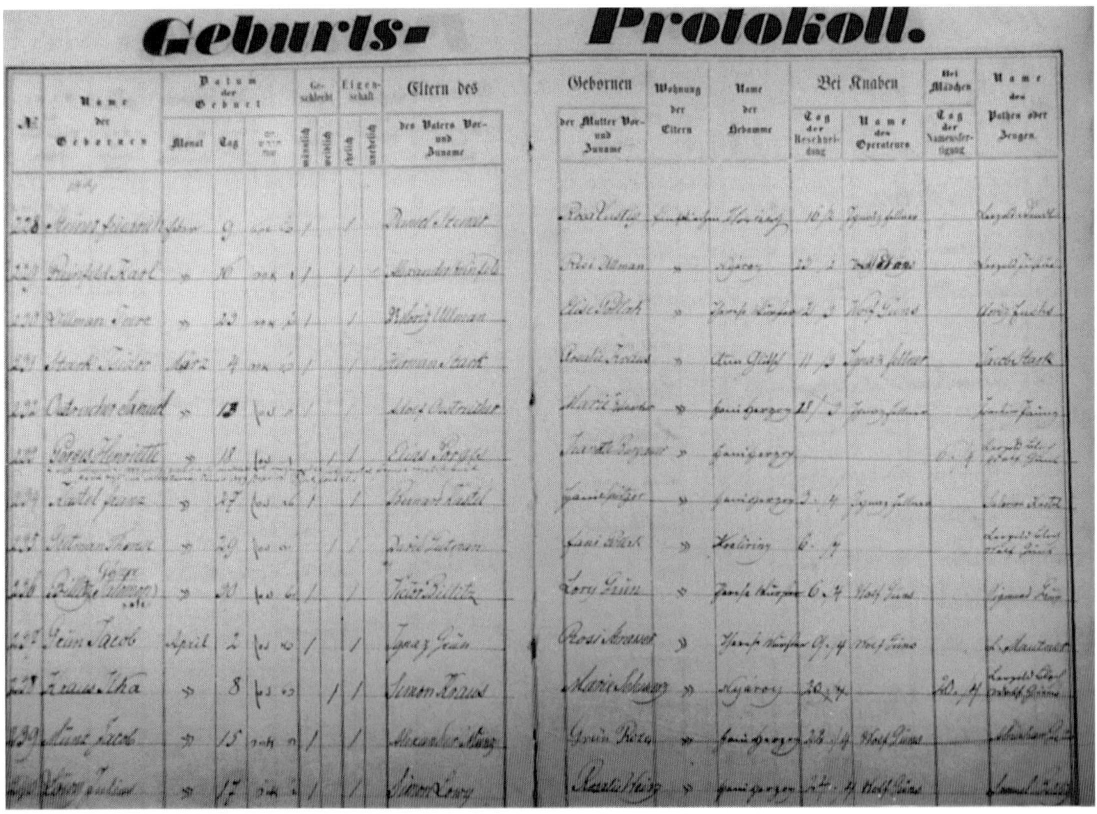

Fig. 6. The registration of the newborn Imre Ullmann in the birth registry.

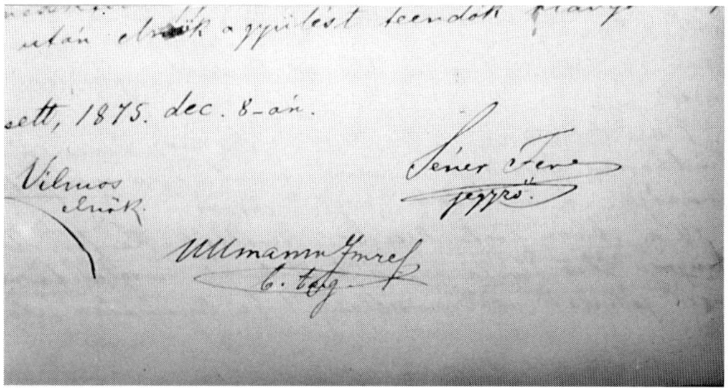

Fig. 7. The signature of Ullmann on minutes of the meeting of the schoolboy's literary society.

book was written in German. Fünfkirchen is the German name of Pécs, which is the translation of the original name Quinque Ecclesiae given during the Roman Age. His father, Moritz Ullmann, was a well-know general practioner of medicine in Pécs [9].

When the young Imre attended elementary school in Pécs his name was entered in the Golden Book of the school as one of the three best pupils in his class. Having completed his elementary education Imre entered the Gymnasium of the Cictercian Order in Pécs. The Cictercians ran a famous Gymnasium, where Imre became a member of its literary society (fig. 7). On the basis of one of his certificates he was rated excellent in Latin, Greek, Hungarian, German, Geography and History, but only satisfactory in mathematics and the natural science, biology.

In 1880 Ullmann went to Vienna to attend its world-famous medical university. At that time Vienna was the capital of the Austrian-Hungarian Empire. There was also a well-known medical school in Buda; however, from Pécs, it was much easier to reach the Austrian part of the monarchy because there was a direct railway connection between Vienna and Pécs.

He finished his medical studies at the age of 23, and, because of his interest in the newly born discipline of bacteriology, he went to Paris to work with Pasteur. In Pasteur's lab he received training in animal experimentation and because of his great interest in clinical research successfully volunteered to prove the effectiveness of Pasteur's antisera against rabbit [10].

In 1885 he returned to Vienna and started to practice as a surgeon at the First Department of Surgery of the university. After several attempts, he performed his famous transplant demonstration on March 7, 1902. He did an allotransplantation and removed the kidney of a dog and transplanted it into the neck of another dog, the renal artery being joined to the carotid artery and the renal vein to the external jugular vein by means of special chackles (e.g. Payr's prostheses). The end of the ureter was sutured to the skin and – in the presence of the audience – urine flowed from the ureter. The kidney functioned for 5 days. He published his work [5], and because of the interest it received he continued his transplantation experiments on different animals for some time. He even attempted to transplant the kidney of a pig into the elbow of a young uraemic woman, but failed to resolve the technical difficulties [11].

It has been said that, although he did not succeed in doing a human transplantation, Ullmann gave birth to the era of transplantation, stimulated vascular surgery to solve the problem of vascular anastomoses of transplants and stimulated the development of transplantation immunology [12–14].

References

1 Bollinger RR, Stickel DL: Transplantation. Historical aspects; in Sabiston DC Jr, Lyerly HK (eds): Textbook of Surgery. The Biological Basis of Modern Surgical Practice. Philadelphia, Saunders, 1994, p 383.

2 Klimpel V: Zum 125. Geburtstag von Emerich Ullmann (1861–1937). Z Exp Chir Transplant Künstl Organe 1987;20:177–179.

3 Lagiader F: 72 years of organ transplantation. Eur Surg Res 1974;6:197–208.

4 Lesky E: Die erste Nierentransplantation Emerich Ullmann (1861–1937). Münch Med Wochenschr 1974;116:1081–1084.

5 Ullmann E: Experimentelle Nierentransplantation. Wien Klin Wochenschr 1902;11:281–285.

6 Rajczy Á: Régiekröl röviden. Magyarország 1986;33:31.

7 Rajczy P: Professzorok és diákok Nagy Lajos Király pécsi egyetemén. Baranya-megyei Történelmi Közlemények 1992–1993; V-VI.évf.1-2 szám, pp 131–136.

8 Török B: Egy elfelejtett magyar tudós, Dr. Ullmann Imre (1861–1937). Orvosi Hetilap 1974; 115:2069–2071.

9 Rajczy P: Pécsi diák – bécsi utcanév. Új Dunántúli Napló 1991;12:04.10.

10 Glaser H: Az életért harcoltak. Orvosok híres önkísérletei, Budapest, 1963, pp 93–94.

11 Küss R, Bourget P: An Illustrated History of Organ Transplantation. Laboratoires Sandoz, Rueil-Malmaison, France, 1992.

12 Carrel A: Transplantation in mass of the kidneys. J Exp Med 1908;10:98–141.

13 Hierholzer K, Winau R: Pioneer nephrologists of Berlin. Am J Nephrol 1992;12:442–450.

14 Pichlmayr R, Grotelüschen B: Entwicklung und heutiger Stand der Nierentransplantation. Med Welt 1973;24:26–29.

History of Dialysis and Transplantation

American Journal of Nephrology

Am J Nephrol 1999;19:350–354

The Early Years of Chronic Dialysis: The Seattle Contribution

Christopher R. Blagg

Northwest Kidney Centers and the University of Washington, Seattle, Wash., USA

Key Words
Hemodialysis · Peritoneal dialysis · Scribner · Seattle Artificial Kidney Center

Abstract
Long-term hemodialysis for chronic renal failure first became possible with development of the Teflon shunt by Belding Scribner and coworkers at the University of Washington, Seattle, in 1960. Over the next 4 years, many of the advances in dialysis occurred in Seattle. These included recognition and treatment of complications such as malignant hypertension, gouty episodes due to uric acid accumulation, subcutaneous calcification, anemia, iron overload, and peripheral neuropathy. Technical advances included improving the shunt, and in collaboration with Professor A.L. Babb, development of a proportioning system to make dialysate from concentrate and water and the first automated home hemodialysis machine. Dr. Boen and Dr. Tenckhoff developed automated peritoneal dialysis equipment and peritoneal access devices. The world's first outpatient dialysis center, the Seattle Artificial Kidney Center, was established in 1962, and used an anonymous lay committee to select from medically suitable patients those to be treated by the center. This triage was an important step in the development of biomedical ethics, and in 1964, Scribner's presidential address to the American Society for Artificial Internal Organs discussed the problems of patient selection, termination of treatment, patient suicide, death with dignity, and selection for transplantation.

Dialysis as a treatment for acute renal failure evolved from Kolff's development of the artificial kidney in the early 1940s. However, efforts to do repeated dialysis for the long-term care of patients with chronic uremia failed because the necessary materials were not yet available. A fortunate combination of circumstances in Seattle changed this in 1960, and for the next decade and longer, many of the technical developments of dialysis occurred there. This paper is a brief chronology of the events that occurred.

Hemodialysis

1953
Dialysis for acute renal failure in Seattle began with the appointment of Belding Scribner (fig. 1) as an Associate in Medicine at the recently established University of Washington Medical School.

KARGER
Fax +41 61 306 12 34
E-Mail karger@karger.ch
www.karger.com

© 1999 S. Karger AG, Basel
0250–8095/99/0192–0350$17.50/0

Accessible online at:
http://BioMedNet.com/karger

Christopher R. Blagg, MD
Northwest Kidney Centers
700 Broadway
Seattle, WA 98122 (USA)
Tel. +1 206 292 2941, Fax +1 206 860 5821, E-Mail blagg@u.washington.edu

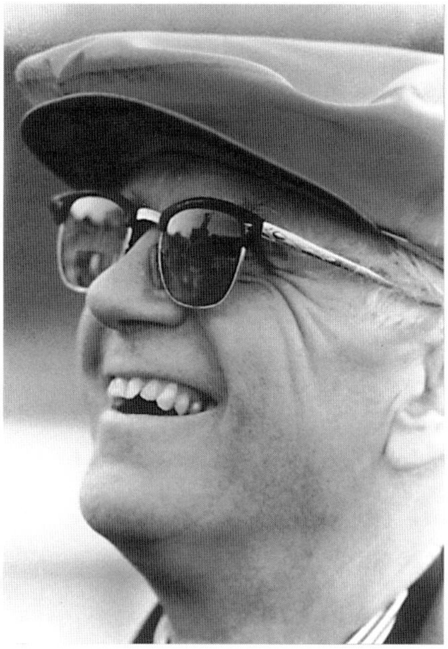

1

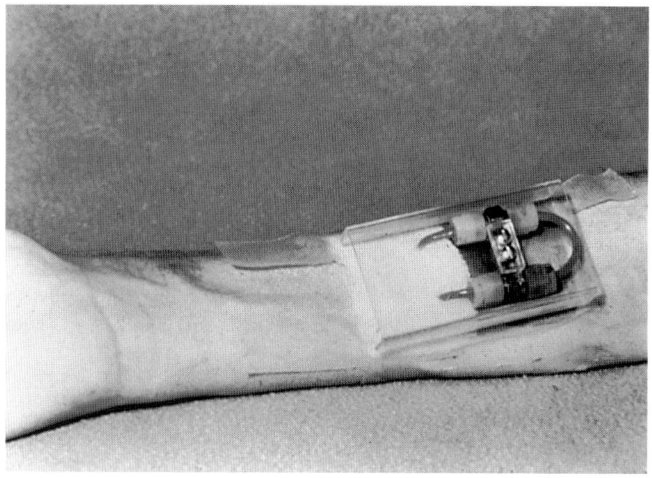

2

Fig. 1. Belding H. Scribner.
Fig. 2. Teflon shunt.

1957

Scribner and his team studied gastrodialysis as a treatment for uremia, using equipment developed to cycle dialysis fluid in and out of a large intragastric cellophane balloon [1]. This removed very little nitrogenous material, although enough hydrochloric acid was removed to require replacement to prevent alkalosis. The publication on this technique resulted in an invitation to Scribner to join the recently founded American Society for Artificial Internal Organs (ASAIO).

1960

A patient thought to have acute renal failure was found on biopsy to have irreversible chronic renal disease and had to be sent home to die. As a result, Scribner cogitated on how to provide the blood access for long-term hemodialysis using a shunt between a forearm artery and vein. This had been tried before, notably by Nils Alwall in Sweden, but had always failed because of clotting, bleeding or infection. Fortuitously, Teflon tubing had just become available and, because of its tissue nonreactivity, was being used to cover pacemaker leads. Scribner and Wayne Quinton, an engineer at the University of Washington Hospital, devised a shunt using this tubing and commercially available plumbing supplies. Only later was it realized that this remained patent between dialyses because of the nonstick properties of Teflon.

March 9, 1960

With Wayne Quinton bending Teflon tubing at the bedside, David Dillard, a pediatric heart surgeon, placed the first shunt in the left forearm of Clyde Shields, a local machinist with chronic renal failure (fig. 2). It worked, allowing repeated hemodialysis, and so on March 20 a similar shunt was placed in a second patient, a 22-year-old shoe salesman. This was also successful, and so a third patient soon was started on dialysis. Initially, all were treated with one 24-hour dialysis weekly and a 40-gram protein low-potassium diet, and as a result developed lethargy, pruritus, nausea and vomiting some 24–36 h before the next dialysis. Two four-layer Skeggs-Leonards dialyzers in parallel were used, and up to 450 liters of dialysate was made from preweighed bags of chemicals and tap water mixed with a canoe paddle in a Sears Roebuck chest-type freezer and refrigerated to 4 °C to retard bacterial growth.

April 1960

Scribner's team was anxious to show off their success at the ASAIO meeting but had not submitted an abstract. Consequently, they took Clyde Shields and his wife, Emmy, to the meeting in Chicago, and showed Clyde, his shunt, and the preliminary data to selected individuals at a special breakfast meeting. That evening in his hotel room, Quinton showed them how to bend Teflon and make cannulas. George Schreiner, the editor of the ASAIO Transactions saw the importance of this development and was kind enough to allow manuscripts to be submitted and published [2, 3].

1961

During a trip to Scandinavia, Scribner was given a Kiil dialyzer by Claus Brun. Originally designed as a membrane oxygenator, this made an admirable dialyzer because of its reproducible performance and low blood flow resistance, and it had a higher solute clearance than the Skeegs-Leonards dialyzer. As a result, the Kiil became the standard dialyzer in Seattle until cheap low-resistance disposable dialyzers became available some ten years later.

Within a few months of starting dialysis, the first patients began to develop problems. Clyde developed malignant hypertension resistant to reserpine and hydralazine but that was controlled, without drugs, by effective ultrafiltration [4], although this caused cramps and hypotension late in dialysis. The patients also developed gout-like episodes due to uric acid accumulation [5] and subcutaneous lumps that proved to be metastatic calcification. In addition, Clyde began to have difficulty in walking, and the third patient developed severe peripheral neuropathy. All these problems were improved by increasing the frequency of dialysis to 12 h twice a week. In addition, because aluminum-containing antacids used by ulcer patients were known to cause phosphate depletion, they were tried and found to be very successful in treating the calcifications. Iron overload also developed as a result of the need for repeated transfusions to treat anemia. Studies of bone marrow kinetics by Joe Eschbach and others [6] showed that by stopping transfusions the suppressed marrow would slowly become active again to provide acceptable hematocrit levels.

1961

The all-Teflon cannula was rigid, and so arm movements caused the tip to damage the vessel intima. Despite the fact that Dow Corning said it could not be done Quinton discovered how to extrude silicone rubber as tubing. A segment of this was inserted in the shunt to act as a shock absorber, so extending cannula life [7].

1963

Scribner began a collaboration with A.L. Babb, professor of Nuclear Engineering, which led to the development of the first proportioning pump system for dialysate production – 'the monster' [8]. This mixed water and concentrated electrolyte solution to make dialysate for four dialysis stations. The use of a 34:1 mix required the use of something other than bicarbonate in the concentrate, and Charles Mion came up with acetate [9]. This became part of all dialysate concentrates for many years.

1963–1964

Babb [10] and his staff miniaturized the proportioning system to make a single-patient automated home hemodialysis machine – 'the minimonster' – for use by a 15-year-old girl with renal failure. This proved safe, effective and economical, was the prototype for single-patient equipment generally, and made home hemodialysis feasible [11, 12].

1965

Scribner proposed the square meter-hour hypothesis based on the observation that peritoneal dialysis patients rarely developed neuropathy [13]. Over the next 10 years this evolved into the middle molecule hypothesis [14, 15] which became a major stimulus to further research on uremic toxicity, membrane technology and dialysis techniques.

Peritoneal Dialysis

1962

Fred Boen, the Dutch peritoneal dialysis pioneer, came to Seattle and modified the gastrodialysis equipment to make a closed peritoneal dialysis system using 40-liter jugs of dialysate sterilized by autoclaving [16].

1963

Boen was joined by Henry Tenckhoff, who continued to work on peritoneal dialysis after Boen returned to The Netherlands. Over the next 9 years, Tenckhoff developed the peritoneal catheter that bears his name [17], devised home peritoneal dialysis equipment using heat sterilization at the bedside to prepare the dialysate [18] and a home peritoneal dialysis system using reverse osmosis and ultraviolet light for sterilization [19]. The latter was used extensively until the development of continuous ambulatory peritoneal dialysis by Popovich and Moncrieff – the former having been a graduate student with Babb.

The Seattle Artificial Kidney Center and Bioethics

1961

When it became obvious that long-term hemodialysis worked, Scribner approached Dr. James Haviland, president of the King County Medical Society, to ask for help in establishing a community-based, free-standing outpatient dialysis unit.

January 1962

With assistance from the Seattle Area Hospital Council and funding from the John A. Hartford Foundation and the US Public Health Service, the Seattle Artificial Kidney Center (SAKC) was established in the basement of the Swedish Hospital's nurses home as the first out-of-hospital freestanding dialysis unit [20]. It opened with three beds, three patients, two nurses, one technician and a physician. Patients were dialyzed for 12–16 h twice weekly with Skeggs-Leonards (later Kiil dialyzers), using Sweden Freezer batch tanks for the dialysate [21].

1962

Based on a survey and from life insurance data it was estimated there would be 5–20 ideal candidates for dialysis per million population per year. As this was beyond the capacity of the SAKC, a selection process had to be implemented. A Medical Advisory Committee was established to review potential patients by strict medical criteria – emotional stability, age less than 45 years, disabled by uremic symptoms, without long-standing hypertension and its complications, especially coronary artery and cerebrovascular disease, and demonstrated willingness to cooperate with the treatment and dietary restrictions. Children, young adults who were not self-supporting and non-residents of the state of Washington were excluded. Medically acceptable candidates were then referred to an anonymous Admissions and Policy Committee consisting of two physicians who were not nephrologists, a lawyer, a housewife, a businessman, a labor leader and a minister. They attempted to assess the relative worth of candidates to their family and the community in terms of degree of dependence of others upon the candidate's continuing existence, and their rehabilitation potential and moral value or worth. The minister who chaired the committee has since described his experience [22].

November 1962

This committee became notorious as a result of a *Life* magazine article on Scribner and the Seattle program [23]. Subsequently, it became the subject of many articles and discussions [24–27], and has been regarded as responsible for the birth of bioethics as a separate discipline [28]. This is discussed elsewhere in more detail [29].

April 1964

Scribner's presidential address to the ASAIO discussed the ethical lessons learned from the Seattle experience: the problems of patient selection, overt termination of treatment, patient suicide, death with dignity, and selection for organ transplantation [30]. These issues are just as relevant today, as is his comment that 'scientists are also members of society and have an obligation to be concerned about the effect of their discoveries on society'.

Acknowledgements

I would like to thank Dr. Babb for his help with information and, as always, Dr. Scribner for his support and friendship over the years.

References

1 Marr TA, Burnell JM, Scribner BH: Gastrodialysis in the treatment of acute renal failure. J Clin Invest 1960;39:653–661.
2 Quinton We, Dillard DH, Scribner BH: Cannulation of blood vessels for prolonged hemodialysis. Trans Am Soc Artif Intern Organs 1960;6:104–113.
3 Scribner BH, Buri R, Caner JEZ, Hegstrom R, Burnell JM: The treatment of chronic uremia by means of intermittent hemodialysis: A preliminary report. Trans Am Soc Artif Intern Organs 1960;6:114–122.
4 Hegstrom RM, Quinton WE, Dillard DH, Cole JJ, Scribner BH: One year's experience with the use of indwelling Teflon cannulas and bypass. Trans Am Soc Artif Intern Organs 1961;7:47–56.
5 Caner JEZ, Hegstrom RM, Decker JD: Recurrent acute (gouty?) arthritis in chronic renal failure treated with periodic hemodialysis. JAMA 1964;36:571–582.
6 Eschbach JW, Funk D, Adamson J, Kuhn I, Scribner BH, Finch CA: Erythropoiesis in patients with renal failure undergoing chronic dialysis. N Engl J Med 1967;276:653–658.
7 Quinton WE, Dillard DH, Cole JJ, Scribner BH: Eight months' experience with Silastic-Teflon bypass cannulas. Trans Am Soc Artif Intern Organs 1962;8:236–243.
8 Grimsrud L, Cole JJ, Lehman GA, Babb AL, Scribner BH: A central system for the continuous preparation and distribution of dialysis fluid. Trans Am Soc Artif Intern Organs 1964;10:107–109.
9 Mion CM, Hegstrom RM, Boen ST, Scribner BH: Substitution of sodium acetate for sodium bicarbonate in the bath fluid for hemodialysis. Trans Am Soc Artif Intern Organs 1964;10:110–113.

10 Babb AL: Design and construction of a portable, single patient dialysate proportioning machine at the University of Washington 1964–65. ASAIO J 1995;41:1–10.
11 Curtis FK, Cole JJ, Fellows BJ, Tyler LL, Scribner BH: Hemodialysis in the home. Trans Am Soc Artif Intern Organs 1965;11:7–10.
12 Eschbach JW Jr, Wilson WE, Peoples RW, Wakefield AW, Babb AL, Scribner BH: Unattended overnight home hemodialysis. Trans Am Soc Artif Intern Organs 1966;12:346–356.
13 Scribner BH: Discussion. Trans Am Soc Artif Intern Organs 1965;11:29.
14 Babb AL, Popovich RP, Christopher TG, Scribner BH: The genesis of the square meter-hour hypothesis. Trans Am Soc Artif Intern Organs 1971;17:81–91.
15 Scribner BH, Babb AL: Evidence for toxins of 'middle' molecular weight. Kidney Int 1975; 7(suppl 2):S349–S351.
16 Boen ST, Mion CM, Curtis FK, Shilipetar G: Periodic peritoneal dialysis using the repeated puncture technique and an automatic cycling machine. Trans Am Soc Artif Intern Organs 1964;10:409–414.
17 Tenckhoff H, Schecter H: A bacteriologically safe peritoneal access device. Trans Am Soc Artif Intern Organs 1968;14:181–187.
18 Tenckhoff H, Shilipetar G, van Paaschen WH, Swanson E: A home peritoneal dialysate delivery system. Trans Am Soc Artif Intern Organs 1969;15:103–107.
19 Tenckhoff H, Meston B, Shilipetar G: A simplified automatic peritoneal dialysis system. Trans Am Soc Artif Intern Organs 1972;18: 436–439.
20 Haviland JW: Experiences in establishing a community artificial kidney center. Trans Am Clin Climatol Assoc 1966;72:125–136.
21 Murray JS, Tu WH, Albers JB, Burnell JM, Scribner BH: A community hemodialysis center for the treatment of chronic uremia. Trans Am Soc Artif Intern Organs 1962;8:315–320.
22 Darrah JB: The committee. Trans Am Soc Artif Intern Organs 1987;33:791–793.
23 Alexander S: They decide who lives, who dies: Medical miracle puts moral burden on small committee. Life 1962;53:102–125.
24 Schreiner GE: Problems of ethics in relation to hemodialysis; in Wolstenholme GEW, O'Connor M (eds): Ethics in Medical Progress: With Special Reference to Transplantation. Boston, Little, Brown 1996, p 128.
25 Sanders D, Dukermenier J Jr: Medical advance and legal lag: Hemodialysis and kidney transplantation. UCLA Law Rev 1968;15:366–380.
26 Rescher N: The allocation of exotic medical lifesaving therapy. Ethics 1969;79:173–186.
27 Childress JF: Who shall live when not all can live? Surroundings 1970;53:339–355.
28 Jonsen AR: The Birth of Bioethics. New York, Oxford University Press, 1998.
29 Blagg CR: Development of ethical concepts in dialysis: Seattle in the 1960s. Symposium on the History of Dialysis. Nephrology 1998;4: 235–238.
30 Scribner BH: Presidential address: Ethical problems of using artificial organs to sustain human life. Trans Am Soc Artif Intern Organs 1964;10:209–213.

American Journal of Nephrology

History of Dialysis and Transplantation

Am J Nephrol 1999;19:355–362

Artificial Dialysis Membranes: From Concept to Large Scale Production

Jörg Vienken[a] Michael Diamantoglou[b] Werner Henne[b] Bernd Nederlof[a]

[a]Fresenius Medical Care, Bad Homburg, and [b]Akzo Nobel Membrana, Wuppertal, Germany

Key Words

Historical dialysis membranes · Collodion · Cellophane · Cellulose · Modified cellulose membranes · Polysulfone-membrane modifications

Abstract

The development of hemodialysis from an experimental concept to a routine medical therapy is closely related to research, manufacturing and availability of dialysis membranes. Collodion, a cellulose-trinitrate derivative, was the first polymer to be used as an artificial membrane and played a central role in further investigations and applications. Basic studies on the mechanism of solute transport through membranes, like diffusion, were done by A. Fick and T. Graham using collodion as a membrane material. In vivo dialysis in animals and humans was performed with collodion by J. Abel in the USA and G. Haas in Germany. Cellophane and Cuprophan membranes replaced collodion later, because of their better performance and mechanical stability. However, due to its alleged lack of hemocompatibility, membranes made from unmodified cellulose lost their market share. They have been replaced by modified cellulosic and synthetic dialysis membranes which show a better hemocompatibility than unmodified cellulose membranes. Most of the new membrane materials are also available in high-flux modifications and for this reason suitable as well for more effective therapy modes, such as hemodiafiltration and hemofiltration. The success of hemodialysis as a routine therapy is also the success of membrane development, because both, a reproducible membrane production and an unlimited availability of dialysis membranes have increased the number of dialyzed patients to about 1 million patients worldwide in 1999.

Introduction

The realization of hemodialysis as a routine therapy for several hundred thousands of patients does not depend on research in physiology and medicine alone. Industrial achievements in terms of production technology and economic availability contribute considerably to new medical therapies such as hemodialysis. The search for appropriate membrane materials, their identification and assessment of chemical and performance properties are essential when membrane properties are adapted to the needs of dialysis patients. Further, membrane materials must be able to undergo standard sterilization processes and should be available in large and reproducible quantities.

KARGER

Fax + 41 61 306 12 34
E-Mail karger@karger.ch
www.karger.com

© 1999 S. Karger AG, Basel

0250–8095/99/0192–0355$17.50/0

Accessible online at:
http://BioMedNet.com/karger

Dr. Jörg Vienken
Fresenius Medical Care, Else Kroener Strasse 1
D–61352 Bad Homburg (Germany)
Tel. +49 6172 609 2463, Fax +49 6172 609 2468
E-Mail joerg.vienken@fmc-ag.de

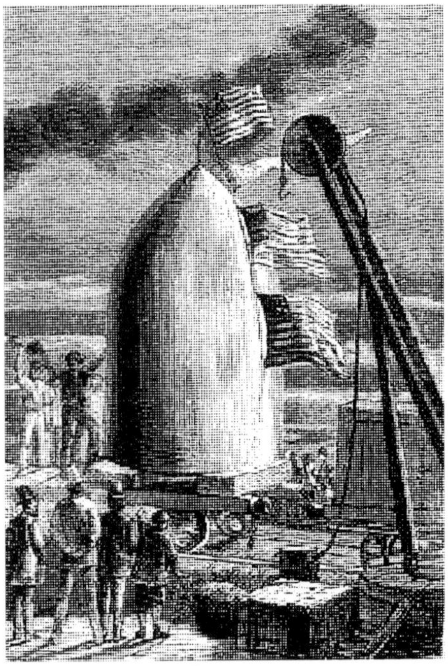

Fig. 1. Collodion or cellulose nitrate is highly explosive and also called guncotton. Jules Verne reported in his story *'From the Earth to the Moon'* published in 1865 about its use for launching a space rocket.

The beginning of research on dialysis membranes in modern times can be attributed to a Scotsman from Glasgow. The chemist Thomas Graham [1] (1805–1869) used the term 'dialysis' in the literature in 1854, when he described the movement of various types of solutes through a membrane forced by osmotic pressures. Graham had fashioned his first membranes from an ox bladder, he later used membranes made from parchment paper. Adolph Fick (1829–1901) from Kassel, Germany, published his famous laws on diffusion in 1855, 1 year after Thomas Graham. His fundamental experiments had been stimulated by earlier observations of Robert Brown in 1827 on the movements of gas molecules, these effects being later called 'Brownian movement'. Fick attributed the passive transport of solutes through membranes to diffusional processes as a consequence of differences in their concentration on either side of the membrane [2].

Both, Thomas Graham and Adolph Fick, would certainly never have dreamt that their principal observations led to a medical therapy called hemodialysis, which has become a routine treatment mode for blood purification about 150 years later and that currently more than 1 million uremic patients owe their lives to this therapy.

In this paper we concentrate on the advent of artificial dialysis membranes, their first application, manufacturing and characterization. A short perspective on membranes in modern dialysis is presented at the end of this short review.

Artificial Membranes in Dialysis: The Early Observations

Natural membranes, like ox bladder, sheep peritoneum or parchment paper, have several disadvantages: their permeability and performance are not always reproducible. The performance and stability of membranes from animal sources depends on their origin and on their preparational processes. With artificial membranes fabricated from chemical polymers these problems are overcome, because these materials can be manufactured by controlled physical and chemical processes. Depending on these processes membranes with specific performance characteristics can be prepared, such that material properties according to therapeutic needs are obtained.

The historical starting point of such an artificial membrane was collodion. Collodion is a syrupy liquid that forms a porous film when dried. In chemical terms collodion is equivalent to cellulose-trinitrate, the cellulose ester of nitric acid. It was first synthesized by H. Branconnot in France in 1833. Under standard preparational conditions collodion has a degree of substitution of 2.7, which means that more than 90% of the free hydroxyl groups of cellulose are substituted. Due to its high content of nitrate groups, cellulose nitrate or nitrocellulose has explosive properties. It explodes at 186 °C, which explains its common name of guncotton. In his book *From the Earth to the Moon,* published in 1865, Jules Verne described the launch of a space rocket with the help of such guncotton material (fig. 1). Later in 1889, Alfred Nobel mixed collodion with nitrated glycerol and through this procedure obtained the famous nitroglycerin. The application of colloidon was not restricted to its function as guncotton. Cellulose-trinitrate was used for wound covering in medicine in 1848 and later for the development of films in photography.

Membranes from cellulose nitrate are easily produced. When dissolved in either acetone or ether/ethanol mixtures, cellulose nitrate precipitates under drying conditions and forms a porous film with the properties of a membrane. Adolph Fick [2] used such flat films in his in vitro studies on diffusion, however, only with limited success: he was not able to produce flat collodion membranes which were thin enough to allow diffusion of solutes under controlled conditions.

W. Schumacher [3] in Bonn, Germany confirmed Fick's observations and applied the term 'membrane diffusion' in 1860 to the transport of solutes through membranes and used this term in the title of his publication. Similar to A. Fick, W. Schumacher started his experiments with natural membranes obtained from beans and algae *(Caulerpa prolifera),* but he did not succeed because of their weak mechanical stability. Collodion was finally the material of choice for him:

> 'Mit den Häuten, welche sich aus Collodium bilden, beim Verdampfen des Aethers und Alkohols, habe ich ausgezeichnete Erfolge gehabt und habe sie bei allen Versuchen, die später mitgetheilt werden, in Anwendung gebracht. Sie besitzen eine ausgezeichnete Permeabilität, besonders wenn sie vor dem völligen Verdampfen des Aethers unter Wasser gebracht werden; sie erleiden durch Wasser, die meisten Salze, verdünnte Säuren, bei gewöhnlicher Temperatur keine Veränderungen und sind in beliebige Form zu bringen. Übrigens wird der Zweck der Arbeit oft auch über das Material entscheiden' [3].
>
> (I have obtained excellent results with the skins from collodion after the evaporation of ether and alcohol and used these skins in all experiments reported later. They possess an excellent permeability, mainly when exposed to water before the complete evaporation of ether. At standard temperatures, they are not modified by either water, salts or diluted acids and can be fabricated into any geometric shape. By the way, the target of an experimental work determines the type of material to be used.)

Schumacher started with collodion sacs, but did the major part of his experiments on osmotic forces and membrane diffusion with 80-mm-long collodion tubes with an internal diameter of 17–18 mm [3]. Collodion was also used in the first experiments in immunology by E. Metschnikoff, the father of the concept of cellular immunity. Metschnikoff [4] started his investigations on cellular phagocytosis with reed membranes in 1887, but switched to collodion membranes later because of their better performance and reproducibility [5]. Similar to Metschnikoff, B. Richardson [6] in London elaborated on the function of collodion membranes in contact with body liquids, such as blood and lymph in 1889. Richardson differentiated between structures in the body that were 'crystalline' and those that were 'colloidal' in nature, the latter being composed of large molecules or aggregations of smaller ones suspended in a continuous liquid medium.

In conclusion, collodion membranes served as the first, but perfect vehicles for the in vitro investigations of membrane diffusion and immunological processes.

Hemodialysis as an Experimental in vivo Therapy: Collodion Membranes

While Thomas Graham's and W. Schumacher's devices for studying diffusional processes could already be considered a rudimentary dialyzer, the first device incorporating all the basic elements common to today's dialyzers was developed in the early 1900s by John Abel and his colleagues [7] at the John Hopkins University in Baltimore. They published their first article on the technique of 'vividiffusion' in dogs and, not surprisingly, used collodion tubes in their device which was conceptually very similar to the modern hollow-fiber dialyzers of today, and for which they coined the name 'artificial kidney'.

The credit for pioneering the first dialysis on human patients goes, however, to the German physician Georg Haas from Giessen, who lived from 1886 to 1971. Haas was educated by the famous physiologist Franz Hofmeister in Strassburg, where he started his first animal experiments in 1914 [8–11] with membranes from reed stalks which he prepared according to a procedure described by P. Philippson [12] in 1902. Philippson had shown that reed membranes were superior to parchment paper in their performance, due to a faster separation of colloid and crystalline solutes. Typical dimensions of reed stalk membranes at that time were 15 cm in length with a volume of 8–10 ml [12]. However, as shown above for other biological materials, membranes from reed stalks were not suitable for the separation of large quantities of solutes because of their small size and high mechanical sensitivity.

Independent of the data reported by Abel et al. [7], in 1913, which were not available for Haas at that time due to communication problems during World War I, Haas later used collodion membranes, which he prepared according to prescriptions of two chemists: the Austrian Chemist Fritz Pregl (1869–1930, Nobel prize winner 1923 [13]) and Arnold Eggerth, who worked at that time at the Hoagland Laboratories in New York [14]. Haas described the vast difficulties he had to overcome in his experiments and stated in one of his first reports:

> 'Ich möchte sagen, es war ein Leidensweg, denn kaum, dass ein Hindernis beseitigt war, so folgte sofort ein weiteres auf dem Fuss.' ... Zunächst galt es die geeignete Dialysemembran zu finden. Ich habe eine Reihe von Dialysatoren aus dem verschiedenartigsten Material, tierische Membranen, pflanzliche Membranen, papierne Dialysatoren, ausprobiert. Weitaus am besten, sowohl mit Rücksicht auf die Herstellung, die sichere Sterilisierung und den Dialyseeffekt, bewährten sich mir die Dialysatoren aus Collodium, denen man jede gewünschte Form zu geben in der Lage ist' [10].
>
> (I'd like to say, it was a way of the Cross, because once one obstacle had been removed another followed ... Above all, it was necessary

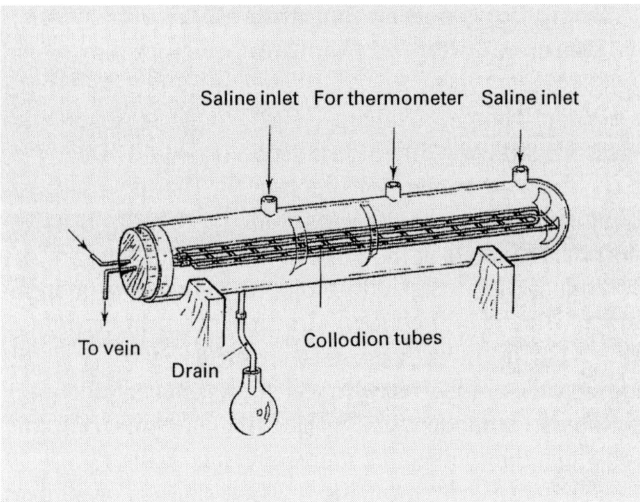

Fig. 2. Scheme of the first artificial kidney used for dialysis in humans by Georg Haas, Giessen. A glass cylinder of 160 cm length and 8 cm width contained a pair of collodion tubes which were located on a glass support inside the glass tube. Blood entry and exit ports were positioned at one end and connected to the membranes by small glass tubes. Every unit had two dialysate ports and an additional port for a temperature probe. At the bottom of the glass cylinder, there was also a drain for dialysate sampling. Haas used as many as six of these cylinders in parallel during his dialysis sessions. The length of his collodion tubes added up to 756 cm giving rise to a membrane surface area of 1,530 cm^2.

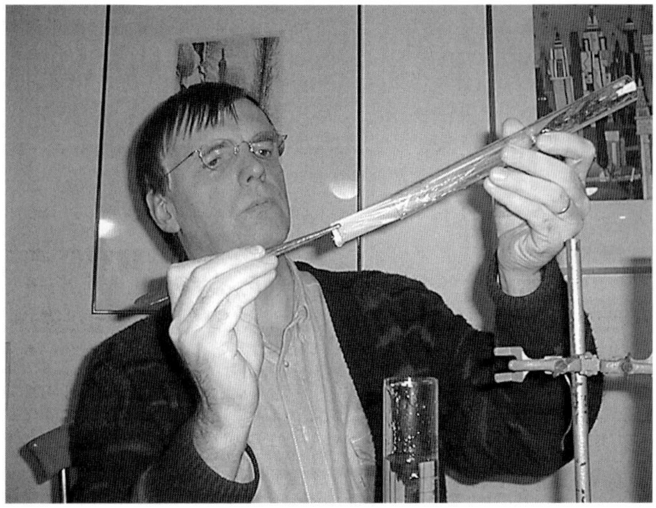

Fig. 3. When collodion membrane has formed at the inner surface of the glass tube, the glass cylinder is rinsed with water whereby membranes slightly shrink. A careful manipulation with a pincette allows the removal of the tubular membrane.

Table 1. Dimensions of the Haas dialyzer (year 1924) [10]

	Specification
Cylindric glass tube	
Length	160 cm
Diameter	8 cm
Volume	15 liters Ringer solution
Collodion tubes	
Pairs of tubes	3
Total tube length	756 cm
Tube diameter	2 cm
Membrane surface area	1,530 cm^2
Total volume	2,373 ml
Anticoagulants	Hirudin, later heparin
Hemodialysis	1st patient (summer 1924); dialysis time: 15 min

to find a suitable dialysis membrane. I have tried a series of different dialyzers from a variety of materials, animal and vegetable membranes and paper dialyzers. The best performance was obtained with dialyzers made from collodion with respect to fabrication, dialysis effects, safe sterilization and because they can be obtained in any geometric shape.)

It is beyond the scope of this review to go into the details of the Haas dialyzer shown in figure 2. However, it might be useful for the interested reader to learn more about the dimensions of the Haas dialyzer, which are shown in table 1. They indicate the technological achievements of George Haas. Compared to Schumacher's collodion tubes with a length of 8 cm, the length of the individual collodion tubes prepared by G. Haas was 126 cm, which indicates his enormous skill in producing these membranes.

We tried to repeat the experiments of G. Haas by preparing collodion tubes in an actual experiment. Here are the experimental details. (1) Preparation of cellulose trinitrate: 600 g of sulfuric acid were mixed with 600 g nitric acid and added to 25 g of cellulose during permanent cooling at 5 °C for a further 24 h. The resulting product was poured into cool water and washed until the solution had a neutral pH. Collodion was then dried over P_2O_5 at 40 °C. (2) Preparation of collodion tubes: Collodion was dissolved as a 6% solution in either a mixture of ether/ethanol or acetone. This solution was poured into a vertically positioned glass tube which had been closed by a silicone rubber plug at its lower end (dimensions of the glass tube in our experiment: length: 30 cm, width: 2 cm). After some minutes, all gas bubbles in the solution had disappeared and the collodion solution leaked out of the glass tube into a beaker as a result of carefully having removed the plug. A thin collodion membrane layer was formed at

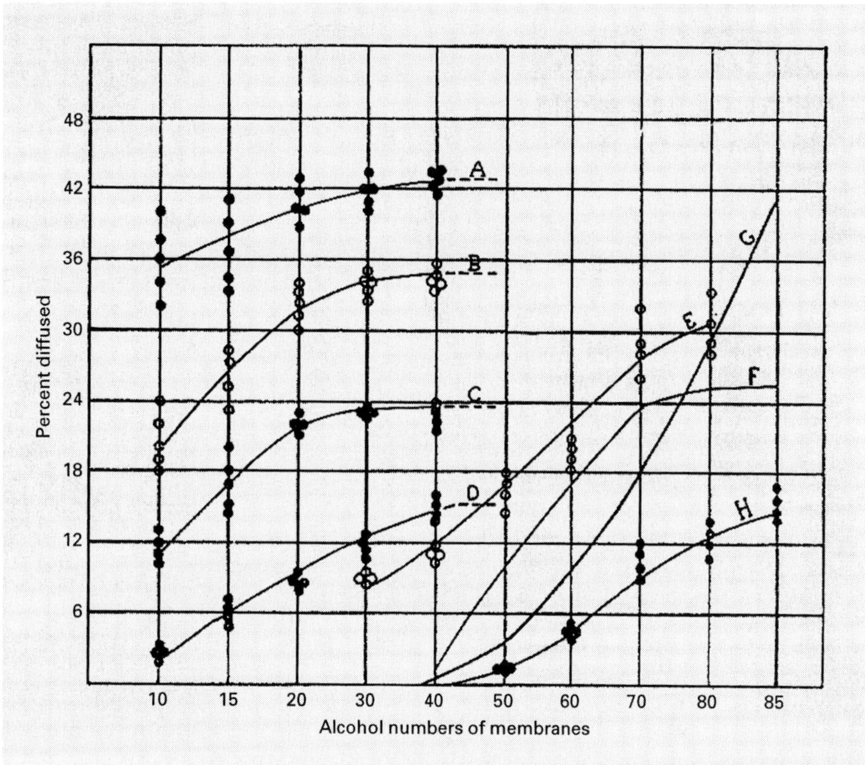

Fig. 4. A. Eggerth [14] analyzed the permeability of collodion membranes for different solutes in 1921. His results show that membrane permeability depends on the type of solvent used for the dissolution of collodion. The higher the content of alcohol in the ethanol/ether solvent mixture, the higher the permeability of the resulting membrane. A = Sodium chloride, 10 min at 20 °C; B = potassium dihydrogen phosphate, 10 min at 20 °C; C = saccharose, 30 min at 20 °C; D = indigo carmine, 20 min at 20 °C; E = primary proteose, 2.5 h at 20 °C; F = methemoglobin, 3 h at 35 °C; G = Congo red, 3 h at 35 °C; H = dialyzed serum, 3 h at 35 °C.

the inner surface of the glass tube which became opaque through the evaporation of the solvent after about a further 15 min. The glass cylinder was then filled with water whereby the collodion membrane tube slightly shrank away from the glass wall. By carefully pulling the resulting tube with a pincette (fig. 3), the membrane could be removed from the glass tube and dried on air.

Membranes like this were characterized by A. Eggerth [14], who was able to show in 1921 that the permeability of collodion membranes for different solutes only depended on the composition of the solvent. The content of alcohol (ethanol) in the mixture with ether determined membrane performance for small and large solutes, like NaCl, KH_2PO_4, indigo, methemoglobin, Congo red and dialyzed serum. This proves that it is possible to vary and determine membrane properties through changes in manufacturing processes (fig. 4).

Writing at a later time [10], Haas noted the lack of support for his work by both his colleagues and the hospital, and stated in a review in 1952 [15] that despite his complete description of a dialyzing system in the early 1920s, hemodialysis as a therapeutic procedure had to be reinvented after World War II. He showed a high level of respect for the work done 'by Kolff in Holland, Alvall in Sweden, Murray in Canada, Skeggs, Leonards, Heister, Muerhead, Merill, etc in the USA' [15]. In the same publication, Haas pointed out that the most important contribution to the progress in dialysis research was the application of a new membrane material [15], because the above mentioned authors successfully introduced a new material to their dialysis research, namely cellophane membranes, which from that time on dominated the market of dialysis membranes for the next 20 years.

Hemodialysis as Standard Therapy: Cellophane® and Cuprophan®

In 1937, W. Thalhimer [16] discovered that a membrane used in the sausage industry could be employed in removing solutes from the blood. This man-made cellulose-hydrate material, called cellophane, was manufactured by either the Visking Company in Chicago, Ill., USA or the Kalle Company in Wiesbaden, Germany. Cellophane membranes turned out to be uniform in thickness, strong and could be produced in large quantities. Thalhimer experimented with dog blood and used for the first time in hemodialysis heparin as an anticoagulant [17].

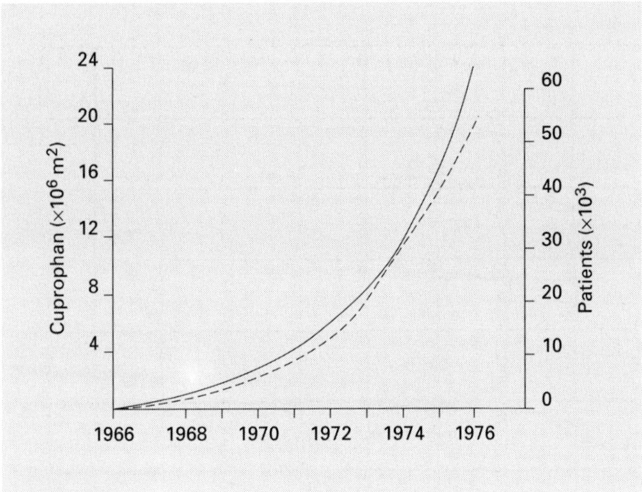

Fig. 5. The number of dialyzsed patients (---) worldwide directly depended on the availability of dialysis membranes (——). A sharp increase could be observed after an industrialized production of Cuprophan membranes was initiated [19].

Cellophane was employed by W. Kolff in his rotating drum artificial kidney. In this very effective device however, high mechanical stress was exerted on the membrane material with the consequence of frequent leaks and ruptures. Kolff and his coworkers were able to locate and repair them, but were still looking for an alternative material. This was identified in the late 1950s by Frederik Kiil [18] of Norway when he developed his parallel-plate dialyzser. Kiil was interested in producing a dialyzer with a large surface area that required a lower blood priming volume and could be used without a blood pump. The first Kiil device was a one square meter kidney made up of two layers of flat membranes that were bolted together to prevent blood path expansion. It appears that Kiil was the first to use a new cellulose membrane, called Cuprophan. Cuprophan membranes had a greater porosity for solutes and water than other materials. Further, there were only very few incidences of membrane rupture in Kiil's system.

At that time, Cuprophan, like cellophane, was produced for the sausage and packaging industry and available only in flat sheet form.

Parallel to F. Kiil and based on the experience with Visking cellophane, B. Watchinger and W. Kolff experimented with a twin-coil artificial kidney in a hospital in Wuppertal, Germany. This hospital was close to the production site of the Enka company, which was the manufacturer of Cuprophan® [19] and it is not surprising that a fruitful cooperation started. As a result, Enka, represented by its general manager Dr. Werner Bandel, decided to invest in the production of dialysis membranes. The company could profit from its chemical and technological expertise on large scale production of textile fibers and started the first standardized industrial production of dialysis membranes (flat sheet) in the world in 1966 [19, 20]. A year later a worldwide sales volume of DEM 1.0 million was achieved. This success stimulated the beginning of the Cuprophan tubular membrane production in 1969.

Do we overestimate these achievements, if we assume that the rise in the number of dialysis patients during the following years is closely related to the standardized mass production and thus to the general availability of Cuprophan dialysis membranes (fig. 5)? Membranes used in dialyzers after World War II were all in tubular or flat sheet form. A major breakthrough in the development of modern artificial kidneys came with the introduction of ultrathin capillary fibers, where the fiber wall represented the dialysis membrane. The availability of hollow fiber membranes represents another milestone of dialyzer mass production. The inner diameter of 200 μm and membrane wall thickness down to 5.0 μm of capillary membranes allow the production of rather handy devices with a small priming volume. The credit for the development of the first capillary dialyzer goes to Richard Stewart from Michigan, USA and to the Dow Chemical Company for their first dialyzer with cellulose acetate hollow fiber membranes. The version finally used in the first clinical trial in 1967 comes very close to the design of our dialyzers today. It contained 11,000 fibers, which provided a surface area of approximately 1 m^2. The ends of the fibers were encased in silicone rubber near the ports, which provided a barrier between blood entry and exit pathways. Enka followed the Dow Chemical Company and started its Cuprophan capillary membrane production in 1974 with great success: in 1976 a turnover in membrane sales of DEM 54 million was achieved.

Today we know that the idea of a capillary membrane dialyzer was the right concept for modern dialysis therapy. Filtering uremic toxins through membranes was not always considered to be sufficiently effective in removing all uremic toxins. Observations that clearance values for small solutes never add up to 100% and large molecules whose molecular weight does not allow membrane removal due to a too small average pore size led to new concepts: what about combining filter properties with adsorbing features by using additional adsorber materials, e.g. charcoal?

Consequently, devices incorporating both, membranes and adsorbing particles have been developed and produced [21]. A cross-sectional scheme of such a capillary membrane, designed as a sandwich of two membranes which are filled with activated carbon particles, is shown in figure 6. This black dialysis membrane was marketed for several years. Although the idea of an 'all-in-one filter and adsorber' is fascinating, the production of these systems was abandoned in the early 1980s due to manufacturing difficulties.

Cellulosic membranes in all configurations have considerably contributed to the perfection of dialysis therapy and represent the major prerequisites for the rise in the patient number from the 1960s to the 1980s of this century.

Hemodialysis as Routine Therapy: Modified Cellulosic and the Synthetic Membranes

From the late 1970s to the 1980s of this century hemodialysis has developed from an experimental treatment mode to a routine therapy. However, intensive research on physiological consequences of blood-material interaction revealed that the classical Cuprophan membrane suffered from two major disadvantages, i.e. a lack of hemocompatibility and its availability in low-flux configuration only.

Cellulosic membranes activate the complement cascade and stimulate blood-cell activation. Research on blood-material interaction has shown that the chemical surface may trigger detrimental physiological events and that a modification of the chemical surface structure of such a dialysis membrane reduces these effects. Consequently, cellulosic membrane modifications, such as several types of cellulose esters (e.g. cellulose-acetate) membranes and cellulose-ethers, like Hemophan®, have been developed. Clinical studies have proven that these materials show a better hemocompatibility pattern than unmodified cellulose.

Parallel to the development of improved production technology of cellulosic dialysis membranes other types of materials have been selected to serve as membrane polymers. The underlying concept of this development was to imitate the properties of the human glomerular basement which has a higher permeability and a larger ultrafiltration coefficient than the classical cellulosic membranes. The polymer polysulfone (PSu) was selected for this purpose. The Berghoff and Fresenius companies collaborated to produce the first hemofiltration membrane and hemofilter in 1978 and in the same year, first clinical tests with such a membrane were performed in Stuttgart, Germany. Further improvements followed when Fresenius bought all rights from Berghoff and continued to manufacture PSu membrane in its own laboratories. The advantages

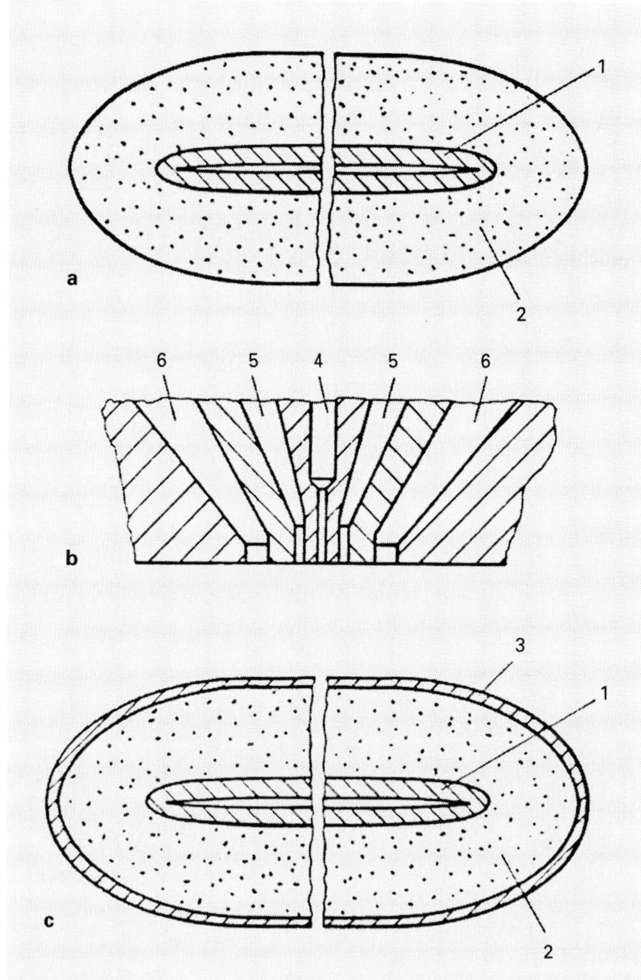

Fig. 6. All-in-one capillary membranes showing both, filtering and adsorbing capacity for uremic toxins. Two capillary membranes were concentrically arranged and filled with activated carbon particles. This black dialysis membrane was marketed for several years before production was abandoned [modified from 21]. **a** Cross section of a tubular membrane. 1 = Cuprophan membrane; 2 = support structure made up of a mixture of cellulose and charcoal absorbent. **b** Cross section of a spinning gap for tubular membranes used for preparing adsorbing tubular membranes. 4 = Exit port for gas or liquids serving as bore solution; 5 = gap for the Cuoxam solution; 6 = ring-like gap to spin a mixture of adsorbent suspended in Cuoxam. **c** Tubular membrane with two cellulosic membranes on either blood and dialysate side. The intermediate gap is filled with the adsorbing suspension of charcoal.

and positive clinical effects of this new membrane polymer in terms of high ultrafiltration, large sieving coefficients for inulin and β_2-microglobulin were reported in a short article by Streicher and Schneider [22] in 1983. The authors concluded that dialysis with PSu membranes further did not induce complement activation and leukopenia and thus overcame the concerns of a lack of hemocompatibility. In parallel to the development of a PSu hemofilter new types of dialysis machines were produced which allowed for volume-controlled ultrafiltration with the help of a balancing chamber. With this technology, hemofilter PSu membranes could also be applied to standard hemodialysis and hemodiafiltration. Two years later in 1985, the PSu family was enlarged by a new member, a low-flux membrane which successfully underwent clinical trials in 1987.

Apart from the advantageous hemocompatibility pattern, this PSu material also exhibited an adsorptive capacity for endotoxins and its molecular fragments and is, therefore, in line with the actual requirements for modern dialyzers. The use of a single polymer for multiple purposes explains its success in the marketplace as more than 55% of all dialyzers sold in the USA in 1997 were made of PSu.

Conclusion

The history of hemodialysis from an experimental to a routine therapy is closely related to the development of dialysis membranes. Industrial manufacturing under reproducible conditions made it possible to overcome the pitfalls of early membrane selection from animal and vegetable sources; this supported a rise in patient numbers worldwide also in future years.

References

1 Graham T: The Bakerian lecture: On osmotic force. Phil Trans R Soc Lond 1854;144:177–228.
2 Fick A: Über Diffusion. Ann Phys Chem 1855; 94:59–86.
3 Schumacher W: Über Membrandiffusion. Ann Phys Chem 1860;110:337–370.
4 Metschnikoff E: Sur la lutte des cellules de l'organisme contre l'invasion des microbes. Ann Inst Pasteur 1887;1:322–336.
5 Metschnikoff E, Roux E, Taurelli-Salimbeni: Toxine et antitoxine cholérique. Ann Inst Pasteur 1896;10:261–279.
6 Richardson B: Practical studies in animal dialysis. Asclepiad (Lond) 1889;6:331–332.
7 Abel J, Rowntree L, Turner B: On the removal of diffusible substances from the circulating blood of living animals by means of dialysis. J Pharmacol Exp Ther 1913;5:275–283.
8 Haas G: Dialysieren des strömenden Blutes am Lebenden. Klin Wochenschr 1923;2:1888.
9 Haas G: Versuche der Blutauswaschung am Lebenden. Klin Wochenschr 1925;4:13–14.
10 Haas G: Über Blutwaschung. Klin Wochenschr 1928;7:1356–1362.
11 Wizemann V, Benedum J: Nephrology, dialysis, transplantation: 70th anniversary of haemodialysis – The pioneering contribution of Georg Haas (1886–1971). Nephrol Dial Transplant 1994;9:1829–1831.
12 Philippson P: Über die Verwendbarkeit der Schilfschläuche zur Dialyse. Beitr Chem Physiol Pathol 1902;1:80–82.
13 Pregl F: Beiträge zur Methodik des Dialysierverfahrens von E. Abderhalden. Fermentforschung 1914;1:7–12.
14 Eggerth A: The preparation and standardisation of collodion membranes. J Biol Chem 1921;18:203–221.
15 Haas G: Über die künstliche Niere. Dtsch Med Wochenschr 1952;77:1640–1641.
16 Thalhimer W: Experimental exchange transfusions for reducing azotemia: Use of artificial kidney for this purpose. Proc Soc Exp Biol Med 1938;37:641–643.
17 Thalhimer W, Solandt D, Best C: Experimental exchange transfusion using purified heparin. Lancet 1938;ii:554–556.
18 Kiil F: Development of a parallel flow artificial kidney in plastics. Acta Chir Scand Suppl 1960; 253:140–142.
19 Von Sengbusch G, Henne W: Pioniere der Dialyse; in Yearbook 125 Years Ferdinand Sauerbruch Klinikum. Wuppertal, Born, 1988, pp 135–139.
20 Stewart R, Cerny J, Mahon H: An artificial kidney made from capillary fibers. Invest Urol 1966;5:614–624.
21 Henne W, Dünweg G, Schmitz W: Dialysemembran, insbesondere für die Hämodialyse. German Patent, 1982, DE 27 05 734 C3.
22 Streicher E, Schneider H: Polysulfone membrane mimicking human glomerular basement membrane. Lancet 1983;ii:1136.

Author Index Vol. 19, No. 2, 1999

American Journal of Nephrology

KARGER

Fax + 41 61 306 12 34
E-Mail karger@karger.ch
www.karger.com

© 1999 S. Karger AG, Basel

Accessible online at:
http://BioMedNet.com/karger

American Journal of Nephrology

Subject Index Vol. 19, No. 2, 1999

KARGER
Fax + 41 61 306 12 34
E-Mail karger@karger.ch
www.karger.com

© 1999 S. Karger AG, Basel

Accessible online at:
http://BioMedNet.com/karger